Orthopedics: Research and Advances

Orthopedics: Research and Advances

Edited by **Sharlton Pierce**

Callisto Reference
New York

Published by Callisto Reference,
106 Park Avenue, Suite 200,
New York, NY 10016, USA
www.callistoreference.com

Orthopedics: Research and Advances
Edited by Sharlton Pierce

International Standard Book Number: 978-1-63239-689-1 (Hardback)

Printed in China.

Contents

Preface

Orthopedics is a part of medical science which deals with treating the problems of the musculoskeletal system which consists of skeleton, ligaments, joints, cartilage, tendons, etc. Infections, tumours, and congenital disorders are popularly treated under this branch by surgical or non-surgical ways. It uses recent techniques like radiology and x-rays to diagnose and treat the problems such as broken bones or limbs. This book elucidates new researches and advances in a multidisciplinary approach about this subject. It includes some of the vital pieces of work being conducted across the world on various topics related to this field. Those with an interest in this area will find this book very helpful. It will serve as a valuable reference guide for students and orthopedicians alike.

This book has been the outcome of endless efforts put in by authors and researchers on various issues and topics within the field. The book is a comprehensive collection of significant researches that are addressed in a variety of chapters. It will surely enhance the knowledge of the field among readers across the globe.

It gives us an immense pleasure to thank our researchers and authors for their efforts to submit their piece of writing before the deadlines. Finally in the end, I would like to thank my family and colleagues who have been a great source of inspiration and support.

Editor

Biomechanical testing of distal femur osteotomy plate fixation techniques: the role of simulated physiological loading

Justus-Martijn Brinkman[1*], Christof Hurschler[2], Jens Agneskirchner[3], Philip Lobenhoffer[3], René M Castelein[4] and Ronald J van Heerwaarden[1]

Abstract

Background: Implants for fracture and/or osteotomy fixation are often tested according to basic mechanical test models such as open gap tests or 4-point-bending tests. These may be suitable to test and compare different implants for safety and clinical approval, but are not always representative of the post-operative situation, which is decisive when it comes to bone healing. In the current study the Knee Expert Group of the Association for the Study of Internal Fixation has compared the available open gap test results of the latest version of the TomoFix Medial Distal Femoral Plate and the antecedent plate design, with the test results of a more physiological and life-like test model. In the open gap test model the antecedent plate design was found to have superior stiffness and fatigue strength.

Methods: In the current study simulated postoperative conditions for medial closing wedge supracondylar osteotomies were used. The constructs were subjected to cyclical axial and torsional loading and were subsequently tested to failure.

Results: The more life-like tests in this study showed that the latest version was either more or equally stable and stiff than the antecedent version of the plate, in all of the tests. It is argued that the difference in results between the two loading models is due to differences in test design.

Conclusions: These test results stress the importance of not only using standard open gap and 4-point-bending tests, but also to use as life-like as possible test conditions for any form of biomechanical testing of new implants.

Keywords: Plate fixation; Biomechanical testing; Femur osteotomy; Fracture; Stability

Background

Implants for fixation of fractures and osteotomies have since long been tested for safety and clinical approval and have been compared to each other in so called open gap or 4-point-bending biomechanical test models [1–6]. The biomechanical loading protocols used aim at testing construct stability and fixation strength to bone and include in general axial and torsion loading, stiffness and fatigue testing. Although the open gap model purposely represents a worst case scenario of implant loading in unstable fractures, for many fractures and closing wedge osteotomies however this model represents a non-physiological test situation. The reduced fracture fragments or closed osteotomy gap are likely to improve the overall stability and stiffness of the construct [7–9].

In recent years so called Locking Compression Plates (LCP) have been developed specifically for fixation of osteotomies around the knee. Various factors have been identified to influence construct stability of LCP in plate fixation techniques; working length (i.e. distance of the first screw to the fracture), number of screws, distance of the plate to the bone, gap size and plate length [2]. Increased working length, fewer screws, a greater distance of the plate to the bone, an increased gap size and a shorter plate all negatively influenced the stability of the construct [2]. These parameters have been investigated using composite cylinders and finite element analysis (FEA) under simulated non-physiological loading conditions [2].

The latest version of the TomoFix Medial Distal Femoral Plate (MDF) (Synthes GmbH, Switzerland), has shown

* Correspondence: m.brinkman@maartenskliniek.nl
[1]Department of Orthopaedics, Limb deformity reconstruction unit, Sint Maartensclinic, Woerden, The Netherlands
Full list of author information is available at the end of the article

equal static strength but inferior stiffness and fatigue strength when compared to the antecedent plate design under these non-physiological testing conditions (Figure 1A and B), performed in house by the plates manufacturer.

These results were evaluated by a group of osteotomy experts involved in the development of plates for fixation of osteotomies around the knee; the Knee Expert Group (KNEG) of the Association for the Study of Internal Fixation (AO/ASIF). They questioned the validity and the clinical relevance of the open gap model in the testing of closing wedge osteotomy techniques. It was argued that open gap and 4-point-bending tests, while being necessary from a safety standpoint, test the material and design properties of the implant, but are not a representation of the stability of the whole construct, once it is implanted in the patient.

A validated biomechanical testing model with life-like simulated loading conditions has been previously used to compare the construct stability of different types of plate fixation techniques for distal femur osteotomies, one of which was the antecedent version of the MDF plate [7,8]. The new design MDF plate has a different shape than its predecessor; it has a more anatomical pre-formed shape resulting in an improved fit to the distal femur which reduces the distance of the plate to the bone, subsequently reducing leverage forces resulting on the plate (Figure 2). It has an optimized screw-hole orientation, providing a better fit for the screws in the femur. It has also been made slightly shorter and slimmer in favor of reduced prominence, while the thickness of both plates is the same.

In this study both designs were tested under axial and torsion loads in a material testing machine (MTS) in a composite replicate femur model, under simulated physiological loading conditions. The composite bone model provided reproducible bone properties and avoided the availability problems and variability associated with cadaver specimens. The mechanical properties of these bones have been validated [10]. The study hypothesis was that, in contrast to the open gap model test results, there is no difference in stability and stiffness between the two designs using a simulated physiologic post-operative test model for comparison.

Methods

The same test protocol as has been previously used by Brinkman et al. was used in the current study [7,8]. Fourteen femurs in total were available; 7 for each plate type ('NEW', anatomical MDF plate and 'OLD', antecedent MDF plate, Table 1). Bi-plane closing wedge distal femur osteotomies were performed, and the plates implanted according to standard surgical technique [11]. All femurs were aligned in a standardized way using an alignment jig and a femur saw guide (Balansys, Mathys Medical, Bettlach, Swiss), the closing wedge osteotomy was directed 20° oblique to the distal femur condylar line, a wedge of 10° was removed. The bone deformation needed for the closing of the wedge and the implant fixation were performed without producing a fracture in the opposite bone bridge. The femur head and trochanter and the distal femur end were thereafter embedded in a polyurethane-based cold-curing resin (Ureol FC 53,

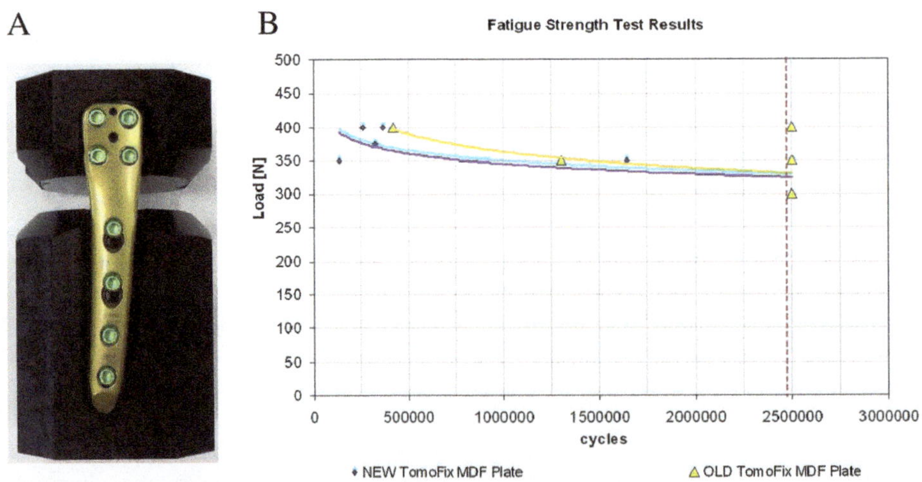

Figure 1 Open gap test setup and results. A. Anatomical MDF plate fixated in composite cylinder blocks for open gap model testing. **B.** Condensed schematic representation of the open gap fatigue tests as provided by the manufacturer (Synthes GmbH). Both plates were setup to be tested over 2500000 cycles (vertical line = end point of test runs), 2 of 5 antecedent MDF plate design plates (triangle symbol) and 5 of 5 anatomical MDF plate design plates (diamond symbol) failed before reaching the tests end at the various loading levels used (300, 350 and 400 N, antecedent MDF plate and 350,375 and 400 N, anatomical MDF plate plate). Trend lines for both are also shown (bottom line = anatomical MDF plate, top line = antecedent MDF plate).

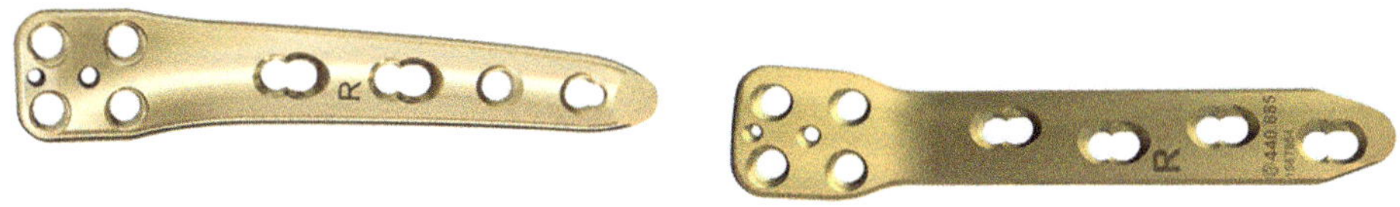

Figure 2 Both the anatomical MDF plate, left, and the antecedent MDF plate, right. The anatomical MDF plate has an optimized shape, to better fit the distal femur; it has improved screw-hole directions, and is shorter and slimmer, but equally thick.

Vantico GmbH, Wehr, Germany) in a specially constructed fixture; the fixture allowed for mounting of the femur in a materials testing machine (MTS) (Mini Bionix, MTS Systems Corporation, Eden Prairie, MN, USA) (Figure 3). The fixture was designed in such a way that the axis of loading of the replicate femur in the MTS was through the centre of the femur head proximal and through a point 18-mm medial from the mid-condylar distance, creating a mechanical femur axis of 2°; reproducing loading in the normally aligned human knee after a supra-condylar femur osteotomy (SCO) for valgus osteoarthritis.

Measuring system

The principles of rigid body motion were used to measure (micro) motion across the SCO. Reference point pairs, relative to which motion was measured, were defined on the replicate femur both proximal and distal to the osteotomy gap; two points across the midpoint of the intact cortical bone bridge, two points midway across the osteotomy and two points just posterior of the plate on the femur. Motion (displacement) of the diaphysis of the femur proximal to the osteotomy was measured relative to the femur condyles distal to the osteotomy using an ultrasound 3D motion-analysis system (CMS20S, Zebris Medizintechnik, GmbH, Isny, Germany). This system is based on the travel time measurement of ultrasonic pulses that are emitted by miniature speakers on a marker-triplet to microphones on a second marker-quartet (Figure 2). It has been previously used by Brinkman et al. in biomechanical testing of various osteotomy techniques [7,8].

Loading protocol

The replicate femurs were subjected to axial and torsional loading protocols designed to simulate physiological loading (Table 1). Cyclical axial loading was performed at two loading levels (150 and 800 N) on all femurs, during 100 cycles for each load at a rate of 0.5 Hz. Cyclical torsional loading was thereafter performed in all femurs. Internal rotation around the Z-axis with a cyclical moment loading of 5 Nm at a rate of 0.25 Hz was applied during 100 cycles, with an increasing axial pre-load (Table 1). The different axial preloads were used to simulate no, partial and full weight bearing.

Four femurs were subsequently tested to failure under axial compression, with displacement control at a rate of 0.1 mm per second. Failure was defined by a drop of actuator loading, either because of failure of the bone, bone–implant construct, or of the implant itself. Three femurs were tested to failure under torsion, with displacement control at a rate of 0.25° per second. Criteria for failure were the same as used for the axial loading failure tests.

Data analysis

The displacement data recorded was computed using a custom-written program in Mathematica (version 5.0, Wolfram research, Inc, Champaign, IL, USA); the change in position and the angle of rotation around all axes for each measuring point and the change in absolute distance between the measuring points was calculated. Displacement at the SCO was calculated using the change in the (absolute) distance between the measuring points per loading cycle. The amount of motion that occurs at the

Table 1 Overview of the configurations and test protocols

	Implant type	Axial loading Axial loads		Torsional loading 5NM torsion load With axial pre load		
Total no	Test runs	1	2	3	4	5
Femurs		150 N	800 N	0 N	150 N	800 N
7	MDF OLD	100	100	100	100	100
7	MDF NEW	100	100	100	100	100
14						

Overview of the test runs: axial tests at 150 N and 800 N both 100 cycles per test run, torsion tests at 5 Nm, with 0 N, 150 N and 800 N axial pre-load, again 100 cycles per test run. 'MDF NEW' = anatomical MDF plate, 'MDF OLD' = antecedent MDF plate.

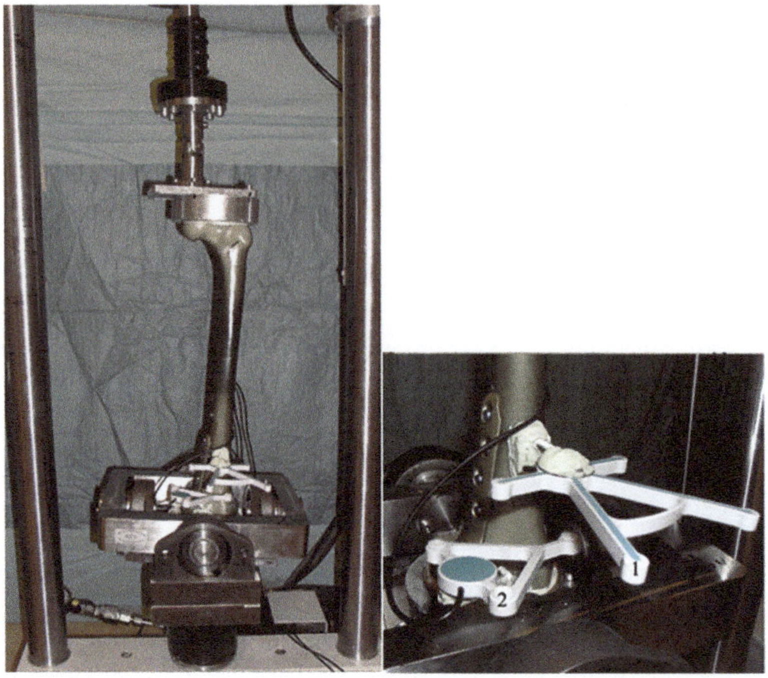

Figure 3 Overview of the test setup used. Left: the entire setup, the femur loaded in the MTS. Right: Close-up of the measuring system; 1 and 2, microphone and speaker templates.

SCO was defined as the difference between the maximum increase and maximum decrease in the distance between measuring points; determined for each cycle and per measuring point. A greater mean difference calculated over 100 cycles and 3 measuring points indicates more motion allowed by the bone–implant construct. Stability was subsequently defined as the amount of motion allowed by the construct. A similar approach was used in the torsional tests. The amount of motion was calculated by determining the amount of rotation around the Z-axis that is allowed by the bone–implant construct during each cycle. Stability in torsion was defined as the amount of rotation allowed by the construct. The stiffness under axial compression of the construct was calculated by plotting displacement at the SCO during the failure test, defined as the average amount of movement on the Z-axis of the 3 previously defined point pairs, against the force data. Stiffness of the bone–implant construct was defined as the slope of the linear portion of the force - deformation curve (i.e. the force required per millimeter of displacement). Stiffness under torsion loading was calculated by plotting the rotation around the Z-axis over time against the moment (Nm) applied by the MTS and defined as Nm required for one degree of rotation.

Statistical analysis

Statistical analysis was performed using SPSS statistical software (Version 11.5, SPSS, Inc, Chicago, IL, USA); the independent sample T-test was used to measure statistical differences between the motion data that was recorded and subsequently computed for the two configurations, P values < 0.05 were considered significant using a 95% confidence interval (CI95).

Results

Axial tests

No visible damage to bone, bone-implant construct or implant was found in any of the test runs. During each cycle of loading and unloading, a corresponding movement at the osteotomy was observed to occur. At 800 N the anatomical MDF plate allowed statistically significantly less motion than the antecedent MDF plate, at 150 N there was no difference (Table 2).

Torsion tests

Again no visible damage to bone, bone-implant construct or implant was found in any of the test runs. In the test run with no axial preload the anatomical MDF plate allowed statistically significantly less motion than the antecedent MDF plate; in the other runs there was no difference between the two (Table 2).

Axial failure tests

Seven failure tests (4 antecedent MDF plate, 3 anatomical MDF plate) resulted in a per-trochanteric femoral neck failure, *i.e.,* failure occurred proximally to the osteotomy in the replicate femurs. In one femur with the anatomical MDF plate a two level femur fracture occurred; a femoral

Table 2 Axial and torsion test results

			Total runs	Mean	SD
Axial tests	150 N	NEW plate	700	0.085651	0.054997
		OLD plate	700	0.087737	0.056193
	800 N	NEW plate	700	0.088803	0.048292
		OLD plate	700	0.096411	0.044069*
Torsion tests	0 N	NEW plate	700	0.077263	0.022999
		OLD plate	700	0.080334	0.025255*
	150 N	NEW plate	700	0.076817	0.02146
		OLD plate	700	0.078167	0.023
	800 N	NEW Plate	700	0.076932	0.021548
		OLD plate	700	0.077137	0.02275

*Statistically significantly less motion with the anatomical MDF plate design. Results for the axial and torsion test runs, movement is in mm for the axial tests and in degrees for the torsion tests. 'NEW plate' = anatomical MDF plate, 'OLD plate' = antecedent MDF plate.

neck fracture as in the other tests, but a femur shaft fracture just proximal to the plate occurred as well. No macroscopically observable failure at the bone-implant interface or of the implant itself was observed in any of the tests. No fractures of the opposing lateral cortex bone-bridge were observed with both plates. During the axial failure tests, the force time course of loading typically demonstrated increasing motion with increasing axial compression load with a sudden drop in load at failure. Calculated stiffness was similar in both plate types (Table 3).

Torsion failure tests

In the 6 femurs that were tested to failure under torsion loads, different patterns of failure were observed. Two femurs (one anatomical MDF plate, one antecedent MDF plate) did not fail, the test ended because the drive-shaft of the MTS itself came loose, which became apparent by a sudden drop in load on the femur. In those two there was no visible damage to the construct, their calculated stiffness did not differ from the other femurs. In two (again one anatomical MDF plate, one antecedent MDF plate) the test ended because of a fracture at the biplane hinge on the lateral cortex bone-bridge. And in two (one anatomical MDF plate, one antecedent MDF plate) a spiral fracture occurred just proximal of the osteotomy, just anterior of the proximal screw-bone interface. Calculated stiffness again was similar in both plates (Table 3).

Table 3 Axial and torsion failure test results

Femur	NEW axial	OLD	NEW Torsion	OLD
1	4313.10	4240.50	31.00*	32.10*
2	4242.90	4193.50	33.40	37.20
3	4011.20	5002.10	29.50	26.50
4	3607.60	4084.80		
Average	4043.70	4380.23	31.30	31.93
Significance	P = 0.27		P = 0.78	
(p < 0.05 = sign)				

Results for the axial and torsion failure tests, axial force is in N/mm, torsion force is Nm/°; differences are not statistically significant.
*Femurs in which the drive-shaft of the MTS came loose.
'NEW' = anatomical MDF plate, 'OLD' = antecedent MDF plate.

Discussion

The most important finding in this study was that in contrast to the results of the open gap tests, the anatomical MDF plate was not found to be statistically significantly less stable and stiff than the antecedent MDF plate. In two test runs the anatomical MDF plate allowed statistically significantly less motion than the antecedent MDF plate (800 N axial test and the torsion test with no axial pre-load). In all the other tests there was no statistically significant difference between the two. Again as in previous studies the axial failure tests ended because of per-trochanteric femoral neck fractures, not because of failure at the osteotomy[7]. Stiffness in the current tests also was very similar in both plates, with the antecedent MDF plate on average showing a slightly higher stiffness, but not statistically significant. In the torsion failure tests, the failure modes differed somewhat between femurs, but again there was no difference between the two plates. Again the antecedent MDF plate showed a slightly higher stiffness on average, but not statistically significant.

In these tests, as in previous tests by Brinkman et al., the post-operative situation after medial closing wedge SCO was reproduced as "life-like" as possible, with simulated partial and full weight bearing and simulated leg alignment as in patients that undergo SCO [7,8].

In the open gap model which is often used to compare the mechanical strength of osteosynthesis implants, a composite cylinder is cut in half and both ends are fixated with a plate (Figure 1A). That construct is then tested under axial and torsion loads, with motion measured across the gap. As documented by Stoffel et al. gap size and plate length are important factors in the overall stability [2]. It is therefore not unexpected that under these circumstances a shorter and slimmer plate has a lower stiffness and fatigue strength than a plate that is longer and that has an expanded shaft.

Various authors have compared different types of plates and nails, and different types of screw configurations, using sawbones or human cadaver bones, in distal femur and proximal tibia fracture models [1,3–6,9]. Almost all use some form of gap model; with the gap representing the unstable fracture [1,3–6]. David et al. used anatomic reduction without fracture gaps in a cadaver study testing a locked nail and an angled blade plate [9]. They stated that direct bony opposition more closely approximates the clinical situation, in which fracture fragments are reduced anatomically before placement of the fixation device. So as a consequence of the fracture reduction in most fractures stability is likely to be increased, which is not simulated in gap models. Similarly in closing wedge SCO there is no gap, both ends of the osteotomy are rigidly compressed against each other. And because of the controlled nature in which the SCO is created, closed and fixated there is inherent stability of the construct. Furthermore because of the gap in gap model testing the loading conditions at the plate are completely different, in a gap model the plate is loaded under tension, in the current setup under compression, because it is on the medial side of the femur. In SCO the load at the knee is shifted from lateral to medial, therefore after SCO the compressive forces will be on the medial side, as is the case in the current test setup.

The above arguments can also be made against concerns over the inferior results of the anatomical MDF plate in the fatigue tests using an open gap test model; they were not performed under simulated post-operative conditions. Fatigue testing with an open gap model may give a better understanding of the plate's failure mode. However it is questionable whether fatigue test results are representative of the clinical situation in SCO, because ongoing bone-healing will stabilize the construct as the implant fatigues, i.e., load sharing takes place decreasing the loading on the plate. Closing wedge SCO typically heal in 6 – 12 weeks, specific postoperative rehabilitation protocols provide for partial and full weight-bearing tailored to stability of fixation construct and time to full bone healing [12]. In our experience bone healing using a bi-plane osteotomy technique is fast and increased stability through bone healing occurs quickly [11]. This whole process is not simulated in any biomechanical test setup and can only be documented in in-vivo bone healing studies.

Limitations of the study are that, because of the small number of femurs available, the failure data set is small in size. No fatigue tests were performed, due to data size collection and time limitations. The MTS is not able to reliably load the construct quickly therefore fatigue testing of a single femur would have taken weeks. No power calculations were performed and no test- re-test reliability measurements were performed.

As with all experimental tests, the test setup used does not account for the variation in host biology and is a representation of what could happen in vivo and is for sure a simplification. The forces that are exerted on a leg during flexion and extension were not simulated; simple axial and torsional loading was used. These limitations are true however for most if not all types of biomechanical testing models. Furthermore the data is not comparable to the two previously published biomechanical studies by Brinkman et al., because 4th generation sawbones were used instead of 3rd as the 3rd generation sawbones are no longer commercially available [7,8]. According to Heiner the 4th generation bones mirror human bones more closely than the 3rd [10]. Tests with the 4th generation bones should therefore, if anything, be more representative of the post-operative situation after SCO.

Conclusions

The current test results show that under simulated physiological loading conditions there is no difference in stability between the two plates; the latest design Tomofix MDF provides as much, if not more, stability and equal stiffness compared to the antecedent design. These test results stress the importance of not only using standard open gap and 4-point-bending tests, but also to use as life-like as possible test conditions for any form of biomechanical testing of new implants.

Competing interests

A grant was provided by Synthes GmbH and received by the Medizinischen Hochschule Hannover, Germany, to perform the current study. They had no influence whatsoever on its outcome and the data published in this study.

Authors' contributions

JMB performed the tests, computed the results and drafted the manuscript. CH wrote the custom software and was one of the primary developers of the measuring method, he supervised the laboratory work. CH, JA and PL conceptualized the original as-life-like as possible test setup for testing of osteotomies, they supervised the project and helped draft the manuscript. RMC helped draft the manuscript. RJvH was the main supervisor of the project and was one of the KNEG members that came up with the idea of challenging the open gap tests. All authors read and approved the final manuscript.

Acknowledgments

We would like to thank Hans Radenborg for his help with performing the osteotomies.

J.M. Brinkman would like to thank the Marti- Keuning Eckhardt Foundation for their support of his scientific work.

Author details

[1]Department of Orthopaedics, Limb deformity reconstruction unit, Sint Maartensclinic, Woerden, The Netherlands. [2]Labor für Biomechanik und Biomaterialien, Orthopädische Klinik der Medizinischen Hochschule Hanover, Hanover, Germany. [3]Sportsclinic Germany, Hanover, Germany. [4]Department of Orthopedics, University Medical Centre Utrecht, Utrecht, The Netherlands.

References

1. Ito K, Grass R, Zwipp H (1998) Internal fixation of supracondylar femoral fractures: comparative biomechanical performance of the 95-degree blade plate and two retrograde nails. J Orthop Trauma 12:259–266
2. Stoffel K, Dieter U, Stachowiak G, Gachter A, Kuster MS (2003) Biomechanical testing of the LCP–how can stability in locked internal fixators be controlled? Injury 34(Suppl 2):11–19
3. Zlowodzki M, Williamson S, Cole PA, Zardiackas LD, Kregor PJ (2004) Biomechanical evaluation of the less invasive stabilization system, angled blade plate, and retrograde intramedullary nail for the internal fixation of distal femur fractures. J Orthop Trauma 18:494–502
4. Crist BD, Khalafi A, Hazelwood SJ, Lee MA (2009) A biomechanical comparison of locked plate fixation with percutaneous insertion capability versus the angled blade plate in a subtrochanteric fracture gap model. J Orthop Trauma 23:622–627
5. Cullen AB, Curtiss S, Lee MA (2009) Biomechanical comparison of polyaxial and uniaxial locking plate fixation in a proximal tibial gap model. J Orthop Trauma 23:507–513

6. Heiney JP, Barnett MD, Vrabec GA, Schoenfeld AJ, Baji A, Njus GO (2009) Distal femoral fixation: a biomechanical comparison of trigen retrograde intramedullary (i.m.) nail, dynamic condylar screw (DCS), and locking compression plate (LCP) condylar plate. J Trauma 66:443–449
7. Brinkman JM, Hurschler C, Agneskirchner JD, Freiling D, van Heerwaarden RJ (2011) Axial and torsional stability of supracondylar femur osteotomies: biomechanical comparison of the stability of five different plate and osteotomy configurations. Knee Surg Sports Traumatol Arthrosc 19:579–587
8. Brinkman JM, Hurschler C, Staubli AE, van Heerwaarden RJ (2011) Axial and torsional stability of an improved single-plane and a new bi-plane osteotomy technique for supracondylar femur osteotomies. Knee Surg Sports Traumatol Arthrosc 19:1090–1098
9. David SM, Harrow ME, Peindl RD, Frick SL, Kellam JF (1997) Comparative biomechanical analysis of supracondylar femur fracture fixation: locked intramedullary nail versus 95-degree angled plate. J Orthop Trauma 11:344–350
10. Heiner AD (2008) Structural properties of fourth-generation composite femurs and tibias. J Biomech 41:3282–3284
11. Freiling D, van Heerwaarden R, Staubli A, Lobenhoffer P (2010) The medial closed-wedge osteotomy of the distal femur for the treatment of unicompartmental lateral osteoarthritis of the knee. Oper Orthop Traumatol 22:317–334
12. Freiling D, Lobenhoffer P, Staubli A, van Heerwaarden RJ (2008) Medial closed-wedge varus osteotomy of the distal femur. Arthroskopie 21:6–14

2

Intratendinous injections of platelet-rich plasma: feasibility and effect on tendon morphology and mechanics

John J Wilson[1*], Kenneth S Lee[3], Connie Chamberlain[1], Ryan DeWall[2,3], Geoffrey S Baer[1], Marcus Greatens[1] and Nicole Kamps[1]

Abstract

Background: Intratendinous injections may have important effects on the properties of collagen microarchitecture, morphology, and subsequent mechanical properties of the injected tendon. The purpose of this study was to examine the effects of intratendinous PRP injections; the injectant retention within tendons, the distribution of intratendinous injectant, and whether intratendinous injection or needle fenestration alters tendon morphology or mechanics.

Methods: Design: Controlled Laboratory Study.
Interventions: In the first part of the study, 18 lamb extensor tendons were selected to receive methylene blue-containing PRP injection (PRP/MB), methylene blue only injection (MB), or needle fenestration. The volume of retained injectant was measured and injectant distribution and tendon morphology were examined microscopically. In the second portion of the study, 18 porcine flexor tendons were divided into control, needle fenestration, or saline injection groups. Young's Modulus was then determined for each tendon under 0-4% strain.
Main outcome measures: 1) Injectant volume retained; 2) Injectant distribution; 3) Post-injection/fenestration alterations in morphology, biomechanics.

Results: Intratendinous injectant is retained within the tendon. The difference between PRP and PRP/MB groups was not significant ($p = 0.78$). Intratendinous spread of the injectant solution within the tendon occurs primarily in the proximodistal direction, with very little cross-sectional penetration. Intratendinous injections resulted in microscopic morphology disruption (e.g., separation and disorganization of both the collagen bundles and cellular distribution). There were significant differences in Young's Modulus between control ($E_{ctrl} = 2415.48$) and injected tendons ($E_{inj} = 1753.45$) at 4% strain ($p = 0.01$). There were no differences in Young's Modulus between fenestrated and control tendons.

Conclusions: Intratendinous PRP injections are retained within the tendon, and primarily distributes longitudinally with minimal cross-sectional spread. Intratendinous injections may alter tendon morphology and mechanics.

Keywords: Platelet-rich plasma; Intratendinous injections; Tendon mechanics

* Correspondence: wilson@ortho.wisc.edu
[1]Division of Sports Medicine, Department of Orthopedics and Rehabilitation, University of Wisconsin School of Medicine and Public Health, 1685 Highland Avenue, Madison, Wisconsin 53705, USA
Full list of author information is available at the end of the article

Background

Tendinopathy is a common source of pain and functional impairment, accounting for 30-50% of sports-related overuse injuries and affecting large numbers of laborers who perform repetitive movements (Scott and Ashe 2006; Forde et al. 2005). Most tendinopathies develop gradually as a result of repeated physical strain (Kazemi et al. 2010; Kraushaar and Nirschl 1999). The strenuous and repetitive nature of recreational and occupational activities can lead to degenerative tendon alterations, characterized by collagen fiber disorganization, neovascularity, tendon thickening, increased cellularity, matrix disorganization, tenocyte apoptosis, and the clinical manifestations of pain and dysfunction (Sharma and Maffulli 2006; Jozsa and Kannus 1997; Cook and Purdam 2009). There is generally a paucity of inflammatory cells (Khan et al. 1999). Tendinopathies are often refractory to conservative treatment modalities (e.g. rest, non-steroidal anti-inflammatory drugs, physical therapy, bracing, corticosteroids) and such treatments have not been proven to affect healing at the cellular level (Mishra and Pavelko 2006).

Platelet-rich plasma (PRP) injection therapy has shown promise as an effective therapy for chronic tendinopathy (Mishra and Pavelko 2006; Filardo et al. 2010; Barrett 2004; Thanasas et al. 2011; Peerbooms et al. 2010; Gosens et al. 2011; Mishra et al. 2014). Platelets, which are small fragments of megakaryocytes that are essential for normal coagulation, also play a vital role in tissue healing via their release of platelet-derived growth and differentiation factors at the site of injury (Lee et al. 2011). PRP injections are proposed to stimulate and augment regenerative healing of degenerative tissue through the coordinated action of the PRP growth factors and cytokines (Sampson et al. 2008; Anitua et al. 2006; Anitua et al. 2005; Molloy et al. 2003). After intratendinous injection, platelets are activated upon exposure to collagen and local release of thrombin induced by needle fenestration. Upon platelet activation, platelet-derived growth factors (PDGFs) are released locally where they exert various responses through local cellular and cytokine signaling pathways necessary for cell proliferation and remodeling at the cellular level (Everts et al. 2006).

Recent studies have demonstrated beneficial results of PRP therapy in chronic tendinopathies, including those refractory to conventional treatment modalities (Mishra and Pavelko 2006; Filardo et al. 2010; Barrett 2004; Thanasas et al. 2011; Peerbooms et al. 2010; Gosens et al. 2011; Mishra et al. 2014). Other research has demonstrated beneficial effects of saline injections or simple percutaneous tendon fenestration for tendinopathy (Housner et al. 2009; McShane et al. 2006; McShane et al. 2008; Testa et al. 2002; Testa et al. 1999; Chan et al. 2008; Crisp et al. 2008). Despite the emerging evidence for the efficacy of PRP therapy, it is not known whether the beneficial effects of PRP injection therapy are a result of the PRP and its inherent growth factors, or simply due to the controlled tendon trauma and localized bleeding caused by the tendon fenestration. Therefore, it is important to understand whether it is technically feasible for an injectant to remain within the tendon after intratendinous injection in order for the hypothesized clinical benefits of the injectant (e.g., PRP and PDGFs) to be realized.

Similarly, little is known regarding the effects intratendinous injections may have on the properties of collagen microarchitecture, morphology, and subsequent mechanical properties of the injected tendon. Tendons do not act as rigid structures, but rather demonstrate viscoelastic properties that allow them to stretch, store, and release energy transmitted from their associated muscle group (Maganaris 2002; Alexander 1988; Zajac 1989). Several studies have demonstrated that tendinopathy alters these mechanical properties in affected tendons, resulting in increased cross-sectional area, less tendon stiffness, and lower Young's Modulus (Helland et al. 2013; Arya and Kulig 2010). The mechanical alterations due to tendinopathy result in an inherently weakened tendon structure. Intratendinous injections or fenestration may have additional important short-term and long-term effects on the mechanical properties of tendons. Understanding these consequences is necessary for optimizing the tendinopathy treatments while minimizing complications.

The goals of this study are to determine the effects of intratendinous PRP injections including, (1) the retention of injectant within the tendon, (2) the distribution of PRP after intratendinous injection, (3) whether intratendinous injection or tendon needle fenestration alters tissue morphology, and (4) whether intratendinous injection or tendon needle fenestration alters tendon mechanical properties.

Methods

Part one

Eighteen fresh frozen lamb extensor carpi radialis tendons obtained from a local abattoir were dissected, weighed, and then divided into three subgroups by a single researcher (MG). PRP was first diluted with .014% methylene blue. Six tendons were selected to each receive a single 0.25 mL injection of methylene blue-containing platelet-rich plasma (PRP-MB), six were prepared to each receive a single 0.25 mL injection of methylene blue alone (MB), and six served as controls and received only a needlestick without injection. Platelet-rich plasma was obtained from 20 mL of whole blood, drawn from the investigator (MG) in lab. The whole blood was spun in a benchtop centrifuge (Sorvall Legend, RT+, Thermo Fisher Scientific, Waltham, MA) for 10 minutes at 312 G, yielding 3.5 mL of un-activated (e.g., using thrombin or calcium chloride) PRP. The injections were administered using a 22-gauge, 1.5" needle

(Magellan®). The needle was inserted longitudinally at a 45-degree angle at the junction of the proximal 1/3 and middle 1/3 of each dissected tendon. Immediately following injection or needlestick, each tendon surface was gently dabbed dry to remove any extratendinous fluid. The wet weights of the tendons were obtained before and immediately after injections using a light balance (Mettler Toledo, Columbus, OH) with a repeatability of 0.0001 g. The difference between pre- and post- injection weights was calculated to determine the volume of injectant remaining within the tendon. The tendons were then trimmed to fit into 4.5 cm cassettes, embedded in optimal cutting temperature (OCT) medium and flash frozen in liquid nitrogen. Longitudinal sections of the frozen samples were cut at 10 μm thickness, mounted on Superfrost Plus (Thermo Fisher Scientific, Waltham, MA) microscope slides and used for H&E staining. Representative tendon micrographs of each tendon were collected using a camera-assisted microscope (Nikon Eclipse microscope, model E6000, Nikon Instruments, Inc, Mellville, NY with an Olympus camera, model DP79, Olympus Imaging America, Inc, Center Valley, PA).

The distribution of the injectant in each sample was then measured longitudinally (maximum proximodistal spread) and transversely (maximum diameter of injectant spread within the tendon) using the H&E micrographs. The extent of collagen fiber microarchitecture disruption was also qualitatively assessed.

Tendons embedded in cryostat gel were then sectioned into 10 μm slices, and mounted onto slides for further analysis. An experienced tissue histologist (C.C.) then evaluated injected tendons to measure longitudinal (maximum proximodistal spread) and cross-sectional (maximum diameter of injectant spread within the tendon) distribution of the injectant. The same histologist also qualitatively assessed tendon collagen fiber microarchitecture disruption.

Part two

Eighteen similarly sized porcine flexor digitorum tendons (3rd digit) were excised by a single researcher (NK) from 18 forelimbs obtained from a local abattoir. Specimens were kept hydrated in physiologic buffered saline until loading into the mechanical test system. Porcine flexor tendons, rather than lamb extensor carpi radialis tendons, were utilized for mechanical testing, since they were comparable in size (length, weight, circumference) to the lamb extensor tendons sectioned in part one, and were conveniently available for testing. Six tendons served as controls, six received a single needle fenestration, and six were selected to receive a single 0.25 mL bolus injection of 0.9% saline within the tendon. The injections and fenestrations were performed using a technique identical to part one. Immediately following the tendon treatments, a Mark-10 ESM301 Test Stand (Mark-10 Corp; Copiague, NY) was used to stretch the tendons from 0-4% strain (Figure 1). Force was measured with a MARK-10 Series 5 Force Gauge (Mark-10 Corp; Copiague, NY), and the load and displacement data were recorded with MESUR™ gauge load and travel analysis software (Mark-10 Corp; Copiague, NY). From these data stress (Force/Area) and strain $((l-l_0)/l_0)$ were calculated. The Young's Modulus was calculated as (stress/strain). The measurements obtained for each tendon within each group were then averaged for comparative analysis and paired t-tests were used to examine the effect of increased strain on Young's Modulus (E) for each treatment group.

Results

1) Intratendinous retention of injectant
   Pre-injection tendon weight did not significantly differ among the three groups as determined by one-way ANOVA ($F(2,15) = 0.75$, $p = 0.49$). The post-injection weight of the tendons in the PRP-MB group increased by an average of 0.22 ± 0.03 g (Table 1). Based on the measured density of this fluid (1.40 g/mL), this correlates to an average of 62.7% of the 0.25 mL injectant retained per tendon in this group. The post-injection weights of the MB tendons increased

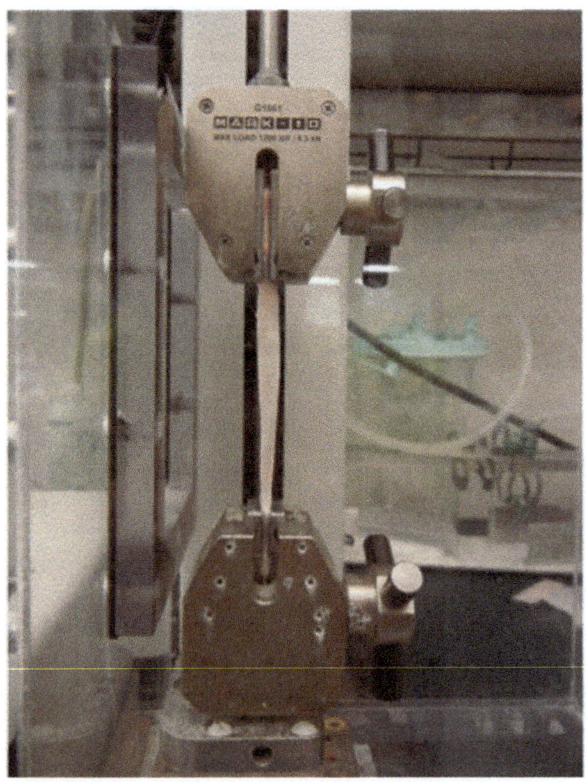

Figure 1 Mark-10 force measurement system.

Table 1 Average volume of injectant retained within tendons of MB only vs. PRP/MB groups

Group	Avg. pre-weight (g)	Avg. post-weight (g)	Avg. increase in weight (g)	% Injectant retained	P-value
MB Only	2.78 ± 0.26	3.00 ± 0.26	0.23 ± 0.04	54.4	0.78
PRP/MB	2.39 ± 0.21	2.39 ± 0.21	0.22 ± 0.01	62.7	

Data are expressed as the mean ± S.E.M.

by an average of 0.23 ± 0.10 g, correlating to 52.4% injectant volume retained, again based on the measured density of the injected fluid (1.76 g/mL). The average retention of MB versus PRP-MB was not significantly different (p = 0.78). As expected, the control needle fenestration tendons did not have a significant change in weight.

2) Distribution of injectant
The mean proximodistal penetration of injectant for the PRP-MB group was 2.91 ± 0.32 cm (Table 2). This was not significantly different from the MB group, which had a mean proximodistal penetration of 2.77 ± 0.40 cm (p = 0.80). The PRP-MB group had a mean cross-sectional penetration of 0.21 ± 0.06 cm, significantly less than the average 0.27 ± 0.04 cm seen in the MB group (p = 0.02).

3) Tissue morphology following injection
Each tendon was examined microscopically after injection or fenestration for evidence of normal tendon morphology disruption. Injected tendons (MB and PRP-MB) consistently demonstrated disruption of normal tendon morphology compared to control tendons (needlestick). Characteristic findings of injected tendons included separation of adjacent collagen bundles and disorganization of both the collagen bundles and cellular distribution (Figure 2).

4) Effect of intratendinous injection and fenestration on tendon mechanical properties
Young's modulus (E), the slope of the stress–strain curve, was used as a measure of the tissue mechanical property in the context of multiple different levels of tensile strain (0-4%) upon the tissue (Table 3). The injection group did show a lower average Young's Modulus (E = 1753.45 kPa) at 4% strain compared to control tendons (E = 2415.48 kPa), demonstrating that injected tendons were significantly less stiff than controls under the highest level of strain tested (p = 0.01).

Table 2 Average proximodistal and cross-sectional distribution of injectant in PRP/MB vs. MB only groups

Proximodistal	Avg. spread (cm)	P-value
MB only	2.77 ± 0.40	0.80
PRP/MB	2.91 ± 0.32	
Cross-sectional		
MB only	0.27 ± 0.04	0.02
PRP/MB	0.21 ± 0.06	

The effect of needle fenestration on the mechanical properties of tendons was then analyzed, again measured as Young's Modulus (E) (Table 4). There was no significant difference in Young's Modulus at any level of strain in the fenestrated group compared to the control group.

Discussion

Intratendinous injections of PRP for tendinopathy are thought to rely on the intrinsic properties and interplay between the growth factors contained within plasma and the platelet alpha granules (Lee et al. 2011). Some of the important growth factors contained within PRP include platelet-derived endothelial growth factor, transforming growth factor-beta, vascular endothelial growth factor, fibroblast growth factor, epidermal growth factor, and insulin-like growth factor-1 (Anitua et al. 2004; Lee et al. 2011). Several *in vitro* and *in vivo* studies have demonstrated the ability of PRP to improve healing at the cellular level (Schnabel et al. 2007; Majewski et al. 2009; Zhang and Wang 2010; de Mos et al. 2008; Kajikawa et al. 2008; McCarrel and Fortier 2009). The rapidly expanding use of PRP clinically, however, has outpaced the scientific understanding of the precise mechanisms by which such treatments influence healing. If the hypothetical benefits of PRP stem from its ability to locally affect cellular healing, then a relevant amount of PRP injectant must remain in the tendon into which it was injected. It is also important to understand what effects, if any, these intratendinous injections have on the integrity and biomechanical properties of tissue. To date, there is limited understanding of the distribution of intratendinous injections, and, just as importantly, the resulting histological and biomechanical effects on tissue. Understanding the behavior of injected PRP and its effects on the tissue have important implications for optimizing patient care and outcomes.

We evaluated the intratendinous retention and distribution of PRP into a tendon using ex vivo laboratory techniques and post-injection histological tissue evaluation. We then examined the biomechanical tissue properties of fenestrated and injected tendons to determine whether these treatments have any immediate detrimental effects on tissue. Our results demonstrate that intratendinous PRP injections are not only feasible, but the majority of injectant remains within the tendon following injection. One study by Wiegerinck and colleagues looked at the distribution of PRP injected into cadaveric

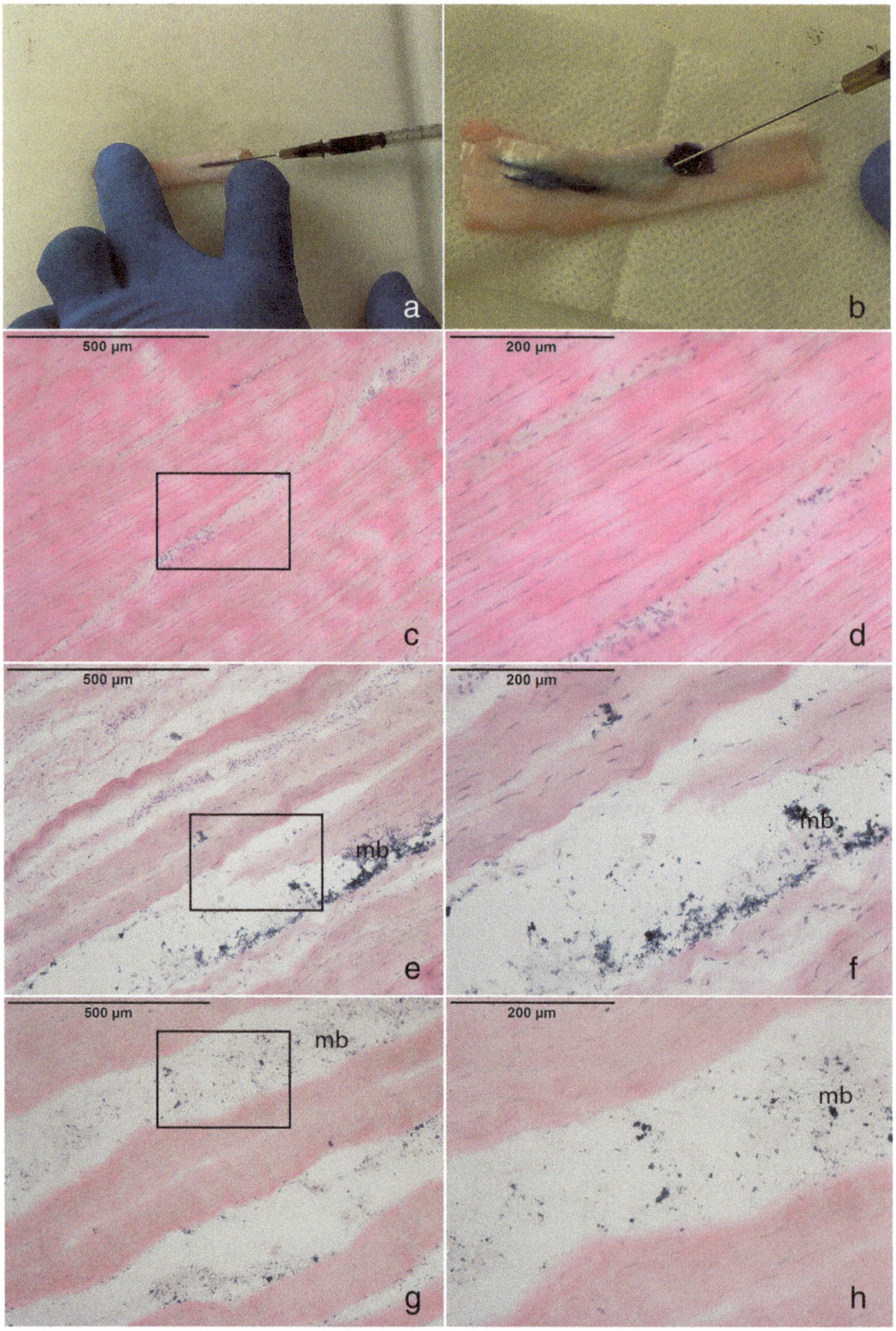

Figure 2 Morphologic changes in injected tendons versus control. Figures 2**a)** and 2**b)** represent the injection process of the PRP/MB and MB into the lamb tendon. The tendon significantly expands as the solution is injected **(2b)**. H&E images of the **2c)** and **2d)** fenestrated tendon, **2e)** and **2f)** MB-injected tendon and 2 g) and 2 h) PRP/MB-injected tendon. Note the methylene blue staining (mb) within the open spaces between the collagen fibers. Rectangles in **2c)**, **2e)**, and **2 g)** represent the area captured in images **2d)**, **2f)**, and **2 h)**.

Achilles tendons. The results demonstrated a wide, poorly localized distribution of injectant upon post-injection dissection and evaluation of the tendon and inscribing tissues (Wiegerinck et al. 2011). The results of our study are similar in that, while the majority of injectant remained within the tendon, there was also a moderate amount of injectant that escaped the tendon substance, resulting in volume retention of less than two-thirds of the injectant in all injected tendons in this trial. A recent retrospective study of pre-and post-injection ultrasound imaging of tendons injected with PRP or autologous blood verified that injectant remained

Table 3 Young's modulus of injected vs. control tendons at various levels of strain

	1% Strain	2% Strain	3% Strain	4% Strain
Average E Control (kPa)	53.68	444.81	1295.60	2415.48
Average E Injection (kPa)	63.43	373.55	893.59	1753.45
P-value	0.66	0.56	0.09	0.01

within the tendon of interest following injection, but injected solution was also visualized in tissues adjacent to the injected area (Loftus et al. 2012). Quantifying the volume of fluid remaining within the tendon immediately after the injection however, was not possible using the aforementioned study methods. Our study agrees with their findings, but quantifies the amount of solution remaining within a tendon after injection. Using histological evaluation, we were also able to quantitatively describe the characteristics of intratendinous spread of the fluid and the qualitative effects on tissue morphology immediately after injection. Loftus and colleagues suggest that the spread of injectant within a tendon proceeds more distally than expected, aligning with our findings of predominantly proximodistal spread. They did not specify, however, the degree of cross-sectional spread within the tissue, and hypothesized that peppering techniques may not be necessary given the non-local spread of injectant within the tissue (Loftus et al. 2012). Our results suggest that cross sectional spread is minimal, which may limit adequate distribution of injectant within tendon. This is consistent with the results demonstrated by van den Belt and colleagues in a similar in vitro study of intratendinous injections into horse flexor tendons (van den Belt et al. 1993). This observation was particularly evident in PRP-injected tendons in our study and the significant difference between PRP and methylene blue only injections limiting cross-sectional spread may be related to platelet activation and clotting upon exposure to tendon collagen, resulting in even further reduced cross-sectional spread across collagen bundles. This may suggest that larger areas or volumes of tendinopathy may require a peppering technique to ensure adequate distribution within the pathologic tissues being treated, in contrast to the conclusions of Loftus. Multiple fenestrations associated with a peppering technique may also provide theoretical benefit in creating local bleeding and exposure to thrombin, a known activator of platelets and stimulus to an acute healing response. The PRP utilized in this study was not activated using thrombin or calcium chloride, and may differ from clinical applications in which activation of PRP is performed.

Table 4 Young's modulus of fenestrated vs. control tendons at various levels of strain

	1% Strain	2% Strain	3% Strain	4% Strain
Average E Control (kPa)	53.68	444.81	1295.60	2415.48
Average E Fenestration (kPa)	60.03	532.03	1333.34	2358.95
P-value	0.82	0.51	0.87	0.76

The morphology of tendon microarchitecture is noticeably altered following intratendinous injection with a fluid bolus, whereas needle fenestration did not appear to have a significant effect on visualized tendon morphology. This may help to explain why intratendinous injections resulted in alterations of biomechanical properties, specifically decreased stiffness (E), with higher strain forces. There was no significant effect of needle fenestration on the biomechanical properties of tendons compared to controls. This demonstrates that injected tendons were significantly less stiff at higher levels of strain than control tendons and suggests that intratendinous injections may weaken the injected tendon, at least immediately following injections.

The use of intratendinous injections of PRP is emerging as a therapy for various chronic tendinopathies (Mishra and Pavelko 2006; Filardo et al. 2010; Barrett 2004; Thanasas et al. 2011; Peerbooms et al. 2010; Gosens et al. 2011; Mishra et al. 2014). While there is optimism surrounding PRP therapy, the feasibility and biomechanical effects of intratendinous injections on the treated tendon tissue is largely unknown and may have important implications for determining the optimal treatment strategy for such tendinopathies. In a letter to the editor by Knobloch, et al. (Knobloch et al. 2008) in response to a published study of intratendinous injections for Achilles tendinopathy (Maxwell et al. 2007), the authors raised concerns regarding the unknown effect of intratendinous level of collagen distribution on the potential adverse effects of intratendinous injections. Our study specifically examined the biomechanical effects, but other deleterious effects on tendon beyond physical disruption and biomechanical detrimental effects are also hypothesized (Abate et al. 2014). Such proposed effects include risk of pressure-induced tissue necrosis and focal infections, as well as focal tendon hypoxia and elevated lactate concentrations in tendons with tendinosis (Knobloch et al. 2008). These effects should be considered for future study as well.

Further study is warranted at a number of levels to increase our understanding of the effects of intratendinous injections. While this study demonstrates that a significant portion of a 0.25 mL injectant can be retained, it is likely to vary considerably with different injection volumes and operator dependent techniques. It is also not known whether the retention and distribution of intratendinous injections performed in vivo would be altered by factors such as blood flow and forces placed on the tendons during normal motion in the extremity (Wiegerinck et al. 2014). These factors may affect the injectant retention and distribution within the tendon. Although injected tendons in this study demonstrated visual disruption of normal morphology and immediately altered mechanical properties at higher levels of strain, it is not known what effect these alterations have on long-term function, morphology, and overall health of tendons in vivo.

A recognized limitation of this study is the fact that two different species and tendon types were analyzed for convenience reasons. Although the tendons were similarly sized, and from the forelimb of the animal, it is plausible that extensor and flexor tendons do not behave similarly in their response to intratendinous injections or tendon strain due to inherent differences in their structural and mechanical properties at baseline. Pollock and Shadwick's study on the relationship between mechanical properties of various limb flexor and extensor tendons in 18 different quadrupedal mammals with different body mass did not significantly differ in their mechanical properties (Pollock and Shadwick 1994). Therefore, for the purposes of this study, tendon similarities were felt to be sufficient to allow for an initial investigation of the potential effects of intratendinous injections.

Given the relatively small sample size in both parts of this study and the fact that all measurements were collected at a single point in time immediately after treatment administration, future studies with larger sample sizes and the ability to measure these variables at multiple points in time would be very beneficial in better characterizing the effects of intratendinous injections and how best to counsel patients receiving this treatment.

Though this study demonstrated alteration of tendon mechanics in injected tendons at 4% strain, it remains unknown whether similar alteration would be seen in vivo or to what significance this type of alteration may have on likelihood of re-injuries or rupture, which obviously must be considered when determining timing for return to activity or sport. Another limitation of this study is the fact that the effect of intratendinous injections and fenestration on mechanical properties of the tendon was only tested to a maximum of 4% strain. In normal movement and activity, tendons typically experience strains of less than 4%, predominantly due to uncrimping of the collagen fibers until reaching roughly 2% strain and then due to actual stretch of the collagen fibers as strains increase beyond that (Kelc Robi et al. 2013). When a tendon is strained beyond 4%, microfailure of individual fibrils begins to occur and macrofailure (e.g., rupture) of the tendon typically occurs when it is stretched to greater than 8-10% its original length (Kelc Robi et al. 2013; Woo et al. 2000). In porcine tendons, irreversible damage generally occurs at or above 6.5% strain (Duenwald-Kuehl et al. 2012). Thus, while our study suggests that intratendinous injections have the potential to alter tendon mechanics at strains on the upper limit of those produced with normal activity, further research is necessary to investigate whether tendon mechanics are also altered at higher levels of strain and whether or not the point of rupture is affected following these treatments. Similarly, further research is necessary to determine whether or not the observed alteration of mechanics is reproducible in an in vivo model and whether the addition of PRP to the injectant results in alterations different than those seen with saline injections. Our results suggest early tendon loading at low strain is likely acceptable, but it may be prudent to exercise caution and avoidance of high strain loading of tendons treated with intratendinous injection in the immediate period following injection. It is not known how long the mechanical effects observed in this study may persist.

Conclusions

Intratendinous PRP injections are retained within the tendon, and primarily distributes longitudinally with minimal cross-sectional spread. Intratendinous injections may alter tendon morphology and mechanics.

Competing interests

The authors declare that they have no competing interests.

Authors' contributions

JW conceived the study, participated in its design and conduct, and helped to draft the manuscript. KL, CC, RD, and GB participated in study design and manuscript preparation. MG and NK conducted the laboratory experimentation on experimental tissues and participated in manuscript preparation. All authors have read and approved the final manuscript.

Acknowledgements

Funding support provided by the Herman and Gwendolyn Shapiro Student Research Foundation, University of Wisconsin School of Medicine and Public Health.

Author details

[1]Division of Sports Medicine, Department of Orthopedics and Rehabilitation, University of Wisconsin School of Medicine and Public Health, 1685 Highland Avenue, Madison, Wisconsin 53705, USA. [2]Department of Biomedical Engineering, University of Wisconsin School of Medicine and Public Health, Madison, Wisconsin 53705, USA. [3]Department of Radiology, University of Wisconsin School of Medicine and Public Health, Madison, Wisconsin 53705, USA.

References

Abate M, Verna S, Di Gregorio P, Salini V, Schiavone C (2014) Sonographic findings during and after Platelet Rich Plasma injections in tendons. Muscles Ligaments Tendons J 4(1):29–34

Alexander RMN (1988) Elastic Mechanisms in Animal Movement. Cambridge University Press. New York, New York, USA

Anitua E, Andia I, Ardanza B, Nurden P, Nurden AT (2004) Autologous platelets as a source of proteins for healing and tissue regeneration. Thromb Haemost 91(1):4–15, Doi: 10.1267/thro04010004

Anitua E, Andia I, Sanchez M, Azofra J, del Mar Zalduendo M, de la Fuente M, Nurden P, Nurden AT (2005) Autologous preparations rich in growth factors promote proliferation and induce VEGF and HGF production by human tendon cells in culture. J Orthop Res 23(2):281–286, Doi: 10.1016/j.orthres.2004.08.015

Anitua E, Sanchez M, Nurden AT, Nurden P, Orive G, Andia I (2006) New insights into and novel applications for platelet-rich fibrin therapies. Trends Biotechnol 24(5):227–234, Doi: 10.1016/j.tibtech.2006.02.010

Arya S, Kulig K (2010) Tendinopathy alters mechanical and material properties of the Achilles tendon. J Appl Physiol (1985) 108(3):670–675, Doi: 10.1152/japplphysiol.00259.2009

Barrett SES (2004) Growth factors for chronic plantar fasciitis. Podiatry Today 17(11):36–42

Chan O, O'Dowd D, Padhiar N, Morrissey D, King J, Jalan R, Maffulli N, Crisp T (2008) High volume image guided injections in chronic Achilles tendinopathy. Disabil Rehabil 30(20–22):1697–1708, Doi: 10.1080/09638280701788225

Cook JL, Purdam CR (2009) Is tendon pathology a continuum? a pathology model to explain the clinical presentation of load-induced tendinopathy. Br J Sports Med 43(6):409–416, Doi: 10.1136/bjsm.2008.051193

Crisp T, Khan F, Padhiar N, Morrissey D, King J, Jalan R, Maffulli N, Frcr OC (2008) High volume ultrasound guided injections at the interface between the patellar tendon and Hoffa's body are effective in chronic patellar tendinopathy: a pilot study. Disabil Rehabil 30(20–22):1625–1634, Doi: 10.1080/09638280701830936

de Mos M, van der Windt AE, Jahr H, van Schie HT, Weinans H, Verhaar JA, van Osch GJ (2008) Can platelet-rich plasma enhance tendon repair? a cell culture study. Am J Sports Med 36(6):1171–1178, Doi: 10.1177/0363546508314430

Duenwald-Kuehl S, Kondratko J, Lakes RS, Vanderby R Jr (2012) Damage mechanics of porcine flexor tendon: mechanical evaluation and modeling. Ann Biomed Eng 40(8):1692–1707, Doi: 10.1007/s10439-012-0538-z

Everts PA, Knape JT, Weibrich G, Schonberger JP, Hoffmann J, Overdevest EP, Box HA, van Zundert A (2006) Platelet-rich plasma and platelet gel: a review. J Extra Corpor Technol 38(2):174–187

Filardo G, Kon E, Della Villa S, Vincentelli F, Fornasari PM, Marcacci M (2010) Use of platelet-rich plasma for the treatment of refractory jumper's knee. Int Orthop 34(6):909–915, Doi: 10.1007/s00264-009-0845-7

Forde MS, Punnett L, Wegman DH (2005) Prevalence of musculoskeletal disorders in union ironworkers. J Occup Environ Hyg 2(4):203–212, Doi: 10.1080/15459620590929635

Gosens T, Peerbooms JC, van Laar W, den Oudsten BL (2011) Ongoing positive effect of platelet-rich plasma versus corticosteroid injection in lateral epicondylitis: a double-blind randomized controlled trial with 2-year follow-up. Am J Sports Med 39(6):1200–1208, Doi: 10.1177/0363546510397173

Helland C, Bojsen-Moller J, Raastad T, Seynnes OR, Moltubakk MM, Jakobsen V, Visnes H, Bahr R (2013) Mechanical properties of the patellar tendon in elite volleyball players with and without patellar tendinopathy. Br J Sports Med 47 (13):862–868, Doi: 10.1136/bjsports-2013-092275

Housner JA, Jacobson JA, Misko R (2009) Sonographically guided percutaneous needle tenotomy for the treatment of chronic tendinosis. J Ultrasound Med 28(9):1187–1192

Jozsa L, Kannus P. (1997) Human Tendons: Anatomy, Physiology, and Pathology. Human Kinetics. Champaign, Illinois, USA

Kajikawa Y, Morihara T, Sakamoto H, Matsuda K, Oshima Y, Yoshida A, Nagae M, Arai Y, Kawata M, Kubo T (2008) Platelet-rich plasma enhances the initial mobilization of circulation-derived cells for tendon healing. J Cell Physiol 215 (3):837–845, Doi: 10.1002/jcp.21368

Kazemi M, Azma K, Tavana B, Rezaiee Moghaddam F, Panahi A (2010) Autologous blood versus corticosteroid local injection in the short-term treatment of lateral elbow tendinopathy: a randomized clinical trial of efficacy. Am J Phys Med Rehabil 89(8):660–667, Doi: 10.1097/PHM.0b013e3181ddcb31

Kelc Robi NJ, Kuhta Matevz, Vogrin Matjaz (2013) The Physiology of sports injuries and repair processes. Curr Issues Sports Exerc Med. doi: 10.5772/54234

Khan KM, Cook JL, Bonar F, Harcourt P, Astrom M (1999) Histopathology of common tendinopathies. update and implications for clinical management. Sports Med 27(6):393–408

Knobloch K, Spies M, Vogt PM (2008) Adverse effects of intratendinous injection. AJR American J Roentgenol 190 (5):W316. author reply W317. doi:10.2214/ajr.07.3380

Kraushaar BS, Nirschl RP (1999) Tendinosis of the elbow (tennis elbow). clinical features and findings of histological, immunohistochemical, and electron microscopy studies. J Bone Joint Surg Am 81(2):259–278

Lee KS, Wilson JJ, Rabago DP, Baer GS, Jacobson JA, Borrero CG (2011) Musculoskeletal applications of platelet-rich plasma: fad or future? AJR Am J Roentgenol 196(3):628–636, Doi: 10.2214/ajr.10.5975

Loftus ML, Endo Y, Adler RS (2012) Retrospective analysis of postinjection ultrasound imaging after platelet-rich plasma or autologous blood: observational review of anatomic distribution of injected material. AJR Am J Roentgenol 199(4):W501–W505, Doi: 10.2214/ajr.11.8075

Maganaris CN (2002) Tensile properties of in vivo human tendinous tissue. J Biomech 35(8):1019–1027

Majewski M, Ochsner PE, Liu F, Fluckiger R, Evans CH (2009) Accelerated healing of the rat Achilles tendon in response to autologous conditioned serum. Am J Sports Med 37(11):2117–2125, Doi: 10.1177/0363546509348047

Maxwell NJ, Ryan MB, Taunton JE, Gillies JH, Wong AD (2007) Sonographically guided intratendinous injection of hyperosmolar dextrose to treat chronic tendinosis of the Achilles tendon: a pilot study. AJR Am J Roentgenol 189(4): W215–W220, Doi: 10.2214/ajr.06.1158

McCarrel T, Fortier L (2009) Temporal growth factor release from platelet-rich plasma, trehalose lyophilized platelets, and bone marrow aspirate and their effect on tendon and ligament gene expression. J Orthop Res 27(8):1033–1042, Doi: 10.1002/jor.20853

McShane JM, Nazarian LN, Harwood MI (2006) Sonographically guided percutaneous needle tenotomy for treatment of common extensor tendinosis in the elbow. J Ultrasound Med 25(10):1281–1289

McShane JM, Shah VN, Nazarian LN (2008) Sonographically guided percutaneous needle tenotomy for treatment of common extensor tendinosis in the elbow: is a corticosteroid necessary? J Ultrasound Med 27(8):1137–1144

Mishra A, Pavelko T (2006) Treatment of chronic elbow tendinosis with buffered platelet-rich plasma. Am J Sports Med 34(11):1774–1778, Doi: 10.1177/0363546506288850

Mishra AK, Skrepnik NV, Edwards SG, Jones GL, Sampson S, Vermillion DA, Ramsey ML, Karli DC, Rettig AC (2014) Efficacy of platelet-rich plasma for chronic tennis elbow: a double-blind, prospective, multicenter, randomized controlled trial of 230 patients. Am J Sports Med 42(2):463–471, Doi: 10.1177/0363546513494359

Molloy T, Wang Y, Murrell G (2003) The roles of growth factors in tendon and ligament healing. Sports Med 33(5):381–394

Peerbooms JC, Sluimer J, Bruijn DJ, Gosens T (2010) Positive effect of an autologous platelet concentrate in lateral epicondylitis in a double-blind randomized controlled trial: platelet-rich plasma versus corticosteroid injection with a 1-year follow-up. Am J Sports Med 38(2):255–262, Doi: 10.1177/0363546509355445

Pollock CM, Shadwick RE (1994) Relationship between body mass and biomechanical properties of limb tendons in adult mammals. Am J Physiol 266(3 Pt 2):R1016–R1021

Sampson S, Gerhardt M, Mandelbaum B (2008) Platelet rich plasma injection grafts for musculoskeletal injuries: a review. Curr Rev Musculoskelet Med 1(3–4):165–174, Doi: 10.1007/s12178-008-9032-5

Schnabel LV, Mohammed HO, Miller BJ, McDermott WG, Jacobson MS, Santangelo KS, Fortier LA (2007) Platelet Rich Plasma (PRP) enhances anabolic gene expression patterns in flexor digitorum superficialis tendons. J Orthop Res 25(2):230–240, Doi: 10.1002/jor.20278

Scott A, Ashe MC (2006) Common tendinopathies in the upper and lower extremities. Curr Sports Med Rep 5(5):233–241

Sharma P, Maffulli N (2006) Biology of tendon injury: healing, modeling and remodeling. J Musculoskelet Neuronal Interact 6(2):181–190

Testa V, Capasso G, Maffulli N, Bifulco G (1999) Ultrasound-guided percutaneous longitudinal tenotomy for the management of patellar tendinopathy. Med Sci Sports Exerc 31(11):1509–1515

Testa V, Capasso G, Benazzo F, Maffulli N (2002) Management of Achilles tendinopathy by ultrasound-guided percutaneous tenotomy. Med Sci Sports Exerc 34(4):573–580

Thanasas C, Papadimitriou G, Charalambidis C, Paraskevopoulos I, Papanikolaou A (2011) Platelet-rich plasma versus autologous whole blood for the treatment of chronic lateral elbow epicondylitis: a randomized controlled clinical trial. Am J Sports Med 39(10):2130–2134, Doi: 10.1177/0363546511417113

van den Belt AJ, Keg PR, Kik KJ, Barneveld A (1993) The correlation between the dose and distribution of intratendinous fluid injections in the flexor tendons/ligaments of the horse. Zentralbl Veterinarmed A 40(9–10):713–719

Wiegerinck JI, Reilingh ML, de Jonge MC, van Dijk CN, Kerkhoffs GM (2011) Injection techniques of platelet-rich plasma into and around the Achilles tendon: a cadaveric study. Am J Sports Med 39(8):1681–1686, Doi: 10.1177/0363546511401577

Wiegerinck JI, de Jonge S, de Jonge MC, Kerkhoffs GM, Verhaar J, van Dijk CN (2014) Comparison of postinjection protocols after intratendinous achilles platelet-rich plasma injections: a cadaveric study. J Foot Ankle Surg. doi:10.1053/j.jfas.2014.05.015

Woo SL, Debski RE, Zeminski J, Abramowitch SD, Saw SS, Fenwick JA (2000) Injury and repair of ligaments and tendons. Annu Rev Biomed Eng 2:83–118, Doi: 10.1146/annurev.bioeng.2.1.83

Zajac FE (1989) Muscle and tendon: properties, models, scaling, and application to biomechanics and motor control. Crit Rev Biomed Eng 17(4):359–411

Zhang J, Wang JH (2010) Platelet-rich plasma releasate promotes differentiation of tendon stem cells into active tenocytes. Am J Sports Med 38(12):2477–2486, Doi: 10.1177/0363546510376750

3

Induction of bone formation in abdominal implants constituted by collagen sponges embedded with plant-based human transforming growth factor family proteins in ectopic dog model

Juan Carlos Jacinto-Tinajero[1], Daniel Ascencio[2], Brenda Marquina[1], Jorge Barrios-Payán[1], Maria Concepcion Gutierrez[3], Miguel Gomez Lim[4] and Rogelio Hernández Pando[1,5*]

Abstract

Background: Trauma, osteomyelitis, bone tumour resections and congenital deformities are the main causes of bone deficiency in which autologous graft is the preferred treatment, but usually the bone supplies are limited.

Methods: An experimental model of heterotopic bone formation in the subcutaneous abdominal area of dogs was developed. This model consists in omentum wrapped implants constituted by collagen type 1 sponges embedded with demineralized bone powder, calcium cloride, thrombin and platelet rich plasma; the implant is totally converted in trabecular bone after four months of implantation. This model was improved by accelerating bone production, after the isolation of the most conspicuous histological constituents (inflammatory, bone and adipose tissues) by laser microdisection and purified from them RNA that was used to determine by RT-PCR the gene expression kinetics of the most important growth bone factors. Then, the most abundant and rapidly synthesized factors were produced by genetic engineering in tobacco plants.

Results: Bone morphogenetic proteins 2 and 7 and transforming growth factor-β1were the most rapidly and highly synthesized factors, and they were efficiently produced in a genetic engineering plant based system in tobacco leaves. Their incorporation as recombinant proteins in the scaffold collagen sponge induced in just one month mature heterotopic bone.

Conclusion: This study demonstrates for the first time that this plant system is able to produce recombinant bone growth factors in high amount and at low cost, and they were highly efficient to rapidly induce bone formation in abdominal implants potentially useful for autotransplantation.

Keywords: Heterotopic bone; Tissue engineering; Bone morphogenetic proteins

Background

There are several problems that cause bone defects; the most important are trauma, osteomyelitis, bone tumour resections and development deformities [1]. In cases in which bone reconstruction is associated with bone defect, the traditional therapies are usually not successful and some cases require amputation [2]. Due to these problems the treatment of bone defect has been recently studied, being vascularized bone grafting and distraction osteogenesis the election therapies [3]. Another new perspective in the treatment of this problem is tissue engineering.

Bone tissue engineering is based in part of tissue induction, that can be defined as a process in which a tissue or product derived from it causes a second undifferentiated tissue to differentiate into bone. This process is orchestrated by signaling molecules that govern cell proliferation, migration, and differentiation, which depend on the

* Correspondence: rhdezpando@hotmail.com
[1]Experimental Pathology and Surgery Departments, National Institute of Medical Sciences and Nutrition "Salvador Zubiran", Mexico city, Mexico
[5]Department of Pathology, National Institute of Medical Sciences and Nutrition 'Salvador Zubirán', Section of Experimental Pathology, Mexico city, DF 14000, Mexico
Full list of author information is available at the end of the article

microenvironment and recruitment of progenitor cells, recapitulating embryonic development [4]. Indeed, this process is similar to heterotopic bone formation [5] which usually starts with the proliferation of mesenchymal and perivascular undifferentiated cells, followed by their osteoblastic cell differentiation producing mature bone tissue. Thus, bone induction requires at least of three elements: osteoprogenitor cells, osteoinductive factors and supporting extracellular matrix [6,7]. We developed an experimental model of heterotopic bone formation by the integration of these three elements in the subcutaneous abdominal area of dogs [8]. This model consist in omentum wrapped implants constituted by collagen type I sponges, which is the supportive matrix that have the osteo-inductive factors bone morphogenetic proteins (BMP); platelets rich plasma that is another source of BMP and other growth factors such as transforming growth factor beta I (TGFβ1), platelet derived growth factor (PDGF) and insulin like growth factor I and II (IGF). We also added to the implants thrombin that induces the production of fibrinogen and fibrin which are also osteoinductive factors and promote vascular proliferation after binding vascular endothelial growth factor (VEGF); moreover, both proteins give a soft consistency and moldable condition permitting to give the implant the desired shape and size that is maintained by the neoformed bone. Although this is an efficient model of heterotopic bone formation, it needs a long time for complete bone formation (four months). The aim of the present work was to accelerate a more efficient bone production in this model. In order to do this, we first isolated using laser microdisection the most conspicuous histological constituents and purified from them total RNA, that was used to determine by RT-PCR the gene expression kinetics of the most important growth bone factors. In a second part of the study, the most abundant and early expressed growth factors (BMP-2, BMP-7, TGF-β1) were produced in *Nicotiana benthamiana* as recombinant proteins and added to the implants. We decided to use plants for expressing these factors because plants do not contain animal pathogens, have low production costs and rapid production of recombinant proteins is easily performed [9,10]. We used a transient expression system which does not result in transgenic plants. Our results showed a much more rapid production of heterotopic bone (1 month), which could be useful for auto-transplantation.

Methods

Experimental model of heterotopic bone formation

Fourteen mongrel dogs, 4–6 months old and weighing 15-20 kg, free of evident infectious or parasitic illnesses, were anesthetized with pentobarbital (16 mg/kg) and atropine (0.5 mg/kg). Anesthesia was maintained with 2% Ethrane (enflurane). An abdominal midline incision was performed and the great omentum was dissected tailoring a flap with a pedicle from the right gastro-omental artery, keeping the omentum flap immersed in the subcutaneous tissue. The implant was constituted by a sponge of type I collagen and polyvinylpyrrolidone (Fibroquel; Aspid Laboratory, Mexico), embedded with 5 ml of demineralized bone powder (DBP) (Veterinary Transplant Services, Seattle, WA), 5 ml of dog platelet-rich plasma, 10,000 IU of bovine thrombin (Behring, Mexico), and 2.5 ml of 10% calcium cloride (14.7 mg). The mixture of platelet-rich plasma, DBP, thrombin, and collagen formed a soft material that after 1 or 2 minutes was easily moldable and allowed the formation of a cylinder that was wrapped with the omentum flap. Animals were maintained in conventional room with food and water ad libitum. This protocol was approved by the Animal Research and Ethics Committees of the National Institute of Medical Sciences and Nutrition, according to Mexican and International laws.

Kinetics of growth factors genetic expression from specific histologic compartments

The mosaic expression of growth factors during skeletogenesis indicates that diverse bones have different expression of them and it should have therapeutic significance [5]. We hypothesized that a similar situation should exist during heterotopic bone formation. Thus, abdominal implants were dissected and removed after 7, 14, 28, 60, 90, and 120 days of their implantation. Each implant was divided into quadrants and fixed by immersion in 4% paraformaldehyde diluted in phosphate buffered saline solution. After 3 days of decalcification with formic acid, the tissue was embedded in paraffin, sectioned, and stained with hematoxylin and eosin. At least two sections were obtained from each quadrant. In these slides, the most conspicuous tissues were the connective-inflammatory tissue, adipose tissue, and osteoid or mature bone trabeculae. We laser captured these areas by separate under direct microscopic visualization by melting of the selected regions onto a thermoplastic film mounted on optically transparent LCM caps using the Arcturus XP equipment (Arcturus Engineering, Mountain View, CA, USA). The thermoplastic film containing the microdissected tissue cells was used to isolate total RNA using the RNeasy mini kit (Qiagen, Valencia, CA, USA). Quality and quantity of RNA were evaluated through spectrophotometry (260/280 nm) on agarose gels. Reverse transcription of the mRNA was performed using 5 μg RNA, oligo-dT and the Omniscript kit (Qiagen). Real-time PCR was performed using the 7500 real-time PCR system (Applied Biosystems, Foster City, CA, USA) and Quantitect SYBR Green Master-mix kit (Qiagen). Standard curves of quantified and diluted PCR product, as well as negative controls, were included in each PCR run. Specific primers were designed using the program Primer Express (Applied Biosystems) for the following targets: TGF-β1 F: ATG TCA CTG GAG TCG TGA GGC. TGF-β1 R: CCT CGA CTT CCC CTC CAT G. BMP 2 F: AGC CTG GCC AAC ACC GT. BMP 2 R: CAA AGA TTC TAA TTC TTC GT. BMP 6 F: GCG CCT CAG CCC CAA. BMP 6 R: AGG AGT TCT TCC TCT CTC TA. BMP 7 F: GCA GGA CTT GAT CAT CGC TC. BMP 7 R: CCC TCA CAG TAG TAA GCG CGA. IGF 1 F: CAA TTG CTG TTG GGT CGT CA. IGF 1 R: CGC TGA ACA GGG CTT CTG TA. IGF 2 F: GGA CAG CCT GCT TGC TCA AT. IGF 2 R: TTC ACT TGC TCG CAG TTT TCC HPRT F: GGA CAG TAG GAC TGA GCG GCT. HPRT R: CTA CGA TGT GAT GGC CTC CC.

Production of recombinant growth factors in Nicotiana benthamiana

As shown below our study of gene expression kinetics of growth factors showed that BMP-2 was the most rapid and highest expressed factor, followed by BMP-7 and TGF-β1. Thus, we produced these as recombinant proteins in plants.

The sequences employed (TGFβ1 GenBank: X02812.1 TGFβ1, BMP2 NM_001200.2, BMP7 NM_001719.2) were optimized for expression in plants and synthesized by Genscript.com for cloning. All sequences contained a 6xHis tag at the 3′end and were flanked with BsaI sites and cloned in the pICH31070 vector. Orientation and codon in-frame for all constructs were confirmed by restriction analysis and sequencing. All expression vectors were kindly provided by Dr. Yuri Gleba (Icon Genetics) [11]. The expression vectors were introduced into Agrobacterium tumefaciens GV3101 by electroporation. The infiltration of Agrobacterium into N. benthamiana plants was performed as described [12]. In brief, Agrobacterium overnight cultures were grown in YENB medium to high cell density (OD600 = 0.6) and were diluted into infiltration buffer (10 mM MES, pH 5.5; 10 mM $MgSO_4$) to reach the desired concentration. Bacterial suspensions were infiltrated into plants leaves using vacuum. After infiltration, the plants were grown under glasshouse conditions for 10 days. Leaves were then harvested, frozen in liquid nitrogen and stored at 80°C. Subsequently they were macerated and resuspended in extraction buffer (10 mM PBS pH 7.4, 5 M NaCl, 0.5 M EDTA pH 8.0, 0.01% Triton X-100, 50 mM sodium ascorbate, 100 mM PMSF, 100 mM DTT) at 1:2 (v/w) ratio and centrifuged (8000 × g) for 20 min at 4°C. The supernatant was retained and the concentration of total soluble protein (TSP) was determined by the Bradford method (Bio-Rad) with BSA as standard. For purification of the growth factors, the extracts were loaded on a HisTrap HP column (GE Healthcare Life Sciences), the column washed and the 6xHis tag-containing proteins eluted as described by the manufacturers. Fractions were collected and analyzed by SDS-PAGE. Those fractions showing the factors in the purest form were pooled and stored. The identity of each factor was confirmed by western-blot. Briefly, equal amounts of protein from each factor were separated on a non-reducing 12% SDS-PAGE, transferred to nitrocellulose membrane and blocked with 5% fat free milk in TBS/0.05% Tween 20 for 2 h. The membrane was incubated with anti-TGFβ1 (Santa Cruz Biotechnology), anti-BMP-2 or BMP-7 (Peprotech) polyclonal rabbit antibodies at 4°C overnight. After washing, the membrane was incubated with HRP-conjugated anti-rabbit antibody (Santa Cruz Biotechnology) in Tris-Tween 20 for 1 h. Following several washes, the blot was developed by chemiluminescence (Super Signal West Pico Chemiluminescent Substrate, Thermo Scientific). Control blots were processed without incubation of the primary Ab.

Effect of recombinant BMP2, BMP7 and TGFβ1 in the heterotopic bone production in abdominal implants

In two independent experiments, eight mongrel dogs were used for the evaluation of heterotopic bone formation in implants with recombinant growth factors. Following the same procedure described above, in the right side were made two implants, in the upper implant was added 2 cc (200 mg) of recombinant BMP-2, in the lower implant was added the same amount of BMP-7, while in the left side three implants were produced, in the top implant was added the same concentration of TGF-β1, in the middle implant was added the three growth factors in the same doses and the bottom implant was the control without recombinant factors. Right and left implants were removed after 1 and 4 weeks and evaluated histologically for bone formation in sections stained with hematoxilin and eosin. The percentage of the tissue implant conformed by trabecular bone was determined by automated morphometry. Other sections were stained with Masson trichrome and von Kossa techniques in order to evaluate bone maturation. Cellular proliferation was evaluated by the detection of proliferative cell nuclear antigen (PCNA) using conventional immunohistochemistry [8].

Statistical analysis

Student's T-test was used to determine statistical significance of bone growth factors expression and histomorphometry. $p < 0.05$ was considered significant.

Results

Gene expression kinetics of growth factors during heterotopic bone formation

Figure 1 shows that at 7 days of implantation, BMP-2 was the highest expressed factor in the connective inflammatory tissue around or distant from small areas of

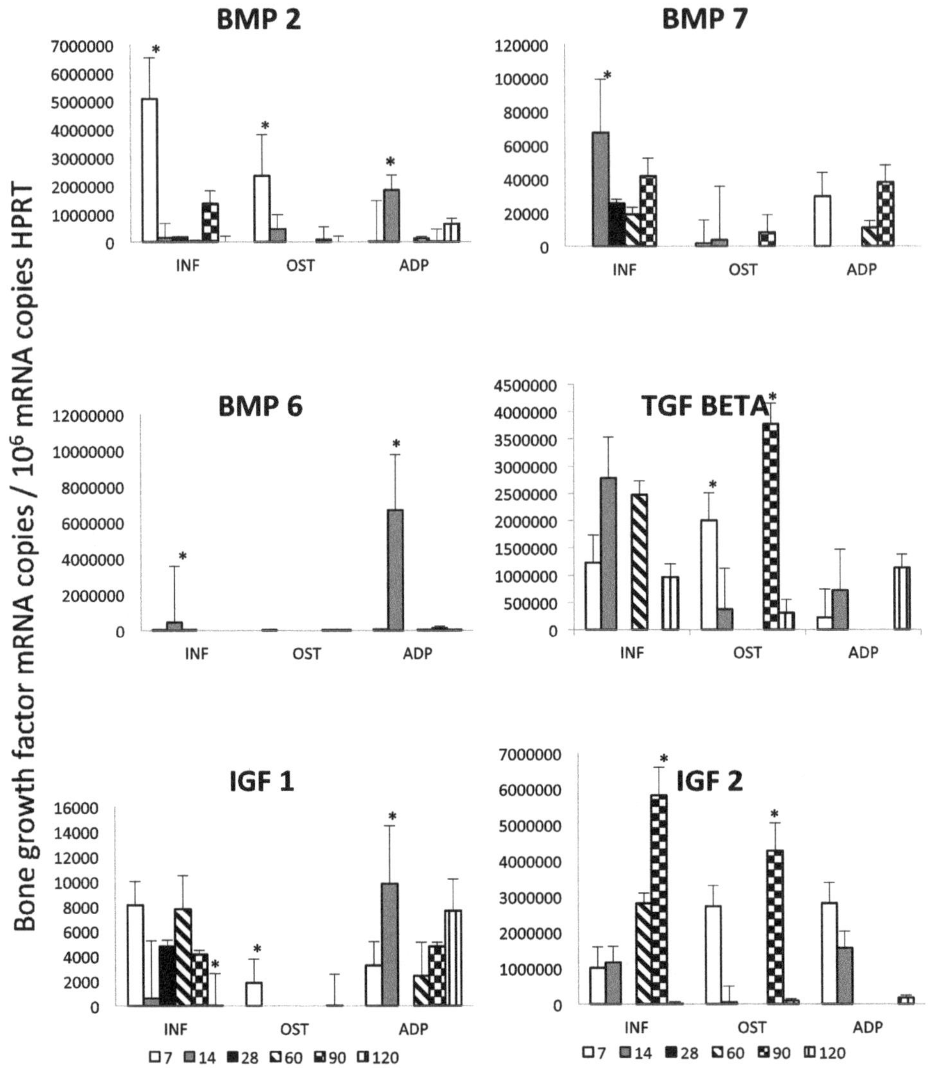

Figure 1 Kinetics of bone growth factors gene expression during heterotopic bone formation. Bone trabeculae (OST), inflammatory tissue (INF) and adipose tissue (ADP) were isolated from the implants using laser microdissection and used to isolate total RNA to determine by RT-PCR the indicated bone growth factor during the heterotopic bone formation. Numbers indicate the day when the implant was obtained after the implantation. Results are present as mean and standard deviation from three dogs in the indicated time points. Two independent experiments were run with similar results. Asterisks represent statistical significance comparing the groups in each time point ($p < 0.05$).

immature bone, in which also was determined a high expression of this growth factor, while in the adipose tissue the expression of BMP-2 raised its peak after two weeks of implantation being the number of transcripts similar than in the osteoid after one week of implantation. Then, the expression of BMP-2 progressively declined in the three different tissues. TGF-β1 was also highly expressed after one week of implantation in immature bone, and this expression was twofold higher after two months when well formed trabecular bone was already produced, while in the connective tissue around bone trabeculae the peak of TGF-β expression was after 2 and 4 weeks of implantation and similarly expressed after 4 months in the three different tissues (Figure 1).

The kinetics of BMP-7 expression was different; this factor showed its highest expression after 2 weeks of implantation in the inflammatory cells located around or distant to bone trabeculae, followed by temporal decrease and increasing again after 60 days showing similar level of expression in the adipose tissue, while a mild and stable expression was detected in the trabecular bone. In contrast, BMP-6 was only expressed after one week of implantation in the inflammatory and adipose tissue (Figure 1). IGF-2 exhibited its highest level after 3 months of implantation in the inflammatory and bone tissue, while in the adipose tissue it raised its peak after one week of implantation. In contrast, IGF-1 exhibited a lower and constant expression (Figure 1).

Production of recombinant BMP-2, BMP-7 and TGF-β1 in tobacco and their effect in heterotopic bone formation

BMP-2, BMP-7 and TGF-β1 were successfully produced in tobacco leaves and their molecular identity was confirmed by western-blotting (Figure 2). After purification, the same amount of each growth factor was added to the implants and the bone production was evaluated after 1 and 4 weeks. All animals survived the surgical procedure. Neither infection nor significant local inflammation was seen. During the surgical resection, the implants showed excellent vascularization without excessive adherences, allowing for an easy surgical extraction and maintained their cylindrical shape. Control implants that did not have the recombinant proteins showed scarce bone formation, less than 5% after one month of implantation (Figures 3 and 4). In contrast, the implants that had recombinant growth factors showed trabecular mature bone since the first week of implantation, being 3%, 12% and 40% in implants with recombinant BMP-2, BMP-7 and TGF-β1 respectively. The percentage of bone formation progressively increased, being more than 80% after one month of implantation with TGF-β1, followed by 60% and 45% in the implants with BMP-2 and BMP-7 respectively. Both factors induced the nuclear expression of PCNA in the mesenchimal cells around the bone trabeculae, and particularly BMP7 induced relatively large areas of osteoid material (Figure 4). Thus, cellular proliferation and differentiation are involved in heterotopic bone production. The addition of the three growth factors in the same implant showed lesser production of heterotopic bone than the implants that received each factor independently, histologically this implants showed numerous small blood vessels and osteoid. This efficient and relatively rapid bone production confirms the effective biological efficiency of these factors produced in plants.

Discussion

The preferred treatment of bone deficiency is autologous graft with bone harvested from sites such as the iliac crest [13], but usually the available autologous bone supplies are limited and harvesting is painful and with risk of infection. Bone allograft is an alternative, but it has limited success because the delayed time to fusion or incomplete graft incorporation due to the elicited immune response [14]. Thus, several novel approaches are currently being explored, such as tissue engineering [7].

Well-vascularised intramuscular sites are highly favorable to the induction of bone formation and this has motivated the manufacturing of heterotopic bone for autologous transplantation [15]. We used another strategy for heterotopic bone formation, producing abdominal implants constituted by a type I collagen sponge embedded with DBP, platelets and calcium cloride wrapped with omentum [8]. We now improved this system by the addition of recombinant BMP-2, BMP-7 or TGF-β1which were the quickest and highest bone growth factors produced in this model.

The induction of bone tissue requires osteoprogenitor cells, osteoinductive factors and a supporting extracellular matrix that must interact in a highly regulated process [5-7]. We wrapped the implants with omentum, which is constituted by adipose cells, fibrous tissue and a blood vessels network. Adipose tissue is a mesodermally derived organ that has a stromal population containing endothelial, smooth muscle and stem cells [16]. Adipose tissue-derived stem cells share many characteristics of its counterpart in bone marrow including multilineage differentiation [17]. Thus, the omentum adipose tissue is a good source of mesenchymal stem cells for heterotopic bone formation.

Adequate vascularization is another important attribute for heterotopic bone production [18], and the omentum has an extensive blood vessels network that is a good source of nutrients, oxygen, and growth factors, creating a proper microenvironment for bone induction. We added platelet rich plasma to our implants because these cells are a source of growth factors that induce blood vessels production [19]. High vascularization is also related with an adequate inflammatory response with numerous macrophages that induce chemotaxis of mesenchymal stem cells and promote their differentiation to bone cells through production of osteogenic

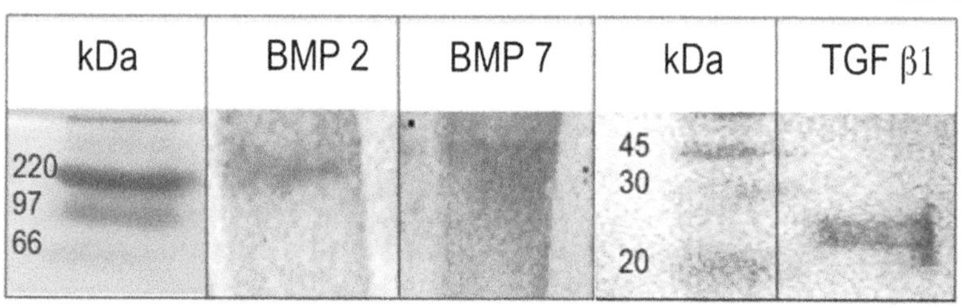

Figure 2 Identification by western-blot of recombinant BMP-2, BMP-7 and TGF-β1 from *Nicotiana benthamiana* leaves. Crude extracts from plants containing each factor and obtained as described in the text were filtered on 0.2 μm membranes and loaded on a HisTrap HP column. Each factor was loaded separately. Fractions were dialyzed against PBS, loaded on a SDS-PAGE gel, transferred to nitrocellulose membranes and incubated with specific rabbit policlonal antibodies to confirm its identity. Molecular weight markers (kDa) are indicated on the left.

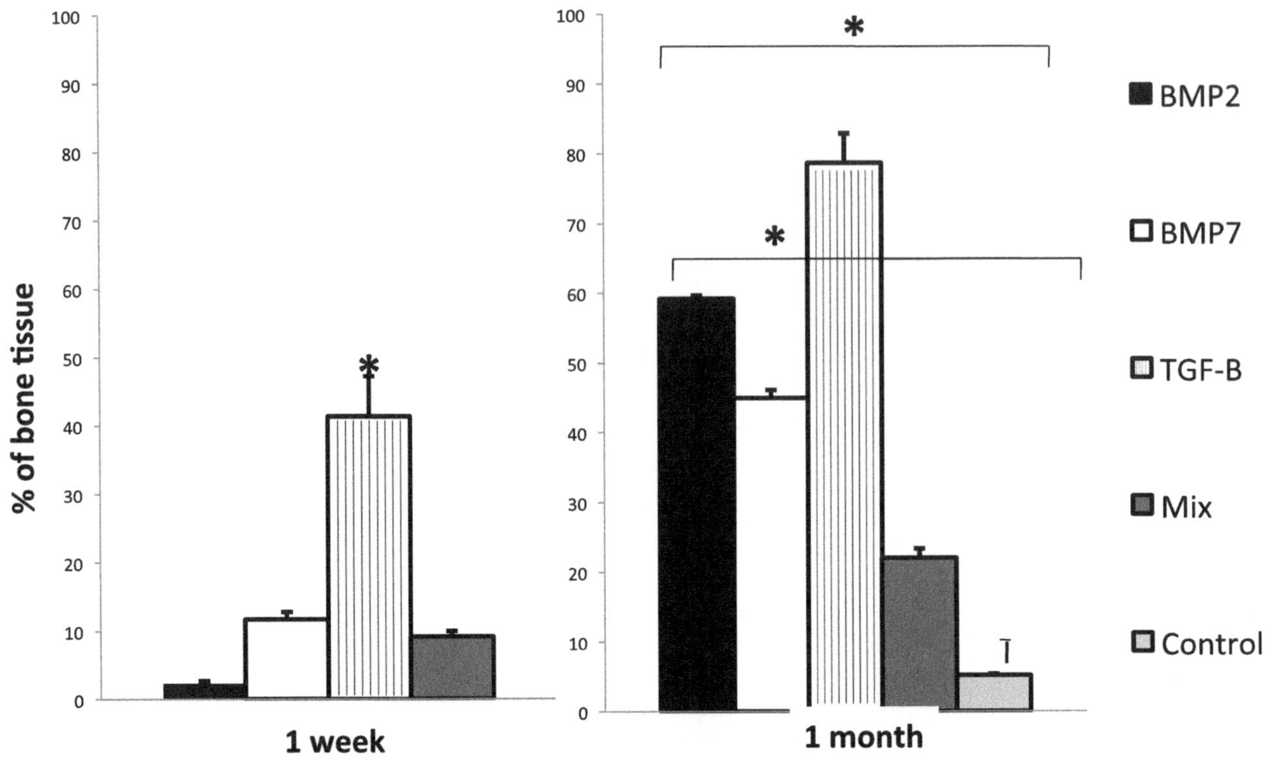

Figure 3 Determination of the percentage of bone tissue by automated morphometry after one and four weeks of implantation adding the indicated growth factors. Results are presented as means and standard deviation of three different dogs in the indicated time points. Mix means implants with the three factors in the same concentration. Asterisk represent statistical difference ($p < 0.005$) among the indicated groups. Two independent experiments were run with similar results.

factors [8]. This was clearly demonstrated by our gene expression kinetics study which showed the inflammatory tissue as the site of the highest expression of BMP and TGF-β1.

A significant focus of research on tissue engineering has been the developing of ideal carriers for bone growth factors [20]. The carrier should act as three-dimensional space scaffolding across which de novo bone formation can occur; and also should maintain an effective concentration of growth factors and containing them in order to avoid extraneous bone formation. Collagen is considered a good carrier, because it is a good source of adhesion-signaling molecules and is also a support for blood vessels and parenchymal cells. We used a type I collagen sponge as carrier, because it is also osteoinductive and favored vascular growth due to its physical characteristics. There is also a good amount of fibrous tissue in the omentum, which contributed to the confinement of the implant and growth factors, avoiding the bone production outside the implant and facilitates its surgical resection avoiding the formation of adherences.

Other essential elements in bone formation are specific growth factors, such as BMP, FGF, PDGF, IGFs [21,22]. BMP is the largest sub group of growth factors that belong to the TGF-β superfamily; they are pleiotropic regulators that mediate various sequential cellular responses such as: chemotaxis and proliferation of progenitor cells, differentiation into osteoblast, vascular invasion, bone formation, remodeling and bone marrow differentiation [6,21]. For bone induction, the most commonly utilized BMPs are BMP2 and 7. BMP2 acts upstream inducing global cellular mobilization (day 1 to 3), whereas BMP7 acts on bone differentiation (day 2 to 5) [2]. These kinetics patterns were also observed in our model, during the first week of implantation BMP2 was highly expressed, while BMP7 raised its maximal expression during the second week. We produced both factors in tobacco leaves as recombinant proteins and added into the implants. After one month, 60% and 45% of the implant was constituted by trabecular bone when added BMP-2 or BMP-7 respectively. The induction of cell proliferation by both BMPs was demonstrated by the immunohistochemistry detection of the cell proliferation marker PCNA, which showed numerous positive cells in the mesenchymal tissue around bone trabeculae. Thus both recombinant proteins are efficient inducing a more rapid bone production in this model. Indeed, both BMPs are now available in the clinical setting [2], and recent evidence has shown that heterodimeric BMPs may have a greater effect than homodimers alone [23]. However in our experimental conditions, we did not

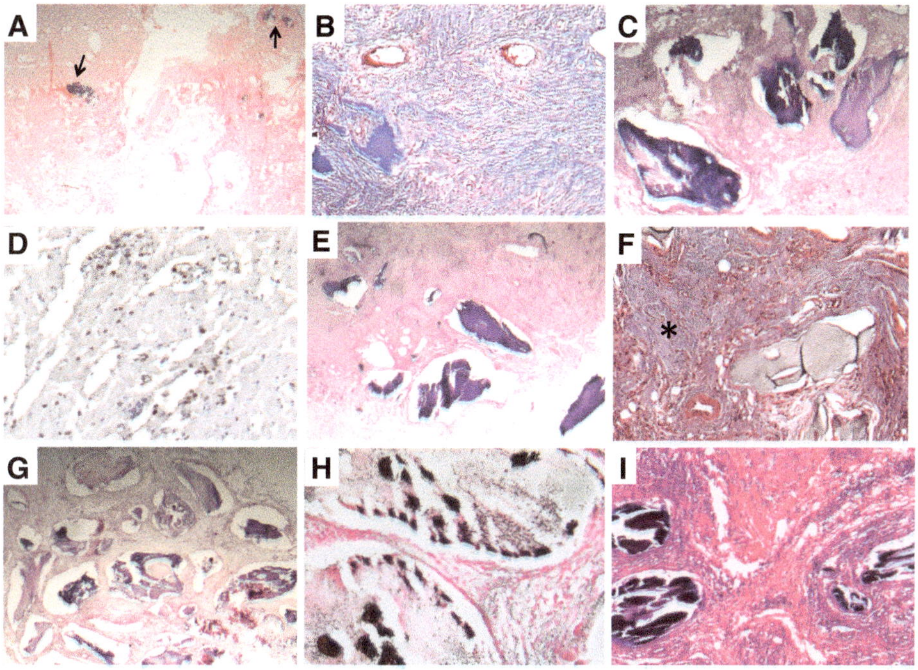

Figure 4 Representative histology of implants after 4 weeks of abdominal implantation. A) Control implant without any factor is essentially constituted of fibroadipose tissue with small areas of bone (arrows). **B)** Fibrous tissue in control implant is well demonstrated by Masson trichromic staining. **C)** In contrast, implant with recombinant BMP-2 shows large mature bone trabeculae surrounded by fibrous or mesenchymal tissue. **D)** This mesenchymal tissue shows numerous cells with PCNA positive immunostaining. **E)** Similar bone production is observed in implant with BMP-7. **F)** This implant with BMP7 shows extensive areas of osteoid in section stained with Masson technique (asterisk). **G)** Even more bone trabeculae are seen in an implant with addition of TGF-1. **H)** They are mature trabeculae constituted by well calcified bone as show by Von Kossa staining. **I)** In comparison, fewer bone trabeculae were induced in implant with all the TGF family factors.

observe this better effect when both factors were added in the same implant at the same amount; perhaps because the dose, proportions and the timing for their administration. More investigation should be done exploring this important issue, which we consider an easy procedure considering that the implant is below the abdominal skin facilitating the direct BMP administration by injection.

The most efficient factor to induce bone formation in our model was TGF-β1. This cytokine increases bone formation mainly by recruiting osteoblast progenitors and stimulating their proliferation, as well as by promoting the early stages of bone differentiation [24]. Results from *P. ursinus* have shown that low doses of TGF-β1 combined with recombinant human osteogenic protein-1 result in the induction of massive ossicles in heterotopic sites (rectus abdominis muscle) as early as 15 days [25]. In our model, 80% of the abdominal implants were constituted by trabecular bone with only one dose of TGF-β1 administered alone. However, there are some potential disadvantages of this procedure. First, TGF-β1 not only modulates bone formation but can also stimulate osteoclast formation, which can be prevented by its administration during early implantation. Second, the half-life of TGF-β1 is short (2 min), implying the need for a matrix to allow for its slow release, we believe that collagen matrix can do this function, as well as containing it avoiding other activities of TGF-β outside the bone.

Although both BMP-2 and BMP-7 are potent osteoinductive agents, very large doses are required to produce an adequate biologic response. Indeed, the concentration of BMPs used in clinical trials are more than one million times greater than that found in human bone [26], and recombinant BMP is quite expensive. In this sense, plants represent an ideal alternative for production of recombinant proteins as they lack mammalian pathogens and the proteins produced are identical to the native ones and highly cost effective [9,10,27].

Conclusion

Implants constituted by collagen type 1 sponge embedded with DBP, calcium cloride, thrombin, platelets and recombinant TGFβ1 wrapped with omentum efficiently induce heterotopic bone formation in the subcutaneous abdominal area in dogs. It was demonstrated for the first time that growth factors produced in plants in high amounts and at low cost were highly efficient to rapidly induce heterotopic bone formation potentially useful for autotransplantation.

Competing interests
Authors declare that there are not competing interests.

Authors' contributions
JCJT carried out the surgical work, tissue laser microdisection and bone growth factor kinetics. AD designed the experimental model of heterotopic bone production. BM supervised and performed the molecular work. JBP carried out the histological work. MCG analyzed and interpreted the results. MGL designed and performed the production of recombinant bone growth factors in plants. RHP designed the improvement of the experimental model, supervised the experimental work and wrote the paper. All authors read and approved the final manuscript.

Acknowledgments
This study was supported by the Mexican Council of Science and Technology CONACyT (contract no 2006-C01-45386). JCJT was recipient of a postdoctoral scholarship from CONACyT.

Author details
[1]Experimental Pathology and Surgery Departments, National Institute of Medical Sciences and Nutrition "Salvador Zubiran", Mexico city, Mexico. [2]Plastic Surgery, Angeles Hospital, Mexico city, Mexico. [3]Experimental Biology Department, Metropolitan University, Mexico city, Mexico. [4]Department of Genetic Engineering in Plants, National Politechnique Institute Center of Research and Advanced Studies, Irapuato, Mexico. [5]Department of Pathology, National Institute of Medical Sciences and Nutrition 'Salvador Zubirán', Section of Experimental Pathology, Mexico city, DF 14000, Mexico.

References
1. Reichert JC, Saifzadeh S, Wullschleger ME, Epari DR, Schütz MA, Duda GN, Schell H, van Griensven M, Redl H, Hutmacher DW (2009) The challenge of establishing preclinical models for segmental bone defect research. Biomaterials 30:2149e63
2. Obert L, Deschaseaux F, Garbuio P (2005) Critical analysis and efficacy of BMPs in long bones non-union. Injury Int J Care Injured 365:538–542
3. Giotakis N, Narayan B, Nayagam S (2007) Distraction osteogenesis and nonunion of the docking site: is there an ideal treatment option? Injury 38: S100e7
4. Boden SD (1999) Bioactive factors for bone tissue engineering. Clin Orthop 367:S84–S94
5. Ekelund A, Brosjo¨ O, Nilsson O (1991) Experimental induction of heterotopic bone. Clin Orthop 263:102–12
6. Urist MR (1965) Bone formation by autoinduction. Science 150:893–9
7. Caplan AI, Goldberg VM (1999) Principles of tissue engineered regeneration of skeletal tissue. Clin Orthop 367:S12–S16
8. Ascencio D, Hernàndez Pando R, Berrios JP, Ridaura SC, Lopez Corella E, Carrasco D, Frenck S (2004) Experimental induction of heterotopic bone in abdominal implants. Wound Repair Regen 12:643–649
9. Kirk DD, Webb SR (2005) The next 15 years: taking plant-made vaccines beyond proof of concept. Immunol Cell Biol 83:248–256
10. Yusibov V, Streatfield SJ, Kushnir N (2011) Clinical development of plant-produced recombinant pharmaceuticals: vaccines, antibodies and beyond. Hum Vaccine 7:313–21
11. Marillonnet S, Thoeringer C, Kandzia R, Klimyuk V, Gleba Y (2005) Systemic agrobacterium tumefaciens – mediated transfection of viral replicons for efficienttransient expression in plants. Nat Biotechnol 23(6):718–23
12. Coconi Linares N, Ortega Dávila E, García Machorro J, García Cordero J, Cedillo-Barrón L, Gómez Lim MA (2013) Targeting of envelope domain III protein of DENV type 2 to DEC-205 receptor elicits neutralizing antibodies in mice. Vaccine 31:2366–2371
13. Lasanianos NG, Kanakaris NK, Giannoudis PV (2009) Current management of long bone defects. Orthopaedics and Trauma 24(2):149–162
14. Burchardt H, Enneking W (1978) Transplantation of bone. Surg Clin North Am 58:403–427
15. Heliotis M, Lavery KM, Ripamonti U, Tsiridis E (2006) Transformation of a prefabricated hydroxyapatite/osteogenic protein-1 implant into a vascularised pedicled bone flap in the human chest. Int J Oral Maxillofac Surg 35:265–269
16. Zuk PA, Zhu M, Mizuno H, Huang J, Futrell JW, Katz AJ, Benhaim P, Lorenz HP, Hedrick MH (2001) Multilineage cells from human adipose tissue: implications for cell-based therapies. Tissue Eng 7:211–228
17. Strem BM, Hicok KC, Zhu M, Wulur I, Alfonso Z, Schreiber RE, Fraser KJ, Hedrick HM (2005) Multipotential differentiation of adipose tissue-derived stem cells. Keio J Med 54:132–141
18. Moore MAS (2002) Putting the neo into neoangiogenesis. J Clin Invest 109:313–5
19. Sahni A, Francis CW (2000) Vascular endothelial growth factor binds to fibrinogen and fibrin and stimulates endothelial cell proliferation. Blood 96:3772–8
20. De Bruijn JD, Yuan H, Dekker R, Layrolle P, de Groot K, van Blitterswijk CA (2000) Osteoinductive biomimetic calcium-phosphate coatings and their potential use as tissue-engineering scaffolds. In: Davies JE (ed) Bone Engineering. Em squared, Toronto, Canada, pp 421–431
21. Samartzis D, Khanna N, Shen HF, An HS (2005) Update on bone morphogenetic proteins and their application in Spine surgery. J Am Coll Surg 200:236–248
22. Fakhry A, Ratisoontorn C, Vedhachalam C (2005) Effects of FGF-2/-9 in calvarial bone cell cultures: differentiation stage-dependent mitogenic effect, inverse regulation of BMP-2 and noggin, and enhancement of osteogenic potential. Bone 36:254–66
23. Zhu W, Rawlins BA, Boachie-Adjei O (2004) Combined bone morphogenetic protein-2 and –7 gene transfer enhances osteoblastic differentiation and spine fusion in a rodent model. J Bone Miner Res 19:2021–32
24. Janssens K, ten Dijke P, Janssens S, Van Hul W (2005) Transforming Growth Factor-β1 to the Bone 26:743–774
25. O'Kane S, Ferguson MW (1997) Transforming growth factor β's and wound healing. Int J Biochem Cell Biol 29:63–78
26. Baltzer AW, Lieberman JR (2004) Regional gene therapy to enhance bone repair. Gene Ther 11:344e50
27. Gomez Lim MA (2011) Plants as platform for production of pharmaceutical compounds. In: Liong MT (ed) Bioprocess Sciences and Technology. Nova Science Publishers, New York, p 295

4

Bulk effect of the deltoid muscle on the glenohumeral joint

Claudio Rosso[1,2,5], Andreas M Mueller[1,2], Brett McKenzie[1], Vahid Entezari[1], Andrea Cereatti[4], Ugo Della Croce[4], Arun J Ramappa[3], Ara Nazarian[1] and Joseph P DeAngelis[3*]

Abstract

Background: There remains controversy on the role of the deltoid on glenohumeral translations during basic and pitching motions. We thus studied the passive effect of the deltoid on the deltoid glenohumeral joint center (GHJC).

Methods: Six shoulders were tested using an automated mechanical system. A baseline motion pattern of the intact specimen was contrasted with glenohumeral translation after removal of the deltoid. Each condition was evaluated in abduction (ABD) and an abbreviated throwing motion (ATM) using retro-reflective, bone-embedded markers. The absolute trajectory and the area under the curve (AUC) for each motion were calculated and glenohumeral kinematics with respect to the GH translation were compared.

Results: The removal of the deltoid resulted in significant changes of the GH translation. During 30-60° of ABD, it resulted in a superior and more anterior GH translation, while in the 60-90° segment in a more inferior and medial GH translation. During 90-120°, the GH translation was medialized. In the pitching motion from maximum external rotation to 90° of external rotation (ER), the removal of the deltoid resulted in a more superior, anterior and lateral GH translation. The deltoid thus limits anterior translation in the abduction-external rotation position. In the remaining segments (90-80° and 80-45° of ER), it resulted in a lateralization of the GH translation.

Conclusions: Modelling the throwing shoulder, the deltoid has a significant influence on glenohumeral motion. Athletes with deltoid dysfunction and limited range of motion are at risk for injury due to the resulting change in their throwing mechanics.

Keywords: Bulk effect; Shoulder; Biomechanics; Pitching; Deltoid muscle; Motion analysis

Background

The shoulder has the greatest range of motion of all joints in the human body. It benefits from mobility at the glenohumeral, sternoclavicular, acromioclavicular joints and scapulothoracic articulation and functions to position the hand in space (An et al. 1991). However, since the glenohumeral joint (GH) has little bony stability, its supporting passive (labral and ligamentous) and dynamic (muscular) restraints help to preserve shoulder function.

While a number of muscles are central to the function of the shoulder in *in-vivo* settings, the deltoid together with the supraspinatus muscle have a significant role in initiating abduction and flexion when the arm is at rest (Reed et al. 2013). The deltoid muscle makes up approximately 20% of the shoulder muscles (Bassett et al. 1990; Lee and An 2002), where its most important function is humeral elevation due to its largest moment arm in comparison to all shoulder muscles (Kuechle et al. 1997). Additionally, in patients with rotator cuff arthropathy, the deltoid serves as the primary source of arm elevation. In this condition, the three main segments of the deltoid (anterior, middle and posterior) are crucial, such that the success of a reverse total shoulder arthroplasty hinges on the health and function of the deltoid (Ackland et al. 2010, 2011; Gulotta et al. 2012). Moreover, the deltoid muscle has been shown to passively affect the superior-inferior translation of the humeral head and limit anterior glenohumeral translation when the arm is abducted and externally rotated and thus is said to

* Correspondence: jpdeange@bidmc.harvard.edu
[3]Department of Orthopaedic Surgery, Beth Israel Deaconess Medical Center, Harvard Medical School, 330 Brookline Avenue, Stoneman 10, Boston, MA 02215, USA
Full list of author information is available at the end of the article

contribute to glenohumeral stability (Halder et al. 2001; Kido et al. 2003).

In passive *ex-vivo* studies, the deltoid has extensively been studied in conjunction with reverse shoulder arthroplasty but not in the intact joint (Ackland et al. 2011; Henninger et al. 2012). It has been proposed that its muscle bulk creates pressure that may increase joint stability and thus decrease glenohumeral translation ("bulk effect") (Ovesen and Nielsen 1986; Ackland et al. 2011; Kido et al. 2003). The "bulk effect" has never been clearly defined but it is commonly accepted that the passive weight of the deltoid could be considered as the "bulk effect". As a result of its superficial position, the deltoid may have an important role as a passive restraint (Howell and Galinat 1988). Both, Colachis et al. and Markhede et al. found that loss of function of the deltoid did not increase glenohumeral translation (Colachis et al. 1969; Markhede et al. 1985). Colachis et al. rendered the deltoid muscle inactive using an axillary nerve block, while Markhede et al. assessed the remaining function of the upper limb after removal of the deltoid muscle following tumor resection. While the removal of the deltoid muscle resulted in a decrease in strength, the loss was less than predicted with *a priori* calculations.

However, there is no universally accepted dogma

We thus hypothesized that the *removal of the deltoid muscle would not affect glenohumeral translation* in our validated model (Rosso et al. 2013; Entezari et al. 2012; Mueller et al. 2014). The aim of the study was to prove this.

Methods

Testing apparatus

Our validated and published robotic testing system that generates automated motion segments for a cadaveric torso over a designated trajectory was used in this study (Rosso et al. 2013; Entezari et al. 2012). The robotic system consists of lower (torso) and an upper (hand) frames that provide linear as well as rotational motion along seven axes. The lower frame generates motion along X, Y, Z axes and around the Z axis, while the upper frame generates motion along the X, Y and Z axes, as highlighted in Figure 1. Motion was generated using linear and rotary closed loop actuators that are controlled via a centralized programmable system to generate any motion trajectory within the actuators' limits. Limits and home switches were combined with encoders to produce closed loop feedback for each axis, ensuring safety for the cadaver/operator and precision. A detailed description of the apparatus has recently been published (Entezari et al. 2012). Also, the precision and accuracy of the testing system in reproducing pure and complex trajectories has been established in a separate publication (Rosso et al. 2013). Torsos were mounted onto a rod fixture while held in place with volume expanding foam and were mounted onto the lower frame. The end effector of the upper frame was secured to the radius and the ulna using a Schanz pin.

Cadavers and motion analysis

Experiments were carried out on six fresh-frozen human torsos acquired from Medcure Anatomical Tissue Bank (Orlando, FL, USA). All specimens had intact shoulders with no history of shoulder pain. During dissection, we found all rotator cuffs to be intact while the status of the long head of the biceps could not be evaluated as the rotator cuff was not removed. More demographic data can be found in Table 1.

Motion data, consisting of three dimensional positions of reflecting markers in the global coordinate system, were

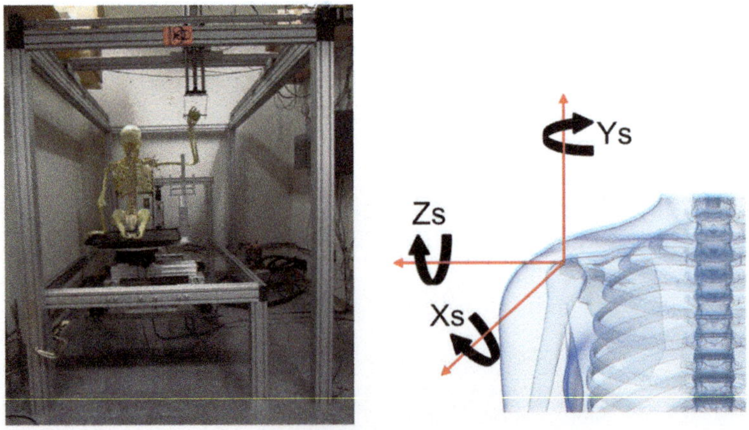

Figure 1 Left side: Testing apparatus with a lower (small) frame and an upper (large) frame. The upper frame can move in X, Y and Z directions, while the lower frame can move in X, Y, Z directions and rotate around the Y axis. Right side: An illustration of the system axes according to the ISB (International Society of Biomechanics) standards. The Z axis represents the medio-lateral axis while Y represents the supero-inferior axis and the X axis the antero-posterior axis. (Wu et al. 2005).

Table 1 Demographic data

Age	Cause of death	Height [m]	Weight [kg]	BMI	Gender	Race
64	Lung Cancer w/mets	1.88	125	35.3	m	Caucasian
57	Respiratory Failure	1.88	139	39.4	m	Caucasian
60	Esophageal Cancer w/Mets	1.93	109	29.2	m	Caucasian
64	Prostate Cancer	1.78	61	19.4	m	Caucasian
50	Myocardial Infarction	1.70	64	21.9	m	Caucasian
49	Glioblastoma	1.78	95	30.1	m	Caucasian
67	Myocardial Infarction	1.85	84	24.4	m	Caucasian

acquired using a five-camera stereo-photogrammetric system (ProReflex Cameras®, Qualisys, Gothenburg, Sweden, 120 frames/s). The acquisition volume was a 1.5-m-sided cube. This system has been validated and can resolve differences in glenohumeral translations as little as 0.5 mm (Rosso et al. 2013; Entezari et al. 2012).

While the specimen was secured to the robotic system, a steel pin equipped with a four marker cluster (transosseous bi-cortical) was implanted into the humeral diaphysis (Figure 2). An acromion marker cluster, equipped with four markers was directly attached to the acromion using three screws (4 mm × 10 mm). The acromion marker cluster was made of an alloy triangular base specifically shaped to be positioned over the flat part of the acromion (Cereatti et al. 2014). Before starting the dynamic acquisitions, with the arm hanging along the side of the torso, the positions of the following anatomical landmarks [28] were measured and registered with respect to the relevant bone marker clusters using a pointer equipped with a four-marker cluster according to the Calibration Anatomical System Techniques (CAST) [22]: the most caudal point on lateral epicondyle (LE), the most caudal point on medial epicondyle (ME), the trigonum spinae scapulae (TS), the angulus inferior (AI), the angulus acromialis (AA), the most ventral point of processus (PC) and the most dorsal point on the acromioclavicular joint (AC).

The poses of the marker cluster coordinate system of the humerus and the scapula, relative to the global coordinate system, were estimated using a SVD (singular value decomposition) technique (Soderkvist and Wedin 1993). The anatomical coordinate systems of humerus and scapula were defined according to the ISB (International Society of Biomechanics) recommendations (Figure 1) [21] and were registered relative to the corresponding marker cluster coordinate systems according to [22].

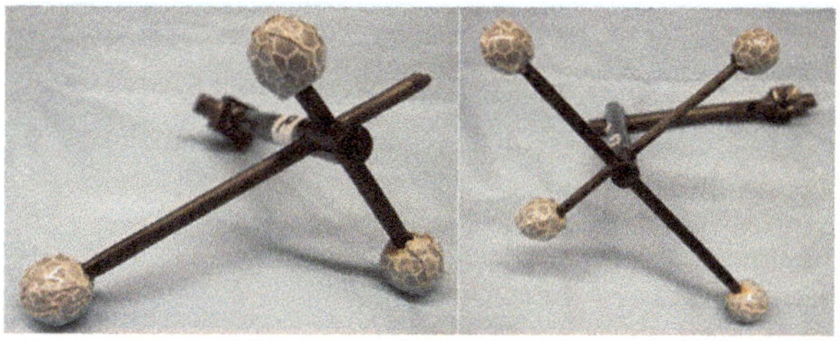

Figure 2 Marker cluster. This figure depicts the four marker cluster used.

The position of the glenohumeral joint center was determined according to the regressive equation described by Meskers et al. (Meskers et al. 1998). In particular, while the arm was hanging along the side of the torso, this position with respect to the scapula marker cluster was identified as the baseline neutral position. The position was then expressed with respect to this neutral position. This procedure allowed to define two glenohumeral joint center positions for the scapula and humerus, respectively. These two positions were assumed to coincide in the reference shoulder position (arm hanging along the side of the torso).

In order to recreate every day and sport-specific motions, two different types of motion segments were chosen for this study: 1) humeral elevation in the coronal plane (abduction, ABD) from 30° to 150° (120° range) and 2) abbreviated throwing motion (ATM). According to the definition of the baseball pitching motion (Meister 2000), we defined an abbreviated throwing motion ranging from the late cocking (maximal external rotation of the humerus) to the deceleration phase. The ATM motion was tested from maximal external rotation in 90° of abduction of the humerus (abduction- external rotation (ABER) position) into approximately 45° of external rotation (75° range). This would also recreate the abduction-external rotation moment as published by Kido et al. (Kido et al. 2003).

Abduction was chosen as a basic motion of the arm, and the abbreviated throwing motion was chosen as a uniquely human motion (Roach et al. 2013), where maximal external rotation removes laxity from passive restraints, thereby further increasing motion repeatability.

Figure 3 depicts the range of each motion segment, while Figure 4 depicts the posterior restraint needed to attain maximal external rotation in the abbreviated throwing motion. For each of the abovementioned trajectories (ABD and ATM), two shoulder conditions were tested in triplicates: 1) cadaver with deltoid on (DON), and 2) cadaver with deltoid off (DOFF). For the DON configuration, only the skin was removed prior to data acquisition. Prior to DOFF data acquisition, the entire deltoid muscle was identified and dissected exposing the subacromial space and rotator cuff. The remaining tissue was kept moist with physiologic 0.9% saline throughout the experiment, and no other restraints were introduced into any anatomic locations (i.e. no rigid fixation of scapula). External rotation of the arm during the ATM motion was ensured by using a posterior restraint to the humerus. The posterior restraint had to be implemented as else a posterior motion of the arm would result in horizontal abduction and not in external rotation of the humerus (Figure 4). The posterior restraint was applied to the humerus while the robotic device moved posteriorly. In this way, the arm was forced into external rotation (Figure 4). As the calculation of the removal of the deltoid was done in comparison to the motion with deltoid (DON) using the same posterior restraint, its effect can be neglected. Testing was conducted with no resting time between each repetition.

A total of 12 (2 conditions × 2 shoulder motion × 3 trials) data sets were acquired for each specimen, and for each trial at each instant of time, the position vectors of the humerus GHJC were expressed in the scapular reference system. Glenohumeral translation was defined as the displacement vector of the humerus GHJC with respect to its position at the beginning of the motion under analysis expressed in the scapula anatomical frame.

Data analysis

The absolute trajectory and the area under the curve (AUC) for each specimen at each motion segment were generated. AUC was calculated for each condition on each axis using the trapezoidal rule in order to appropriately assess the path-dependent motion (Matlab version 12, Mathworks, Natick, MA, USA). Given the real time data acquisition capability of the testing system used in this study, the motion trajectory itself could be compared between different testing conditions. To that end, the area under the curve of the motion trajectory was used as a quantitative surrogate for variations in the motion path across different conditions. Area under the curve, averaged across the three trials per condition, was used to compare differences in the motion paths between different conditions (DON and DOFF) for each motion segment and each motion (ABD and ATM).

Motion segments were divided into discrete steps to facilitate statistical comparison of data between different conditions (DON and DOFF). The ABD motion was discretized into five 30° increments ($ABD^{30°, 60°, 90°, 120°, 150°}$). Similarly, the ATM motion was discretized into 4 increments to match pitching phases $ABER^{MAX}$ (maximum external rotation in 90° of abduction, early cocking), $ABER^{90°}$ (mid acceleration), $ABER^{80°}$ and $ABER^{45°}$ (ball

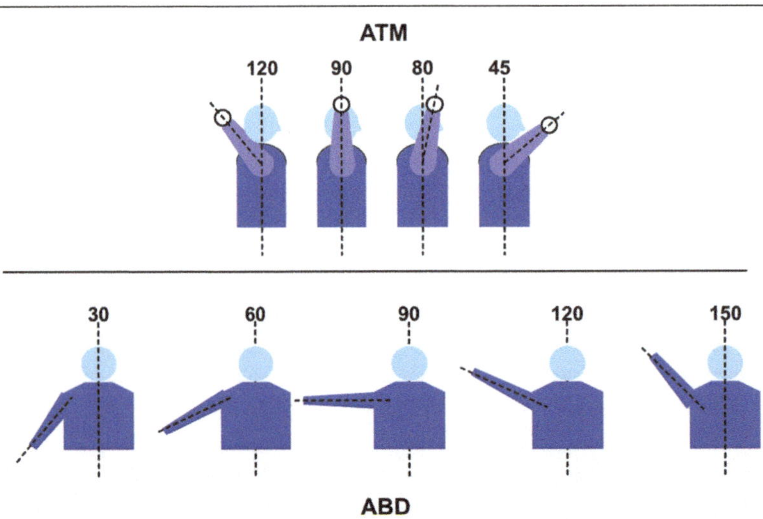

Figure 3 Illustration of the range of motion of the abbreviated throwing motion (ATM, top) and abduction (ABD, bottom). The ATM segments were defined according to the phases of the pitching motion as published by Meister.(Meister 2000): Segment I ranged from maximal external rotation at 90° of humeral abduction to 90° of external rotation, segment II ranged from 90° or ER to 80° of external rotation of the humerus, and segment III ranged from 80° of external rotation to 45° of external rotation and was at the same time the end of the motion (end of acceleration phase). The abduction was segmented into 30-60-90-120-150 degrees of abduction.

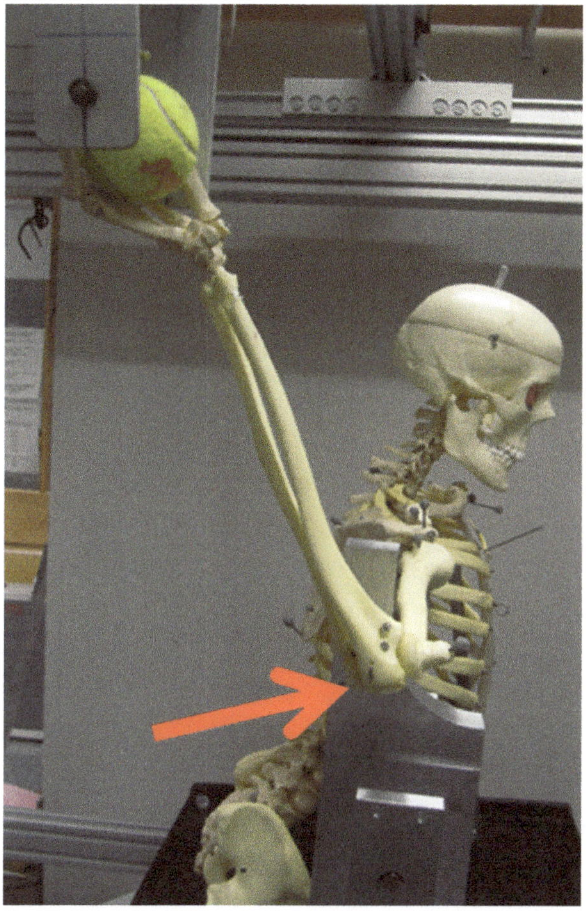

Figure 4 The posterior restraint (red arrow) permits the humerus to externally rotate, while the hand is pulled dorsally. This was used for the abbreviated throwing motion (ATM) for creating the external rotation needed for replicating the late cocking phase of baseball pitching.

release). In the ATM motion, the arm was at 90° of abduction and pivoted around the humeral axis. Repeated measures Analysis of Variance (ANOVA) with arm angle and test repetition (3 per specimen per condition) as within-subject factors and group as between-subject factor was conducted for X, Y and Z translations. For cases were the assumption of sphericity was not met, the Huynh-Feldt correction was used to adjust the degrees of freedom of the F test. The Wilcoxon Signed–Rank test was used to compare the areas under the curves (AUC) between the conditions. The AUC comparisons were conducted for the entire curve and for each curve segment between arm angles (Figure 3. ABD: $ABD^{30°-60°}$, $ABD^{60°-90°}$, $ABD^{90°-120°}$, $ABD^{120°-150°}$ and $ABD^{30°-150°}$ and ATM: $ABER^{MAX-90°}$, $ABER^{90°-80°}$, $ABER^{80°-45°}$ and $ABER^{MAX-45°}$). Data analysis was performed using SPSS (version 21.0, IBM-SPSS, Armonk, NY, USA) and MedCalc (MedCalc, Ostend, Belgium) statistical software packages, and statistical significance level was set at P value < 0.05.

Ethics statement

The study has been conducted in conjunction with current ethical standards on the use of human tissue. An approval by the IRB was not needed due to the use of cadavers and not live human subjects.

Results

Statistical analysis revealed that all data was distributed normally in the study (P values greater than 0.05 for all cases). In absolute GH translation, the ABD motion segment (X, Y and Z axes) did not significantly differ between DON and DOFF conditions at the abduction range of $ABD^{30°}$ to $ABD^{150°}$ [Figure 5a, b and c] (Huynh-Feldt within subject effect P values 0.87, 0.88 and 0.92, respectively). Similarly, in the ATM motion segment, the absolute GH translation components (X, Y and Z) did not differ significantly between DON and DOFF conditions at the ATM range of $ABER^{MAX}$ to $ABER^{45°}$ [Figure 6a, b, c] (Huynh-Feldt within subject effect P values 0.62, 0.75 and 0.85 respectively).

There were differences in motion trajectories as revealed by AUC analysis of the two conditions for both the ABD and the ATM motion segments. In case of the ABD segment, there were differences in the X axis ($ABD^{30°-60°}$ segment ($P < 0.001$)), Y axis ($ABD^{30°-60°}$ ($P = 0.04$) and $ABD^{60°-90°}$ ($P = 0.02$)) and Z axis ($ABD^{60°-90°}$ ($P = 0.01$), $ABD^{90°-120°}$ ($P = 0.04$) and $ABD^{30°-150°}$ ($P = 0.02$)) [Figure 5d, e, f]. These results suggest that at 30-60° abduction, the removal of the deltoid resulted in a more superior (X axis) and anterior GH translation (Y axis), while at 60-90° of abduction, the removal of the deltoid resulted in a more inferior (Y axis) and medial displacement of the GH translation (Z axis). From 90° to 120°, the removal of the deltoid resulted in a medialization of the GH translation (Z axis). Overall, the removal of the deltoid resulted in a medialization of the GH translation in abduction ($ABD^{30°-150°}$).

In case of the ATM segment, there were differences in X axis ($ABER^{MAX-90°}$ segment ($P < 0.001$)), Y axis ($ABER^{MAX-90°}$, ($P < 0.001$) and Z axis ($ABER^{MAX-90°}$, $ABER^{90°-80°}$, $ABER^{80°-45°}$, $ABER^{MAX-45°}$ ($P < 0.01$ for all cases)) [Figure 6d, e and f]. These results suggest that from $ABER^{MAX}$ to $ABER^{90°}$ all axes are affected by the removal of the deltoid resulting in a more superior, anterior and more lateral positioning of the glenohumeral translation. However, in the remaining ATM motion segments, only the medio-lateral (Z axis) was involved: the removal of the deltoid resulted in a lateralization of the glenohumeral translation in the $ABER^{90°-80°}$ and $ABER^{80°-45°}$ segments as well as the overall ATM range of motion ($ABER^{MAX-45°}$ segment). It thus limits anterior translation in the ABER (abduction-external rotation position).

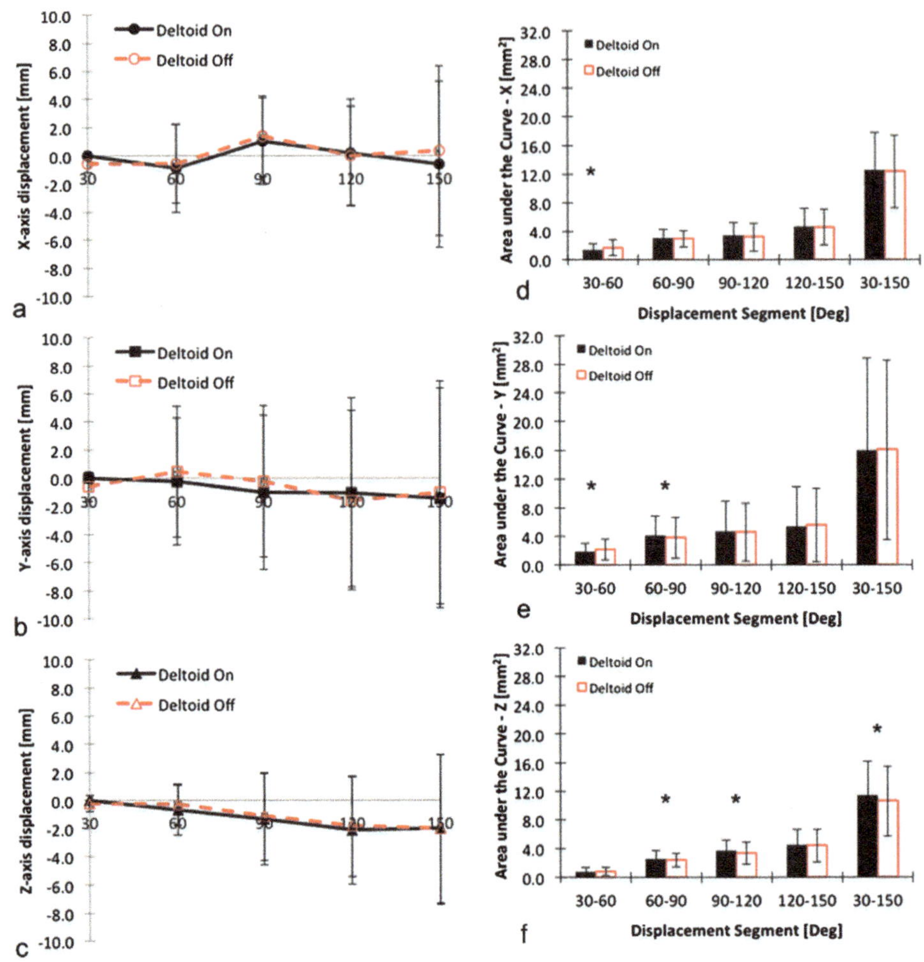

Figure 5 Presentation of absolute curves per condition for the ABD motion segment in X (a), Y (b) and Z (c) axes, and presentation of AUC curves per condition for ABD motion in X (d), Y (e) and Z (f) axes. The star (*) highlights significant differences between DON and DOFF (please see text for details). *Legend: ABD = abduction; DON = deltoid intact; DOFF = deltoid removed.*

Discussion

The purpose of this investigation was to study the passive effect of the deltoid on glenohumeral translations in abduction and abbreviated throwing motion using an intact cadaveric torso. In biomechanical testing, the deltoid is often removed to gain access to the underlying rotator cuff. While this technique is believed to be an acceptable compromise, little data are available to justify this decision, because the passive role of the deltoid has not been described. To improve upon prior descriptions of shoulder kinematics, this investigation employed a novel system designed to evaluate the shoulder using an intact cadaveric torso, rather than an isolated glenohumeral joint.

In this investigation, the removal of the deltoid resulted in significant effects on glenohumeral translation and the center of rotation and thus glenohumeral stability, affirming the importance of the deltoid as a passive restraint with its bulk effect. Its main influence was on the medio-lateral axis (Z axis) in both motions (ABD and ATM). We could also show a stabilization effect of the deltoid in the segment of $ABER^{MAX}$ to $ABER^{90°}$ as advocated in prior dynamic studies (Halder et al. 2001; Kido et al. 2003).

The effect of shoulder muscles such as the rotator cuff or deltoid muscles on glenohumeral translation has been debated for decades (Markhede et al. 1985; Ovesen and Nielsen 1986; Lee and An 2002; Kido et al. 2003; Colachis et al. 1969; Lee et al. 2000). Since deltoid muscle activity helps to stabilize the glenohumeral articulation, its role as a passive restraint has been attributed to the deltoid's ability to produce an abduction moment and stabilize the humeral head (Billuart et al. 2007). While describing the 'bulk effect' in cadaveric studies, no clear definition of the phenomenon has been developed, even though it is agreed upon that an increase in translation occurs with the removal of tissues that are not directly related to the joint capsule. In an *ex-vivo* study, Ovesen and Nielsen showed

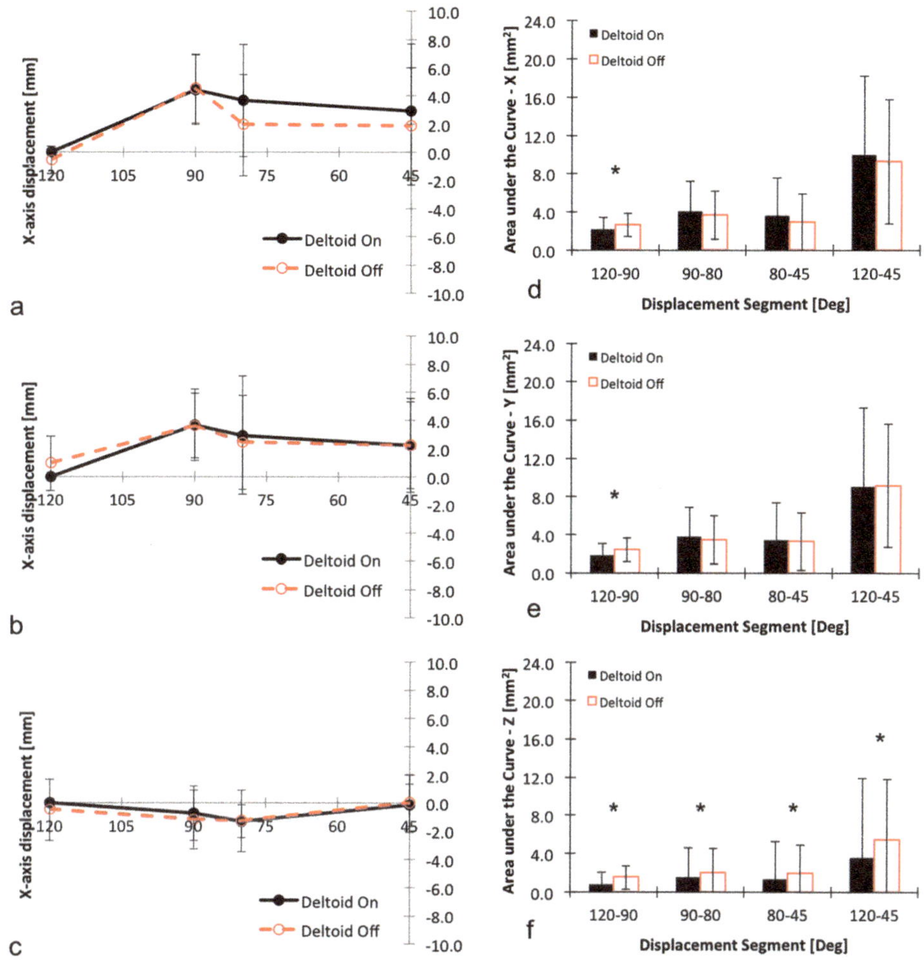

Figure 6 Presentation of absolute curves per condition for the ATM motion segment in X (a), Y (b) and Z (c) axes, and presentation of AUC curves per condition for ABD motion in X (d), Y (e) and Z (f) axes. The star (*) highlights significant differences between DON and DOFF (please see text for details). *Legend: AUC = area under the curve; ATM = abbreviated throwing motion; DON = deltoid intact; DOFF = deltoid removed; 120=MAX.*

increased anterior-posterior glenohumeral translation after removal of the skin and soft-tissues around the shoulder (Ovesen and Nielsen 1986). In another study assessing the effect of muscle volume, the bulk effect was shown when increased muscle volume was correlated with diminished laxity (Howell and Galinat 1988).

Weiner et al. studied plain radiographs showing superior migration of the humeral head (increased superior glenohumeral translation) in static rotator cuff-deficient shoulders, thus supporting the fact of superior pull by the deltoid on the humerus (Weiner and Macnab 1970). An EMG study by Hawkes et al. described the deltoid as a glenohumeral stabilizer in different every-day tasks. The authors studied 13 groups of muscles in healthy subjects including the three parts of the deltoid (anterior, middle and posterior) and studied their activity in a FIT-HaNSA protocol representing different every-day tasks (Hawkes et al. 2012). In an anatomic study, the deltoid functioned to oppose the inferior shear of the latissimus dorsi and the inferior part of the subscapularis muscles (Ackland and Pandy 2009). Moreover, Itoi et al. found that the rotator cuff did not cause a significant bulk effect in a cadaveric study comparing stability at different scapular inclination angles before and after removal. Its removal did not significantly increase glenohumeral translation (Itoi et al. 1993).

Current thinking suggests that scapular positioning might have a much more important role in this motion as described by Itoi et al. (Motzkin et al. 1994; Itoi et al. 1993).

Our model of the throwing shoulder is designed to quantify the passive effects of the shoulder's supporting soft tissues on glenohumeral motion. Recognizing that the rotator cuff and the glenohumeral ligaments (joint capsule) provide passive stability to the joint at the end range of motion, our cadaveric model does not actively load the joint. For this reason, we have intentionally limited the scope of our investigation to the end range of glenohumeral motion.

The passive effect of the soft tissues is isolated when the humerus is abducted ninety-degrees from the thorax and the humerus is maximally externally rotated. This position coincides with the late cocking/early acceleration phases of the throwing motion, when the throwing athlete's shoulder experiences the greatest strain, is most vulnerable to injury, and passively stabilized. For the clinical and sports biomechanics community, understanding the forces at this extreme range of motion offers the greatest opportunity for injury prevention, improved rehabilitation, and advancing surgical treatments of shoulder pathology.

As our model does not actively load the glenohumeral joint, we did not evaluate the mid-range of motion, where dynamic muscle contractions are essential for normal glenohumeral mechanics. Flexion and extension are central to the normal range of motion, but do not rely on the passive stability best studied in our model. The results from this study attribute a significant passive role to the deltoid muscle and its dynamic importance in co-contraction and enhancement of the concavity-compression on the glenohumeral joint must also be emphasized (McMahon et al. 2003; Hawkes et al. 2012). The deltoid is a key player in *active* glenohumeral stability (Hawkes et al. 2012; Billuart et al. 2008; Kido et al. 2003; Halder et al. 2001) and appears to additionally add stability to the glenohumeral joint by its mere presence, thus supporting the bulk effect theory.

As with any work, this study has certain limitations. This investigation was designed to test a range of motion, but the technique did not control for the forces applied to the cadaver. For this reason, in applying the same trajectories, native differences in range of motion and other inter-specimen variability were not addressed. Secondly, we used a posterior restraint in order to recreate external rotation, which might alter glenohumeral joint kinematics. This was the only way to recreate sufficient external rotation without horizontal abduction.

An important advantage of this study was the use of whole torsos in order to account for the whole shoulder girdle with its surrounding soft-tissues (muscles, tendons, ligaments, skin). The shoulder girdle was allowed to move freely in all axes and was not restricted by any tension wires.

Conclusions

Results of this cadaveric study indicate that removal of the deltoid muscle significantly affects the center of rotation for the glenohumeral joint during abduction and abbreviated throwing motion. In this way, the deltoid appears to have an important passive role in lateralization of the GH translation in the pitching motion and its medialization in the GH translation in abduction. Additionally, removal of the deltoid appears to limit anterior translation in the Abduction external rotation position.

Competing interests

There is no conflict of interest announced from the authors regarding this study or this manuscript.

Authors' contributions

All authors have contributed to writing and correcting this manuscript. CR: principal author, writing manuscript, conducting study, analyzation, study planning. AMM: writing manuscript, conducting study, analyzation. BM: writing manuscript, conducting study. VE: writing manuscript, conducting study. AC: writing manuscript, conducting study, study planning. UDC: writing manuscript, study planning. AJR: writing manuscript, study planning, analyzation. AN: writing manuscript, study planning, analyzation. JPD: writing manuscript, study planning, analyzation. All authors read and approved the final manuscript.

Acknowledgments

The authors would like to acknowledge the Medical Advisory Committee for Major League Baseball (AN and AJR) and the Department of Orthopaedic Surgery at the Beth Israel Deaconess Medical Center for funding this project. The authors gratefully acknowledge the Swiss Society of Orthopaedic Surgery and Traumatology (CR and AMM), the Swiss National Science Foundation (CR and AMM) and the Lichtenstein Foundation Basel, Switzerland (CR) for providing financial support. They would also like to acknowledge Dr. Glenn Fleisig and his team from the American Sports Medicine Institute for their help with the motion analysis component of the project. Lastly, the authors would like to thank Mr. William Dow for providing help with the figures.

This work was awarded the 'Poster Prize Basic Research' from the Swiss Society of Orthopaedics and Traumatology in 2012.

Author details

[1]Center for Advanced Orthopaedic Studies, Beth Israel Deaconess Medical Center and Harvard Medical School, Boston, MA, USA. [2]Orthopaedic Department, University Hospital Basel and University of Basel, Basel, Switzerland. [3]Department of Orthopaedic Surgery, Beth Israel Deaconess Medical Center, Harvard Medical School, 330 Brookline Avenue, Stoneman 10, Boston, MA 02215, USA. [4]Information Engineering Unit, POLCOMING Department, University of Sassari, Sassari, Italy. [5]Altius Swiss Sportsmed Center, Rheinfelden, Switzerland.

References

Ackland DC, Pandy MG (2009) Lines of action and stabilizing potential of the shoulder musculature. J Anat 215(2):184–197, doi:10.1111/j.1469-7580.2009.01090.x

Ackland DC, Roshan-Zamir S, Richardson M, Pandy MG (2010) Moment arms of the shoulder musculature after reverse total shoulder arthroplasty. J Bone Joint Surg Am 92(5):1221–1230, doi:10.2106/JBJS.I.00001

Ackland DC, Roshan-Zamir S, Richardson M, Pandy MG (2011) Muscle and joint-contact loading at the glenohumeral joint after reverse total shoulder arthroplasty. J Orthop Res 29(12):1850–1858, doi:10.1002/jor.21437

An KN, Browne AO, Korinek S, Tanaka S, Morrey BF (1991) Three-dimensional kinematics of glenohumeral elevation. J Orthop Res 9(1):143–149, doi:10.1002/jor.1100090117

Bassett RW, Browne AO, Morrey BF, An KN (1990) Glenohumeral muscle force and moment mechanics in a position of shoulder instability. J Biomech 23(5):405–415

Billuart F, Devun L, Gagey O, Skalli W, Mitton D (2007) 3D kinematics of the glenohumeral joint during abduction motion: an ex vivo study. Surg Radiol Anat 29(4):291–295, doi:10.1007/s00276-007-0208-2

Billuart F, Devun L, Skalli W, Mitton D, Gagey O (2008) Role of deltoid and passives elements in stabilization during abduction motion (0 degrees-40 degrees): an ex vivo study. Surg Radiol Anat 30(7):563–568, doi:10.1007/s00276-008-0374-x

Cereatti A, Rosso C, Nazarian A, DeAngelis JP, Ramappa AJ, Della Croce U (2014) Scapular motion tracking using an acromion skin marker-cluster: in vitro accuracy assessment. J Med Biol Engin (Mar 20, 2014), doi: 10.5405/jmbe.1723

Colachis SC Jr, Strohm BR, Brechner VL (1969) Effects of axillary nerve block on muscle force in the upper extremity. Arch Phys Med Rehabil 50(11):647–654

Entezari V, Trechsel BL, Dow WA, Stanton SK, Rosso C, Muller A, McKenzie B, Vartanians V, Cereatti A, Della Croce U, Deangelis JP, Ramappa AJ, Nazarian A (2012) Design and manufacture of a novel system to simulate the biomechanics of basic and pitching shoulder motion. Bone Joint Res 1(5):78–85, doi:10.1302/2046-3758.15.2000051

Gulotta LV, Choi D, Marinello P, Wright T, Cordasco FA, Craig EV, Warren RF (2012) Anterior deltoid deficiency in reverse total shoulder replacement: a biomechanical study with cadavers. J Bone Joint Surg Br 94(12):1666–1669, doi:10.1302/0301-620X.94B12.29116

Halder AM, Halder CG, Zhao KD, O'Driscoll SW, Morrey BF, An KN (2001) Dynamic inferior stabilizers of the shoulder joint. Clin Biomech (Bristol, Avon) 16(2):138–143

Hawkes DH, Alizadehkhaiyat O, Fisher AC, Kemp GJ, Roebuck MM, Frostick SP (2012) Normal shoulder muscular activation and co-ordination during a shoulder elevation task based on activities of daily living: an electromyographic study. J Orthop Res 30(1):53–60, doi:10.1002/jor.21482

Henninger HB, Barg A, Anderson AE, Bachus KN, Tashjian RZ, Burks RT (2012) Effect of deltoid tension and humeral version in reverse total shoulder arthroplasty: a biomechanical study. J Shoulder Elbow Surg 21(4):483–490, doi:10.1016/j.jse.2011.01.040

Howell SM, Galinat BJ (1988) The containment mechanism: the primary stabilizer of the glenohumeral joint. Orthop Trans 12:458

Itoi E, Motzkin NE, Morrey BF, An KN (1993) Bulk effect of rotator cuff on inferior glenohumeral stability as function of scapular inclination angle: a cadaver study. Tohoku J Exp Med 171(4):267–276

Kido T, Itoi E, Lee SB, Neale PG, An KN (2003) Dynamic stabilizing function of the deltoid muscle in shoulders with anterior instability. Am J Sports Med 31(3):399–403

Kuechle DK, Newman SR, Itoi E, Morrey BF, An KN (1997) Shoulder muscle moment arms during horizontal flexion and elevation. J Shoulder Elbow Surg 6(5):429–439

Lee SB, An KN (2002) Dynamic glenohumeral stability provided by three heads of the deltoid muscle. Clin Orthop Relat Res 400:40–47

Lee SB, Kim KJ, O'Driscoll SW, Morrey BF, An KN (2000) Dynamic glenohumeral stability provided by the rotator cuff muscles in the mid-range and end-range of motion. A study in cadavera. J Bone Joint Surg Am 82(6):849–857

Markhede G, Monastyrski J, Stener B (1985) Shoulder function after deltoid muscle removal. Acta Orthop Scand 56(3):242–244

McMahon PJ, Chow S, Sciaroni L, Yang BY, Lee TQ (2003) A novel cadaveric model for anterior-inferior shoulder dislocation using forcible apprehension positioning. J Rehabil Res Dev 40(4):349–359

Meister K (2000) Injuries to the shoulder in the throwing athlete. Part one: Biomechanics/pathophysiology/classification of injury. Am J Sports Med 28(2):265–275

Meskers CG, van der Helm FC, Rozendaal LA, Rozing PM (1998) In vivo estimation of the glenohumeral joint rotation center from scapular bony landmarks by linear regression. J Biomech 31(1):93–96

Motzkin NE, Itoi E, Morrey BF, An KN (1994) Contribution of passive bulk tissues and deltoid to static inferior glenohumeral stability. J Shoulder Elbow Surg 3(5):313–319, doi:10.1016/S1058-2746(09)80076-1

Mueller AM, Rosso C, Entezari V, McKenzie B, Hasebroock A, Della Croce U, Nazarian A, Ramappa AJ, DeAngelis JP (2014) The effect of supraspinatus tears on glenohumeral translations in passive pitching motion. Am J Sports Med 42(10):2455-62. doi: 10.1177/0363546514547348

Ovesen J, Nielsen S (1986) Anterior and posterior shoulder instability. A cadaver study. Acta Orthop Scand 57(4):324–327

Reed D, Cathers I, Halaki M, Ginn K (2013) Does supraspinatus initiate shoulder abduction? J Electromyogr Kinesiol 23(2):425–429, doi:10.1016/j.jelekin.2012.11.008

Roach NT, Venkadesan M, Rainbow MJ, Lieberman DE (2013) Elastic energy storage in the shoulder and the evolution of high-speed throwing in Homo. Nature 498(7455):483–486, doi:10.1038/nature12267

Rosso C, Muller AM, Entezari V, Dow WA, McKenzie B, Stanton SK, Li D, Cereatti A, Ramappa AJ, DeAngelis JP, Nazarian A, Della Croce U (2013) Preliminary evaluation of a robotic apparatus for the analysis of passive glenohumeral joint kinematics. J Orthop Surg Res 8(1):24, doi:10.1186/1749-799X-8-24

Soderkvist I, Wedin PA (1993) Determining the movements of the skeleton using well-configured markers. J Biomech 26(12):1473–1477

Weiner DS, Macnab I (1970) Superior migration of the humeral head. A radiological aid in the diagnosis of tears of the rotator cuff. J Bone Joint Surg Br 52(3):524–527

Wu G, van der Helm FC, Veeger HE, Makhsous M, Van Roy P, Anglin C, Nagels J, Karduna AR, McQuade K, Wang X, Werner FW, Buchholz B, International Society of B (2005) ISB recommendation on definitions of joint coordinate systems of various joints for the reporting of human joint motion–Part II: shoulder, elbow, wrist and hand. J Biomech 38(5):981–992

5

Changes in synovial fluid biomarkers and clinical efficacy of intra-articular injections of hyaluronic acid for patients with knee osteoarthritis

Yoshihiro Kusayama*, Yasushi Akamatsu, Ken Kumagai, Hideo Kobayashi, Masato Aratake and Tomoyuki Saito

Abstract

Background: The changes in synovial fluid biomarkers after intra-articular injection of hyarulonic acid (IA HA) remain controversial. We investigate the changes in the properties of synovial fluid (SF) and clinical symptoms before the first and fifth IA HA.

Methods: A total of 73 patients (73 knees) with symptomatic knee osteoarthritis were treated with five weekly intra-articular injections of HA and 55 patients (55 knees) were analyzed. The SF total volume, viscosity, and levels of HA, chondroitin 4-sulfate (C4S), chondroitin 6-sulfate (C6S), keratin sulfate, and interleukin (IL)-6 were measured before the first and fifth injections. Clinical evaluations were performed using the American Knee Society score for physician-based outcome measurements and Knee injury and Osteoarthritis Outcome Score for patient-based outcome measurements before the first and fifth injections.

Results: The SF viscosity and levels of HA were significantly increased, and the total SF volume and levels of chondroitin 4-sulfate, chondroitin 6-sulfate, and interleukin-6 were significantly decreased. The physician-based and patient-based outcome scores were improved.

Conclusions: Our findings speculate that HA injections significantly modulate levels of intra articular biomarkers which may indicate beneficial effect for articular cartilage and synovium membrane.

Keywords: Intra-articular hyaluronic acid; Knee osteoarthritis; Biomarker; Viscosity; Synovial fluid; Interleukin-6

Background

Knee osteoarthritis (OA) is a common disease in aging people. The characteristics of OA are degeneration and destruction of the articular cartilage, with secondary induction of hydrarthrosis and synovitis by inflammatory cytokines and growth factors from the destroyed cartilage and synovial membrane [1]. In advanced OA, hyaluronic acid (HA) is decreased in the synovial fluid (SF) [2], and the SF viscosity and chondroprotective function are also reduced. These changes cause further destruction of the articular cartilage.

The theoretical basis of intra-articular injection of HA (IA HA) is to improve the joint lubrication and SF viscosity [3]. The efficacy of IA HA is controversial in the past randomized control trials or meta-analysis [4-12].The American Academy of Orthopaedic Surgeons stated that IA HA is no longer recommended in the 2nd edition of their guideline for knee OA treatment published in 2013 [13]. The Osteoarthritis Research Society International commented that the treatment appropriateness of IA HA is uncertain in their guidelines for the management of knee OA [14]. HA drug for intra-articular injection was produced in Japan at 1987, IA HA was still widely used for treatment of knee OA to this day and we have confidence in this therapy. Therefore, the efficacy and safety of IA HA remain controversial between Japan and other countries.

Many biomarkers are reported to be related with this pathogenesis. Some types of biomarkers reflect cartilage degeneration, others reflect inflammation condition of synovium. The destruction of joint cartilage associated with OA degeneration leads to the release of chondroitin 6-sulfate (C6S), chondroitin 4-sulfate (C4S), and keratin sulfate (KS) from proteoglycan molecules into the SF, which can also be measured as biomarkers of joint

* Correspondence: kusayama@hotmail.co.jp
Department of Orthopaedic Surgery, Yokohama City University School of Medicine, 3-9 Fukuura, Kanazawa-ku, Yokohama 236-0004, Japan

cartilage turnover [15,16]. We used biomarkers in SF for evaluation of IA HA, because these factors directly reflect the states of the articular cartilage and synovial membrane. Inflammation is one of the factors associated with OA changes [17,18]. Synovitis, which is secondarily induced, is related to joint destruction and OA progression [19]. Inflammatory cytokines are released from the synovial membrane under the synovitis condition. Interleukin-1-β (IL-1β), tumor necrosis factor-α (TNF-α), matrix metalloproteases (MMP-1, MMP-3, MMP13) are known for proinflamatory mediators [20]. IL-6 is also one of the inflammatory cytokines that is especially elevated in rheumatoid arthritis [21,22]. IL-6 is also detected in SF from patients with knee OA, and high levels of IL-6 are associated with the development of OA and pain severity [23-27]. We measured the IL-6 concentrations as a biomarker for inflammatory reactions in knee OA treated by IA HA. The first therapeutic purpose of IA HA is supplementation of the decreased HA concentration and viscosity in SF induced by OA changes, but few researchers have measured the HA concentration and viscosity in SF after IA HA [3,28-30]. We evaluated the HA concentration and viscosity of SF to evaluate the practical changes in the SF properties after IA HA treatment.

We performed five weekly IA HA treatments. We hypothesize that HA has condroprotective effect and inhibitory effect for synovitis, and that biomarkers which indirectly reflect cartilage metabolism and inflammation condition would be changed after IA HA treatment. No studies have measured biomarkers of cartilage degeneration products, inflammation, and viscosity in SF and clinical results at the same time. The main purpose of this study was to investigate the changes in SF viscosity, HA, C4S, C6S, and KS as cartilage degenerative biomarkers, IL-6 as an inflammatory biomarker, and also we assessed clinical symptoms before and after IA HA treatments.

Methods

Patients

The study subjects were all patients who fulfilled the American College of Rheumatology criteria for knee OA [31] and visited our outpatient clinic between January 2010 and August 2013. The inclusion criteria for the study were: (1) age above 40 years; (2) radiographic classification of knee OA of Kellgren–Lawrence (K/L) grade 2 or 3 [32]; and (3) hydroarthrosis detected by clinical examination. The exclusion criteria were: (1) previous treatment with IA HA or corticosteroid; (2) opioid or non-steroidal anti-inflammatory drug administration within the previous 6 weeks; (3) knee arthritis caused by rheumatoid arthritis, gout, pseudogout, avascular necrosis, injury, or joint infection; and (4) surgical treatment including arthroscopy or high tibial osteotomy. All patients provided informed consent and agreed to participate in the study. This study was approved by the ethics committee of our hospital. Ethical committee approval number is B1000902020.

Intra-articular injection and sample collection

Patients were treated with five weekly intra-articular injections of 1% HA (low molecular weight: approximately 900 kDa) solution with a dosage of 2.5 ml/injection (Artz; Seikagaku Corporation, Tokyo, Japan). The SF samples were collected as much as possible through a lateral suprapatellar approach using a 21-gauge needle before each HA injection, and centrifuged at 15,000 × *g* for 15 minutes at room temperature. The supernatants were collected and immediately stored at −80°C until analysis. The biomarkers in SF were analyzed before the first and fifth IA HA treatments.

Measurement of joint biomarkers

The C6S and C4S levels in SF were measured by high performance liquid chromatography according to the method reported by Shinmei et al. [15]. The SF samples were diluted 10-fold and subjected to a series of digestions with chondroitinase ABC and chondroitinase AC-II (Seikagaku Corporation). The chondroitinase digestions produced the unsaturated disaccharides Δdi-6S and Δdi-4S from the CS chain structures in C6S and C4S, respectively. After ultrafiltration of the digested solutions, the levels of Δdi-6S and Δdi-4S in the filtrates were analyzed, and the area of the peak corresponding to each unsaturated disaccharide was calculated.

The KS levels in SF were measured by high performance liquid chromatography according to the method reported by Yamada et al. [33]. The SF samples were diluted 10-fold and treated with keratanase II (Seikagaku Corporation) for digestion into two disaccharide isomers, β-galactosyl-(1–4)-6-0-sulfo-N-acetylglucosamine (L2) and β-6-0-sulfo-galactosyl-(1–4)-6-0-sulfo-N-acetylglucosamine (L4). The concentrations of these disaccharide isomers were determined and the sum of their levels was considered to be the KS level. The HA levels in SF were measured by the Morgan–Elson method [34]. The SF samples were digested with HAase SD (Seikagaku Corporation), and the concentration of the resulting unsaturated disaccharides was determined as the HA level.

The IL-6 levels in SF were measured by chemiluminescent enzyme immunoassay (CLEIA) using mouse monoclonal antibodies against recombinant IL-6 (Fujirebio Inc., Tokyo, Japan) [35]. The assay format was based on a two-step sandwich CLEIA method. Briefly, 160 μl of SF was added to 50 μl of a suspension of ferrite microparticles coated with a monoclonal antibody against IL-6 as a solid phase and incubated for 10 minutes at 37°C. The particles were separated magnetically and washed, and 250 μl of another monoclonal antibody against IL-6 conjugated with alkaline phosphate was added to the particles. After incubation at 37°C for 10 minutes, the particles were washed again. Subsequently, the substrate solution [AMPPD; 3-(2′-spiroadamantane)-4-methoxy-4-(3″-phosphoryloxy) phenyl1,2-dioxetane disodium] was added at 37°C. After incubation for 5 minutes, the chemiluminescent signals were photon-counted. The assay was performed using a Lumipulse *f* system (Fujirebio Inc.), which is a fully automated CLEIA analyzer.

Measurement of SF viscosity

Viscosity measurements were performed using a cone-flat plate-type rotational viscometer in the same way which was reported by the XIV Japanese Pharmacopeia [36]. SF was introduced to fill the gap between a flat disc and a cone forming an angle, α (rad). When either the flat disc or the cone was rotated at a constant angular velocity or constant torque, the torque acting on the disc or cone surface rotated by the viscous flow and the corresponding angular velocity in the steady state were measured. The viscosity of the SF, η, was calculated using the following equation:

$$\eta = \frac{3\alpha}{2\pi R^3} \cdot \frac{100\boldsymbol{T}}{\omega}$$

where η is the viscosity of the liquid (mPa · S), π is the circumference/diameter ratio, R is the radius of the cone (cm), α is the angle between the flat disc and the cone (rad), ω is the angular velocity (rad/s), and T is the torque acting on the flat disc or cone surface (10^{-7} N · m).

Radiographs

A weight-bearing anteroposterior knee radiograph was acquired at the first outpatient clinic visit for assessing inclusion or exclusion criteria. The degree of knee degeneration was classified according to the K/L grade [32]. All patients were graded by two observers (YK and YA) to avoid differences in incomplete radiographic grading. The femorotibial angle was measured by one of the observers (YK).

Evaluation of clinical symptoms

We examined the clinical symptoms before the first and fifth IA HA treatments. Clinical efficacy was evaluated by the American Knee Society (AKS) score for physician-based outcomes and Knee injury and Osteoarthritis Outcome Score (KOOS) for patient-based outcomes [37,38]. We used the AKS knee and function scores. The KOOS is a questionnaire that covers five patient-related dimensions: pain; other disease-specific symptoms; activities of daily living; sport/recreation functions; and knee-related quality of life. For each question, five alternatives are presented, with a score range from 0 to 4 points. The KOOS questionnaires were filled out by the patients before the first and fifth IA HA treatments.

Statistical analysis

All statistical analyses were performed using SPSS for Windows (SPSS, Chicago, IL, USA). Data were expressed as mean ± standard deviation. Biomarkers were compared using Wilcoxon's rank-sum test. For correlation analyses, Spearman's rank correlation was used. Values of $P < 0.05$ were considered significant.

Results

Characteristics of the patients

A total of 73 outpatients (73 knees) with symptomatic knee OA who had indications for IA HA treatment were enrolled in this study. Eighteen patients (18 knees) became dry knee before the five weekly IA HA treatments were completed and they were excluded. Therefore, 55 knees (27 right knees and 28 left knees) were registered. The study subjects comprised 40 females and 15 males with a mean age and body mass index of 66.7 ± 9.0 years and 23.7 ± 2.8 kg/m^2, respectively. The K/L grades were grade 2 in 34 knees, grade 3 in 21 knees. The mean femorotibial angle was 178.3 ± 3.3°.

Changes in biomarkers after injections

The mean total SF volume, which was 15.9 ml before the first injection and 8.7 ml before the fifth injection, was significantly decreased by the IA HA treatments ($P < 0.001$) (Figure 1). The mean HA level was significantly increased from 1.48 mg/ml to 1.73 mg/ml ($P <$ 0.001). The mean C6S and C4S levels were significantly decreased from 62.2 nmol/ml to 49.6 nmol/ml ($P < 0.05$) and from 18.2 nmol/ml to 15.9 nmol/ml, respectively ($P < 0.05$). The mean KS level was not significantly changed from 6.70 μg/ml to 6.18 μg/ml. The mean IL-6 level was significantly decreased from 3458 pg/ml to 486 pg/ml ($P < 0.05$). The mean SF viscosity was significantly increased from 48.6 mPa · S to68.7 mPa · S ($P < 0.001$) (Table 1).

Clinical results

No complications or side effects (e.g. hematoma, infection, allergic reaction, secondary arthritis) were observed. The mean range of motion, which was 129° before the first injection and 140° before the fifth injection, was significantly improved by the IA HA treatments ($P < 0.001$). The mean AKS knee score, which was 63 points before the first injection and 79 points before the fifth injection, was significantly improved by the IA HA treatments ($P < 0.001$). The mean AKS function score, which was 72 points before the

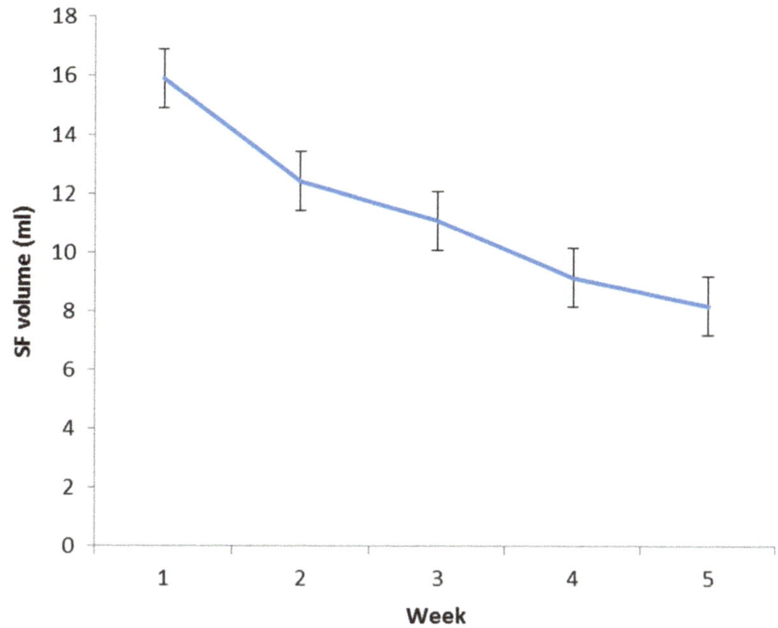

Figure 1 Time-course changes of mean SF volume before each injection.

first injection and 92 points before the fifth injection, was significantly improved by the IA HA treatments (P < 0.001). The mean values of all KOOS subscale scores and total KOOS score were significantly improved by the IA HA treatments (P < 0.001) (Table 2).

Correlations among the biomarkers and the clinical scores

Correlation analyses were performed between the biomarkers (HA, C6S, C4S, KS, IL-6, SF viscosity) and SF volume and the clinical scores before the first and fifth injections. Significant positive correlations were observed between the SF viscosity measurement and the KOOS symptom score (r = 0.466, P = 0.001) before the fifth injection (Figure 2). A significant negative correlation was observed between the SF volume measurement and the KOOS symptom score (r = −0.449, P = 0.001) before the fifth injection (Figure 3). No significant correlations were found between the other biomarkers and the clinical scores.

Table 1 Levels of biomarkers and volume in SF before the first HA injection (week 0) and fifth injection (week 5)

	Week 0	Week 5	*P* value
HA (mg/ml)	1.48 ± 0.40	1.72 ± 0.36	<0.001
C6S (nmol/ml)	62.2 ± 30.4	49.6 ± 18.4	0.001
C4S (nmol/ml)	18.2 ± 6.3	15.9 ± 4.6	0.001
KS (μg/ml)	6.68 ± 4.25	6.18 ± 3.81	0.172
IL-6 (pg/ml)	3458 ± 9094	486 ± 1294	0.013
Viscosity (mPa · S)	48.1 ± 26.7	67.8 ± 35.2	<0.001
SF (ml)	15.9 ± 12.5	8.2 ± 8.7	<0.001

SF: synovial fluid. HA: hyaluronic acid. C6S: chondroitin 6-sulfate. C4S: chondroitin 4-sulfate. KS: keratin sulfate. IL-6: interleukin-6.
Data are given as mean ± standard deviation.

Discussion

This study showed that biomarkers (C4S, C6S, IL-6) and the SF volume were significantly decreased and HA and viscosity were significantly increased after IA HA treatment. These improvements of SF properties indicated that IA HA had potential of affecting for the joint cartilage and synovium membrane with knee OA.

The factors that determine the development of knee OA are degeneration, abrasion, and destruction of the cartilage, synovitis associated with these cartilage changes, and further joint destruction resulting from decreased viscosity in the SF [1-3]. HA was reported to have inhibitory effects on cartilage destruction, anti-inflammatory effects, and supplementary effects for SF viscosity when used to treat these pathological conditions in OA models in vitro [39-42]. The present study showed that IA HA treatments can exert these three effects clinically by evaluating three types of joint markers.

IA HA caused significant decreases in C6S and C4S, which were used as biomarkers for cartilage degeneration and destruction. CS is bound to the mucopolysaccharide side chains of proteoglycans, which are the main components of joint cartilage [43]. Degeneration and destruction of joint cartilage leads to the release of CS into the SF [15,16]. CS is also related to the amount of articular cartilage, and a previous report described that CS in SF increases at the early stage of OA and

Table 2 Changes in clinical results before the first HA injection (week 0) and fifth injection (week 5)

	Week 0	Week 5	*P* value
Range of motion (degrees)	129 ± 13	140 ± 7	<0.001
AKSKS (points)	63.8 ± 10.8	80.0 ± 10.1	<0.001
AKSFS (points)	72.6 ± 11.8	92.7 ± 7.0	<0.001
KOOS Pain (points)	56.2 ± 17.5	81.3 ± 11.2	<0.001
KOOS Symptoms (points)	62.6 ± 14.8	82.4 ± 12.8	<0.001
KOOS Activity of Daily Living (points)	72.6 ± 17.4	90.3 ± 8.1	<0.001
KOOS Sports (points)	45.1 ± 18.6	73.9 ± 13.6	<0.001
KOOS Quality of Life (points)	35.5 ± 14.8	63.6 ± 16.3	<0.001
Total KOOS score	272.0 ± 73.7	391.6 ± 50.8	<0.001

AKSKS: American Knee Society knee score. AKSFS: American Knee Society function score. KOOS: Knee injury and Osteoarthritis Outcome Score.
Data are given as mean ± standard deviation.

decreases at the advanced stage of OA [44]. HA inhibits cartilage degeneration in vitro, as shown in studies using rabbits [42]. Our subjects were K/L 2 and 3, and they had residual cartilage. The results of C4S and C6S before the 1st injection were influenced by the acceleration of cartilage degeneration. The decrease of C4S and C6S between before the 1st and 5th injection did not indicate that residual cartilage was decreased by progression of OA, but that IA HA suppressed the degeneration of OA. C6S mainly consists joint cartilage and C4S is distributed not only cartilage, but also synovium membrane [15], the decrease of C4S and C6S may have the meaning which IA HA worked for both cartilage and synovium membrane. Some studies investigated the changes in CS after IA HA. Kobayashi et al. [45] showed that C6S and C4S were significantly decreased after IA HA (molecular weight: 800 kDa) treatments conducted for 16 patients with knee OA. Similarly, Hasegawa et al. [46] showed that C6S and C4S were significantly decreased after IA HA (molecular weight: 900 kDa) treatments conducted for 28 patients with knee OA. Meanwhile, Sugimoto et al. [47] showed that there were no significant changes in C6S and C4S

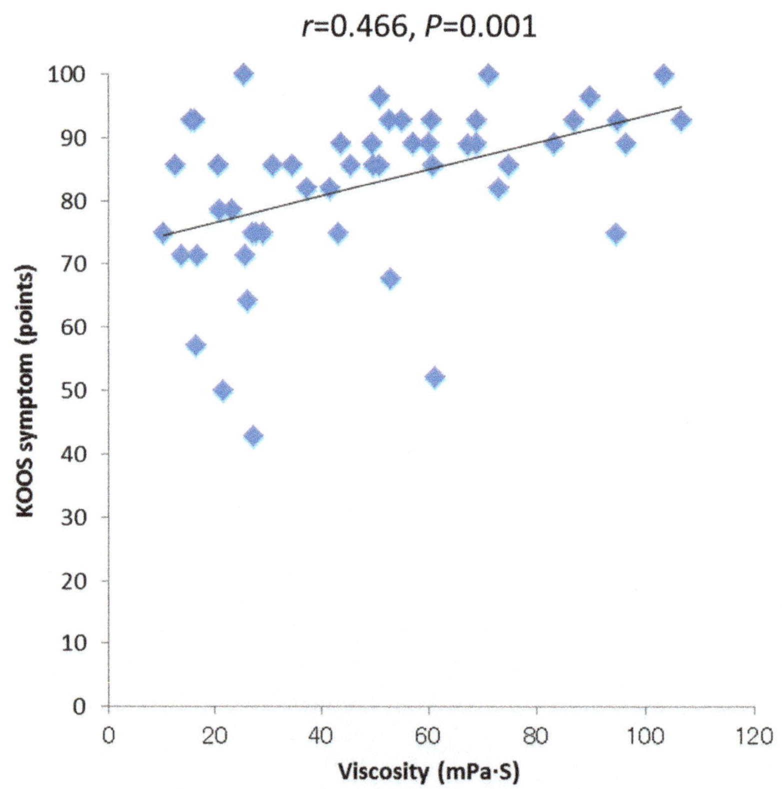

Figure 2 **Correlation between the SF viscosity measurement and the KOOS symptom score before the fifth IA HA treatment.**

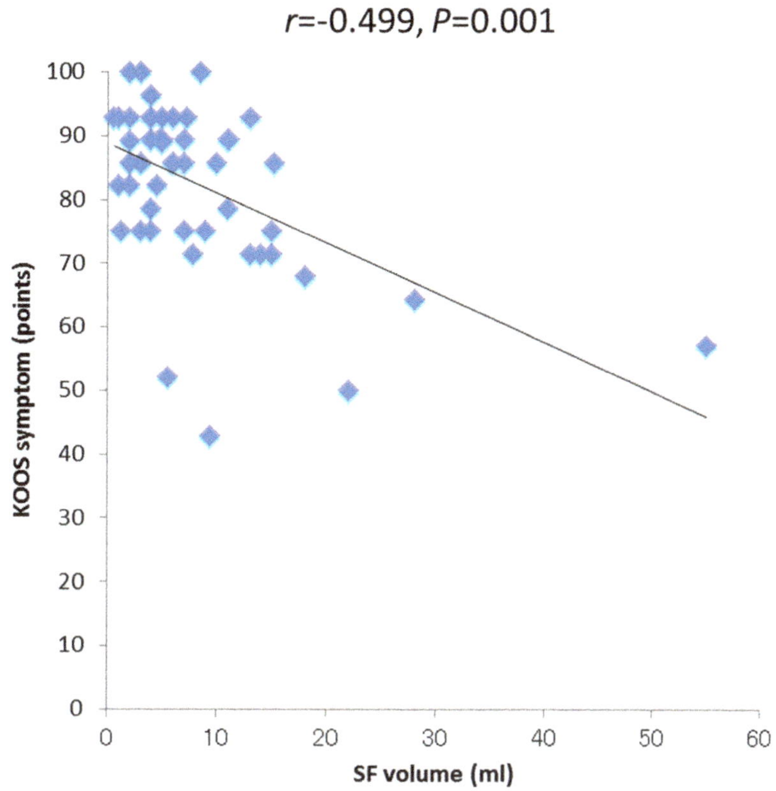

Figure 3 Correlation between the SF volume measurement and the KOOS symptom score before the fifth IA HA treatment.

after IA HA (molecular weight: 900 kDa) treatments conducted for 32 patients with knee OA. These findings demonstrate that there is no consensus about the CS changes after IA HA. Our study, which involved a larger sample size than the other studies, revealed significant decreases in C4S and C6S after IA HA treatments. The decreasing changes in these biomarkers support the possibility which IA HA have inhibitory effects of cartilage degeneration and releasing proteoglycans.

Campion et al. [16] reported that KS is useful biomarker for OA. Hasegawa et al. [46] showed that KS was significantly decreased after 5 weekly IA HA treatments conducted 28 patients with knee OA. We also thought to be useful for measurement of cartilage degeneration and measured KS. However, we were not able to show the significant change of KS. We considered that no significant change of KS also had a meaning. Biomarkers changes in the SF were not simply attenuated by repeated aspiration from the results of no significant change of KS and the decreasing of C4S, C6S and IL-6. The result of no change of KS is important to show no attenuation effect.

OA is known to cause inflammatory conditions and secondary synovitis [19]. IL-1, IL-6, tumor necrosis factor-alpha, and prostaglandin E2 have been reported to act as inflammatory biomarkers for OA [48-50]. Beekhuizen et al. [25] compared the levels of 47 cytokines in OA patients with those in healthy individuals and found that IL-6 was significantly increased. Similarly, Livshits et al. [26] found that IL-6 was a significant predictor of radiographic knee OA. IL-6 has various physiological effects, and causes destruction of cartilage via its angiogenic effects and activation of osteoclasts in joints [51,52]. Suppression of IL-6 has the possibility to be effective in protecting against the cartilage degeneration in OA. Therefore, the levels of IL-6 represent an indicator of the inflammatory conditions caused by OA and secondary synovitis, and were found to be significantly decreased after IA HA treatments in the present study. There are some previous reports about the levels of IL-6 in SF after IA HA treatment. Bianchi et al. [53] reported that oral treatment with non-steroidal anti-inflammatory drugs reduced the levels of IL-6 in SF, and Gallelli et al. [54] showed similar results. However, the changing levels of IL-6 in SF after IA HA treatment were not clear. HA was reported to act on the synovial membrane and inhibit synovitis in dogs [41]. In the present study, the decreased levels of IL-6 after IA HA treatments support our hypothesis that IA HA has inhibitory effects on synovitis and inflammatory reactions. Synovitis increases the SF volume, and we observed a significant decrease in the SF volume after IA HA. Our results support the opinion that HA has anti-inflammatory effects.

The levels of HA and viscosity, which are decreased in SF of patients with OA, are indicators of the therapeutic effects, and our results revealed significant increases in both factors after IA HA treatments. HA is present in the intra-articular SF, cartilage, and synovial membrane. The viscosity and water-holding capacity of HA in SF are responsible for its function as a shock absorber for the joint and provide lubrication to the joint [3]. HA infiltrates the synovial membrane and cartilage in vitro and promotes HA synthesis [41]. There are a few reports regarding the use of HA in actual clinical practice, which showed that HA supplementation through IA HA treatment increases viscosity and HA in SF [28,29,55]. The elimination half-life of HA in the knee joints of rabbits was reported to be approximately 12 hours, and injected HA may not remain in the knee joint beyond 1 week [56]. Contrary to these results, HA in SF was found to be increased after IA HA in this study. Accordingly, we believe that the increased HA reflects not only the injected HA but also newly produced HA, which resulted from improvement in the condition of the synovial membrane and cartilage caused by IA HA. Since the increase in SF viscosity is dependent on the HA level, the significant increase in HA would improve the properties of the SF after IA HA.

The relationships between biomarkers and clinical scores might enable us to identify the biomarkers that act as prognostic factors and indicate therapeutic effects. To date, researchers have reported several correlations between biomarkers and clinical scores. Hasegawa et al. [46] found a negative correlation between C4S or tenascin-C and VAS scores, while Sugimoto et al. [47] found a positive relationship between C6S or aggrecan and the JOA score. However, there are also reports that no correlations were found between biomarkers and clinical scores [45,55]. In the present study, we investigated the correlations between C6S, C4S, HA, IL-6, SF viscosity, or SF volume and each item in the AKS and KOOS scores. Our results indicated a positive correlation between SF viscosity and KOOS symptom scores before the fifth injection. No other positive correlations between biomarkers and clinical scores were observed. These results suggest that SF viscosity is related to the clinical scores. A higher viscosity of SF, which reflects the theoretical basis of IA HA, was found to be the important factor for the clinical scores. Additionally, the SF volume exhibited a negative correlation with the KOOS symptom scores at the fifth visit after IA HA treatment. No other negative correlations between biomarkers and clinical scores were observed. Increased SF volume elevated pressure in the knee joint, worsened range of motion and clinical symptom. The correlation coefficients (r) between viscosity and KOOS symptom, and SF volume and KOOS symptom were 0.466 and –0.499. These correlation coefficients might not be strong. However, these correlations indicate that viscosity and hydrarthrosis are important parameters for IA HA treatment.

Significant improvements were observed in the five subscales of the KOOS, AKS knee, and AKS function scores. The KOOS is a patient-based clinical assessment score, for which the patients themselves input their subjective symptoms. Meanwhile, the AKS score is a physician-based clinical assessment score, in which a physician examines the patient, takes a history, and evaluates the symptoms. Improvements were observed in both the patient-based KOOS and physician-based AKS scores in the present study. The measurements of two different types of clinical score were more reliable in researching for efficacy of IA HA.

This study has several limitations. First, the study did not have a control group, because our hospital decided that it was ethically inappropriate to create such a control group. Without control group, we were not able to deny the possibility of attenuation effect by repeated aspiration. Second, the follow-up period was short. Although there were significant changes in joint biomarkers after IA HA treatments, the results of long-term treatment remain unclear. Third, many patients in this study had early and moderate OA (K/L grade 2 and 3). This is because patients with terminal OA (K/L grade 4) are indicated for surgical treatment rather than conservative treatment. Therefore, there may have been patient bias. Fourth, our results showed biomarkers of C4S, C6S, KS and IL-6. We were not able to mention other biomarkers in the SF.

Conclusion

To the best of our knowledge, this is the first report of simultaneous measurements of HA levels together with SF viscosity and levels of biomarkers C6S, C4S, KS, and IL-6 to evaluate the efficacy of IA HA before first and fifth injection. Also, all of the clinical symptoms were significantly improved. The changes in the levels of biomarkers suggested that IA HA treatments may have cartilage-protective effects, anti-inflammatory effects, and SF viscosity-replenishing effects.

Competing interests

The authors declare that they have no competing interests.

Authors' contributions

YK carried out the measurement of biomarkers, radiographs and clinical symptom and drafted the manuscript. YA carried out the measurement of biomarkers, radiographs and clinical symptom and drafted the manuscript. KK carried out the assist with writing the manuscript. HK carried out the assist with writing manuscript. MA carried out the assist with manuscript preparation. TS carried out the assist with manuscript preparation. All authors read and approved the final manuscript.

References

1. Poole AR, Rizkalla G, Ionescu M, Reiner A, Brooks E, Rorabeck C, Bourne R, Bogoch E (1993) Osteoarthritis in the human knee: a dynamic process of cartilage matrix degradation, synthesis and reorganization. Agents Actions Suppl 39:3–13

2. Dahl LB, Dahl IM, Engström-Laurent A, Granath K (1985) Concentration and molecular weight of sodium hyaluronate in synovial fluid from patients with rheumatoid arthritis and other arthropathies. Ann Rheum Dis 44(12):817–822
3. Balzas EA, Denlinger JL (1993) Viscosupplementation: a new concept in the treatment of osteoarthritis. J Rheumatol Suppl 39:3–9
4. Petrella RJ, Petrella M (2006) A prospective, randomized, double-blind, placebo controlled study to evaluate the efficacy of intraarticular hyaluronic acid for osteoarthritis of the knee. J Rheumatol 33(5):951–956
5. Day R, Brooks P, Conaghan PG, Petersen M (2004) A double blind, randomized, multicenter, parallel group study of the effectiveness and tolerance of intraarticular hyaluronan in osteoarthritis of the knee. J Rheumatol 31(4):775–782
6. Wang CT, Lin J, Chang CJ, Lin YT, Hou SM (2004) Therapeutic effects of hyaluronic acid on osteoarthritis of the knee. A meta-analysis of randomized controlled trials. J Bone Joint Surg Am 86-A(3):538–545
7. Bellamy N, Campbell J, Robinson V, Gee T, Bourne R, Wells G (2006) Viscosupplementation for the treatment of osteoarthritis of the knee. Cochrane Database Syst Rev, doi:10.1002/14651858
8. Divine JG, Zazulak BT, Hewett TE (2007) Viscosupplementation for knee osteoarthritis: a systematic review. Clin Orthop Rel Res 455:113–122
9. Lo GH, LaValley M, McAlindon T, Felson DT (2003) Intra-articular hyaluronic acid in treatment of knee osteoarthritis: a meta-analysis. JAMA 290 (23):3115–3121
10. Arrich J, Piribauer F, Mad P, Schmid D, Klaushofer K, Mullner M (2005) Intraarticular hyaluronic acid for the treatment of osteoarthritis of the knee: systematic review and meta-analysis. CMAJ 172(8):1039–1043
11. Medina JM, Thomas A, Denegar CR (2006) Knee osteoarthritis: should your patient opt for hyaluronic acid injection? J Fam Pract 55(8):669–675
12. Rutjes AW, Juni P, da Costa BR, Trelle S, Nuesch E, Reichenbach S (2012) Viscosupplementation for osteoarthritis of the knee: a systematic review and meta-analysis. Ann Intern Med 157(3):180–191
13. Jevsevar DS (2013) Treatment of osteoarthritis of the knee: evidence-based guideline, 2nd edition. J Am Acad Orthop Surg 21(9):571–576
14. McAlindon TE, Bannuru RR, Sullivan MC, Arden NK, Berenbaum F, Bierma-Zeinstra SM, Hawker GA, Henrotin Y, Hunter DJ, Kawaguchi H, Kwoh K, Lohmander S, Rannou F, Roos EM, Underwood M (2014) OARSI guidelines for the non-surgical management of knee osteoarthritis. Osteoarthritis Cartilage 22(3):363–388, doi:10.1016/j.joca.2014.01.003
15. Shinmei M, Miyauchi S, Machida A, Miyazaki K (1992) Quantitation of chondroitin 4-sulfate and chondroitin 6-sulfate in pathologic joint fluid. Arthritis Rheum 35(11):1304–1308
16. Campion GV, McCrae F, Schnitzer TJ, Lenz ME, Dieppe PA, Thonar EJ (1991) Levels of keratan sulfate in the serum and synovial fluid of patients with osteoarthritis of the knee. Arthritis Rheum 34(10):1254–1259
17. Benito MJ, Veale DJ, FitzGerald O, van den Berg WB, Bresnihan B (2005) Synovial tissue inflammation in early and late osteoarthritis. Ann Rheum Dis 64(9):1263–1267
18. Felson DT (2006) Clinical practice: osteoarthritis of the knee. N Engl J Med 354(8):841–848
19. Sellam J, Berenbaum F (2010) The role of synovitis in pathophysiology and clinical symptoms of osteoarthritis. Nat Rev Rheumatol 6(11):625–635
20. Goldring MB, Otero M (2011) Inflammation in osteoarthritis. Curr Opin Rheumatol 23(5):471–478
21. Sack U, Kinne RW, Marx T, Heppt P, Bender S, Emmrich F (1993) Interleukin-6 in synovial fluid is closely associated with chronic synovitis in rheumatoid arthritis. Rheumatol Int 13(2):45–51
22. Houssiau FA, Devogelaer JP, Van Damme J, de Deuxchaisnes CN, Van Snick J (1988) Interleukin-6 in synovial fluid and serum of patients with rheumatoid arthritis and other inflammatory arthritides. Arthritis Rheum 31(6):784–788
23. Kaneko S, Satoh T, Chiba J, Ju C, Inoue K, Kagawa J (2000) Interleukin-6 and interleukin-8 levels in serum and synovial fluid of patients with osteoarthritis. Cytokines Cell Mol Ther 6(2):71–79
24. Doss F, Menard J, Hauschild M, Kreutzer HJ, Mittlmeier T, Müller-Steinhardt M, Müller B (2007) Elevated IL-6 levels in the synovial fluid of osteoarthritis patients stem from plasma cells. Scand J Rheumatol4 36(2):136–139
25. Beekhuizen M, Gierman LM, van Spil WE, Van Osch GJ, Huizinga TW, Saris DB, Creemers LB, Zuurmond AM (2013) An explorative study comparing levels of soluble mediators in control and osteoarthritic synovial fluid. Osteoarthritis Cartilage 21(7):918–922, doi:10.1016/j.joca.2013.04.002
26. Livshits G, Zhai G, Hart DJ, Kato BS, Wang H, Williams FM, Spector TD (2009) Interleukin-6 is a significant predictor of radiographic knee osteoarthritis: The Chingford Study. Arthritis Rheum 60(7):2037–2045, doi:10.1002/art.24598
27. Shimura Y, Kurosawa H, Sugawara Y, Tsuchiya M, Sawa M, Kaneko H, Futami I, Liu L, Sadatsuki R, Hada S, Iwase Y, Kaneko K, Ishijima M (2013) The factors associated with pain severity in patients with knee osteoarthritis vary according to the radiographic disease severity: a cross-sectional study. Osteoarthritis Cartilage 21(9):1179–1184, doi:10.1016/j.joca.2013.05.014
28. Bagga H, Burkhardt D, Sambrook P, March L (2006) Long term effects of intrarticular hyaluronan on synovial fluid in osteoarthritis of the knee. J Rheumatol 33(5):946–950
29. Grecomoro G, La Sala F, Francavilla G (2001) Rheologic changes in the synovial fluid of patients with gonarthritis induced by intraarticular infiltration of hyaluronic acid. Int J Tissue React 23(2):67–71
30. Mensitieri M, Ambrosio S, Iannace S, Nicolais L (1995) Viscoelastic evaluation of different knee osteoarthritis therapies. J Mater Sci Mater Med 6:130–137
31. Altman R, Asch E, Bloch D, Bole G, Borenstein D, Brandt K, Christy W, Cooke TD, Greenwald R, Hochberg M (1986) Development of criteria for the classification and reporting of OA of the knee. Classification of osteoarthritis of the knee. Diagnostic and therapeutic criteria committee of the American Rheumatism Association. Arthritis Rheum 29(8):1039–1049
32. Kellgren JH, Lawrence JS (1957) Radiological assessment of osteoarthrosis. Ann Rheum Dis 16(4):494–502
33. Yamada H, Miyauchi S, Morita M, Yoshida Y, Yoshihara Y, Kikuchi T, Washimi O, Washimi Y, Terada N, Seki T, Fujikawa K (2000) Content and sulfation pattern of keratan sulfate in hip osteoarthritis using high performance liquid chromatography. J Rheumatol 27(7):1721–1724
34. Reissig JL, Storminger JL, Leloir LF (1955) A modifi ed colorimetric method for the estimation of N-acetylamino sugars. J Biol Chem 217(2):959–966
35. Isomura M, Ueno M, Shimada K, Kogaki H, Ashihara Y (1994) Highly sensitive chemiluminescent enzyme immunoassay with gelatin-coated ferrite solid phase. Clin Chem 40:1830–1831
36. The Ministry of Health, Labour and Welfare (2011) The Japanese Pharmacopoeia, Sixteenth Edition: 69., http://jpdb.nihs.go.jp/jp16e/. Accessed 24 Mar 2011
37. Insall JN, Dorr LD, Scott RD, Scott WN (1989) Rationale of the knee society clinical rating system. Clin Orthop Relat Res 248:13–14
38. Roos EM, Roos HP, Lohmander LS, Ekdahl C, Beynnon BD (1998) Knee Injury and Osteoarthritis Outcome Score (KOOS)–development of a self-administered outcome measure. J Orthop Sports Phys Ther 28(2):88–96
39. Shimazu A, Jikko A, Iwamoto M, Koike T, Yan W, Okada Y, Shinmei M, Nakamura S, Kato Y (1993) Effects of hyaluronic acid on the release of proteoglycan from the cell matrix in rabbit chondrocyte cultures in the presenceand absence of cytokines. Arthritis Rheum 36(2):247–253
40. Gotoh S, Onaya J, Abe M, Miyazaki K, Hamai A, Horie K, Tokuyasu K (1993) Effects of the molecular weight of hyaluronic acid and its action mechanisms on experimental joint pain in rats. Ann Rheum Dis 52(11):817–822
41. Asari A, Miyauchi S, Matsuzaka S, Ito T, Kominami E, Uchiyama Y (1998) Molecular weight-dependent effects of hyaluronate on thearthritic synovium. Arch Histol Cytol 61(2):125–135
42. Shimizu C, Kubo T, Hirasawa Y, Coutts RD, Amiel D (1998) Histomorphometric and biochemical effect of various hyaluronans on early osteoarthritis. J Rheumatol 25(9):1813–1819
43. Roughley PJ, Mort JS (1986) Ageing and the aggregating proteoglycans of human articular cartilage. Clin Sci (Lond) 71(4):337–344
44. Uesaka S, Miyazaki K, Ito H (2004) Age-related changes and sex differences in chondroitin sulfate isomers and hyaluronic acid in normal synovial fluid. Mod rheumatol 14(6):470–475
45. Kobayashi K, Matsuzaka S, Yoshida Y, Miyauchi S, Wada Y, Moriya H (2004) The effects of intraarticularly injected sodium hyaluronate on levels of intact aggrecan and nitric oxide in the joint fluid of patients with knee osteoarthritis. Osteoarthritis Cartilage 12(7):536–542
46. Hasegawa M, Nakoshi Y, Tsujii M, Sudo A, Masuda H, Yoshida T, Uchida A (2008) Changes in biochemical markers and prediction of effectiveness of intra-articular hyaluronan in patients with knee osteoarthritis. Osteoarthritis Cartilage 16(4):526–529
47. Sugimoto H, Yamada H, Terada N, Kanaji A, Kato S, Date H, Ichinose H, Miyazaki K (2006) Intraarticular injection of high molecular weight hyaluronan for osteoarthritis of the knee - prediction of effectiveness with biological markers. J Rheumatol 33(12):2527

48. Fernandes JC, Martel-Pelletier J, Pelletier JP (2002) The role of cytokines in osteoarthritis pathophysiology. Biorheology 39(1–2):237–246
49. Henrotin YE, Labasse AH, Simonis PE, Zheng SX, Deby GP, Famaey JP, Crielaard JM, Reginster JY (1999) Effects of nimesulide and sodium diclofenac on interleukin-6, interleukin-8, proteoglycans and prostaglandin E2 production by human articular chondrocytes in vitro. Clin Exp Rheumatol 17(2):151–160
50. Goldring MB (1999) The role of cytokines as inflammatory mediators in osteoarthritis: lessons from animal models. Connect Tissue Res 40(1):1–11
51. Jikko A, Wakisaka T, Iwamoto M, Hiranuma H, Kato Y, Maeda T, Fujishita M, Fuchihata H (1998) Effects of interleukin-6 on proliferation and proteoglycan metabolism in articular chondrocyte cultures. Cell Biol Int 22(9–10):615–621
52. Kwan Tat S, Padrines M, Theoleyre S, Heymann D, Fortun Y (2004) IL-6, RANKL, TNF-α/IL-1: interrelations in bone resorption pathophysiology. Cytokine Growth Factor Rev 15(1):49–60
53. Bianchi M, Broggini M, Balzarini P, Franchi S, Sacerdote P (2007) Effects of nimesulide on pain and on synovial fluid concentrations of substance P, interleukin-6 and interleukin-8 in patients with knee osteoarthritis: comparison with celecoxib. Int J Clin Pract 61(8):1270–1277
54. Gallelli L, Galasso O, Falcone D, Southworth S, Greco M, Ventura V, Romualdi P, Corigliano A, Terracciano R, Savino R, Gulletta E, Gasparini G, De Sarro G (2013) The effects of nonsteroidal anti-inflammatory drugs on clinical outcomes, synovial fluid cytokine concentration and signal transduction pathways in knee osteoarthritis. A randomized open label trial. Osteoarthritis Cartilage 21(9):1400–1408, doi:10.1016/j.joca.2013.06.026
55. Shimizu M, Higuchi H, Takagishi K, Shinozaki T, Kobayashi T (2010) Clinical and biochemical characteristics after intra-articular injection for the treatment of osteoarthritis of the knee: prospective randomized study of sodium hyaluronate and corticosteroid. J Orthop Sci 15(1):51–56
56. Brown TJ, Laurent UB, Fraser JR (1991) Turnover of hyaluronan in synovial joints: elimination of labelled hyaluronan from the knee joint of the rabbit. Exp Physiol 76(1):125–134

6

Biomechanical evaluation of a biomimetic spinal construct

Tian Wang[1,2], Jonathon R Ball[3], Mattew H Pelletier[1] and William R Walsh[1*]

Abstract

Background: Laboratory spinal biomechanical tests using human cadaveric or animal spines have limitations in terms of disease transmission, high sample variability, decay and fatigue during extended testing protocols. Therefore, a synthetic biomimetic spine model may be an acceptable substitute. The goal of current study is to evaluate the properties of a synthetic biomimetic spine model; also to assess the mechanical performance of lateral plating following lateral interbody fusion.

Methods: Three L3/4 synthetic spinal motion segments were examined using a validated pure moment testing system. Moments (±7.5 Nm) were applied in flexion-extension (FE), lateral bending (LB) and axial rotation (AR) at 1Hz for total 10000 cycles in MTS Bionix. An additional test was performed 12 hours after 10000 cycles. A ±10 Nm cycle was also performed to allow provide comparison to the literature. For implantation evaluation, each model was tested in the 4 following conditions: 1) intact, 2) lateral cage alone, 3) lateral cage and plate 4) anterior cage and plate. Results were analysed using ANOVA with post-hoc Tukey's HSD test.

Results: Range of motion (ROM) exhibited logarithmic growth with cycle number (increases of 16%, 37.5% and 24.3% in AR, FE and LB respectively). No signification difference ($p > 0.1$) was detected between 4 cycles, 10000 cycles and 12 hour rest stages. All measured parameters were comparable to that of reported cadaveric values. The ROM for a lateral cage and plate construct was not significantly different to the anterior lumbar interbody construct for FE ($p = 1.00$), LB ($p = 0.995$) and AR ($p = 0.837$).

Conclusions: Based on anatomical and biomechanical similarities, the synthetic spine tested here provides a reasonable model to represent the human lumbar spine. Repeated testing did not dramatically alter biomechanics which may allow non-destructive testing between many different procedures and devices without the worry of carry over effects. Small intra-specimen variability and lack of biohazard makes this an attractive alternative for in vitro spine biomechanical testing. It also proved an acceptable surrogate for biomechanical testing, confirming that a lateral lumbar interbody cage and plate construct reduces ROM to a similar degree as anterior lumbar interbody cage and plate constructs.

Keywords: Synthetic; Lumbar; Sowbones; Biomechanical; Interbody cage; Lateral plate; Anterior plate; Pure moment; Sawbones; Motion segment; Fatigue

* Correspondence: wrwalshau@gmail.com
[1]Surgical & Orthopaedic Research Laboratories, Prince of Wales Clinical School, University of New South Wales, Clinical Science Bldg, Prince of Wales Hospital, Gate 6, Avoca Street, 2031 Sydney, Australia
Full list of author information is available at the end of the article

Background

Development of synthetic replicates has been driven by the challenges associated with using fresh tissues for biomechanical testing. Beyond scarcity and cost considerations, fresh samples are biohazards and require appropriate personal protective equipment as well as the enactment of handling and specimen tracking procedures. There are also social and ethical concerns that must be addressed. Additional limitations that are particularly relevant to the spine include fluctuations in soft and hard tissues properties over time and with exposure to air, which alters the kinematic response of motion segments [1]. During high cycle fatigue tests spinal segments are likely to suffer from tissue putrefaction. Freezing tissues offers an means to hinder decomposition, however initial freezing itself will also influence mechanical properties [2]. With the amount of time between expiration of the donor and subsequent freezing uncontrolled variables, this is likely to further influence the condition of the tissues. Initial tissue quality is also an issue as the majority of the cadaveric specimen is from elderly donors with osteoporosis, or other degenerative pathologies. Inherent inter-specimen variability in size, bone quality and disc pressure [3] will increase data scatter. Animals are a suitable replacement for human cadaveric spines in certain testing protocols [4-11] with well reported anatomical and biomechanical comparisons [12,13] but have limitation in terms of size and angle of lordosis. While these samples may be more easily accessible and more cost effective, they still embody the previously mentioned limitations with human tissues.

The creation of a biomechanically accurate joint complex including soft tissues presents a challenge beyond that of modeling individual bones [14-18]. Further complicating this process in the spine is that intervertebral joints consist two articulating synovial joints (zygapophyseal joints) and one symphysis (intervertebral disc), as well as surrounding syndesmoses (anterior and posterior longitudinal, inter- and supraspinous, intertransverse ligaments and ligamentaflava).

A novel synthetic spinal testing models recently released by Sawbones may have utility in research and development. The current study examined the anatomy and biomechanical aspects of this synthetic biomimetic spine model in cyclic testing; and to evaluate anterior and lateral plating with interbody cages, to address the following questions: 1) is a lateral interbody cage + plate construct mechanically comparable to an anterior interbody cage + plate construct; and 2) is a stand-alone lateral interbody cage construct mechanically comparable to the intact state.

Methods

Evaluation of anatomy

Three L3/4 synthetic spinal motion segments, recently developed by SawBones (Vashon, WA, USA) were evaluated. Samples were examined using clinical computed tomography (CT Aquilion PRIME; Toshiba, Tokyo, Japan) with 0.5 mm slices. 3D models, which were built with Mimics (Materialise, Leuven, Belgium) from the DICOM data, were used to measured anatomy parameters such as end plate depth, end plate width, vertebral body height, spinal canal depth, spinal canal width, pedicle height and pedicle width. Results were compared with anatomical data from the human [19] and sheep [12] lumbar spine.

Cyclic tests

Motion segments were examined with a validated pure moment testing system [20,21]. Moments (±7.5 Nm) were applied in flexion-extension (FE), lateral bending (LB) and axial rotation (AR) at 1Hz for total 10000 cycles in MTS Bionix (MTS Systems, Eden Prairie, MN) with 25 KN axial-torsional load transducer (model number: 662.20D-05, MTS system corporation, Eden Prairie, MN, USA). Motion was assessed at 4, 125, 250, 500, 1000, 2500, 5000 and 10000 cycles. A non-contacting thermometer was used to measure the temperature of disc, endplate and vertebral body at each assessment stage. After a 12 hour rest period, an additional test was run at ±7.5 Nm to determine the influence of temperature (designed as recovery group test). A ±10 Nm cycle was performed to allow additional comparison to the literature, and act as the intact group (INT) for subsequent instrumented tests. A near infrared 3D motion tracking system with retro-reflective markers (Osprey, Motion Analysis, Santa Rosa, CA) was employed to record the motion of the sample. Pretesting calibration found the system accuracy within 0.1 mm in displacement and 0.1° in rotation. Post processing was performed with an in-house written script MATLAB (MathWorks, Natick, MA) to extract the torque-angle curves and resulting range of motion (ROM) and neutral zone (NZ). NZ was calculated based on the Wilke et al. [22].

Implanted conditions

Four cycles (±10 Nm) were applied in the primary anatomical planes. The intact group (INT) results were obtained during the cycle test mentioned above. Each sample was tested in three additional states (Figure 1), 1) lateral interbody cage alone (LIC); 2) lateral interbody cage + plate (LICP); and 3) anterior interbody cage + plate (AICP). PEEK interbody cages (K2M Aleutian, Life Health Care, North Ryde, Australia) were used in this study. The rigid plating system used consisted of a locking plate and four cancellous screws (K2M Cayman, LifeHealthCare, North Ryde, Australia). The implants were sized appropriate to specimen anatomy. Firstly, a box-like incision was made through the lateral annulus followed by discectomy. The disc material was removed using a surgical curette and rongeur. The anterior longitudinal ligament and part

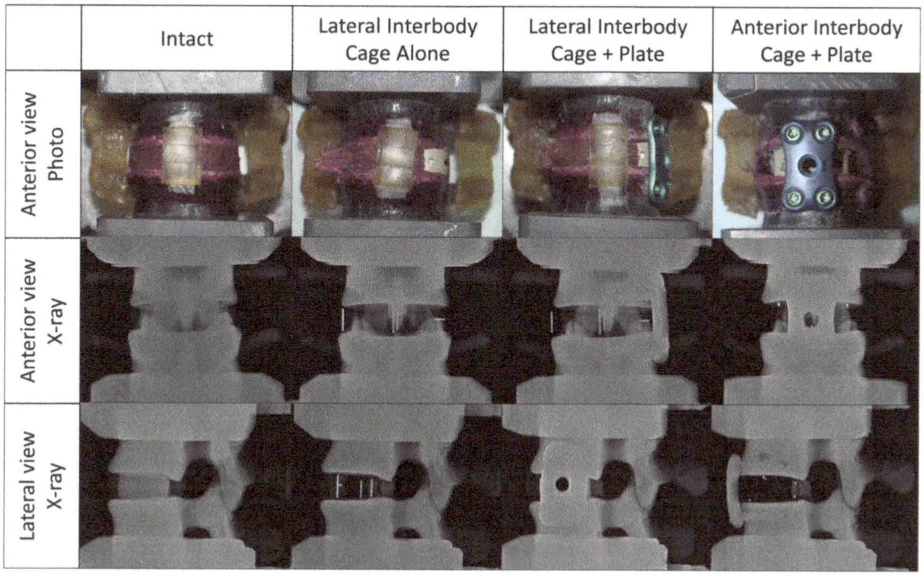

Figure 1 Anterior view photo, anterior view x-ray and lateral view x-ray imaging of different sample conditions.

of anterior annulus was still connected at this stage. The lateral cage (14 mm × 8°) was implanted, and mechanically tested (LIC). A43 mm lateral locking plate was secured with four 6.0/28 mm cancellous screws and mechanically tested (LICP). The lateral interbody cage and plate was removed, the anterior longitudinal ligament and annulus were cut through and a complete discectomy performed. The anterior interbody cage (15 mm × 10°) and plate (38 mm with 6.0/28 mm screws) were then applied and the sample tested (ALCP). Radiographs were taken before and after testing with a high resolution X-ray (MX-20; Faxitron, Tucson, AZ).

Statistical analysis

Data from cyclic tests was analyzed using one way ANOVA with a 0.05 significance level with IBM SPSS Statistics (version 21, IBM, Armonk, NY), followed by a Tukey HSD post hoc analysis. For implanted conditions, ANOVA was again applied followed by Tukey HSD post hoc analysis between test conditions.

Results

Anatomy

L3 and L4 anatomical parameters of the synthetic spine model are compared with published human [19] and sheep [12] L3 and L4 data in Table 1. The synthetic model anatomy showed a close match to the human, while the sheep differs to the other two groups, as expected.

Cyclic tests

Figure 2 shows the individual sample FE, LB and AR ROM results against cycle number. After 10 K cycles, the average ROM of three samples increased 16%, 37.5% and 24.3% in AR, FE and LB respectively. All samples displayed logarithmic growth in ROM with increasing cycle number. However, it was also noted that the absolute value of the ROM differed for sample1against other two, particularly in LB. The mean value for ROM increased from 4 to 10 K cycles and decreased slightly following the recovery period (Figure 3); however no signification differences ($p > 0.1$) were detected between any of these groups. When compared with the 10 Nm cadaveric test results of Panjabi et al. [23] and [24] (Table 2), synthetic ROM were similar to the human data. And for NZ results, most FE NZ and LB NZ were in the range of the cadaveric data, but the AR NZ was smaller than reported human results. Furthermore, compared with human data, the synthetic spine reduced standard deviation by 10%, 30% and 57.5% in AR, FE, and LB ROM respectively.

Implanted conditions

As expected, the ROM of the lateral cage alone group was less than the intact group, and was further reduced with the plate fixation (Figure 4). Quantitative results shown that the ROM of flexion/extension decreased by 51.5% with a lateral cage alone. Further decrease was obtained with a lateral cage + lateral plate (77.8%); this magnitude of reduction was similar to that seen with an anterior cage + plate (81.7%). ROM in lateral bending decreased by 68.2% with a lateral cage alone and further decreased with a lateral cage + plate (87.9%). This magnitude of reduction was greater than that seen with an anterior cage + plate (74.7%). Axial rotation ROM decreased minimally with a lateral cage alone (18.9%), and to a greater

Table 1 Anatomical comparison between synthetic model, human cadaver and sheep; (I) indicates inferior or caudal level; number in brackets indicated the standard deviation

	L3			L4		
	Synthetic model	Human	Sheep	Synthetic model	Human	Sheep
End plate depth(I)	35.48 (0.46)	34.80 (1.24)	20.00 (0.60)	37.09 (1.05)	33.90 (0.85)	20.10 (0.70)
End plate width(I)	49.85 (0.76)	48.00 (1.24)	29.80 (1.30)	52.36 (0.61)	49.50 (1.38)	31.00 (0.60)
Vertebral body height	26.76 (0.03)	23.80 (1.10)	40.20 (1.20)	23.96 (0.86)	24.10 (1.10)	41.10 (0.80)
Spinal canal depth	20.62 (0.19)	17.50 (0.53)	8.60 (0.70)	21.38 (0.45)	18.60 (0.71)	8.80 (0.40)
Spinal canal width	23.53 (0.80)	24.30 (0.64)	12.60 (1.10)	23.37 (1.05)	25.40 (0.49)	12.90 (1.10)
Pedicle height	13.93 (0.90)	14.40 (0.62)	35.70 (1.40)	16.49 (0.44)	15.40 (0.46)	36.30 (1.40)
Pedicle width	12.88 (0.85)	10.20 (0.60)	9.50 (0.90)	11.49 (0.27)	14.10 (0.46)	9.60 (1.00)

extent with a lateral cage + plate (65.6%). This magnitude of reduction was similar to that seen with an anterior cage + plate (66.3%). In addition, cadaveric studies which investigate ROM of lateral interbody cage fusion with and without plate fixation [25-28] (Table 3) correlate well with the current study. Statistical analyses revealed differences between the intact and two cage + plate groups ($p < 0.05$ in AR and $p < 0.01$ in FE and LB). No statistic differences were detected between lateral cage + plate and arterial cage + plate; or between intact and lateral cage alone groups, except in LB ($p < 0.01$).

Discussion

The present study evaluated the response of the novel synthetic spine models to pure moment loading in all three anatomical planes under high cycle testing as well as following implantation with interbody cages and anterior/lateral plates. The anatomy of the synthetic spine compared to published data [12,19] was also reported. Results showed this synthetic spine model presents a better simulation in terms of anatomy than other spine surrogates for the human spine [29-36] (Table 1). The intact synthetic model has comparable biomechanics compared to published results for intact human cadaveric spine segments [23,24] (Table 2). A key measure of spinal kinematics is ROM. When comparing with human spines, ROM results were within the range of the human data, except AR ROM for sample1. NZ represents the lax portion of bending where relatively small loads cause large rotations [23]. Overall, NZ for FE and LB were within the

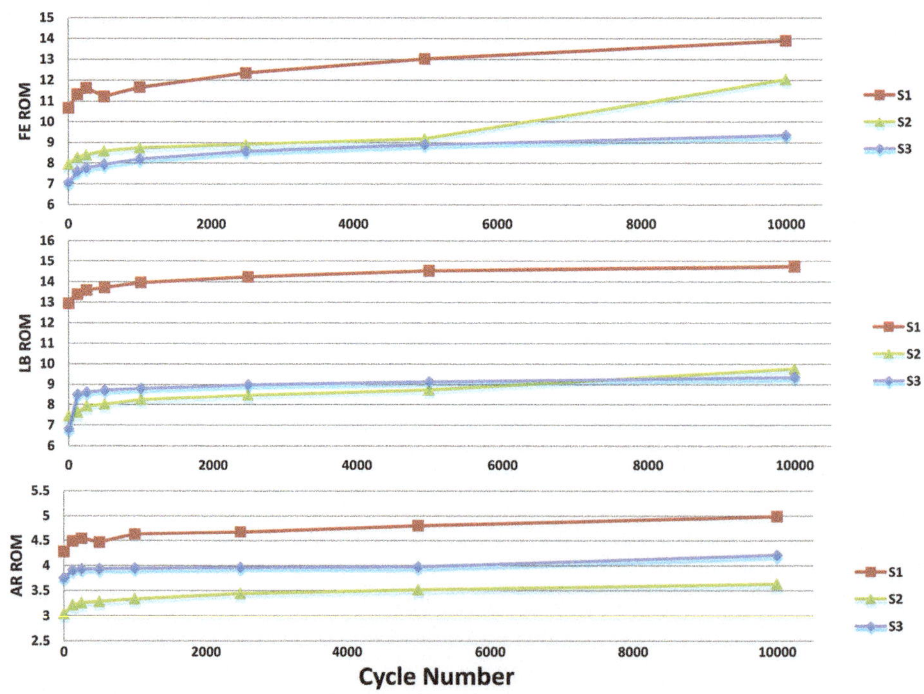

Figure 2 Individual sample ROM results against cycle number. Note the overall logarithm change occurring in relation to cycle number. S1-Sample 1, S2-Sample 2, S3-Sample 3; angle is represented on the Y-axis. FE-flexion/extension; LB-lateral bending; AR-axial rotation.

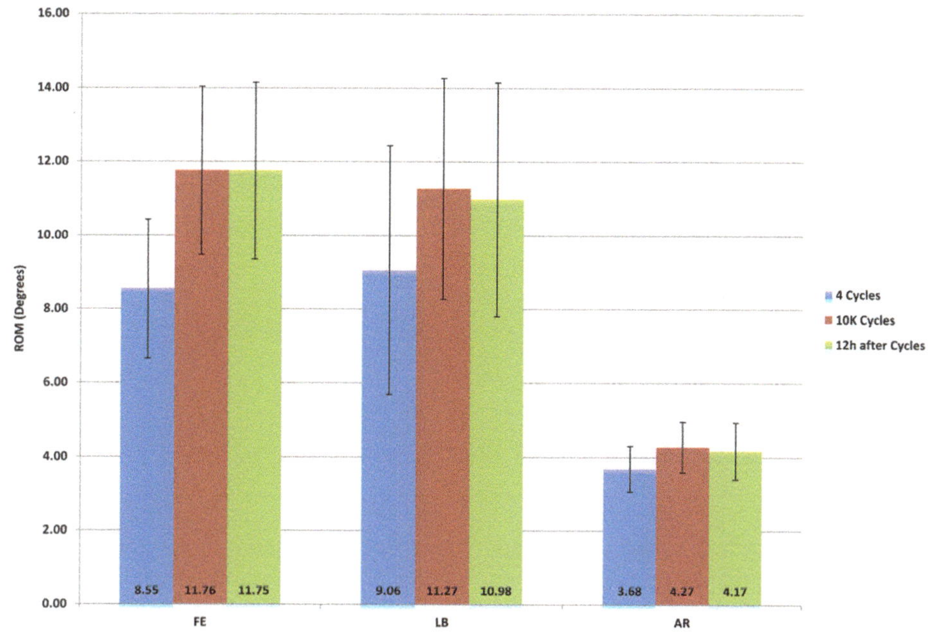

Figure 3 ROM comparison between 4 cycles, 10 K cycles and recovery. FE-flexion/extension; LB-lateral bending; AR-axial rotation.

human data range. In addition, the smaller standard deviation in ROM for all modes of bending, when compared with human data, would be expected to increase repeatability when used for this type of scientific research.

The 10,000 cycle test sequence results represented a long test life of this synthetic model. Although this would not be expected to represent true fatigue testing of implanted constructs in a spine, it is likely to span the working life of the spine in a laboratory environment. Results showed that ROM logarithmically increased with cycle number (Figure 2). Although after 10 K cycles ROM in all three motions had different magnitudes of increase, the final round of tests showed that the ROM was still within range of human.

The decrease in stiffness is likely due to two primary reasons: material property changes and mechanical bonding failure brought by fatigue. Material properties may change permanently due to microscopic failure points induced by cyclic loading, or transiently due to local temperature change. Traditional measures of spinal biomechanics present a torque/angle plot containing a hysteresis curve. This hysteresis area represents the amount of energy that is lost during the cycle. This energy is expended by causing permanent damage or is lost as heat. In the present test, a non-contacting thermometer showed that after 10 K cycles, local temperature increased up to 5°C in FE and LB motions at the intersection between disc and vertebral body. An additional source of heat may have been friction between the different material components. However, the ROM did not change significantly following cooling and recovery over 12 hours (Figure 3). This suggests that the temperature increase may not be the primary driver for changing mechanical properties. Visual inspection found that there were fibers broken in the outer annulus fibrosis, particularly at the intersection between disc and vertebral body. This area represents an abrupt change in material properties which the simulated outer annulus helped to transition. Failure of this construct is likely to have been responsible for a fair portion of the changing biomechanics.

Table 2 10 Nm ROM and NZ results comparing with human cadaveric data

	ROM (degree)				NZ (degree)			
	s1	s2	s3	White [24]	s1	s2	s3	Panjabi [23]
FE	22.9	15.7	12.8	15.0 (7.0)	0.8	0.9	0.9	0.7 (0.6)
LB	18.4	12.7	11.7	16.0 (8.0)	2.3	1.1	1.0	0.9 (0.8)
AR	8.0	5.1	4.8	5.2 (2.0)	0.8	0.8	0.7	1.3 (0.4)

S1-Sample 1, S2-Sample 2, S3-Sample, number in brackets indicated the standard deviation.

Repeated testing with differing implanted conditions showed the influence of interbody cage placement and plating on spinal biomechanics (Figure 4). Compared with the intact state, lateral interbody cage placement did not affect AR, trending towards a significant reduction in FE ($p = 0.06$), and significantly reduced in LB. The geometry and size of the lateral cage provides support in LB via a large footprint and extended lateral dimension, which likely contributed to these findings.

Differences in testing methodology make it difficult to draw exact comparisons with other cadaveric biomechanical

Table 3 Comparison of the current study results with relevant studies

Author/Publication	Applied torque [N · m]	Test conditions	FE ROM [% Intact]	LB ROM [% Intact]	AR ROM [% Intact]
Current study	±10	Lateral cage alone	48.5%	31.4%	81.3%
		Lateral cage and plate	22.2%	11.9%	33.9%
Cappuccino et al., 2010 [26]	±7.5	XLIF cage alone	31.6%	32.5%	69.4%
		XLIF + lateral plate	32.5%	15.9%	53.4%
Bess et al., 2008 [25]	±5	XLIF cage alone	45.8%	41.8%	66.3%
		XLIF + lateral plate	40.0%	24.2%	50.7%
Le Huec et al., 2002 [28]	±7	LLIF cage alone	71.3%	88.5%	107.7%
		LLIF cage + lateral plate	40.3%	27.3%	45.2%
Kim et al., 2005 [27]	±7.5	LLIF graft alone	75.2%	96.9%	71.6%
		LLIF + lateral plate	52.1%	37.9%	41.3%

XLIF-eXtreme Lateral Interbody Fusion; LLIF – Lateral Lumbar Interbody Fusion.

studies. However, similar trends in outcomes can be identified [25] and [26] used a human cadaver model to compare lumbar spine kinematics of a laterally placed interbody device used as a stand-alone construct with various instrumented constructs (Table 3). They tested 5 conditions: (1) intact spine, (2) lateral discectomy and stand-alone lateral interbody device (XLIF), (3) XLIF supplemented by a lateral plate, (4) XLIF supplemented by unilateral pedicle screws, and (5) XLIF supplemented by bilateral pedicle screws. Results revealed that the extreme lateral interbody implant, with or without supplemental fixation, provides primary stabilization in all loading modes compared with intact specimens. The greatest reduction in ROM was observed with lateral bending and flexion-extension in all treatments. Le Huec et al. [28] compared the biomechanics of lateral interbody cage in 8 cadaveric lumbar functional spinal units with 2 additional modes of fixation: a lateral plate and a lateral plate locked to the cage. The laterally placed cage produced a decrease in the ROM compared with intact in flexion extension and lateral bending, but not in axial rotation. The reduction in ROM observed with the plate was significantly reduced relative to the intact spine in all 3 motion planes. Kim et al. [27] evaluated the stability of human cadaveric lumbar spine constructs with interbody reconstruction performed via a traditional ALIF approach or a lateral approach. Specimens

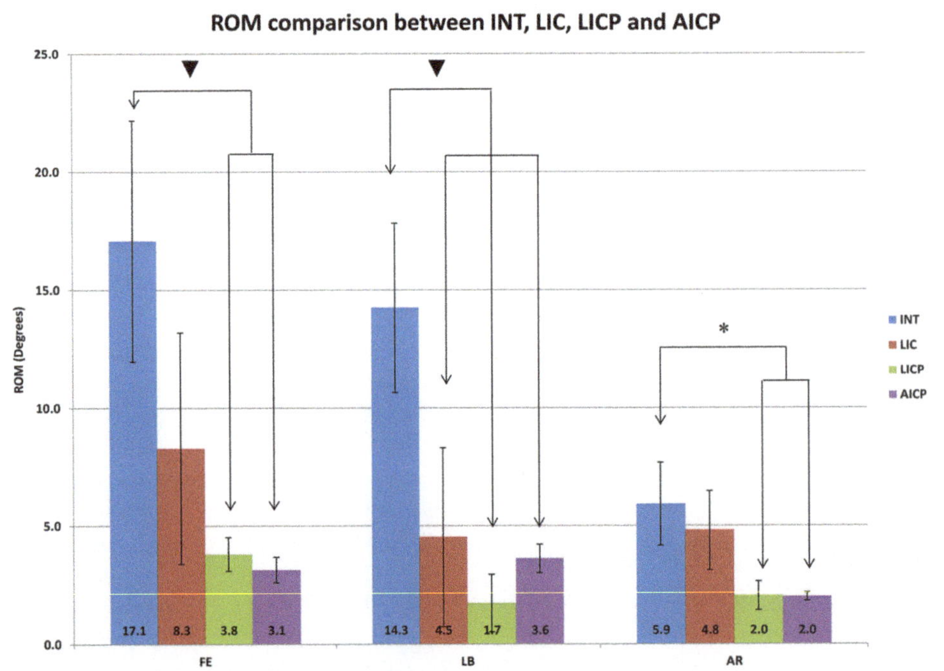

Figure 4 **ROM comparison between intact (INT), lateral interbody cage alone (LIC), lateral interbody cage + plate (LICP), and anterior interbody cage + plate (AICP) group.** ▼ = $p < 0.01$; * = $p < 0.05$.FE-flexion/extension; LB-lateral bending; AR-axial rotation.

were evaluated in 4 conditions: (1) intact spine, (2) destabilization by anterior or lateral discectomy, (3) stand-alone interbody reconstruction and (4) interbody reconstruction supplemented with additional fixation. The stand-alone lateral interbody and ALIF implants restored the ROM and NZ to intact spine values. Compared with the intact spine, supplemental instrumentation significantly reduced the ROM and NZ in all loading modes.

In summary, these cadaveric tests results indicated three primary points. Firstly, the stand-alone lateral interbody cage provided primary stabilization, which is supported by the present study. The present study showed that lateral interbody cage alone can reduce the ROM 48.5% and 31.4% in flexion-extension and lateral bending respectively. Similar reduction can be found in published literature (Table 3). Second, a stand-alone cage did not provide sufficient axial rotational stabilization (66.3%-107.7%), and this was confirmed again by the present study (81.3%). Third, a supplementary lateral plate with screws significantly reinforces the stabilization in all directions. Again, this is supported by the current study. However, a larger reduction in ROM has been found in current study compared to cadaveric data (22.2%, 11.9% and 33.9% in FE, LB and AR respectively vs. 32.5-52.1%, 15.9-37.9%, and 41.3-53.4% with cadaveric sample). This might due to the different loads applied. It also should be noted that the vertebral bodies do not contain simulated cancellous bone. The solid nature of the vertebrae may overestimate the fixation achievable by screws and limit the amount of deformation at the disc/endplate interface.

Limitations

The primary limitation of this study is the small sample size which did not allow robust statistical analysis. Additionally no cadaveric samples were tested for direct comparison. To allow comparison with cadaveric values published results were utilized. This provided mean values but did not allow for any statistical analysis. The destructive nature of the implanted conditions dictated that each sample follow a standard order. Randomized tests with individual samples for each intact and implanted condition may be desirable for future testing.

Conclusion

This study found that based on the anatomy and biomechanical similarities, the synthetic spine tested here provides a reasonable model to represent the human lumbar spine. Repeated testing did not dramatically alter biomechanics which may allow non-destructive testing between many different procedures and devices without the worry of carry over effects. Small intra-specimen variability and lack of biohazard makes this an attractive alternative for in vitro spine biomechanical testing. However, a preconditioning test should be run to check the initial ROM of each sample. It also proved an acceptable surrogate for biomechanical testing, confirming that a lateral lumbar interbody cage and plate construct reduces ROM to a similar degree as anterior lumbar interbody cage and plate constructs. Clearly, more testing is required in the future to evaluate this synthetic model for more complex applications.

Abbreviations

ROM: Range of motion; NZ: Neutral zone; FE: Flexion-extension; LB: Lateral bending; AR: Axial rotation; INT: Intact group; LIC: Lateral interbody cage alone; LICP: Lateral interbody cage with plate; AICP: anterior interbody cage with plate; XLIF: Lateral discectomy and stand-alone lateral interbody device; LLIF: Lateral lumbar interbody fusion; ALIF: Anterior lumbar interbody fusion.

Competing interests

The authors declare that they have no competing interests.

Authors' contributions

TW and MP carried out the mechanical test, performed the statistical analysis and drafted the manuscript. JB participated in the implantation test, also data analysis. WW conceived of the study, and participated in its design and coordination and helped to draft the manuscript. All authors read and approved the final manuscript.

Author details

[1]Surgical & Orthopaedic Research Laboratories, Prince of Wales Clinical School, University of New South Wales, Clinical Science Bldg, Prince of Wales Hospital, Gate 6, Avoca Street, 2031 Sydney, Australia. [2]Graduate School of Biomedical Engineering, University of New South Wales, Sydney, NSW, Australia. [3]Royal North Shore Hospital, St Leonards, NSW, Australia.

References

1. Wilke H-J, Jungkunz B, Wenger K, Claes LE (1998) Spinal segment range of motion as a function of in vitro test conditions: Effects of exposure period, accumulated cycles, angular-deformation rate, and moisture condition. Anat Rec 251(1):15–19. doi:10.1002/(SICI)1097-0185(199805)251:1<15::AID-AR4>3.0.CO;2-D
2. Hongo M, Gay RE, Hsu J-T, Zhao KD, Ilharreborde B, Berglund LJ, An K-N (2008) Effect of multiple freeze–thaw cycles on intervertebral dynamic motion characteristics in the porcine lumbar spine. J Biomech 41(4):916–920. doi:10.1016/j.jbiomech.2007.11.003
3. Cunningham BW, Kotani Y, McNulty PS, Cappuccino A, McAfee PC (1997) The effect of spinal destabilization and instrumentation on lumbar intradiscal pressure: an in vitro biomechanical analysis. Spine 22(22):2655–2663
4. Shono Y, Kaneda K, Abumi K, McAfee PC, Cunningham BW (1998) Stability of posterior spinal instrumentation and its effects on adjacent motion segments in the lumbosacral spine. Spine (Phila Pa 1976) 23(14):1550–1558
5. Kotani Y, Cunningham BW, Abumi K, McAfee PC (1994) Biomechanical analysis of cervical stabilization systems: an assessment of transpedicular screw fixation in the cervical spine. Spine 19(22):2529–2539
6. Bozkus H, Chamberlain RH, Perez Garza LE, Crawford NR, Dickman CA (2004) Biomechanical comparison of anterolateral plate, lateral plate, and pedicle screws-rods for enhancing anterolateral lumbar interbody cage stabilization. Spine (Phila Pa 1976) 29(6):635–641
7. Grubb MR, Currier BL, Shih J-S, Bonin V, Grabowski JJ, Chao EY (1998) Biomechanical evaluation of anterior cervical spine stabilization. Spine 23(8):886–892
8. Richman JD, Daniel TE, Anderson DD, Miller PL, Douglas RA (1995) Biomechanical evaluation of cervical spine stabilization methods using a porcine model. Spine 20(20):2192
9. Schmidt R, Richter M, Claes L, Puhl W, Wilke H-J (2005) Limitations of the cervical porcine spine in evaluating spinal implants in comparison with human cervical spinal segments: a biomechanical in vitro comparison of

porcine and human cervical spine specimens with different instrumentation techniques. Spine 30(11):1275–1282
10. Kanayama MMD, Cunningham BWMS, Weis JCMD, Parker LMMD, Kaneda KMD, McAfee PCMD (1998) The effects of rigid spinal instrumentation and solid bony fusion on spinal kinematics: a posterolateral spinal arthrodesis model. Spine 23(7):767–773
11. Sandén B, Olerud C, Johansson C, Larsson S (2001) Improved bone–screw interface with hydroxyapatite coating: an in vivo study of loaded pedicle screws in sheep. Spine 26(24):2673–2678
12. Wilke HJ, Kettler A, Wenger KH, Claes LE (1997d) Anatomy of the sheep spine and its comparison to the human spine. Anat Rec 247(4):542–555. doi:10.1002/(SICI)1097-0185(199704)247:4<542
13. Wilke HJ, Kettler A, Claes LE (1997) Are sheep spines a valid biomechanical model for human spines? Spine (Phila Pa 1976) 22(20):2365–2374
14. Bertollo N, Gothelf T, Walsh W (2008) 3-Fluted orthopaedic drills exhibit superior bending stiffness to their 2-fluted rivals: Clinical implications for targeting ability and the incidence of drill-bit failure. Injury 39(7):734–741
15. Bertollo N, Gothelf T, Walsh W (2013) In vitro analysis of drill Bit designs: 2 vs 3 flutes. Bone & Joint J Orthopaedic Proc Supple 95(SUPP 15):133–133
16. Bougherara H, Zdero R, Mahboob Z, Dubov A, Shah S, Schemitsch E (2010) The biomechanics of a validated finite element model of stress shielding in a novel hybrid total knee replacement. Proc Inst Mech Eng H J Eng Med 224(10):1209–1219
17. Burroughs BR, Hallstrom B, Golladay GJ, Hoeffel D, Harris WH (2005) Range of motion and stability in total hip arthroplasty with 28-, 32-, 38-, and 44-mm femoral head sizes: an in vitro study. J Arthroplasty 20(1):11–19
18. Harris ML, Morberg P, Bruce WJM, Walsh WR (1999) An improved method for measuring tibiofemoral contact areas in total knee arthroplasty: a comparison of K-scan sensor and Fuji film. J Biomech 32(9):951–958. doi:10.1016/S0021-9290(99)00072-X
19. Panjabi MM, GOEL V, OXLAND T, TAKATA K, DURANCEAU J, KRAG M, PRICE M (1992) Human lumbar vertebrae: quantitative three-dimensional anatomy. Spine 17(3):299
20. Pelletier M, Cordaro N, Lau A, Walsh WR (2012) PEEK versus Ti interbody fusion devices: resultant fusion, bone apposition, initial and 26 week biomechanics. J Spinal Disord Tech. doi:10.1097/BSD.0b013e31826851a4
21. Spenciner D, Greene D, Paiva J, Palumbo M, Crisco J (2006) The multidirectional bending properties of the human lumbar intervertebral disc. Spine J 6(3):248–257. doi:10.1016/j.spinee.2005.08.020
22. Wilke HJ, Wolf S, Claes LE, Arand M, Wiesend A (1995) Stability increase of the lumbar spine with different muscle groups. A biomechanical in vitro study. Spine 20(2):192–198
23. Panjabi M (2003) Clinical spinal instability and low back pain. J Electromyogr Kinesiol 13(4):371–379. doi:10.1016/s1050-6411(03)00044-0
24. White AA, Panjabi MM (1990) Clinical Biomechanics of the Spine, 2nd edition. Lippincott, Philadelphia
25. Bess R, Cornwall G, Vance R, Bachus K, Brodke D (2008) Biomechanics of Lateral Arthrodesis. In: Goodrich JA, Volcan IJ (ed) eXtreme Lateral Interbody Fusion (XLIF). Quality Medical Publishing, St Louis, MO, pp 31–40
26. Cappuccino A, Cornwall GB, Turner AW, Fogel GR, Duong HT, Kim KD, Brodke DS (2010) Biomechanical analysis and review of lateral lumbar fusion constructs. Spine (Phila Pa 1976) 35(26 Suppl):S361–S367. doi:10.1097/BRS.0b013e318202308b
27. Kim SM, Lim TJ, Paterno J, Park J, Kim DH (2005) Biomechanical comparison: stability of lateral-approach anterior lumbar interbody fusion and lateral fixation compared with anterior-approach anterior lumbar interbody fusion and posterior fixation in the lower lumbar spine. J Neurosurg Spine 2(1):62–68. doi:10.3171/spi.2005.2.1.0062
28. Le Huec JC, Liu M, Skalli W, Josse L (2002) Lumbar lateral interbody cage with plate augmentation: in vitro biomechanical analysis. Eur Spine J 11(2):130–136. doi:10.1007/s005860100316
29. Au AG, Aiyangar AK, Anderson PA, Ploeg HL (2011) Replicating interbody device subsidence with lumbar vertebraesurrogates. Proc Inst Mech Eng H 225(10):972–985
30. Dick JC, Zdeblick TA, Bartel BD, Kunz DN (1997) Mechanical evaluation of cross-link designs in rigid pedicle screw systems. Spine 22(4):370–375
31. Murakami HH, Kawahara NN, Tomita KK, Sakamoto JJ, Oda JJ (2002) Biomechanical evaluation of reconstructed lumbosacral spine after total sacrectomy. J Orthop Sci 7(6):658–664
32. Penzkofer R, Hofberger S, Spiegl U, Schilling C, Schultz R, Augat P, Gonschorek O (2011) Biomechanical comparison of the end plate design of three vertebral body replacement systems. Arch Orthop Trauma Surg 131(9):1253–1259. doi:10.1007/s00402-011-1284-7
33. Stanford RE, Loefler AH, Stanford PM, Walsh WR (2004) Multiaxial pedicle screw designs: static and dynamic mechanical testing. Spine 29(4):367–375
34. Tokuhashi Y, Matsuzaki H, Shirasaki Y, Tateishi T (2000) C1—C2 intra-articular screw fixation for atlantoaxial posterior stabilization. Spine 25(3):337–341
35. Wilke H-J, Russo G, Schmitt H, Claes L (1997) A mechanical model of human spinal motion segments-Ein mechanisches modell für humane wirbelsäulenbewegungssegmente. Biomed Tech (Berl) 42(11):327–331
36. Yinger K, Scalise J, Olson SA, Bay BK, Finkemeier CG (2003) Biomechanical comparison of posterior pelvic ring fixation. J Orthop Trauma 17(7):481–487

Platelet-rich plasma to treat ankle cartilage pathology - from translational potential to clinical evidence: a systematic review

Francesca Vannini[1], Berardo Di Matteo[2*] and Giuseppe Filardo[2]

Abstract

Platelet-rich Plasma (PRP) is a fascinating biological treatment showing promising results for the management of cartilage disorders. However, despite the step forwards in this research area and the increasing use of PRP in clinical practice, its use remains still controversial and especially its application as injective treatment for ankle cartilage pathology have been scarcely investigated.

The aim of this paper is to describe the translational evidence for the use of PRP in cartilage treatment and to systematically review all the available evidence regarding the clinical application of PRP for ankle cartilage disorders, in order to understand what is the current state of the art for this specific clinical indication, underlining both limits and potential of this biological strategy.

A systematic review of the clinical literature was performed on the use of PRP to treat ankle cartilage disorders and 7 papers were identified. PRP has been used in two different ways: 5 of the available papers focus on its use as an augmentation procedure to various surgical techniques for cartilage regeneration, while only two studies report its conservative application through intra-articular injections. Based on the limited number of clinical studies available on this topic, this systematic review showed the lack of major adverse events related to PRP and overall good results for the treatment of ankle cartilage pathology, thus confirming the translational potential of this biological treatment suggested by several preclinical studies. Further high quality clinical trials in the ankle are still needed to clarify proper indications and best applicative modalities.

Keywords: PRP; Growth factors; Ankle; Cartilage; Injections; Intra-articular

Introduction

Platelet-rich Plasma (PRP) is a fascinating biological treatment showing promise for the management of cartilage disorders [1,2]. The possibility of using autologous blood to obtain a product rich in growth factors and other bio-active molecules involved in tissue healing has been regarded as an innovative approach that could be sided to classical "on-the shelf" products from pharmaceutical companies.

The first reports in this field of application were published 10 years ago and since then many studies have been made in order to understand the biological effects of PRP and the potential and limits of this approach, not just as a therapeutic strategy for cartilage pathology [3,4] but more in general for a wide range of musculo-skeletal disorders, such as ligament and tendon pathologies [5-7]. However, despite the step forwards in this research area and the increasing use of PRP in the clinical practice, its use remains still controversial, especially its application as a treatment for ankle cartilage pathology [6].

In fact, under a clinical point of view, the vast majority of the studies already published is focused on the application of PRP in the knee joint, whereas only a smaller number of studies deals with other joints such as hip and ankle, either as a conservative injective approach or as an augmentation during surgical procedures for cartilage repair [8-11]. Thus, the rationale for the use of PRP in the ankle is currently mainly derived from the knee application. Among the available knee focused studies, 4 double blind randomized controlled trials show promising

* Correspondence: berardo.dimatteo@gmail.com
[2]II Orthopaedic Clinic and Biomechanics Laboratory, Rizzoli Orthopaedic Institute, Via di Barbiano n. 1/10, 40136 Bologna, Italy
Full list of author information is available at the end of the article

results and an overall support for the therapeutic potential of PRP [12-15]. PRP has been shown to provide a superior clinical outcome with respect to placebo (saline solution), thus proving a real clinical benefit [15]. More controversial is the superiority of the results obtained compared to other treatments: when compared to viscosupplementation, results are not that promising and there is some support but no conclusive evidence that PRP is significantly better than hyaluronic acid (HA) for the treatment of cartilage pathology [12]. The overall literature suggests that PRP is at least as effective as HA and should be therefore considered one of the available options for knee cartilage treatment. While knee pathology can be considered a bench test for all articular locations, other joints have been less enquired by researchers.

The aim of this paper is to describe the translational evidence for the use of PRP in cartilage treatment and to systematically review all the available evidence regarding the clinical application of PRP for ankle cartilage disorders, in order to understand what is the current state of the art for this specific clinical indication, underlining both limits and potential of this biological strategy.

Review

Materials and methods

A systematic review of the literature was performed on the use of PRP to treat ankle cartilage disorders. The search was made on the PubMed database on October 10th, 2014 using the following formula: (PRP OR platelet rich plasma OR platelet concentrate OR PRGF OR platelet gel OR platelet derived growth factors) AND (ankle or tibio-talar or talar) AND (osteoarthritis OR chondropathy OR chondral lesions OR osteochondral lesion). The guidelines for Preferred Reporting Items for Systematic Reviews and Meta-analysis (PRISMA) were used [16]. The screening process and analysis were performed separately by 2 independent researchers (Figure 1).

First, the articles were screened by title and abstract. The following inclusion criteria for relevant articles were used during the initial screening of titles and abstracts: clinical reports of any level of evidence, written in the English language, with no time limitation, on the use of PRP to treat ankle cartilage disorders. Other exclusion criteria were: case reports, articles written in other languages, animal trials, and reviews. In the second step, the full

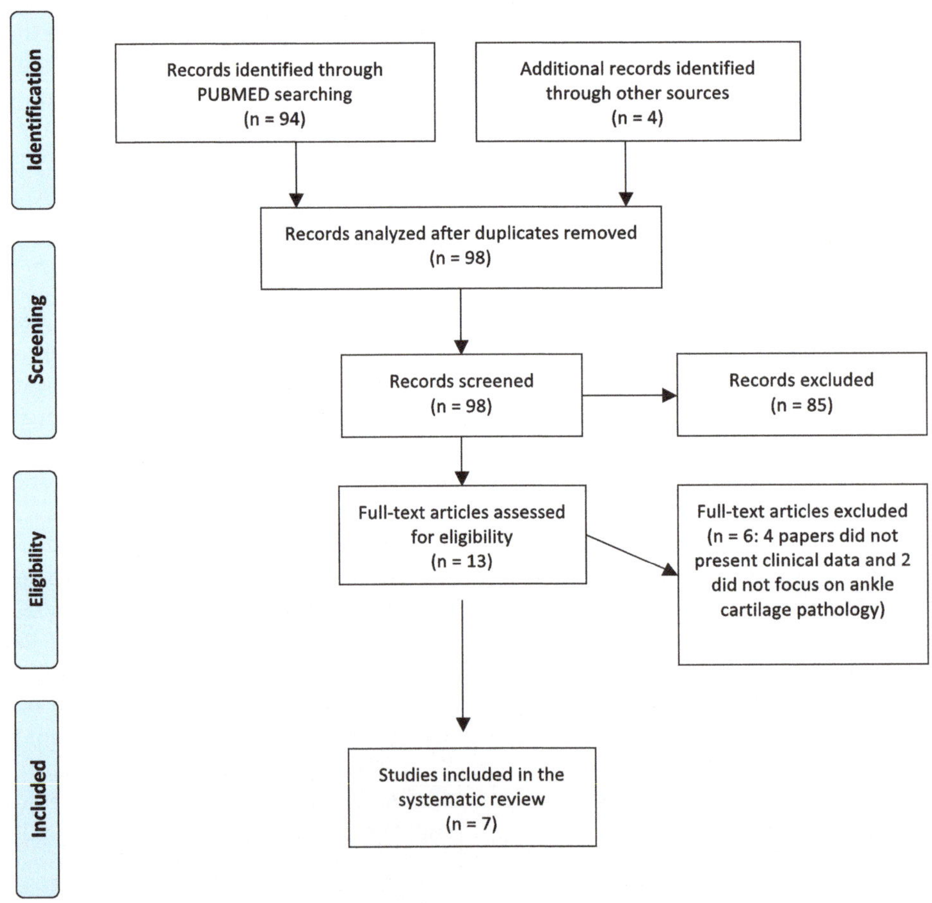

Figure 1 Prisma 2009 flow diagram describing the papers selection process.

texts of the selected articles were screened, with further exclusions according to the previously described criteria. Moreover, articles not reporting clinical results were excluded. Reference lists from the selected papers were also screened. Relevant data were then extracted and collected in a single database with consensus of the two observers to be analyzed for the purposes of the present manuscript. At the end of the process, 7 papers fulfilled the selection criteria and have been described in the following paragraph.

Results

PRP application, as reported in the literature for cartilage disease treatment in the ankle joint, can be summarized in two treatment strategies. Five papers focus on its use as an augmentation procedure to various surgical techniques for cartilage regeneration, while only two studies report its conservative application through intra-articular injections (Table 1).

Conservative application

Conservative application of PRP was firstly reported in a prospective randomized study by Mei-Dan et al. [17], who compared the efficacy of hyaluronic acid (HA) and PRP in 30 patients (15 per group) affected by talar osteochondral lesions not responsive to previous conservative management. Patients were divided into 2 groups: one to receive 3 weekly intra-articular injections of HA (2 ml each); the other one to receive PRP (2 ml each) with the same administration protocol. They were evaluated for up to 28 weeks of follow-up: AHFS (Ankle Hindfoot Score), AOFAS (American Orthopaedic Foot and Ankle Score), and VAS (Visual Analogue Scale) were used to test pain, stiffness and function, showing that PRP was significantly more effective at controlling pain and re-establishing function.

The conservative approach was also described by Angthong et al. [18], who applied PRP to different foot and ankle diseases and, among them, to low grades of ankle OA. PRP was injected under fluoroscope or ultrasound guidance and results were evaluated by VAS-FA (VAS Foot and Ankle) score. Patients with OA were also studied radiographically and scored for the OA grade. The 5 patients with OA included in this study presented a significant improvement in their clinical conditions according to VAS-FA score at a mean follow-up of 16 months (calculated on the whole series of patients). Despite the improved clinical condition, no changes in the degree of OA was evident on MRI 5 months after PRP injection.

Surgical application

The surgical application of PRP as augmentation to microfractures in full thickness osteochondral lesions of the talus has been investigated by Guney et al. [19] in the only randomized comparative study available on this specific application modality: 35 patients were scheduled to receive either microfracture alone or microfracture in association with PRP (a single injection after 6–24 hours from arthroscopic microfractures), and were assessed at 16.2 (12–24) months follow-up using the AOFAS scoring system, Foot and Ankle Ability Measure (FAAM), and the VAS for pain. At baseline, AOFAS and FAAM scores were similar in the two groups, whereas pain scores (VAS) were higher in those who were assigned to the combined treatment. Despite the latter finding, the combined treatment with PRP resulted in significantly better outcomes in terms of functional scores (AOFAS, FAAM overall pain domain, FAAM 15-min walking domain, and pain-related scores) when compared to bone marrow stimulation alone. The authors concluded that PRP as an adjunct to arthroscopic microfracture surgery for the treatment of osteochondral lesions of the talus resulted in improved functional score status in the medium-term evaluation.

The most common surgical application of PRP involved its use as augmentation to scaffold implantation. This strategy for the treatment of full thickness talar osteochondral lesions has been documented by Giannini and his group in four different studies [20-23]. They described the clinical application of an arthroscopic one-stage technique involving autologous mesenchymal stem cells (MSCs), PRP, and either porcine collagen powder or HA membrane. The procedure consisted of harvesting bone-marrow-derived cells from the posterior iliac crest of the patients through a traditional marrow needle. Sixty ml of bone marrow-aspirate were collected and immediately put into a cell separator-concentrator to obtain a final 6-ml concentrate of MSCs. A collagen powder or a HA membrane could then be used. In the former cases, 2 ml of MSCs concentrate was added to 1 g of collagen powder and 1 ml of platelet-rich fibrin gel (obtained the day before surgery). In the latter cases, HA membrane was cut to match the size of the talar ostechondral lesion and then covered with 2 ml of MSCs concentrate and 1 ml of platelet-rich fibrin gel. The entire procedure was performed via ankle arthroscopy and, after the preparation of the lesion, the biological composite was placed in the defect site through a cannula and using a probe to obtain the best possible fit.

The first prospective single-arm clinical trial [20] involved 48 patients (mean age = 28.5 years) affected by focal lesions (mean size = 2.1 cm^2) and evaluated at 6, 12, 18, and 24 months of follow-up using the AOFAS score. A significant increase in this parameter was recorded 6 months after the surgical procedure, and this outcome was confirmed up to the final follow-up. The rate of return to high impact sport activity was satisfactory: more than 75% of the patients returned to sport at 11 months of follow-up. The investigators found a correlation between clinical outcome and lesion size: poorer results

Table 1 Synopsis of all the clinical studies on PRP application in ankle cartilage pathology

AUTHORS, JOURNAL AND YEAR	LEVEL OF EVIDENCE	PATHOLOGY	PRP features	PROTOCOL	PATIENTS	FOLLOW- UP	OUTCOME
Mei-Dan et al. AJSM 2012 [17]	I – Randomized trial	Osteochondral lesions of the talus	Leukocyte-poor PRP Single centrifugation Platelet count: 2-3x basal value Activation: Ca-chloride	3 injections of 2 ml PRP, at two-weeks interval	30 (15 PRP vs 15 HA)	7 months	Statistically significant better clinical outcome for PRP group
Angthong et al. J Foot Ankle Surg 2013 [18]	IV – Case series	Ankle OA	Low platelet concentrate, leukocyte poor PRP Single centrifugation Activation: No	One injection of 3 ml PRP	5	16 months	Significant clinical improvement without any change in OA grade
Guney et al. KSTTA 2013 [19]	II – Randomized trial	Osteochondral lesion of the talus	Platelet count: 5.4x basal value Leukocyte: n.a. 10% NAHCO3 addition before PRP injection	One PRP injection (6–24 hours after performing microfractures)	35 (19 microfractures + PRR vs 15 microfractures alone)	16 months	Combined treatment with PRP determined significantly better outcomes in terms of functional scores with respect to bone marrow stimulation alone.
Giannini et al. Clin Orthop Rel Res 2009 [20]	IV – case series	Osteochondral lesion of the talus	Double centrifugation, leukocyte rich PRF Platelet count 5x basal value	PRP added intra-operatively to the biomaterial during the osteochondral lesion repair	48	24 months	Significant improvement in the AOFAS score of the patietns treated at final FU. 75% of the patients were able to resume sports activity. Cartilage with hyaline appearance in the 2 second look biopsies performed.
Giannini et al. Injury 2010 [21]	III – retrospective comparative trial	Osteochondral lesion of the talus		PRP added intra-operatively to the biomaterial during the osteochondral lesion repair	81 (25 one step technique with PRP vs 10 open ACI vs 46 arthroscopic ACI)	36 months	All the 3 groups had similar patterns of clinical improvement. The one step technique was cheaper.
Battaglia et al. Eur J Radiol 2011 [22]	IV – case series	Osteochondral lesion of the talus		PRP added intra-operatively to the biomaterial during the osteochondral lesion repair	20	24 months	Regenerated tissue with a T2 relaxation time value comparable to hyalinecartilage was found in all the treated cases, covering a mean of 78% of the repaired lesion area.

Table 1 Synopsis of all the clinical studies on PRP application in ankle cartilage pathology *(Continued)*

Giannini et al. Am J Sports med 2013 [23]	IV – case series	Osteochondral lesion of the talus	PRP added intra-operatively to the biomaterial during the osteochondral lesion repair	49	48 months	A significant relationship between the AOFAS score at 48 months' follow-up and the percentage of regenerated cartilage with hyaline features (T2 value of 35–45 ms). Patients with hyaline-like regenerated cartilage in more than 80% of the treated area had a more predictable and stable result.

were found for larger lesions, and previous surgery was also shown to affect the outcome negatively. Conversely, the outcome was not influenced by the lesion depth or by the type of scaffold used (collagen powder or HA membrane). Five second-look arthroscopies were performed at 1 year follow-up: in 2 cases biopsies were taken, revealing, after histologic and immune-histologic analysis, the presence of new cartilage tissue with varying degrees of tissue remodeling towards a hyaline aspect. The overall findings suggested that this novel approach could stimulate tissue regeneration with promising clinical efficacy, thus providing results that may even be comparable to those of autologous chondrocyte implantation (ACI) while avoiding the double surgical time and the inherent stress for the patient.

The same authors performed a further study [21] to compare MSCs + PRP + scaffold with open and arthroscopic ACI. Eighty-one patients were included in this analysis, and three different treatments were compared: 10 patients were treated by open ACI, 46 by arthroscopic ACI, and 25 by the bone-marrow-derived mesenchymal cells "one-step" technique. The clinical results were compared for up to 3 years of follow-up. AOFAS was the test chosen for clinical evaluation and radiographic analysis was performed as well. The clinical improvement in each subgroup was significant and no inter-group difference was observed, thus confirming the possibility of matching the effectiveness of chondrocyte transplantation by a single-step procedure. X-Rays showed no sign of OA progression and MRI revealed a good rate of defect filling and integration of the newly regenerated tissue within the surrounding tissue. Another aspect worth considering is the economic one: in fact, the authors pointed out that their novel one-step regenerative technique costs less than a half than traditional arthroscopic ACI.

An MRI evaluation was performed by Battaglia et al. [22] at 2 years' follow-up from surgery in a selection of 20 patients operated by this one-step technique. MRI images were acquired using, beside a protocol suggested by the International Cartilage Repair Society and the MOCART scoring system, a T2 mapping qualitative sequence. Results were then correlated with AOFAS clinical score, which showed a significant improvement from pre-operatively to 2 years of follow-up. The T2 relaxation time value of 35–45 ms was derived from healthy ankles evaluation and assumed as normal hyaline cartilage value and used as a control. Regenerated tissue with a T2 relaxation time value comparable to hyaline cartilage was found in all the treated cases, covering a mean of 78% of the repaired lesion area. A high clinical score was directly correlated to iso-intense signal in DPFSE fat sat and to the percentage of regenerated hyaline cartilage, and inversely correlated to the percentage of newly formed fibrocartilage. Lesion's depth was negatively correlated to the integrity of the repaired tissue's surface and to the percentage of regenerated hyaline cartilage.

Finally, the same original case series of 49 patients was clinically evaluated at a further follow-up of 4 years [23]. The overall AOFAS score improved significantly, with best results at the 24-month follow-up. A significant decrease in the clinical score was observed between 24 and 36 months postoperatively and between 24 and 48 months in the general case series. Nevertheless, while evaluating the 20 patients who performed T2 mapping MRI 2 years before, it was evident a significant relationship between the AOFAS score at 48 months' follow-up and the percentage of regenerated cartilage with hyaline features (T2 value of 35–45 ms). Patients with hyaline-like regenerated cartilage in more than 80% of the treated area had a more predictable and stable result.

Discussion

The results of this systematic review show the lack of major adverse events related to PRP, and overall good results for the treatment of ankle cartilage pathology, either as conservative approach or as augmentation to surgical procedures, thus confirming the translational potential of this biological treatment suggested by several preclinical studies and also in this limited number of clinical trials regarding the ankle joint.

The literature exploring the potential of PRP in the preclinical setting underlined different aspects that could explain the positive clinical findings obtained with this blood derivative (Table 2).

In vitro studies investigating the effect of PRP on chondrocytes showed various and heterogeneous mechanisms of action [24-26]. Most of these studies agreed in reporting an increased chondrocyte proliferation rate, while the maintenance of chondrocyte marker expression has been observed in several papers but not unanimously confirmed. Other effects ranged from the matrix production stimulation to the inflammation modulation, and some findings even suggested a potential role of PRP as analgesic compound by modulating cannabinoid receptors in chondrocytes [27].

Beside the direct effects on chondrocytes, to understand the translational potential of PRP it is also important to consider the overall role played by PRP in affecting the entire joint homeostasis, as demonstrated by studies focused on different cell types. Platelet concentrates may significantly enhance synoviocyte HA secretion and switch synovial angiogenesis to a more balanced status, even though some reports also suggest some potential drawbacks, likely related to the leukocyte content, due to the metallo-proteinases production and therefore a possible pro-inflammatory response that could lead to an accelerated cartilage catabolism [28].

Table 2 Summary of the findings from in vitro and in vivo evidence concerning the application of PRP in cartilage pathology

IN VITRO EVIDENCE		
PRP EFFECTS ON...	**Chondrocytes culture [3,25-27]**	- Increase chondrocyte proliferation rate
		- Stimulate chondrocyte phenotype expression and mainteinance
		- Increase matrix molecules production
		- Overall reduction of inflammatory response
	Condrocytes + MSC culture [3,29]	- Promotion of MSCs proliferation, adhesion and migration
		- Increased expression of Collagen II
	Synovial Cells culture [3,28]	- Anti or pro-flogistic effects demonstrated, according to the particular PRP formulation used
	Meniscal cells culture [3,30]	- Increase in meniscal cell proliferation rate
		- Stimulation of GAG synthesis
	Stem Cells culture [3,24,29]	- Stimulation of migration and chondrogenic differentiation of cortico-spongious bone cells
		- Superior chondrogenic differentiation of BMSCs
		- Enhanced proliferation rate and retained chondrogenic differentiation potential of ADMSCs
		- Increase in proliferation and migration induction of peripheral blood and umbilical cord blood MSCs
	Bacterial culture [40]	- PRP is able to provide an early protection against bacterial contamination due to the release of antimicrobial proteins
ANIMAL MODELS		
PRP EFFECTS ON...	**Rats [31]**	- In chondral lesion model: PRP improves tissue healing and collagen II expression
		- In OA model: controversial results regarding chondroprotective effects
	Rabbit [32,33,36]	- In Osteochondral lesion: no macroscopic, microscopic and biomechanical benefit after PRP administration
		- In OA model: positive influence on cartilage degeneration process (especially in moderate OA)
	Sheep [35]	- In chondral lesion model: improvement in macroscopic, histologic, and biomechanical cartilage scores. Beneficial effects also when applied together with microfractures
	Pig [37]	- In Rheumatoid Arthritis model: overall reduction in pro-flogistic enzymes and molecules; chondroprotective effect
	Horse [34]	- In OA model: positive modulation of joint homeostasis, with reduction of lameness and joint effusion up to middle term evaluation

Since the overall PRP effect in the articular environment derives from an interaction with the pre-existing environment and other cells, and since some surgical protocols involve the application of both platelets and cells, several studies also investigated the effect of PRP on MSCs of different origin. In all cases an overall stimulatory effect was documented, ranging from a chemotactic action to an increased proliferation, and from the chondrogenic differentiation to the production of molecules specific of the articular cartilage [29,30].

Preclinical studies also explored the rational for PRP use and tested its translational potential in the animal model, with interesting findings in both an acute and chronic lesion setting. Induced OA was treated with PRP injections showing heterogeneous results in different experimental models: while some authors showed no significant effects in the rat model, others suggested an indirect effect through the induction of other cells and a final better histological appearance [29,31]. More concordant and favorable results have been seen in bigger animal models, with a suppression of OA progression or even tissue regeneration in rabbits [32,33], and a significant improvement of degree of lameness and joint effusion treating OA in horses [34].

The treatment of acute chondral or osteochondral lesions has also been documented [35,36]. In these experimental settings, PRP seemed to provide an overall beneficial effect when used as an injective approach or even when applied after microfracturing. The findings emerged from these animal studies showed that PRP was able to increase macroscopic, histologic and biomechanical scores, although a full restoration of hyaline cartilage has not been shown. Furthermore, PRP was also tested in the pig rheumatoid arthritis model [37], revealing an anti-inflammatory potential and a chondroprotective effect that would be worthy of more studies to understand the contribution of PRP as topical therapy even in this more complex immunological disease.

Beside the positive effects of this therapy demonstrated by most of the preclinical in vitro and animal studies, many questions remain still open and how to manage the numerous variables that could optimize PRP translational potential is still controversial.

In fact, the final outcome could be influenced by variables related to the product, such as dose, cell content, activation method and storage procedures, as well as application modality and concomitant procedures [38]. First of all, PRP dose could be of particular importance for the outcome since it is strictly linked to the amount of growth factors and bioactive molecules administered. Both *in vitro* and animal studies showed a time-dependent regulation and the dose-dependency effect of PRP, suggesting that a better clinical outcome can be achieved in function of the platelet count [26,39]. However, beside the amount of platelets, another and more debated aspect could play a major role for the intra-articular application of PRP: cell content, which is the most controversial aspect, especially with regard to the presence of leukocytes. In fact, even though leukocyte presence could contribute to an anti-microbial effect [40], some in vitro studies have shown that leukocyte rich PRP stimulates expression of pro-inflammatory molecules and enzymes detrimental for joint homeostasis [41]. Nonetheless, from a clinical point of view there is a lack of studies addressing this question with a proper methodology and, looking at the current evidence, it has not been demonstrated any significant clinical difference according to PRP formulation, with the exception of post-injective adverse events (more pain and swelling after leukocyte-rich PRP administration) [42]. Activation methods and storage procedures are also aspects under examination: in particular, activation has been demonstrated to affect the physical properties and growth factors release kinetics of PRP [43], even if no data have been reported about differences in clinical results. For what regards storage methods, a recently published *in vitro* trial revealed that freeze thawing is a safe procedure, which sufficiently preserves PRP quality and its ability to induce proliferation and the production of extra cellular matrix (ECM) components in both chondrocytes and synoviocytes [44]. The possibility to preserve PRP could be relevant in the clinical setting since multiple injections of PRP can be required in case of poor response or symptom relapse, and this strategy is therefore attractive: a single blood harvesting can contribute to reduce costs and patient's discomfort. However, therapeutic protocols (i.e.: number of PRP injections and their timing) are still a controversial point, where poor evidence is available, and clinicians tend to adopt very personal approaches, mainly based to their personal experience with other injective products [38].

In conclusion, the translational evidence currently available is overall supporting the application of PRP as a treatment option for both focal chondral/osteochondral lesion and for joint degenerative pathology, due to the milieau of effects exerted by PRP on all the articular tissues. For sure the great variability among PRP formulations, reported by in vitro studies, still remains the main issue to address in order to develop the best product for specific clinical use.

Looking at the available evidence on the clinical benefit obtained with this blood derivative, the application of PRP to treat ankle cartilage pathology is supported by 7 studies: 5 of them dealing with surgical treatment and two with an injective approach [17-23]. The randomized trial by Mei-Dan et al. [17] revealed significant results in favor of PRP but the low number of patients and the short-term follow-up evaluation are weak points, while the study by Angthong et al. [18] deals with the use of PRP in different foot and ankle pathologies and just 5 patients were actually affected by ankle OA. Conversely, the studies testing the surgical application of MSCs + PRP + biomaterials (collagen powder or HA membrane) [19-23] are well documented but the value in determining the actual role of PRP is limited because in all of them it is described the combined use of multiple biological autologous and bio-engineered substances, without control groups, so that it is impossible to determine the actual contribution of PRP itself to the success of the procedure [9].

Conclusion

PRP is certainly a fascinating area of pre-clinical and clinical research. Nonetheless, at present, there is a very limited number of studies regarding the use of PRP for ankle cartilage pathology, since only one Level I trial is available and the surgical application, although particularly successful, relies in the majority of the cases on a combination of different factors.

Many "shadow lines" must be addressed: PRP cannot still be univocally defined and, up to now, there are too many different PRP formulations applied in clinical practice. The many inter-products differences previously discussed and related to preparation methods, cell content, activation and storage procedures, therapeutic protocols and others, reflect the complexity of this biological treatment and justify the difficulties in data comparison among studies and the inherent lack of clear indications about PRP therapy. Despite these limitations, this variability has stimulated a large interest of basic scientists and clinicians to explore what are the best characteristics of PRP to treat specific diseases, and many studies are ongoing to further improve this biological treatment approach. However, regardless of the golden aura around its therapeutic potential, until further studies will prove the real translational potential of the promising results suggested by preclinical *in vitro* and animal studies, thus optimizing its use and identifying the best indications in the clinical practice, PRP should be considered a second line treatment and applied in humans within well controlled studies.

Competing interests
The authors declare that they have no competing interests.

Authors' contributions
FV and BDM carried out the selection of the papers included in the present review. FV, BDM and GF were responsible for writing the paper. GF carried out the final editing of the paper. All authors read and approved the final manuscript.

Author details
[1]I Orthopaedic Clinic and Movement Analysis Laboratory, Rizzoli Orthopaedic Institute, Via di Barbiano n. 1/10, 40136 Bologna, Italy. [2]II Orthopaedic Clinic and Biomechanics Laboratory, Rizzoli Orthopaedic Institute, Via di Barbiano n. 1/10, 40136 Bologna, Italy.

References

1. Boswell SG, Cole BJ, Sundman EA, Karas V, Fortier LA (2012) Platelet-rich plasma: a milieu of bioactive factors. Arthroscopy 28(3):429–439
2. Kon E, Filardo G, Di Martino A, Marcacci M (2011) Platelet-rich plasma (PRP) to treat sports injuries: evidence to support its use. Knee Surg Sports Traumatol Arthrosc 19(4):516–527
3. Filardo G, Kon E, Roffi A, Di Matteo B, Merli ML, Marcacci M (2013). Platelet-rich plasma: why intra-articular? A systematic review of preclinical studies and clinical evidence on PRP for joint degeneration. Knee Surg Sports Traumatol Arthrosc. doi:10.1007/s00167-013-2743-1
4. Kon E, Filardo G, Di Matteo B, Marcacci M (2013) PRP for the treatment of cartilage pathology. Open Orthop J 3(7):120–128
5. Di Matteo B, Filardo G, Kon E, Marcacci M (2014). Platelet-rich plasma: evidence for the treatment of patellar and Achilles tendinopathy-a systematic review. Musculoskelet Surg. doi:10.1007/s12306-014-0340-1
6. Filardo G, Kon E, Di Matteo B, Pelotti P, Di Martino A, Marcacci M (2013) Platelet-rich plasma for the treatment of patellar tendinopathy: clinical and imaging findings at medium-term follow-up. Int Orthop 37(8):1583–1589
7. Filardo G, Presti ML, Kon E, Marcacci M (2010) Nonoperative biological treatment approach for partial Achilles tendon lesion. Orthopedics 33(2):120–123
8. Filardo G, Kon E, Di Matteo B, Di Martino A, Tesei G, Pelotti P, Cenacchi A, Marcacci M (2014) Platelet-rich plasma injections for the treatment of refractory Achilles tendinopathy: results at 4 years. Blood Transfus 12(4):533–540
9. Vannini F, Di Matteo B, Filardo G, Kon E, Marcacci M, Giannini S (2014) Platelet-rich plasma for foot and ankle pathologies: a systematic review. Foot Ankle Surg 20(1):2–9
10. Battaglia M, Guaraldi F, Vannini F, Rossi G, Timoncini A, Buda R, Giannini S (2013) Efficacy of ultrasound-guided intra-articular injections of platelet-rich plasma versus hyaluronic acid for hip osteoarthritis. Orthopedics 36(12):e1501–1508
11. Battaglia M, Guaraldi F, Vannini F, Buscio T, Buda R, Galletti S, Giannini S (2011) Platelet-rich plasma (PRP) intra-articular ultrasound-guided injections as a possible treatment for hip osteoarthritis: a pilot study. Clin Exp Rheumatol 29(4):754
12. Filardo G, Kon E, Di Martino A, Di Matteo B, Merli ML, Cenacchi A, Fornasari PM, Marcacci M (2012) Platelet-rich plasma vs hyaluronic acid to treat knee degenerative pathology: study design and preliminary results of a randomized controlled trial. BMC Musculoskelet Disord 23(13):229
13. Sánchez M, Fiz N, Azofra J, Usabiaga J, Aduriz Recalde E, Garcia Gutierrez A, Albillos J, Gárate R, Aguirre JJ, Padilla S, Orive G, Anitua E (2012) A randomized clinical trial evaluating plasma rich in growth factors (PRGF-Endoret) versus hyaluronic acid in the short-term treatment of symptomatic knee osteoarthritis. Arthroscopy 28(8):1070–1078
14. Cerza F, Carnì S, Carcangiu A, Di Vavo I, Schiavilla V, Pecora A, De Biasi G, Ciuffreda M (2012) Comparison between hyaluronic acid and platelet-rich plasma, intra-articular infiltration in the treatment of gonarthrosis. Am J Sports Med 40(12):2822–2827
15. Patel S, Dhillon MS, Aggarwal S, Marwaha N, Jain A (2013) Treatment with platelet-rich plasma is more effective than placebo for knee osteoarthritis: a prospective, double-blind, randomized trial. Am J Sports Med 41(2):356–364
16. Moher D, Liberati A, Tetzlaff J, Altman DG, The PRISMA Group (2009) Preferred reporting items for systematic reviews and meta-analyses: the PRISMA statement. Open Med 3(3):123–130
17. Mei-Dan O, Carmont MR, Laver L, Mann G, Maffulli N, Nyska M (2012) Platelet-rich plasma or hyaluronate in the management of osteochondral lesions of the talus. Am J Sports Med 40(3):534–541
18. Angthong C1, Khadsongkram A, Angthong W (2013) Outcomes and quality of life after platelet-rich plasma therapy in patients with recalcitrant hindfoot and ankle diseases: a preliminary report of 12 patients. J Foot Ankle Surg 52(4):475–480
19. Guney A, Akar M, Karaman I, Oner M, Guney B (2013). Clinical outcomes of platelet rich plasma (PRP) as an adjunct to microfracture surgery in osteochondral lesions of the talus. Knee Surg Sports Traumatol Arthrosc. doi:10.1007/s00167-013-2784-5
20. Giannini S, Buda R, Vannini F, Cavallo M, Grigolo B (2009) One-step bone marrow-derived cell transplantation in talar osteochondral lesions. Clin Orthop Relat Res 467(12):3307–3320
21. Giannini S, Buda R, Cavallo M, Ruffilli A, Cenacchi A, Cavallo C, Vannini F (2010) Cartilage repair evolution in post-traumatic osteochondral lesions of the talus: from open field autologous chondrocyte to bone-marrow-derived cells transplantation. Injury 41(11):1196–1203
22. Battaglia M, Rimondi E, Monti C, Guaraldi F, Sant'Andrea A, Buda R, Cavallo M, Giannini S, Vannini F (2011) Validity of T2 mapping in characterization of the regeneration tissue by bone marrow derived cell transplantation in osteochondral lesions of the ankle. Eur J Radiol 80(2):e132–139
23. Giannini S, Buda R, Battaglia M, Cavallo M, Ruffilli A, Ramponi L, Pagliazzi G, Vannini F (2013) One-step repair in talar osteochondral lesions: 4-year clinical results and t2-mapping capability in outcome prediction. Am J Sports Med 41(3):511–518
24. Hildner F, Eder MJ, Hofer K, Aberl J, Redl H, van Griensven M, Gabriel C, Peterbauer-Scherb A (2013). Human platelet lysate successfully promotes proliferation and subsequent chondrogenic differentiation of adipose-derived stem cells: a comparison with articular chondrocytes. J Tissue Eng Regen Med. doi:10.1002/term.1649
25. Muraglia A, Ottonello C, Spanò R, Dozin B, Strada P, Grandizio M, Cancedda R, Mastrogiacomo M (2013). Biological activity of a standardized freeze-dried platelet derivative to be used as cell culture medium supplement. Platelets. doi:10.3109/09537104.2013.803529
26. Park SI, Lee HR, Kim S, Ahn MW, Do SH (2012) Time-sequential modulation in expression of growth factors from platelet-rich plasma (PRP) on the chondrocyte cultures. Mol Cell Biochem 361(1–2):9–17
27. Lee HR, Park KM, Joung YK, Park KD, Do SH (2012) Platelet- rich plasma loaded hydrogel scaffold enhances chondrogenic differentiation and maturation with up-regulation of CB1 and CB2. J Control Release 159(3):332–337
28. Assirelli E, Filardo G, Mariani E, Kon E, Roffi A, Vaccaro F, Marcacci M, Facchini A, Pulsatelli L (2014). Effect of two different preparations of platelet-rich plasma on synoviocytes. Knee Surg Sports Traumatol Arthrosc. doi:10.1007/s00167-014-3113-3
29. Mifune Y, Matsumoto T, Takayama K, Ota S, Li H, MeszarosLB UA, Nagamune K, Gharaibeh B, Fu FH, Huard J (2013) The effect of platelet-rich plasma on the regenerative therapy of muscle derived stem cells for articular cartilage repair. Osteoarthritis Cartil 21(1):175–185
30. Moreira Teixeira LS, Leijten JC, Wennink JW, Chatterjea AG, Feijen J, van Blitterswijk CA, Dijkstra PJ, Karperien M (2012) The effect of platelet lysate supplementation of a dextran-based hydrogel on cartilage formation. Biomaterials 33(14):3651–3661
31. Guner S, Buyukbebeci O (2012). Analyzing the effects of platelet gel on knee osteoarthritis in the rat model. Clin Appl Thromb Hemost. doi:10.1177/1076029612452117
32. Kwon DR, Park GY, Lee SU (2012) The effects of intra-articular platelet-rich plasma injection according to the severity of collagenase-induced knee osteoarthritis in a rabbit model. Ann Rehabil Med 36(4):458–46
33. Saito M, Takahashi KA, Arai Y, Inoue A, Sakao K, Tonomura H, Honjo K, Nakagawa S, Inoue H, Tabata Y, Kubo T (2009) Intraarticular administration of platelet-rich plasma with biodegradable gelatin hydrogel microspheres prevents osteoarthritis progression in the rabbit knee. Clin Exp Rheumatol 27(2):201–207
34. Carmona JU, Arguelles D, Climent F, Prades M (2007) Autologous platelet concentrates as a treatment of horses with osteoarthritis: a preliminary pilot clinical study. J Equin Vet Sci 27(4):167–170

35. Milano G, Deriu L, Sanna Passino E, Masala G, Saccomanno MF, Postacchini R, Fabbriciani C (2011) The effect of autologous conditioned plasma on the treatment of focal chondral defects of the knee. An experimental study. Int J Immunopathol Pharmacol 24(1 Suppl 2):117–124
36. Serra CI, Soler C, Carillo JM, Sopena JJ, Redondo JI, Cugat R (2013) Effect of autologous platelet-rich plasma on the repair of full-thickness articular defects in rabbits. Knee Surg Sports Traumatol Arthrosc 21(8):1730–1736
37. Lippross S, Moeller B, Haas H, Tohidnezhad M, Steubesand N, Wruck CJ, Kurz B, Seekamp A, Pufe T, Varoga D (2011) Intraarticular injection of platelet-rich plasma reduces inflammation in a pig model of rheumatoid arthritis of the knee joint. Arthritis Rheum 63(11):3344–3353
38. Tschon M, Fini M, Giardino R, Filardo G, Dallari D, Torricelli P, Martini L, Giavaresi G, Kon E, Maltarello MC, Nicolini A, Carpi A (2011) Lights and shadows concerning platelet products for musculoskeletal regeneration. Front Biosci (Elite Ed) 1(3):96–107
39. Torricelli P, Fini M, Filardo G, Tschon M, Pischedda M, Pacorini A, Kon E, Giardino R (2011) Regenerative medicine for the treatment of musculoskeletal overuse injuries in competition horses. Int Orthop 35(10):1569–1576
40. Mariani E, Filardo G, Canella V, Berlingeri A, Bielli A, Cattini L, Landini MP, Kon E, Marcacci M, Facchini A (2014) Platelet-rich plasma affects bacterial growth in vitro. Cytotherapy 16(9):1294–1304
41. Cavallo C, Filardo G, Mariani E, Kon E, Marcacci M, Pereira Ruiz MT, Facchini A, Grigolo B (2014). Comparison of platelet-rich plasma formulations for cartilage healing: an in vitro study. J Bone Joint Surg Am. 5;96 (5):423–429.
42. Filardo G, Kon E, Pereira Ruiz MT, Vaccaro F, Guitaldi R, Di Martino A, Cenacchi A, Fornasari PM, Marcacci M (2012) Platelet-rich plasma intra-articular injections for cartilage degeneration and osteoarthritis: single- versus double-spinning approach. Knee Surg Sports Traumatol Arthrosc 20(10):2082–2091
43. Dohan Ehrenfest DM, Bielecki T, Jimbo R, Barbé G, Del Corso M, Inchingolo F, Sammartino G (2012) Do the fibrin architecture and leukocyte content influence the growth factor release of platelet concentrates? An evidence-based answer comparing a pure platelet-rich plasma (P-PRP) gel and a leukocyte- and platelet-rich fibrin (L-PRF). Curr Pharm Biotechnol 13(7):1145–1152
44. Roffi A, Filardo G, Assirelli E, Cavallo C, Cenacchi A, Facchini A, Grigolo B, Kon E, Mariani E, Pratelli L, Pulsatelli L, Marcacci M (2014). Does platelet-rich plasma freeze-thawing influence growth factor release and their effects on chondrocytes and synoviocytes? Biomed Res Int. doi:10.1155/2014/692913

In vivo retention and bioactivity of IL-1ra microspheres in the rat intervertebral disc: a preliminary investigation

Deborah J Gorth[1,2,3], John T Martin[2,3], George R Dodge[2,3], Dawn M Elliott[4], Neil R Malhotra[1,2], Robert L Mauck[2,3] and Lachlan J Smith[1,2,3*]

Abstract

Background: Inflammatory cytokines such as interleukin-1 beta (IL-1β) contribute to the progression of intervertebral disc degeneration. Previously we demonstrated, *in vitro*, that by delivering interleukin-1 receptor antagonist (IL-1ra) from poly(lactic co-glycolic acid) (PLGA) microspheres, we could attenuate the degradative effects of IL-1β on the nucleus pulposus (NP) for up to 20 days. The objective of this study was to undertake a preliminary investigation into whether microspheres could be successfully delivered to and retained in the disc *in vivo*, and whether IL-1ra released from those microspheres remained biologically active. For retention studies, fluorescently-labeled microspheres were delivered to the NPs of rat caudal discs. Rats were sacrificed at time points up to 56 days, and microspheres were localized using fluorescent microscopy. To investigate whether IL-1ra microspheres could effectively inhibit the effects of IL-1β *in vivo*, four disc levels were allocated to the following treatment groups: intact; saline; IL-1β; or IL-1β + IL-1ra microspheres. Rats were sacrificed after seven days and NP glycosaminoglycan content was measured.

Findings: Microspheres were visible in the disc at all time points up to 28 days, and localized to the NP, the annulus fibrosus (AF), or both. Glycosaminoglycan content for discs injected with IL-1β alone was significantly lower than for intact controls. For discs injected with IL-1β along with IL-1ra microspheres, glycosaminoglycan content was not significantly different from intact controls.

Conclusions: Microspheres can successfully be delivered to the disc *in vivo* and retained for a clinically relevant time frame. IL-1ra released from microspheres can effectively prevent IL-1β-induced NP glycosaminoglycan loss *in vivo*.

Keywords: Intervertebral disc degeneration; Inflammation; Interleukin-1 receptor antagonist; PLGA microspheres; Rat; *In vivo*

Introduction

Intervertebral disc degeneration is a cascade beginning with changes to the local cellular microenvironment and progressing over years to structural breakdown and functional impairment [1,2]. Changes to the central nucleus pulposus (NP) are implicated in the early stages of disc degeneration, where decreasing proteoglycan content and an associated reduction in hydrostatic pressure impair the ability of the disc to evenly distribute and transfer compressive loads between the vertebrae [3]. Inflammation plays a key role in the progression of disc degeneration. Interleukin-1 beta (IL-1β), in particular, is more highly expressed in the degenerate NP than in the healthy NP [4]. Elevated IL-1β induces catabolic protease activity, which degrades the disc extracellular matrix and contributes to structural failure [5]. Interleukin-1 receptor antagonist (IL-1ra) is an endogenous inhibitor of IL-1β, where it acts by competitively blocking the binding of IL-1β to receptors on IL-1 responsive cells [6]. While IL-1β is upregulated with disc degeneration, there is no concomitant upregulation of IL-1ra [4],

* Correspondence: lachlans@mail.med.upenn.edu
[1]Department of Neurosurgery, Perelman School of Medicine, University of Pennsylvania, 424 Stemmler Hall, 3450 Hamilton Walk, Philadelphia, PA 19104, USA
[2]Department of Orthopaedic Surgery, Perelman School of Medicine, University of Pennsylvania, 424 Stemmler Hall, 3450 Hamilton Walk, Philadelphia, PA 19104, USA
Full list of author information is available at the end of the article

resulting in an imbalance between catabolic and anabolic signaling. In our previous *in vitro* work, we demonstrated that soluble IL-1ra effectively inhibited the degradative effects of IL-1β on NP cells [7]. Further, by delivering IL-1ra from poly(lactic-co-glycolic acid) (PLGA) microspheres, inhibition could be maintained for up to 20 days [8]. Key advantages of PLGA microspheres for drug delivery include that they are biodegradable and biocompatible, already FDA approved for other clinical indications, and most importantly, can be easily tuned to alter degradation and protein release kinetics [9,10].

The objective of this study was to advance this encouraging *in vitro* work to towards clinical translation, by undertaking a preliminary *in vivo* study to demonstrate, firstly, that PLGA microspheres could be delivered to the disc and retained for a clinically relevant time frame *in vivo*; and, secondly, that IL-1ra delivered from these microspheres maintained bioactivity in the *in vivo* space.

Materials and methods

Microsphere fabrication

PLGA microspheres were fabricated as described previously, using the water/oil/water double emulsion technique [8,9]. As in our previous work, we used the pharmaceutical form of IL-1ra, anakinra (Amgen, Thousand Oaks, CA). The initial water/oil emulsion was formed by combining 225μL of IL-1ra (0.15 g/ml) with 1 ml of 75:25 PLGA (0.1 g/ml) (Durect Corporation, Pelham, AL). For fluorescent microsphere studies, the PLGA was supplemented with 3 mg/ml coumarin-6 (Sigma Aldrich; $\lambda_{emission}$ =505 nm; $\lambda_{absorption}$ =444 nm), and saline was substituted for IL-1ra. Fabricated microspheres were lyophilized until required for surgeries, and sterilized via exposure to ultraviolet light for 10 min prior to injection. The release profile of IL-1ra from these microspheres was described previously, and is characterized by an initial burst release, decreasing to an approximately linear and sustained release over the initial 10 days. *In vitro*, bioactive IL-1ra continues to be released for up to 20 days [8].

In vivo microsphere retention study

The Animal Studies Subcommittee of the Philadelphia VA Medical Center approved all animal studies. We first performed a study to confirm that microspheres could be successfully delivered to the rat caudal intervertebral disc, and retained for a clinically relevant time period. Six, male, retired breeder, Sprague-Dawley rats aged 8 months were anesthetized via isoflurane inhalation. Caudal disc levels for injection (C7-8, C8-9 and C9-10) were identified fluoroscopically (Orthoscan HD; Orthoscan, Scottsdale, USA) by counting spine levels caudally from the sacrum. Each disc was exposed via a 5 mm dorsal incision through the skin. Under fluoroscopic guidance, fluorescent microspheres (20 mg/ml in sterile saline, total volume 1.5 μl) were injected into the NP of each of the three disc levels using custom 33-gauge needles designed to restrict the depth of needle insertion to 2.5mm (Figures 1A and B). Each injection was performed carefully over the course of 2-3 s. Animals were euthanized via carbon dioxide inhalation at each of 6 time points post-surgery: 1, 3, 7, 14, 28 and 56 days. Following euthanasia, spine segments containing injected discs were isolated from the tail by bisecting the adjacent vertebral bodies. These segments were snap frozen and sectioned (undecalcified) progressively through the vertebral bone on a cryostat microtome in the transverse plane until the disc was exposed. Sections 20 μm thick were then obtained through the entire thickness of the disc, and captured on glass microscope slides. Sections were immediately imaged on a fluorescence microscope (Eclipse 90i; Nikon, Tokyo, Japan) to determine the presence or absence of microspheres, and their location in the disc (NP or annulus fibrosus (AF)) by overlaying fluorescence images on differential interference contrast (DIC) images of the same region.

In vivo bioactivity study

Next, we performed a study to confirm the *in vivo* bioactivity of IL-1ra microspheres delivered to the rat NP. Four caudal disc levels per animal were utilized (C7-8, C8-9, C9-10 and C10-11), and randomly allocated to one of four study groups: intact (non-injected) controls; sham (vehicle only) injection; IL-1β injection; or IL-1β + IL-1ra microspheres (20 mg/ml) injection. The study was performed for each of two IL-1β doses: 100 ng and 500 ng (each n = 4 animals). All injection volumes were 1.5 μl with sterile saline as the vehicle, delivered using modified 33-gauge needles. Surgeries were performed as described above. All animals were euthanized 7 days post-surgery. Following euthanasia, spine segments containing injected or control discs were isolated, and NP regions analyzed for GAG content. To overcome the challenges associated with accurate determination of GAG content in very small tissue specimens, we developed a dissection technique to accurately isolate NP samples of known volume. Spine segments were snap frozen and mounted in a cryostat microtome. Sections of vertebral bone were progressively removed until the transverse face of the disc was exposed. Four 100 μm-thick sections of disc were then cut and transferred, frozen, to a glass microscope slide. A 1 mm biopsy punch was then used to isolate the NP from the AF. Isolated NP samples were then digested in papain and assayed to determine total sulfated GAG content (expressed as absolute GAG per sample) using the dimethylmethylene blue technique [11]. Differences in GAG content between groups were established using ANOVAs followed by post-hoc, pairwise Tukey's tests. Results were expressed as mean ± standard deviation, with significance defined as $p < 0.05$.

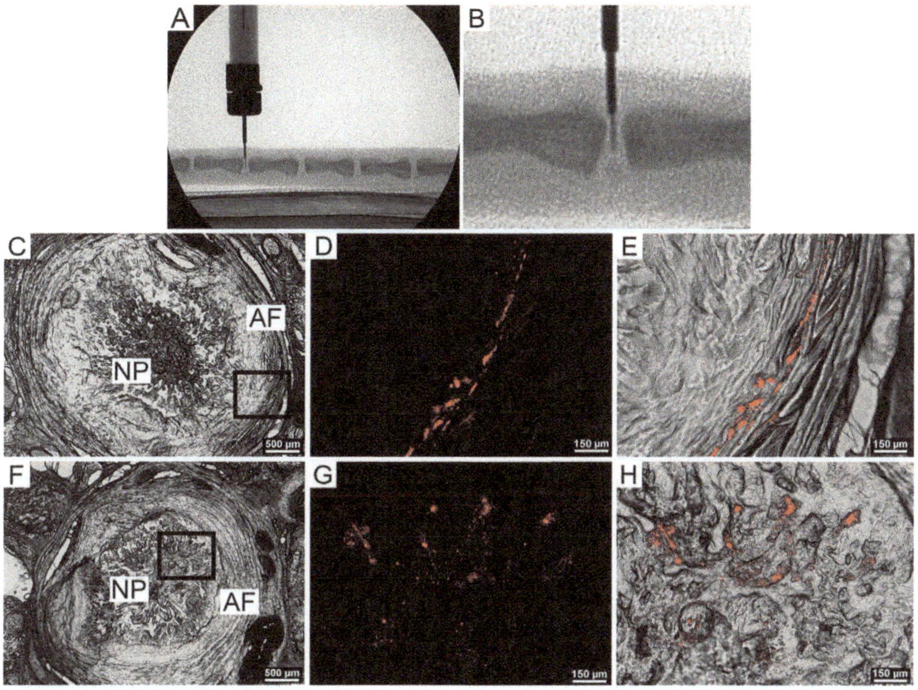

Figure 1 ***In vivo*** **delivery and localization microspheres. A**. Delivery of microspheres to the rat NP from a custom 33-gauge needle under fluoroscopic guidance (lateral aspect). **B**. Higher magnification view of A. **C**. Differential interference contrast (DIC), axial image of entire disc 1 day post injection, showing NP and AF regions. **D**. Higher magnification view of the AF (inset from C.) showing microspheres (red). **E**. Microspheres (red, overlaying DIC image) embedded in the inner lamellae of the AF. **F**. Differential interference contrast, axial image of entire disc 14 days post injection, showing NP and AF regions. **G**. Higher magnification view (inset from F.) showing microspheres (red). **H**. Microspheres (red, overlaying DIC image), embedded in the NP.

Findings

In vivo retention of microspheres

To determine whether microspheres could be successfully delivered to the rat disc and retained for a clinically relevant time frame, fluorescent microspheres were injected into rat caudal discs, and their presence or absence and localization (AF or NP) investigated at six post-surgical timepoints up to 8 weeks. Fluorescence microscopy confirmed the presence of microspheres in all discs and at all time points up to 28 days post-surgery. In discs where microspheres were present, their localization varied between the AF only (63% of discs, Figures 1C-E), the NP only (13% of discs, Figures 1F-H), or both the NP and the AF (25% of discs). There was no apparent association between time point and location of microspheres in the disc. Cryostat sections were also examined for evidence of microsphere leakage along the injection track, but no such leakage was observed.

In vivo bioactivity of IL-1ra microspheres

To confirm that the bioactivity of IL-1ra released from microspheres was maintained following *in vivo* delivery, we investigated the efficacy of IL-1ra microspheres in mitigating GAG loss induced by injection of exogenous IL-1β into rat caudal discs. No statistically significant effect of IL-1β dosage (100 ng or 500 ng) on GAG content was found, so results for both dosages were pooled for subsequent analyses. IL-1β injection alone (Figure 2), resulted in a significantly lower NP GAG content compared to intact controls (65% of intact, $p < 0.05$). For the combined IL-1β and IL-1ra microspheres injection, NP GAG content was maintained, and not significantly different from intact controls (102% of intact, $p > 0.05$). For the saline sham injection, NP GAG content was lower

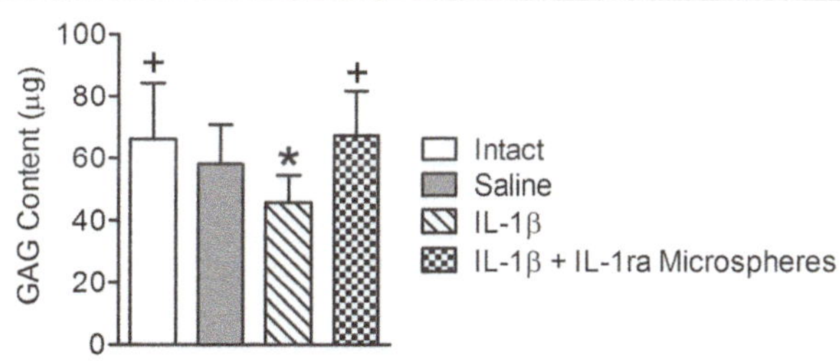

Figure 2 ***In vivo*** **bioactivity of microspheres.** IL-1β injection alone resulted in a significantly lower NP GAG content compared to intact controls. For the combined IL-1β and IL-1ra microspheres injection, NP GAG content was not significantly different from intact controls. For the saline sham injection, NP GAG content was lower than intact controls, but not significantly, and not significantly different from IL-1β alone or combined IL-1β and IL-1ra microspheres. *$p < 0.05$ vs. intact controls; +$p < 0.05$ vs. IL-1β alone.

(87%) than intact, but not significantly, and not significantly different from IL-1β alone or combined IL-1β and IL-1ra microspheres.

Discussion and conclusions

IL-1ra has successfully been used clinically for the treatment of rheumatoid arthritis for a number of years [12], and has recently been investigated as a potential treatment for osteoarthritis [13]. In previous work we demonstrated that soluble IL-1ra can effectively inhibit the degradative effects of IL-1β on the NP at the mechanical, compositional and molecular levels [7]. Another study showed that IL-1ra delivered both directly in solution and by gene therapy inhibited mRNA expression and activity of catabolic enzymes upregulated by IL-1β in disc tissue explants [14]. Further, IL-1ra knockout mice exhibit degenerative changes consistent with human disc degeneration [15].

The avascular nature of the disc, along with the short half-life and required high therapeutic concentrations of IL-1ra [16], suggest that *in vivo*, systemic delivery for treatment of disc degeneration is unlikely to be successful. Repeated intradiscal injections of IL-1ra that would be necessary to sustain high local concentrations, are impractical and may induce further degenerative changes via structural damage to the AF resulting from repetitive delivery. Therefore, to enhance the therapeutic efficacy of IL-1ra for treating disc degeneration, we developed a sustained release delivery vehicle for IL-1ra. Using biodegradable PLGA microspheres, we demonstrated previously that, *in vitro*, we could inhibit the degradative effects of IL-1β on the NP for up to 20 days. Building on these results, in this study we demonstrated that PLGA microspheres can be delivered to the disc *in vivo* and be retained for up to 28 days. Importantly, retention time in the disc (analogous to the time it takes for microspheres to fully degrade), is longer than the time period over which microspheres continue to release active IL-1ra at therapeutic concentrations [8]. In our microsphere retention study, variability was apparent with respect to the location of microspheres in the disc (NP, AF or both). One possible explanation for this is that, with time, microspheres diffuse away from the NP towards the AF where they are caught in the dense, fibrocartilaginous lamellae. However, as there was no apparent association between time point and location of microspheres in the disc, a more likely explanation may have been minor inconsistencies in injection location. We hypothesize that active IL-1ra released from microspheres is likely to diffuse throughout the entire disc structure, irrespective of the location of microspheres. The results of the *in vivo* bioactivity study reported here support this contention: IL-1ra microspheres successfully inhibited NP GAG loss induced by IL-1β.

This study represents a preliminary investigation into the *in vivo* efficacy of using anti-inflammatory microspheres in the intervertebral disc, and is not without limitations. Additional study groups should be investigated as part of future work, such as injection of blank (non-IL-1ra loaded) microspheres, specifically to determine if acidic microsphere degradation products exert any inflammatory effect. Clearance of these degradation products must occur via passive diffusion to vasculature outside the NP. Our previous *in vitro* work suggests that any such effects are likely quite mild [8]. Future studies should also confirm that these microspheres are active for long periods *in vivo*, in the presence of chronic inflammation, and are more effective under such circumstances than a single, bolus injection of IL-1ra. The small sample size was an addition limitation of this study, although it was sufficient to detect significant changes in GAG content.

Attenuation of inflammation in the degenerate disc is only one component of a potential biological therapy for disc degeneration. A stem cell-based component may be required to potentiate tissue regeneration. In addition to preventing further degenerative changes, IL-1ra microspheres may foster a microenvironment that is anti-inflammatory and more conducive to stem cell survival, differentiation and biosynthesis [17]. Pursuant to the encouraging findings reported here, we are now designing combined anti-inflammatory and stem cell-based therapeutics for disc regeneration and evaluating their efficacy in large animal models.

Ethics board approval

This work was conducted with the approval of the Animal Ethics Subcommittee of the Philadelphia VA Medical Center, project number 01251.

Competing interests

The authors declare that they have no competing interests.

Authors' contributions

LJS contributed to study conception and design, drafted the manuscript and contributed to data analysis and interpretation; DJG contributed to study conception and design performed microsphere fabrication and characterization, biochemical assays and histology, assisted with surgeries, and critically revised the manuscript for important intellectual content; JTM contributed to study conception and design, performed surgeries, and critically revised the manuscript for important intellectual content; DME, NRM, RLM and GRD contributed to study conception and design, and critically revised the manuscript for important intellectual content. All authors approved the final manuscript prior to submission.

Acknowledgements

This study was funded by a Department of Veterans Affairs Merit Grant (I01RX000211) and supported by the Penn Center for Musculoskeletal Disorders.

Author details

[1]Department of Neurosurgery, Perelman School of Medicine, University of Pennsylvania, 424 Stemmler Hall, 3450 Hamilton Walk, Philadelphia, PA 19104, USA. [2]Department of Orthopaedic Surgery, Perelman School of Medicine, University of Pennsylvania, 424 Stemmler Hall, 3450 Hamilton Walk, Philadelphia, PA 19104, USA. [3]Translational Musculoskeletal Research Center,

Veterans Affairs Medical Center, 3900 Woodland Avenue, Philadelphia, PA 19104, USA. [4]Department of Biomedical Engineering, College of Engineering, University of Delaware, 125 E. Delaware Ave, Newark, DE 19716, USA.

References

1. Freemont AJ (2009) The cellular pathobiology of the degenerate intervertebral disc and discogenic back pain. Rheumatology 48(1):5–10
2. Smith LJ, Nerurkar NL, Choi KS, Harfe BD, Elliott DM (2011) Degeneration and regeneration of the intervertebral disc: lessons from development. Dis Model Mech 4(1):31–41
3. Adams MA, McNally DS, Dolan P (1996) 'Stress' distributions inside intervertebral discs. The effects of age and degeneration. J Bone Joint Surg (Br) 78(6):965–972
4. Le Maitre CL, Freemont AJ, Hoyland JA (2005) The role of interleukin-1 in the pathogenesis of human intervertebral disc degeneration. Arthritis Res Ther 7(4):R732–745
5. Le Maitre CL, Pockert A, Buttle DJ, Freemont AJ, Hoyland JA (2007) Matrix synthesis and degradation in human intervertebral disc degeneration. Biochem Soc Trans 35(Pt 4):652–655
6. Arend WP (1991) Interleukin 1 receptor antagonist. A new member of the interleukin 1 family. J Clin Invest 88(5):1445–1451
7. Smith LJ, Chiaro JA, Nerurkar NL, Cortes DH, Horava SD, Hebela NM, Mauck RL, Dodge GR, Elliott DM (2011) Nucleus pulposus cells synthesize a functional extracellular matrix and respond to inflammatory cytokine treatment following long term agarose culture. Eur Cells Mater 20(22):291–301
8. Gorth DJ, Mauck RL, Chiaro JA, Mohanraj B, Hebela NM, Dodge GR, Elliott DM, Smith LJ (2012) IL-1ra delivered from poly(lactic-co-glycolic acid) microspheres attenuates IL-1beta-mediated degradation of nucleus pulposus in vitro. Arthritis Res Ther 14(4):R179
9. Cohen S, Yoshioka T, Lucarelli M, Hwang LH, Langer R (1991) Controlled delivery systems for proteins based on poly(lactic/glycolic acid) microspheres. Pharm Res 8(6):713–720
10. Pisal DS, Kosloski MP, Balu-Iyer SV (2010) Delivery of therapeutic proteins. J Pharm Sci 99(6):2557–2575
11. Farndale RW, Buttle DJ, Barrett AJ (1986) Improved quantitation and discrimination of sulphated glycosaminoglycans by use of dimethylmethylene blue. Biochim Biophys Acta 883(2):173–177
12. Mertens M, Singh JA (2009) Anakinra for rheumatoid arthritis: a systematic review. J Rheumatol 36(6):1118–1125
13. Chevalier X, Goupille P, Beaulieu AD, Burch FX, Bensen WG, Conrozier T, Loeuille D, Kivitz AJ, Silver D, Appleton BE (2009) Intraarticular injection of anakinra in osteoarthritis of the knee: a multicenter, randomized, double-blind, placebo-controlled study. Arthritis Rheum 61(3):344–352
14. Le Maitre CL, Hoyland JA, Freemont AJ (2007) Interleukin-1 receptor antagonist delivered directly and by gene therapy inhibits matrix degradation in the intact degenerate human intervertebral disc: an in situ zymographic and gene therapy study. Arthritis Res Ther 9(4):R83
15. Phillips KL, Jordan-Mahy N, Nicklin MJ, Le Maitre CL (2013) Interleukin-1 receptor antagonist deficient mice provide insights into pathogenesis of human intervertebral disc degeneration. Ann Rheum Dis 72(11):1860–1867
16. Amgen (2009) Prescribing Information: Kineret (Anakinra). Thousand Oaks, CA,
17. Felka T, Schafer R, Schewe B, Benz K, Aicher WK (2009) Hypoxia reduces the inhibitory effect of IL-1beta on chondrogenic differentiation of FCS-free expanded MSC. Osteoarthritis Cartilage 17(10):1368–1376

9

The amplitude of pulse-synchronous oscillations varies with the level of intramuscular pressure in simulated compartment syndrome

Andreas Nilsson[1*], Qiuxia Zhang[1,2] and Jorma Styf[1,2]

Abstract

Background: Patients with compartment syndromes have elevated intramuscular pressure (IMP) due to increased volume in the affected muscle. However, the accuracy of IMP as a parameter in diagnosing chronic compartment syndrome has been questioned. It has been observed that arterial pulsations create oscillations in the IMP in patients with abnormally elevated IMP. The amplitude of the IMP oscillations appears to be related to a pathogenic mechanism of elevated IMP. Therefore, the purpose of the present study was to investigate the relation between the amplitude of pulse-synchronous IMP oscillations and the absolute level of IMP with a high-end fiber-optic system in a human experimental model of abnormally elevated IMP (simulated compartment syndrome) of the leg. The hypothesis that the amplitude of the IMP oscillations is correlated to the absolute level of IMP was tested.

Methods: IMP was measured at rest in the anterior tibial muscle in 12 legs of 7 healthy subjects (4 females and 3 males) with a mean age of 28 (range 23–38) years. The subject lay supine with his/her heel placed in a footrest. The foot was kept in a neutral position to avoid biased IMP readings. Measurements were performed at baseline and during 10 minutes with a model of abnormally elevated IMP (simulated compartment syndrome) applied. The abnormally elevated IMP was created by venous obstruction induced by a thigh tourniquet (65 mmHg) of a casted leg. Placement of the pressure-recording catheter was verified by sonography.

Results: The IMP increased from 4.7 (SD = 1.8) mmHg at baseline to 48.6 (SD = 7.1) mmHg when the model of elevated IMP was applied. The amplitude of the pulse-synchronous oscillations was undetectable at baseline. It increased to 3.9 (SD = 1.4) mmHg with increasing IMP when the model was applied. The amplitude of the oscillations showed a positive correlation ($r = 0.59$) with the absolute level of IMP.

Conclusions: The amplitude of the pulse-synchronous IMP oscillations is correlated with the absolute level of IMP during abnormally elevated IMP. The oscillations of IMP may therefore be an additional parameter assuring the abnormally elevated IMP in the diagnosis of compartment syndromes.

Keywords: Intramuscular pressure; Pulse-synchronous oscillations in intracompartmental pressure; Compartment syndrome; Intramuscular arterial pulsations; Fiber-optic technique

* Correspondence: andreas.nilsson@orthop.gu.se
[1]Department of Orthopaedics, Institute of Clinical Sciences, Sahlgrenska Academy, University of Gothenburg, Sahlgrenska University Hospital, Guldhedsgatan 10 A, 413 46 Gothenburg, Sweden
Full list of author information is available at the end of the article

Background

Intramuscular pressure (IMP) is often regarded as the gold standard in the diagnosis of compartment syndromes (Matsen et al. 1976; Hargens et al. 1977; Hargens et al. 1989), since clinical findings without the support of IMP measurements have low sensitivity (Balduini et al. 1993). IMP measurements may be acquired at rest before, during, and at rest after exercise (Styf and Körner 1987). However, several IMP criteria have been suggested and the validity and the evidence for the commonly used pressure criteria in diagnosing chronic compartment syndrome have recently been under question (Tiidus 2014; Aweid et al. 2012; Franklyn-Miller et al. 2012).

Patients with compartment syndrome have an elevated IMP due to increased volume in the affected muscle (Eliassen et al. 1974; Styf and Körner 1987). The volume load reduces the compliance of the compartment. Reduced compliance implies that a small increase in volume in the muscle causes a large increase in IMP. Arterial pulsations create oscillations in the IMP in patients with decreased compliance and abnormally elevated IMP (Styf and Körner 1986). The amplitude of the IMP oscillations appears to be related to a pathogenic mechanism of elevated IMP and it varies with the arterial pulsations and the change in the compliance of the compartment (Styf 1995; Garabekyan et al. 2009; Lynch et al. 2009, Nilsson et al., 2014). The mean amplitude of the IMP oscillations has been reported to be approximately 5 mmHg in patients with chronic anterior compartment syndrome and less than 1 mmHg in patients without chronic anterior compartment syndrome at rest after an exercise test (Styf and Korner 1986). There are, however, no reports establishing the potential relationship between the amplitude of the oscillations and the absolute level of IMP. Therefore, the purpose of the present study was to investigate the amplitude of pulse-synchronous IMP oscillations relation to the absolute IMP with a high-end fiber-optic pressure measurement system in an experimental model of elevated IMP (simulated compartment syndrome) in the human leg. The hypothesis that the amplitude of the IMP oscillations is correlated to the absolute level of IMP was tested.

Methods

Subjects

Seven healthy subjects (four females and three males) with a mean age of 28 (range 23–38) years and a mean body mass index (BMI) of 23 (range 20–26) kg/m^2 volunteered to participate in the study. The study was performed on 12 legs of these subjects. All the subjects gave their informed written consent prior to participation. The study protocol was approved by the regional Research Ethics Committee.

IMP recordings

IMP was recorded for 5 minutes for baseline data, 10 minutes during a model of abnormally elevated IMP (simulated compartment syndrome), followed by 5 minutes of recovery after the model was removed. The subject lay supine with his/her heel placed in a padded footrest. The function of the footrest was to keep the leg at heart level and to ensure that no external compression from the bed was applied to the calf. The heart level was defined as 5 cm below the manubrium sterni. The foot was kept in a relaxed neutral position to avoid effects on the IMP (Weiner et al. 1994). Measurements were made in both legs in five subjects but on different occasions. In two subjects, measurements were only made in one leg.

IMP measurement systems

A fiber-optic pressure transducer with a diameter of 0.42 mm and an estimated volume of 0.072 mm^3 (Samba 420 LP, Samba Sensors AB, Göteborg, Sweden) was used for the IMP measurement. The sensing area is placed at the distal end of the fiber and is forward sensing. The transducer was connected to a Samba 3200 control unit (Samba Sensors AB, Göteborg, Sweden) set to measure relative pressure in mmHg. The transducer was calibrated at room temperature before insertion. The Samba control unit was connected to a computer (PC) equipped with data acquisition hardware from National Instruments (National Instruments, Austin, TX, USA) and custom-made LabView based software. All units were turned on at least 30 minutes before the start of IMP measurements to minimize internal temperature drift. Data were collected at 20 Hz. In addition, a Stryker Intra-Compartmental Pressure Monitor was used with a 1.3 × 60 mm disposable needle with a sideport and interconnected with tubing. The 20 cm long tubing and a 3 ml syringe were prefilled with room-tempered saline. During measurements, the transducer of the monitor was kept at the same level as the tip of the needle to avoid hydrostatic offset. The IMP values from the Stryker system were used as a reference and were not analyzed further.

Model of abnormally elevated IMP (simulated compartment syndrome)

The IMP was abnormally elevated by venous obstruction induced by a thigh tourniquet on a casted leg. The plaster cast was applied over two layers of cotton padding extending from slightly below the knee joint to the distal part of the leg. The proximal part of the plaster was modified to make sufficient room for two catheters used for IMP measurements. A 145 mm wide pneumatic tourniquet was placed around the thigh and inflated to 65 mmHg to obstruct venous return from the leg.

This method of elevating IMP has previously been evaluated in healthy subjects (Styf and Wiger 1998) and used to simulate compartment syndromes in the human leg (Zhang et al. 2001; Wiger and Styf 1998; Wiger et al. 2000; Styf and Wiger 1998). The model elevated IMP to levels that are seen in patients with compartment syndromes and elicited sensory dysfunction, muscle weakness, a mild throbbing pain and oscillations of the IMP (Styf and Wiger 1998). In this study, the model was applied for only 10 minutes to elevate the IMP without provoking any additional symptoms associated with compartment syndromes.

Measurement catheter insertion

A local anesthetic (1–2 ml of xylocain 10 mg/ml with epinephrine, 5 μg/ml) was injected subcutaneously approximately 7 cm below the knee joint and 2 cm lateral to the tibial tuberosity of the test leg. Under sterile conditions, a Venflon introducer (1.3 × 45 mm) was inserted through the skin into the anterior tibial muscle fascia in a distal direction at an angle of 30 degrees from the plane of the skin, while the subject kept his/her ankle joint dorsiflexed. The tip of the needle was then retracted into the sheath of the introducer and the set was bluntly advanced parallel to the muscle fibers in the relaxed muscle with the foot in a neutral position. The angle of insertion was kept as parallel to the muscle fibers as possible to reduce pain, trauma to the muscle and local edema that may affect pressure measurements (Styf 1989). The needle was then removed and the optic fiber was inserted 45 mm into the Venflon tubing. The sensor element of the optic fiber was thereby positioned at the end of the tubing. A Luer lock Tuohy Borst Adapter with a gasket ensured sealing and fixation of the optic fiber. The Stryker needle was inserted using the same procedure but 10 mm lateral or medial (every other time) and parallel to the optic fiber. Since IMP varies with depth (Nakhostine, 1993), both transducers were introduced to the same depth. The depth of the catheter tip and the angle between the catheter and the overlying fascia were measured by sonography (Acuson CV-70, Siemens Medical Solutions USA, Inc., CA, USA).

Blood pressure and pulse rate

Blood pressure and pulse rate were measured repeatedly with a non-invasive blood pressure manometer (NAIS, Matsushita, Electronic Works, Japan) in the left arm. Mean arterial pressure (MAP) was calculated by adding one third of the pulse pressure to the diastolic blood pressure. Local perfusion pressure was calculated as MAP minus IMP.

Statistical method

Wilcoxon signed rank test was used for comparisons and significance was set at $p < 0.05$. Correlations are given with Pearson's r. Unless otherwise stated, all results are given as the mean and standard deviation (SD).

Results

The IMP at baseline was 4.7 (SD = 1.8) mmHg and no oscillations that were synchronous with the arterial pulse could be detected. When the plaster cast was applied, the IMP increased to 15 mmHg and when the tourniquet was inflated to 65 mmHg, the IMP increased to over 40 mmHg within two minutes. The peak-to-peak amplitude of the IMP oscillations was analyzed for IMP values between 20 and 40 mmHg (Figure 1). The amplitude of the oscillations showed a positive correlation ($r = 0.59$, $p < 0.01$) to the level of the IMP. After 10 minutes with the model of abnormally elevated IMP (simulated compartment syndrome) applied, the IMP was 48.6 (SD = 7.1) mmHg and the amplitude of the IMP oscillations was 3.9 (SD = 1.4) mmHg (Figure 2). During recovery, the IMP returned to baseline and the amplitude was no longer detectable.

The local perfusion pressure decreased to 33 mmHg (44% of the baseline value) during the model of abnormally elevated IMP ($p < 0.01$), while the mean arterial pressure and pulse rate were essentially unchanged throughout the experiment ($p > 0.05$) (Table 1).

The distance between the muscle fascia and the tip of the fiber-optic catheter was 6.6 (SD = 1.7) mm and the pennation angle was 9.4 (SD = 2.4) degrees.

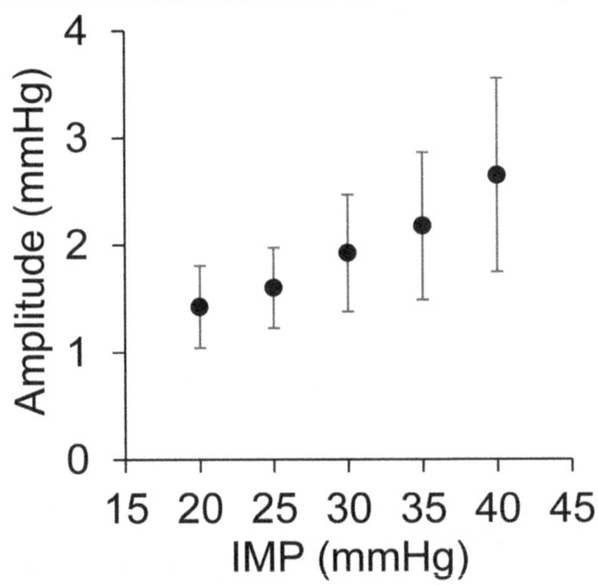

Figure 1 The amplitude of the pulse-synchronous oscillations. The mean amplitude of the pulse-synchronous oscillations increased with the absolute level of the intramuscular pressure (IMP) when the model of abnormally elevated IMP (simulated compartment syndrome) was applied. Error bars = standard deviation.

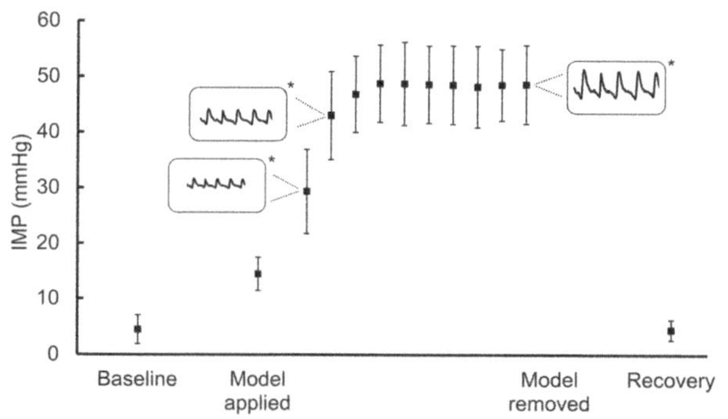

Figure 2 Intramuscular pressure during a model of simulated compartment syndrome. Mean intramuscular pressure (IMP) and standard deviation during a model of abnormally elevated IMP that was induced by venous obstruction of a casted leg. Oscillations in the IMP are schematically visualized (*). The peak-to-peak amplitude of the oscillations increased as a function of the IMP.

Discussion

Our study shows that the amplitude of the pulse-synchronous IMP oscillations is associated with the absolute level of IMP during abnormally elevated IMP. No pulse-synchronous IMP oscillations were detected at baseline or during recovery (normal IMP).

The amplitude of the IMP oscillations has been reported to decrease significantly from 4.9 (SD = 2.7) mmHg before surgery to 1.0 (SD = 0.6) mmHg following fasciotomy in patients with chronic anterior compartment syndrome (Styf and Korner 1986). The amplitude has been reported to be 5.8 (SD = 2.7) in patients with chronic anterior compartment syndrome and less than 1 mmHg or not detectable in patients without chronic anterior compartment syndrome (Styf and Körner 1987). The recorded amplitudes in the present study are in line with the above-mentioned studies on abnormally elevated IMP. The positive correlation between the amplitude and the absolute IMP level found in the current study indicates that the amplitude may be used to verify the diagnosis of compartment syndromes.

The increased IMP during simulated compartment syndrome in the present study reduced the muscle compliance and arterial pulsations were then reflected by pulse-synchronous oscillations in the IMP. The shape of these oscillations was similar to the typical pulsations that are seen in clinical invasive measurements of intra-arterial pressure. The waveform of IMP oscillations has been investigated with non-invasive ultrasound (Lynch et al. 2009). A preliminary report showed that frequency analysis of the fascial displacement waveform revealed a linear correlation between the ratio of the amplitude of the fundamental frequency and the second harmonic frequency and the invasively measured IMP (Wiemann et al. 2006). On the other hand, in an experimental porcine model of acute compartment syndrome, the analysis of the waveform revealed no significant interaction (Garabekyan et al. 2009). Since the amplitude was correlated to the IMP in the present study, the proposal that the proportion of the arterial pressure pulse that transmits through the muscle and affects the displacement of the compartment fascia is a function of the IMP (Garabekyan et al. 2009) is supported. Our results also support the concept that the oscillations might be useful for indirect measurements of the IMP using non-invasive techniques, such as ultrasound (Lynch et al. 2009).

It has been suggested that the thickness and elasticity of the fascia plays a role in the reduction in compartment compliance and the increase in IMP in patients with abnormally elevated IMP (Turnipseed et al. 1995; Hurschler et al. 1994; Detmer et al. 1985; Turnipseed et al. 1989). On the other hand, the stiffness and thickness did not differ between chronic compartment syndrome patients and healthy subjects in a recent study (Dahl 2011). Regardless of how the properties of the fascia influence compliance, the oscillations in the IMP may induce fascial displacement oscillations.

Local perfusion pressure around and below 30 mmHg has been reported to induce transient muscle ischemia (Heppenstall et al. 1988). During simulated compartment syndrome in our study, the local perfusion pressure decreased to 33 mmHg from 75 mmHg at baseline, while the mean arterial pressure and pulse rate were unchanged. Garabekyan and co-authors (Garabekyan et al. 2009) showed that fascial displacement was significantly larger in compartments with decreased perfusion pressure. These findings indicate that the oscillations increase with decreased perfusion pressure, since the perfusion pressure is a function of the IMP.

The experimental model of abnormally elevated IMP (simulated compartment syndrome) was chosen because it elevates the IMP by increasing the volume in the muscle compartment rather than by external compression. The IMP increased to approximately 50 mmHg, similar to previously reported values using this model (Styf and Wiger 1998; Wiger and Styf 1998; Zhang et al. 2001). This magnitude of IMP is also seen in patients with acute compartment syndrome (Taylor et al. 2012)

Table 1 Mean arterial pressure, local perfusion pressure and pulse rate

	MAP		PP		Pulse rate	
	mmHg	SD	mmHg	SD	bpm	SD
Baseline	80	5	75	5.1	62	7
Elevated IMP	82	5	33	9.5	61	9
Recovery	82	7	78	7.6	59	7

Mean arterial pressure (MAP), local perfusion pressure (PP) calculated from the intramuscular pressure (IMP) and pulse rate measured at baseline, during a model of abnormally elevated IMP (simulated compartment syndrome) and recovery.

and at rest after exercise in patients with chronic compartment syndrome (Aweid et al. 2012; Roberts and Franklyn-Miller 2012). By applying the model for only 10 minutes the IMP was abnormally elevated but no other symptoms of compartment syndrome were provoked.

One limitation of this study is that the amplitude of the oscillations was not studied when the local perfusion pressure approached zero, as the IMP was only elevated to approximately 50 mmHg. One strength of this study is that the IMP was measured with a pressure recording system with excellent dynamic properties in a validated model of simulated compartment syndrome in the human leg. Nevertheless, our results need to be confirmed in patients with compartment syndromes.

Conclusions

The amplitude of the pulse-synchronous IMP oscillations increases with increasing absolute level of IMP during a model of abnormally elevated IMP in the human leg. Since the amplitude is correlated with the absolute level of IMP, it may be an additional parameter in both research and in diagnosing compartment syndromes.

Competing interests
Stryker AB, Sweden, paid for the disposable Samba sensors from Samba AB, Sweden, and provided disposable kits for the Stryker pressure monitor. All funding was from internal sources. The authors have no affiliation with Stryker AB or Samba AB.

Authors' contributions
AN collected, processed and interpreted data, performed the statistical analysis and drafted the manuscript. QZ coordinated the study, helped to draft the manuscript and with acquisition of data. JS conceived of the study, introduced the measurement catheters and helped to draft the manuscript. All authors participated in the design of the study, read and approved the final manuscript.

Author details
[1]Department of Orthopaedics, Institute of Clinical Sciences, Sahlgrenska Academy, University of Gothenburg, Sahlgrenska University Hospital, Guldhedsgatan 10 A, 413 46 Gothenburg, Sweden. [2]Department of Orthopaedics, Sahlgrenska University Hospital, Gothenburg, Sweden.

References

Aweid O, Del Buono A, Malliaras P, Iqbal H, Morrissey D, Maffulli N et al (2012) Systematic review and recommendations for intracompartmental pressure monitoring in diagnosing chronic exertional compartment syndrome of the leg. Clin J Sport Med 22(4):356–70

Balduini F, Shenton D, O'Connor K, Heppenstall R (1993) Chronic exertional compartment syndrome: correlation of compartment pressure and muscle ischemia utilizing 31P-NMR spectroscopy. Clin Sports Med 12(1):151–65

Dahl M (2011) Stiffness and thickness of fascia do not explain chronic exertional compartment syndrome. Clin Orthop Relat Res 469(12):3495–500

Detmer DE, Sharpe K, Sufit RL, Girdley FM (1985) Chronic compartment syndrome: diagnosis, management, and outcomes. Am J Sports Med 13(3):162–70

Eliassen E, Folkow B, Hilton S, Öberg B, Rippe B (1974) Pressure-Volume Characteristics of the Interstitial Fluid Space in the Skeletal Muscle of the Cat. Acta Physiol Scand 90(3):583–93

Franklyn-Miller A, Roberts A, Hulse D, Foster J (2012) Biomechanical overload syndrome: defining a new diagnosis. Medicine, British Journal of Sports

Garabekyan T, Murphey GC, Macias BR, Lynch JE, Hargens AR (2009) New non-invasive ultrasound technique for monitoring perfusion pressure in a porcine model of acute compartment syndrome. J Orthop Trauma 23(3):186

Hargens AR, Akeson WH, Mubarak SJ, Owen CA, Gershuni DH, Garfin SR et al (1989) Tissue fluid pressures: from basic research tools to clinical applications. J Orthop Res 7(6):902–9

Hargens AR, Mubarak SJ, Owen CA, Garetto LP, Akeson WH (1977) Interstitial fluid pressure in muscle and compartment syndromes in man. Microvasc Res 14(1):1–10

Heppenstall RB, Sapega AA, Scott R, Shenton D, Park YS, Maris J et al (1988) The compartment syndrome: an experimental and clinical study of muscular energy metabolism using phosphorus nuclear magnetic resonance spectroscopy. Clin Orthop Relat Res 226:138–55

Hurschler C, Vanderby R Jr, Martinez DA, Vailas AC, Turnipseed WD (1994) Mechanical and biochemical analyses of tibial compartment fascia in chronic compartment syndrome. Ann Biomed Eng 22(3):272–9

Lynch JE, Lynch JK, Cole SL, Carter JA, Hargens AR (2009) Noninvasive monitoring of elevated intramuscular pressure in a model compartment syndrome via quantitative fascial motion. J Orthop Res 27(4):489–94

Matsen F, Mayo KA, Sheridan GW, Krugmire R (1976) Monitoring of intramuscular pressure. Surgery 79(6):702–9

Nilsson A, Zhang Q, Styf J (2014) Using the Amplitude of Pulse-Synchronous Intramuscular Pressure Oscillations When Diagnosing Chronic Anterior Compartment Syndrome. Orthopaedic J Sport Med 2(11):2325967114556443

Roberts A, Franklyn-Miller A (2012) The validity of the diagnostic criteria used in chronic exertional compartment syndrome: a systematic review. Scand J Med Sci Sports 22(5):585–95

Styf J (1989) Evaluation of injection techniques in recording of intramuscular pressure. J Orthop Res 7(6):812–6

Styf J, Korner L (1986) Chronic anterior-compartment syndrome of the leg: results of treatment by fasciotomy. J Bone Joint Surg (Am Vol) 68(9):1338–47

Styf J, Körner L (1986) Microcapillary infusion technique for measurement of intramuscular pressure during exercise. Clin Orthop Relat Res 207:253

Styf J, Wiger P (1998) Abnormally increased intramuscular pressure in human legs: comparison of two experimental models. J Trauma Acute Care Surg 45(1):133–9

Styf JR (1995) Intramuscular pressure measurements during exercise. Oper Tech Sports Med 3(4):243–9

Styf JR, Körner LM (1987) Diagnosis of chronic anterior compartment syndrome in the lower leg. Acta Orthop 58(2):139–44

Taylor RM, Sullivan MP, Mehta S (2012) Acute compartment syndrome: obtaining diagnosis, providing treatment, and minimizing medicolegal risk. Cur Rev Musculoskeletal Med 5(3):206–13

Tiidus PM (2014) Is intramuscular pressure a valid diagnostic criterion for chronic exertional compartment syndrome? Clin J Sport Med 24(1):87–8

Turnipseed W, Detmer DE, Girdley F (1989) Chronic compartment syndrome: an unusual cause for claudication. Ann Surg 210(4):557

Turnipseed WD, Hurschler C, Vanderby R Jr (1995) The effects of elevated compartment pressure on tibial arteriovenous flow and relationship of mechanical and biochemical characteristics of fascia to genesis of chronic anterior compartment syndrome. J Vasc Surg 21(5):810–7

Weiner G, Styf J, Nakhostine M, Gershuni DH (1994) Effect of ankle position and a plaster cast on intramuscular pressure in the human leg. J Bone Joint Surg Am 76(10):1476–81

Wiemann JM, Ueno T, Leek BT, Yost WT, Schwartz AK, Hargens AR (2006) Noninvasive measurements of intramuscular pressure using pulsed phase-locked loop ultrasound for detecting compartment syndromes: a preliminary report. J Orthop Trauma 20(7):458–63

Wiger P, Styf JR (1998) Effects of limb elevation on abnormally increased intramuscular pressure, blood perfusion pressure, and foot sensation: An experimental study in humans. J Orthop Trauma 12(5):343–7

Wiger P, Zhang Q, Styf J (2000) The effects of limb elevation and increased intramuscular pressure on nerve and muscle function in the human leg. Eur J Appl Physiol 83(1):84–8

Zhang Q, Styf J, Lindberg LG (2001) Effects of limb elevation and increased intramuscular pressure on human tibialis anterior muscle blood flow. Eur J Appl Physiol 85(6):567–71

10

Role of mesenchymal stem cells in meniscal repair

Peter Angele[1,2*], Richard Kujat[1], Matthias Koch[1] and Johannes Zellner[1]

Abstract

Meniscus integrity is the key for joint health of the knee. Therefore, the main goal of every meniscus treatment should be the maintenance of as much meniscus tissue as possible.
Repair of meniscus tears can be achieved by meniscus suture. However, in a recently published meta-analysis, the long-term outcome of meniscus repair showed a mean failure rate of 24%.
In a preclinical trial, locally applied mesenchymal stem cells produced differentiated meniscus-like tissue in meniscus tears indicating that mesenchymal-based cells, harvested from the bone marrow, enhance meniscus healing in critical-size meniscus tears.
Symptomatic meniscus defects offer the option for meniscus transplantation with porous cell free biomaterials, when a complete meniscus rim is available. Cell-free biomaterials, which are actually in clinical application, reveal variable outcome in mid-term results from complete failure to regeneration with meniscus-like tissue.
In several preclinical studies with different critical-size defects in the meniscus, the application of mesenchymal stem cells could significantly enhance meniscus regeneration compared to empty defects or to cell-free biomaterials. Regenerative treatment of meniscus with mesenchymal stem cells seems to be a promising approach to treat meniscal tears and defects. However it is still not clear, whether the stem cell effect is a direct action of the mesenchymal-based cells or is rather mediated by secretion of certain stimulating factors. The missing knowledge of the underlying mechanism is one of the reasons for regulatory burdens to permit these stem cell-based strategies in clinical practice. Other limitations are the necessity to expand cells prior to transplantation resulting in high treatment costs. Alternative treatment modalities, which use growth factors concentrated from peripheral blood aspirates or mononucleated cells concentrated from bone marrow aspirates, are currently in development in order to allow an attractive one-step procedure without the need for cell expansion in cultures and thus lower efforts and costs.
In summary, Tissue Engineering of meniscus with mesenchymal based cells seems to be a promising approach to treat meniscal tears and defects in order to restore native meniscus tissue. However, advances of the technology are necessary to allow clinical application of this modern regenerative therapy.

Keywords: Mesenchymal stem cells; Meniscus tear; Meniscus suture; Meniscus transplantation; Biomaterial

Introduction

Meniscal lesions represent the most common intra-articular knee injury, and are the most frequent cause of surgical procedures performed by orthopaedic surgeons (Makris et al. 2011). The mean annual incidence of meniscal lesions has been reported to be 66 per 100.000 inhabitants, 61 of which result in meniscectomy (Makris et al. 2011). The changes in "pivoting" sports activities in the past few decades have resulted in increased injury rates of the meniscus (1.5 million injuries in Germany per year) (Stein et al. 2010). Especially in combination with anterior cruciate ligament injuries a high incidence of meniscal lesions (40-80%) can be detected.

Meniscus integrity is the key for joint health of the knee. Untreated meniscus tears cause intermittent pain, joint swelling, recurrent mechanical symptoms (clicking, catching, giving way) and, therefore, significant reduction in quality of life in predominately young and active patients (McDermott 2011).

* Correspondence: peter.angele@ukr.de
[1]University Medical Center Regensburg, Franz-Josef-Strauss-Allee 11, 93053 Regensburg, Germany
[2]Sporthopaedicum Regensburg/Straubing, Hildegard von Bingen Strasse 1, 93053 Regensburg, Germany

In the long-term, meniscus tears can result in the onset of joint degeneration and, finally, knee osteoarthritis with all its consequences including pain, immobility and knee arthroplasty (Lohmander et al. 2007; Stein et al. 2010; Borchers et al. 2011; Jeong et al. 2012; Badlani et al. 2013). In a recent published case–control study (Level of evidence 3) specific meniscus tear morphologies (Meniscus extrusion, complex tears, tears with large radial involvement) have shown to be significantly more common in patients with progressive development of osteoarthritic changes in a 2 year follow-up indicating that these meniscus tears represent a negative prognostic risk factor for later development of osteoarthritis (Badlani et al. 2013).

Removal of meniscus tears lead to short term relief of clinical symptoms, but to knee osteoarthitis in long-term (Salata et al. 2010; Paxton et al. 2011; Papalia et al. 2011; Jeong et al. 2012). Especially the amount meniscus removed, lateral meniscectomy and longer duration of clinical symptoms preoperatively have been identified as negative prognostic risk factors for the onset of osteoarthritis in systematic reviews (Papalia et al. 2011; Jeong et al. 2012). Elevated expression levels of arthritis-related markers in meniscus tears in patients under forty years old, compared to patients over forty years, and in patients with meniscus and anterior cruciate ligament tears, compared to patients with isolated meniscus tears, indicate an increased catabolic response suggesting a higher risk for progression of osteoarthritis following partial meniscectomy (Brophy and Matava 2012).

Knowing the risk for the onset of osteoarthritis after meniscectomy, the majority of meniscus tears are still treated with partial meniscectomy as shown in a huge cohort of more than 1000 young patients undergoing anterior cruciate ligament reconstruction (Fetzer et al. 2009).

Therefore, the main goal of every meniscus treatment should be the maintenance of as much meniscus tissue as possible (Fetzer et al. 2009; Starke et al. 2009; Stein et al. 2010; Abrams et al. 2013). This includes repair of meniscus tears and regeneration of meniscus defects after meniscectomy with regenerative treatment approaches.

In recent years, there has been a growing interest in using mesenchymal stem cells to regenerate damaged tissue such as injured hyaline cartilage or meniscus. These mesenchymal stem cells fulfill a dual role for musculoskeletal repair, because they have the potential to differentiate into the repair cells themselves and to produce special growth factors for its repair (Caplan and Dennis 2006). This review focuses on the present and future treatment options especially for meniscus repair and meniscus regeneration given by the use of intrinsic or exogenous applied mesenchymal stem cells.

Review

Endogenous repair cells of meniscus injury

Currently, a number of potential repair cells for meniscus regeneration are available. Repair cells of meniscus injury can either be located in the meniscus tissue itself or entering the meniscus predominately via circulation. In the following section, we will focus on the availability of repair cells and repair potential of the meniscus.

Endogenous repair of meniscus injury seems to be dependent of the different vascularisation of the outer and the inner zone of the meniscus (Arnoczky 1999). Repair in the vascularized outer zone can be achieved (McDermott 2011), but fail to encourage healing in the avascular inner zone of the meniscus (Hasan et al. 2014; Makris et al. 2011). However, in several studies also regeneration could be seen in the inner zone of the meniscus indicating regenerative potential independently from the vascularization (Nakata et al. 2001; Hennerbichler et al. 2007; Baker et al. 2009; Pabbruwe et al. 2010). Hennerbichler et al. have shown in an experimental setup, that punch defects, which were directly filled with the removed punches, showed no significant difference in healing potential between the vascularized and avascularized meniscus zone (Hennerbichler et al. 2007). Croutze and coworkers could demonstrate equivalent differentiation potential toward chondrogenic phenotype and extracellular matrix production of isolated human meniscus cells from the inner and the outer zone (Croutze et al. 2013). Different studies stated that milieu factors like oxygen tension (Croutze et al. 2013) and growth factors (Pabbruwe et al. 2010) may play a key role in modulating redifferentiation of meniscal fibrochondrocytes at least *in vitro*.

From a clinical standpoint, meniscus cells from meniscectomised tissue would be the ideal cell source for repair. Is this approach applicable? Nakata et al. have shown feasibility of meniscus regeneration by expansion of human meniscus cells from meniscectomised tissue (Nakata et al. 2001). With the same cell source Baker et al. could achieve repair tissue with equivalent mechanical properties than native meniscus tissue (Baker et al. 2009). However the low proliferation rate and matrix production limit the use of this cell type (Nakata et al. 2001). In addition, potential candidates for meniscus transplantation have already undergone partial meniscectomy with the necessity to find alternative cell sources.

Stem cells are characterized by self-renewal capacity and multilineage differentiation potential to a variety of cell types of mesenchymal tissue like bone, cartilage or fat (Caplan 1991; Caplan and Dennis 2006). Recently, the stem cell perspective has changed by identification of pericytes around almost every blood vessel in the body, which contain stem cell characteristics (Bianco et al. 2008;

Bianco 2011; Crisan et al. 2008; Crisan et al. 2011). The existing traditional view, which focuses on the multipotent differentiation capacity of these cells, has been expanded to include their equally interesting role as cellular modulators that bring them into a broader therapeutic scenario (Caplan and Correa 2011).

With this background, it is not surprising that Osawa et al. have identified in the vascularized region of the meniscus more blood-vessel derived stem cells (CD34- and CD146-positive cells) than in the avascular region. These meniscal-derived stem cells were multipotent and contributed to meniscal regeneration, which they proof via transplantation in knee joints of athymic rats (Osawa et al. 2013).

Does also the avascular inner zone of the meniscus contain stem cells? Stem cells have been identified in the surface zone of other avascular tissue, mainly in the articular cartilage (Archer et al. 1994; Dowthwaite et al. 2004; McCarthy et al. 2012), but little is known about meniscus stem cells. Mauck et al. describes regional multilineage differentiation potential of meniscus cells in both zones available, however showed differences in pluripotency between the zones (Mauck et al. 2007). Especially, pluripotent cells from the avascular tissue seem to lack osteogenic differentiation potential, which could be of clinical interest for meniscus regenerative approaches (Mauck et al. 2007; McCarthy et al. 2012).

Besides existence of mesenchymal stem cells in the meniscus, the synovium and the synovial fluid contain stem cells for meniscus regeneration (Sakaguchi et al. 2005; Horie et al. 2009; Matsukura et al. 2014). Matsukura and coworkers found elevated levels of mesenchymal stem cells in the synovium fluid after meniscus injury compared to normal knee joints suggesting that mesenchymal stem cells in the fluid may play a role in regeneration of meniscus (Matsukura et al. 2014). Horie and coworkers showed promotion of meniscal regeneration in rat massive meniscal defects by intra-articular injection of synovial stem cells. The injected cells adhere to the lesion site, directly differentiate in meniscus cells and promote meniscal regeneration without mobilization to distant organs (Horie et al. 2009).

In summary, local or systemic stem cells seem to play a fundamental and essential role in the regeneration of meniscus injury, either as direct repair cells or as a source for secretion of bioactive modulators.

Repair of meniscus tears with meniscus suture

If the meniscus repair succeeds then the patient is left with a normal or near-normal meniscus, and thus no increased risk of osteoarthritis in the future (McDermott 2011; Stein et al. 2010; Paxton et al. 2011). In a cohort study (Level of evidence 3) no osteoarthritic progress was detectable in 80% of the patients after meniscus repair compared with 40% after meniscectomy in a long-term follow-up (mean 9 years) (Stein et al. 2010). In a systematic review meniscal repair showed superior clinical outcome detected by higher Lysholm scores and less radiologic degeneration than meniscectomy (Paxton et al. 2011). However, in a recently published meta-analysis, the long-term outcome of meniscal repair showed a mean failure rate of 23,1% (Nepple et al. 2012).

Augmentation of meniscus suture

Given the low healing potential of meniscus in the avascular zone and the moderate healing rates of meniscus repair in the vascular zone, there is a strong need for true regeneration of viable and biomechanically functional meniscus tissue.

Several methods have been devised to aid the healing of the meniscus, ranging from refreshing the meniscus tears with rasps and creation of access channels in the meniscus base to introduce blood and reparative cells to meniscus tears (Scotti et al. 2013) (Figure 1). The use of fibrin clots, synovial flaps and resorbable scaffolds in or around the tears were also described in the literature in order to enhance meniscus healing potential (Hasan et al. 2013; Starke et al. 2009).

Exogenous fibrin clots seem to improve healing in animal models and in humans (Starke et al. 2009). It is postulated that the clot serves as a chemotactic and mitogenous stimulus. Platelet-rich plasma (PRP), which contains the majority of growth factors in the peripheral blood, seems to promote the clinical healing of meniscus tears even in the white-white zone (Wei et al. 2012) mainly in the earlier period after meniscal suture. However, the clinical use of this intriguing arthroscopically applicable, one-step procedure for meniscus repair is actually not tested in prospective trials due to regulatory burdens.

Augmentation of meniscus suture with mesenchymal stem cells

Preclinical trials have shown enhanced healing of meniscal lesions with the application of mesenchymal based cells (Table 1) (Table 2) (Hasan et al. 2013; Makris et al. 2011; Izuta et al. 2005; Angele et al. 2008; Zellner et al. 2010; Zellner et al. 2013). Locally applied expanded mesenchymal stem cells from the bone marrow have achieved regeneration of longitudinal meniscus tears in the avascular zone in the lateral meniscus of New Zealand White Rabbits. Control groups with untreated tears, treatment with meniscus suture alone or meniscus suture in combination with implanted cell-free biomaterials revealed no recognizable healing indicating the development of a critical size meniscus tear model. In contrast, mesenchymal stem cells from the bone marrow in combination with hyaluronan collagen carriers resulted in meniscal repair

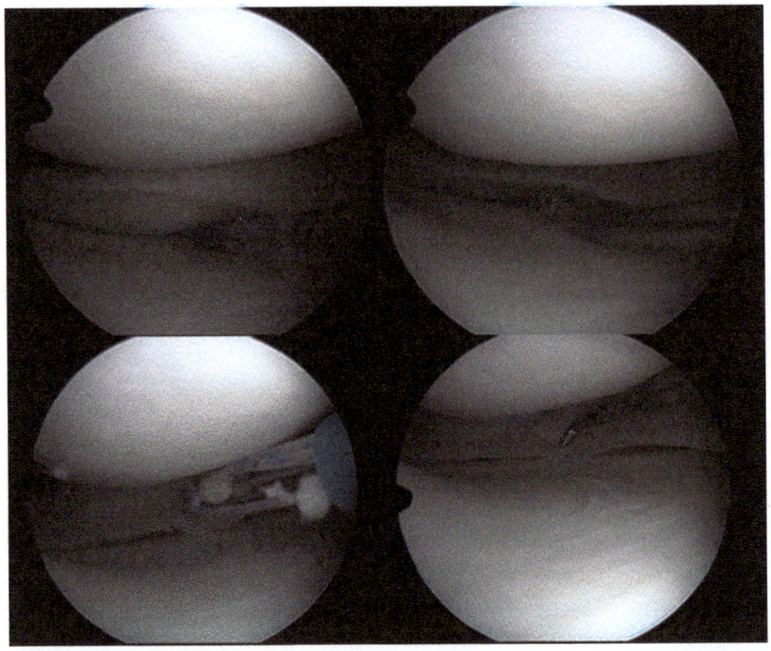

Figure 1 Medial meniscus tear and meniscus repair in a right knee joint: Meniscus tear recognized by a probe (upper left); Meniscus tear preparation with a grasp, which refreshes the tear site (upper right); Meniscus suture with all inside technique (Fast T Fix, Smith nephew) (lower left); Stable meniscus tear after repair (lower right).

with differentiated meniscus-like tissue detected by histology, immunohistochemistry and biomechanical analysis (Figure 2) (Zellner et al. 2013).

It is not clear whether this is a direct action of the mesenchymal-based cells or is rather mediated by secretion of certain stimulating factors (Starke et al. 2009). Despite the fact, that meniscus regeneration seems to be feasible by growth factors and mononucleated cells, none of the cell-based strategies has entered clinical practice to date (Scotti et al. 2013). The implementation of cell-based strategies is mainly limited by regulatory burdens and by the necessity to expand cells prior to transplantation resulting in high treatment costs.

Table 1 Mesenchymal stem cells for meniscus regeneration

Pro/advantages	Cons/disadvantages
• High regenerative potential	• High treatment costs
• Self renewal capacity	• Regulatory burden
• Cellular modulation at lesion site	• Missing knowledge of underlying repair mechanisms
• Potential of differentiation into meniscal repair cells	• Possible need for cell expansions prior to application
• Secretion of bioactive substances like growth factors	
• Support/promotion of intrinsic meniscal healing capacity	

Regeneration of meniscus defects

Searching for optimal restoration of meniscal tissue, biocompatible scaffolds came in the focus for treatment of large meniscal defects in the last decade. The rationale for using cell-free biomaterials after extensive loss of meniscal tissue is based on repopulation of the scaffold by host cells recruited from the synovium or the meniscal remnants (Scotti et al. 2013) (Figure 3).

Two biomaterials are currently in clinical use. The collagen meniscus implant (CMI) was the first scaffold for meniscus replacement. Some authors report satisfactory clinical outcome (Rodkey et al. 1999) while MRI and histological results are controversial. Steadman and Rodkey (2005) saw a tendency of shrinking over time and no histological remnants of the collagen scaffold 5–6 years after implantation (Steadman and Rodkey 2005). Martinek et al. (2006) described predominantly scar tissue formation instead of fibrocartilage after implantation (Martinek et al. 2006). The second biomaterial is a polyurethane based scaffold called Actifit. The first 12 month report showed tissue ingrowth into the scaffold at this time and consistent regeneration in MRI and biopsies (Verdonk et al. 2011).

However, there are no data on the mid- and long term effects of the CMI or the Actifit on the surrounding cartilage in order to prove the beneficial effect on prevention of early onset of osteoarthritis after loss of meniscus tissue. The amount of the developed repair tissue and its quality induced by the cell-free implants still seem to be

Table 2 Regenerative treatment options for meniscal lesions

Treatment	Pro/Cons
Augmentation of meniscal suture and meniscus reconstruction by intraarticular microfracturing	+ Easy to perform + Adhesion of stem cells at lesion site - Uncertain effect - Low concentration of stem cells at defect site
Augmentation of meniscal suture or meniscus cell-free reconstruction (e.g. Actifit) by locally applied growth factors (e.g. PRP)	+ Application directly at meniscal lesion site + High concentration at lesion site + Support of intrinsic healing potential + One-step-procedure - Preparation time - Short term effect at lesion site - Uncertain local effect
Augmentation of meniscal suture by locally applied MSCs (e.g. bone marrow derived)	+ High potential differentiation + Application directly at meniscal lesion site + Support of meniscus regeneration + Use of autologous cells + Potentially one-step-procedure - Preparation time - Regulatory burden - Missing knowledge of repair mechanisms
Intraarticular injection of MSCs/growth factors	+ Adhesion at lesion site + Easy to perform - Uncertain effect - Low concentration of stem cells at lesion site - Harvesting and preparation prior to application - Side effects in the knee joint beside the defect site
Intravascular injection of MSCs	+ Adhesion at lesion site - Uncertain effect - Low concentration of stem cells at lesion site - Harvesting and preparation prior to application - Side effects in other areas besides the defect - No clinical experience
Implantation of MSC loaded carrier/scaffold at meniscal defect site	+ Potential for treatment of meniscal critical size defects + Application directly at meniscal defect site + Option for pre-differentiation of MSC/carrier construct + Use of autologous cells - High costs - Missing knowledge of repair mechanisms - Necessity of cell expansion prior to implantation/two-step-procedure - No clinical experience

crucial and improvable. Scar formation, repair tissue rich of vessels and vascularization into the tip of the new meniscus tissue show the need of improvement of this treatment technique. Additionally the biomechanical stability and the intraoperative handling have to be optimized for better clinical results. At the moment the cell-free meniscus implants are only used in a very selective group of patients. Despite promising short term results of meniscal implants, none of them has currently demonstrated regeneration of a functional, long-lasting meniscal tissue.

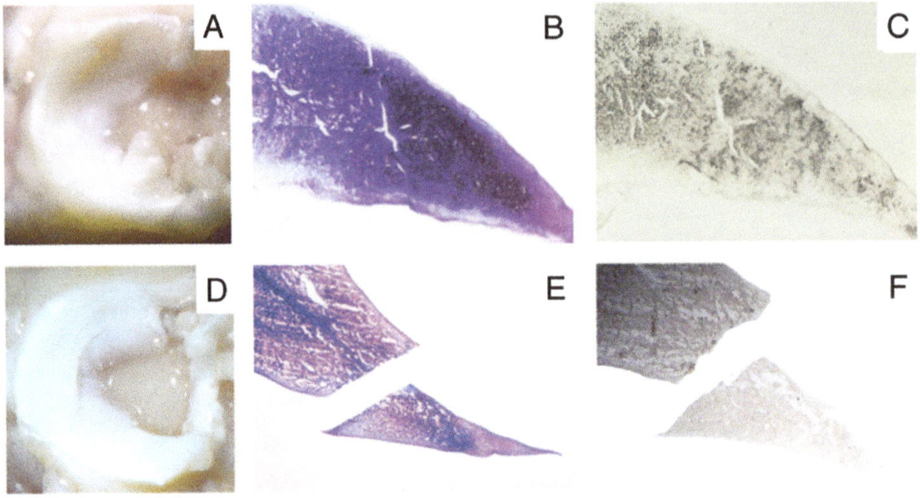

Figure 2 Treatment of meniscal tears (rabbit) in the avascular zone with a mesenchymal stem cell matrix composite resulted in a stable repair compared to implantation of a cell free scaffold: Representative macroscopic views, histological (toluidine blue) and immunohistochemical (collagen type II) slides of menisci and the meniscal repair tissue 3 months after treatment of tears in the avascular zone: A, B, C: treatment with hyaluronan-collagen composite matrices loaded with mesenchymal stem cells; D, E, F: treatment with a cell-free composite matrix (control).

As biomaterials for meniscal substitution need a stable and intact rim of the native meniscus, allogenic meniscal transplantation is actually the only biologic treatment option available for totally meniscectomized knee joints (Lubowitz et al. 2007). A recently published meta-analysis concluded that this procedure is an effective technique for these very selected patients (Elattar et al. 2011). However fixation of the allograft, the limited availability and the frequent mismatch of graft and host tissue (Shaffer et al. 2000) are still problems of this procedure. In addition, long term protection from joint degeneration has not yet been demonstrated (Wirth et al. 2002).

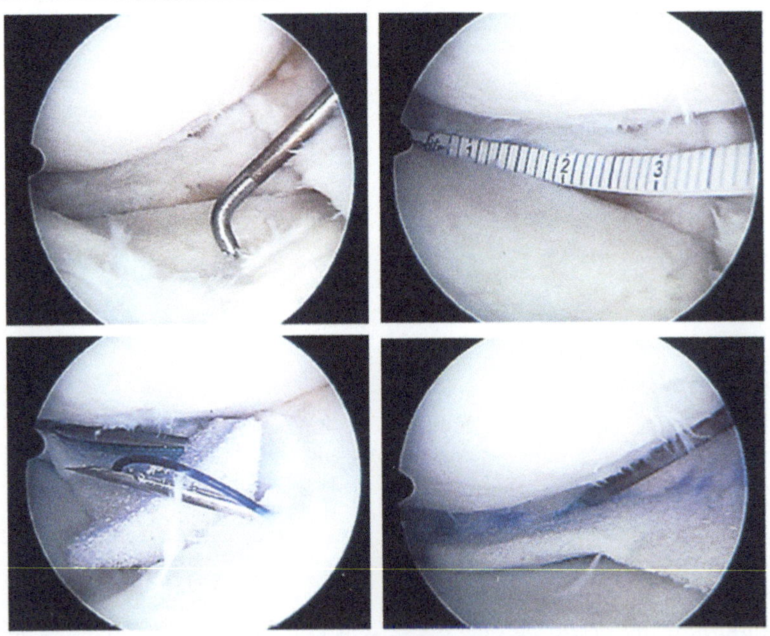

Figure 3 Meniscus transplantation with cell-free biomaterial after subtotal meniscectomy of the medial meniscus (Actifit). Subtotal meniscectomy, note the residual meniscus base (upper left); Measurement of the meniscus defect for preparation of suitable biomaterial (upper right); Insertion of the cell-free biomaterial and fixation with all-inside and outside-in suture techniques (lower row).

Stem cells for regeneration of meniscus defects

In experimental trials different settings have been tested for mesenchymal stem cell based Tissue Engineering approaches for treatment of meniscus defects (Table 1). Stem cells can be administered by different ways of application. In most studies, the local application of mesenchymal stem cells has been used (Table 2).

Ishimura et al. (1991) showed a faster and improved healing of avascular meniscal defects in a rabbit model by using bone marrow fibrin clot constructs compared to fibrin clot alone (Ishimura et al. 1991). They postulated that the benefit of this treatment is due to the pluripotential stem cells in the bone marrow. In a scaffold-free engineered meniscal tissue Aufderheide and Athanasiou (2007) found a high tensile modulus and improved mechanical properties by a high density co-culture of fibrochondrocytes and mesenchymal stem cells in ring shaped moulds (Aufderheide and Athanasiou 2007). Despite these reults, for in vivo application of mesenchymal stem cells, scaffolds seem to be a useful tool to ensure a lasting effect of the cells directly at the defect site. Yamasaki et al. (2008) using cell-seeded rat decellularized meniscus scaffolds, concluded that cell seeded constructs are more effective than scaffolds alone (Yamasaki et al. 2008). Multiple natural and synthetic scaffolds have been used to deliver cells to the meniscal injury (Sweigart and Athanasiou 2001; Buma et al. 2004; Scotti et al. 2013). A hyluronan collagen composite matrix were found to be suitable for chondrogenic differentiation of mesenchymal stem cells (Angele et al. 2009). Treatment of meniscal full size defects with this scaffold seeded with autologous mesenchymal stem cells after resection of the pars intermedia of the medial meniscus in a rabbit model resulted in a complete defect filling after 3 months in vivo. Only treatment with mesenchymal stem cells was able repair this critical size meniscal defects with stable differentiated meniscus like tissue compared to untreated defects or the treatment with a cellfree hyaluronan collagen scaffold (Angele et al. 2008). Similar results were detected for treatment of isolated avascular meniscal punch defects in the pars intermedia of the lateral meniscus in a rabbit model (Zellner et al. 2010). After 3 months in vivo meniscal defects were filled with differentiated repair tissue after treatment with a hyaluronan collagen composite matrix seeded with mesenchymal stem cells (Figure 4). Interestingly precultured stem cell matrix constructs showed a reduced integration in the native meniscus while non precultured stem cell matrix constructs resulted in a completely integrated repair tissue indicating that also the grade of differentiation of the stem cell matrix construct seems to be an important factor for successful treatment of meniscus with stem cell based Tissue Engineering. In the same model growth factors applied by autologous PRP failed to repair the avascular meniscal punch defect. In summary, mesenchymal stem cells seem to play an essential role for treatment of meniscal defects.

Ethical approval

The experimental studies were performed with permission of the Ethical comitee at the University Hospital Regensburg.

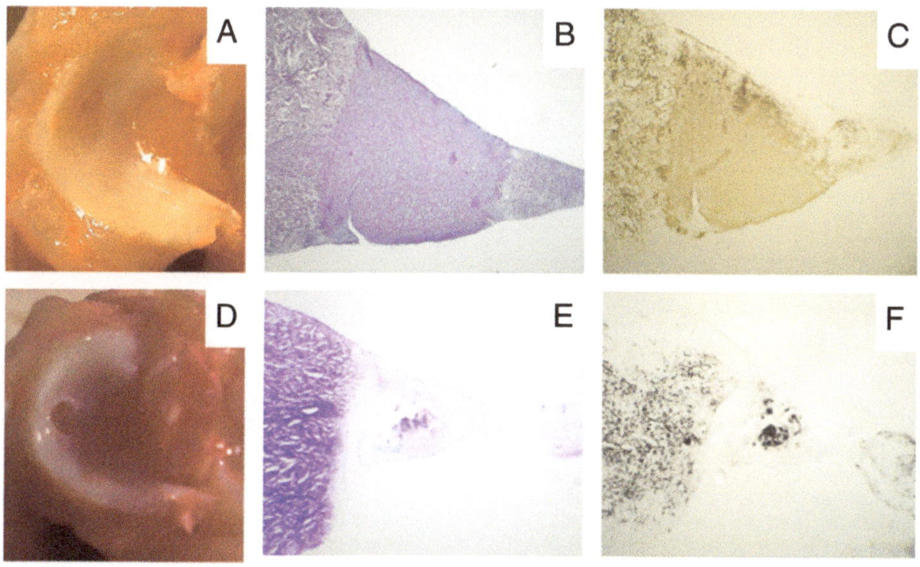

Figure 4 Treatment of meniscal defects (rabbit) in the avascular zone with a mesenchymal stem cell matrix composite resulted in defect filling with a differentiated meniscus like tissue compared to implantation of a cell free scaffold: Representative macroscopic views, histological (toluidine blue) and immunohistochemical (collagen type II) slides of menisci and the meniscal repair tissue 3 months after treatment of circular meniscal punch defects in the avascular zone; A, B, C: treatment with hyaluronan-collagen composite matrices loaded with mesenchymal stem cells; D, E, F: treatment with a cell-free composite matrix (control).

Conclusions

Tissue Engineering of meniscus with mesenchymal based cells seems to be a promising approach to treat meniscal tears and defects in order to restore as much native meniscal tissue as possible. In preclinical trials, treatment of meniscus tears only with suture or meniscus defects with cell-free biomaterials, which both represent the actual clinical practice, fail to show comparable results to mesenchymal cell based approaches.

Despite the fact, that meniscus regeneration seems to be feasible by growth factors and mesenchymal stem cells, none of the cell-based strategies has entered clinical practice to date. The implementation of cell-based strategies is mainly limited by regulatory burdens and by the necessity to expand cells prior to transplantation resulting in high treatment costs.

Consent

Written informed consent was obtained from the patient's for the publication of this report and any accompanying images.

Competing interests

In the past five years one or more authors have received funding from Orteq for research projects, especially for further improvement of the cell-free meniscus implant (Actifit). The company is not financing the manuscript. Otherwise there is no competing interest.

Authors' contributions

PA wrote manuscript, performed surgeries, coordinated basic science projects. RK coordination of basic science projects. MK literature review, help writting the review. JZ performed animal studies, helped writting the manuscript. All authors read and approved the final manuscript.

Acknowledgements

The authors thank Daniela Drenkard and Svetlana Stryshkowa for their technical assistance.

References

Abrams GD, Frank RM, Gupta AK, Harris JD, McCormick FM, Cole BJ (2013) Trends in meniscus repair and meniscectomy in the United States, 2005–2011. Am J Sports Med 41(10):2333–2339, doi:10.1177/0363546513495641

Angele P, Johnstone B, Kujat R, Zellner J, Nerlich M, Goldberg V, Yoo J (2008) Stem cell based tissue engineering for meniscus repair. J Biomed Mater Res A 85(2):445–455, doi:10.1002/jbm.a.31480

Angele P, Muller R, Schumann D, Englert C, Zellner J, Johnstone B, Yoo J, Hammer J, Fierlbeck J, Angele MK, Nerlich M, Kujat R (2009) Characterization of esterified hyaluronan-gelatin polymer composites suitable for chondrogenic differentiation of mesenchymal stem cells. J Biomed Mater Res A 91(2):416–427, doi:10.1002/jbm.a.32236

Archer CW, Morrison H, Pitsillides AA (1994) Cellular aspects of the development of diarthrodial joints and articular cartilage. J Anat 184(Pt 3):447–456

Arnoczky SP (1999) Building a meniscus. Biologic considerations. Clin Orthop Relat Res (367 Suppl):S244–S253

Aufderheide AC, Athanasiou KA (2007) Assessment of a bovine co-culture, scaffold free method for growing meniscus-shaped constructs. Tissue Eng 13(9):2195–2205, doi:10.1089/ten.2006.0291

Badlani JT, Borrero C, Golla S, Harner CD, Irrgang JJ (2013) The effects of meniscus injury on the development of knee osteoarthritis: data from the osteoarthritis initiative. Am J Sports Med 41(6):1238–1244, doi:10.1177/0363546513490276

Baker BM, Nathan AS, Huffman GR, Mauck RL (2009) Tissue engineering with meniscus cells derived from surgical debris. Osteoarthr Cartil 17(3):336–345, doi:10.1016/j.joca.2008.08.001

Bianco P (2011) Minireview: the stem cell next door: skeletal and hematopoietic stem cell "niches" in bone. Endocrinology 152(8):2957–2962, doi:10.1210/en.2011-0217

Bianco P, Robey PG, Simmons PJ (2008) Mesenchymal stem cells: revisiting history, concepts, and assays. Cell Stem Cell 2(4):313–319, doi:10.1016/j.stem.2008.03.002

Borchers JR, Kaeding CC, Pedroza AD, Huston LJ, Spindler KP, Wright RW (2011) Intra-articular findings in primary and revision anterior cruciate ligament reconstruction surgery: a comparison of the MOON and MARS study groups. Am J Sports Med 39(9):1889–1893, doi:10.1177/0363546511406871

Brophy RH, Matava MJ (2012) Surgical options for meniscal replacement. J Am Acad Orthop Surg 20(5):265–272, doi:10.5435/jaaos-20-05-265

Buma P, Ramrattan NN, van Tienen TG, Veth RP (2004) Tissue engineering of the meniscus. Biomaterials 25(9):1523–1532

Caplan AI (1991) Mesenchymal stem cells. J Orthop Res 9(5):641–650, doi:10.1002/jor.1100090504

Caplan AI, Correa D (2011) The MSC: an injury drugstore. Cell Stem Cell 9(1):11–15, doi:10.1016/j.stem.2011.06.008

Caplan AI, Dennis JE (2006) Mesenchymal stem cells as trophic mediators. J Cell Biochem 98(5):1076–1084, doi:10.1002/jcb.20886

Crisan M, Deasy B, Gavina M, Zheng B, Huard J, Lazzari L, Peault B (2008) Purification and long-term culture of multipotent progenitor cells affiliated with the walls of human blood vessels: myoendothelial cells and pericytes. Methods Cell Biol 86:295–309, doi:10.1016/s0091-679x(08)00013-7

Crisan M, Corselli M, Chen CW, Peault B (2011) Multilineage stem cells in the adult: a perivascular legacy? Organogenesis 7(2):101–104

Croutze R, Jomha N, Uludag H, Adesida A (2013) Matrix forming characteristics of inner and outer human meniscus cells on 3D collagen scaffolds under normal and low oxygen tensions. BMC Musculoskelet Disord 14:353, doi:10.1186/1471-2474-14-353

Dowthwaite GP, Bishop JC, Redman SN, Khan IM, Rooney P, Evans DJ, Haughton L, Bayram Z, Boyer S, Thomson B, Wolfe MS, Archer CW (2004) The surface of articular cartilage contains a progenitor cell population. J Cell Sci 117(Pt 6):889–897, doi:10.1242/jcs.00912

Elattar M, Dhollander A, Verdonk R, Almqvist KF, Verdonk P (2011) Twenty-six years of meniscal allograft transplantation: is it still experimental? A meta-analysis of 44 trials. Knee Surg Sports Traumatol Arthrosc 19(2):147–157, doi:10.1007/s00167-010-1351-6

Fetzer GB, Spindler KP, Amendola A, Andrish JT, Bergfeld JA, Dunn WR, Flanigan DC, Jones M, Kaeding CC, Marx RG, Matava MJ, McCarty EC, Parker RD, Wolcott M, Vidal A, Wolf BR, Wright RW (2009) Potential market for new meniscus repair strategies: evaluation of the MOON cohort. J Knee Surg 22(3):180–186

Hasan J, Fisher J, Ingham E (2013) Current strategies in meniscal regeneration. J Biomed Mater Res B Appl Biomater doi:10.1002/jbm.b.33030

Hasan J, Fisher J, Ingham E (2014) Current strategies in meniscal regeneration. J Biomed Mater Res B Appl Biomater 102(3):619–634, doi:10.1002/jbm.b.33030

Hennerbichler A, Moutos FT, Hennerbichler D, Weinberg JB, Guilak F (2007) Repair response of the inner and outer regions of the porcine meniscus in vitro. Am J Sports Med 35(5):754–762, doi:10.1177/0363546506296416

Horie M, Sekiya I, Muneta T, Ichinose S, Matsumoto K, Saito H, Murakami T, Kobayashi E (2009) Intra-articular Injected synovial stem cells differentiate into meniscal cells directly and promote meniscal regeneration without mobilization to distant organs in rat massive meniscal defect. Stem Cells 27(4):878–887, doi:10.1634/stemcells.2008-0616

Ishimura M, Tamai S, Fujisawa Y (1991) Arthroscopic meniscal repair with fibrin glue. Arthroscopy 7(2):177–181

Izuta Y, Ochi M, Adachi N, Deie M, Yamasaki T, Shinomiya R (2005) Meniscal repair using bone marrow-derived mesenchymal stem cells: experimental study using green fluorescent protein transgenic rats. Knee 12(3):217–223, doi:10.1016/j.knee.2001.06.001

Jeong HJ, Lee SH, Ko CS (2012) Meniscectomy. Knee Surg Relat Res 24(3):129–136, doi:10.5792/ksrr.2012.24.3.129

Lohmander LS, Englund PM, Dahl LL, Roos EM (2007) The long-term consequence of anterior cruciate ligament and meniscus injuries: osteoarthritis. Am J Sports Med 35(10):1756–1769, doi:10.1177/0363546507307396

Lubowitz JH, Verdonk PC, Reid JB 3rd, Verdonk R (2007) Meniscus allograft transplantation: a current concepts review. Knee Surg Sports Traumatol Arthrosc 15(5):476–492, doi:10.1007/s00167-006-0216-5

Makris EA, Hadidi P, Athanasiou KA (2011) The knee meniscus: structure-function, pathophysiology, current repair techniques, and prospects for regeneration. Biomaterials 32(30):7411–7431, doi:10.1016/j.biomaterials.2011.06.037

Martinek V, Ueblacker P, Braun K, Nitschke S, Mannhardt R, Specht K, Gansbacher B, Imhoff AB (2006) Second generation of meniscus transplantation: in-vivo study with tissue engineered meniscus replacement. Arch Orthop Trauma Surg 126(4):228–234, doi:10.1007/s00402-005-0025-1

Matsukura Y, Muneta T, Tsuji K, Koga H, Sekiya I (2014) Mesenchymal stem cells in synovial fluid increase after meniscus injury. Clin Orthop Relat Res 472(5):1357–1364, doi:10.1007/s11999-013-3418-4

Mauck RL, Martinez-Diaz GJ, Yuan X, Tuan RS (2007) Regional multilineage differentiation potential of meniscal fibrochondrocytes: implications for meniscus repair. Anat Rec (Hoboken) 290(1):48–58, doi:10.1002/ar.20419

McCarthy HE, Bara JJ, Brakspear K, Singhrao SK, Archer CW (2012) The comparison of equine articular cartilage progenitor cells and bone marrow-derived stromal cells as potential cell sources for cartilage repair in the horse. Vet J 192(3):345–351, doi:10.1016/j.tvjl.2011.08.036

McDermott I (2011) Meniscal tears, repairs and replacement: their relevance to osteoarthritis of the knee. Br J Sports Med 45(4):292–297, doi:10.1136/bjsm.2010.081257

Nakata K, Shino K, Hamada M, Mae T, Miyama T, Shinjo H, Horibe S, Tada K, Ochi T, Yoshikawa H (2001) Human meniscus cell: characterization of the primary culture and use for tissue engineering. Clin Orthop Relat Res (391 Suppl):S208–S218

Nepple JJ, Dunn WR, Wright RW (2012) Meniscal repair outcomes at greater than five years: a systematic literature review and meta-analysis. J Bone Joint Surg Am 94(24):2222–2227, doi:10.2106/jbjs.k.01584

Osawa A, Harner CD, Gharaibeh B, Matsumoto T, Mifune Y, Kopf S, Ingham SJ, Schreiber V, Usas A, Huard J (2013) The use of blood vessel-derived stem cells for meniscal regeneration and repair. Med Sci Sports Exerc 45(5):813–823, doi:10.1249/MSS.0b013e31827d1e06

Pabbruwe MB, Kafienah W, Tarlton JF, Mistry S, Fox DJ, Hollander AP (2010) Repair of meniscal cartilage white zone tears using a stem cell/collagen-scaffold implant. Biomaterials 31(9):2583–2591, doi:10.1016/j.biomaterials.2009.12.023

Papalia R, Del Buono A, Osti L, Denaro V, Maffulli N (2011) Meniscectomy as a risk factor for knee osteoarthritis: a systematic review. Br Med Bull 99:89–106, doi:10.1093/bmb/ldq043

Paxton ES, Stock MV, Brophy RH (2011) Meniscal repair versus partial meniscectomy: a systematic review comparing reoperation rates and clinical outcomes. Arthroscopy 27(9):1275–1288, doi:10.1016/j.arthro.2011.03.088

Rodkey WG, Steadman JR, Li ST (1999) A clinical study of collagen meniscus implants to restore the injured meniscus. Clin Orthop Relat Res (367 Suppl):S281–S292

Sakaguchi Y, Sekiya I, Yagishita K, Muneta T (2005) Comparison of human stem cells derived from various mesenchymal tissues: superiority of synovium as a cell source. Arthritis Rheum 52(8):2521–2529, doi:10.1002/art.21212

Salata MJ, Gibbs AE, Sekiya JK (2010) A systematic review of clinical outcomes in patients undergoing meniscectomy. Am J Sports Med 38(9):1907–1916, doi:10.1177/0363546510370196

Scotti C, Hirschmann MT, Antinolfi P, Martin I, Peretti GM (2013) Meniscus repair and regeneration: review on current methods and research potential. Eur Cell Mater 26:150–170

Shaffer B, Kennedy S, Klimkiewicz J, Yao L (2000) Preoperative sizing of meniscal allografts in meniscus transplantation. Am J Sports Med 28(4):524–533

Starke C, Kopf S, Petersen W, Becker R (2009) Meniscal repair. Arthroscopy 25(9):1033–1044, doi:10.1016/j.arthro.2008.12.010

Steadman JR, Rodkey WG (2005) Tissue-engineered collagen meniscus implants: 5- to 6-year feasibility study results. Arthroscopy 21(5):515–525, doi:10.1016/j.arthro.2005.01.006

Stein T, Mehling AP, Welsch F, von Eisenhart-Rothe R, Jager A (2010) Long-term outcome after arthroscopic meniscal repair versus arthroscopic partial meniscectomy for traumatic meniscal tears. Am J Sports Med 38(8):1542–1548, doi:10.1177/0363546510364052

Sweigart MA, Athanasiou KA (2001) Toward tissue engineering of the knee meniscus. Tissue Eng 7(2):111–129, doi:10.1089/107632701300062697

Verdonk R, Verdonk P, Huysse W, Forsyth R, Heinrichs EL (2011) Tissue ingrowth after implantation of a novel, biodegradable polyurethane scaffold for treatment of partial meniscal lesions. Am J Sports Med 39(4):774–782, doi:10.1177/0363546511398040

Wei LC, Gao SG, Xu M, Jiang W, Tian J, Lei GH (2012) A novel hypothesis: the application of platelet-rich plasma can promote the clinical healing of white-white meniscal tears. Med Sci Monit 18(8):HY47–HY50

Wirth CJ, Peters G, Milachowski KA, Weismeier KG, Kohn D (2002) Long-term results of meniscal allograft transplantation. Am J Sports Med 30(2):174–181

Yamasaki T, Deie M, Shinomiya R, Yasunaga Y, Yanada S, Ochi M (2008) Transplantation of meniscus regenerated by tissue engineering with a scaffold derived from a rat meniscus and mesenchymal stromal cells derived from rat bone marrow. Artif Organs 32(7):519–524, doi:10.1111/j.1525-1594.2008.00580.x

Zellner J, Mueller M, Berner A, Dienstknecht T, Kujat R, Nerlich M, Hennemann B, Koller M, Prantl L, Angele M, Angele P (2010) Role of mesenchymal stem cells in tissue engineering of meniscus. J Biomed Mater Res A 94(4):1150–1161, doi:10.1002/jbm.a.32796

Zellner J, Hierl K, Mueller M, Pfeifer C, Berner A, Dienstknecht T, Krutsch W, Geis S, Gehmert S, Kujat R, Dendorfer S, Prantl L, Nerlich M, Angele P (2013) Stem cell-based tissue-engineering for treatment of meniscal tears in the avascular zone. J Biomed Mater Res B Appl Biomater 101(7):1133–1142, doi:10.1002/jbm.b.32922

11

Measurements of bone tunnel size in anterior cruciate ligament reconstruction: 2D versus 3D computed tomography model

Bernardo Crespo[1], Cathrine Aga[2], Katharine J Wilson[1], Shannon M Pomeroy[1], Robert F LaPrade[1,3], Lars Engebretsen[2,4] and Coen A Wijdicks[5*]

Abstract

Background: Revision anterior cruciate ligament (ACL) reconstruction requires a precise evaluation of previous tunnel locations and diameters. Enlargement of the tunnels, despite not usually affecting primary reconstruction outcomes, plays an important role in revision ACL management. Three dimensional (3D) computed tomography (CT) models are reported to be the most accurate method for identifying the tunnel position and possible conflicts with a revision tunnel placement. However, the ability of 3D CT to measure the tunnel size is still not proven. The goal of this study was to evaluate the ability of measuring the size of the bone tunnels in ACL reconstructed knees with 3D CT compared to the traditional two dimensional (2D) CT method.

Methods: Twenty-four patients had CT scans performed immediately following ACL reconstruction surgery. Their femoral tunnels size were measured by a standard 2D CT measurement and then compared with three novel 3D CT measuring methods: the best transverse section method, the best fit cylinder method and the wall thickness method. The drill size used during surgery was used as a control measure for the tunnel width. Intra-class correlation coefficients were obtained.

Results: The intra-class correlation coefficient and respective 95% confidence interval range (ICC [95% CI]) for the three methods compared with the drill sizes were 0.899 [0.811-0.947] for the best transverse section method, 0.745 [0.553-0.862] for the best fit cylinder method, −0.004 [−0.081 to −0.12] for the wall thickness method and 0.922 [0.713-0.97] for the 2D CT method. The mean differences compared to the drill size were 0.02 mm for the best fit transverse section method, 0.01 mm for the best fit cylinder diameter method, 3.34 mm for the wall thickness method and 0.29 mm for the 2D CT method. The intra-rater agreement (ICC [95% CI]) was excellent for the best transverse section method 0.999 [0.998-0.999] and the 2D CT method 0.969 [0.941-0.984].

Conclusions: The 3D best transverse section method presented a high correlation to the drill sizes and high intra-rater agreement, and was the best method for ACL tunnel evaluation in a 3D CT based model.

Keywords: Anterior cruciate ligament; Tunnel enlargement; Revision ACL; 3D CT model

Background

Tunnel enlargement after an anterior cruciate ligament (ACL) reconstruction is a well-known phenomenon, noticed first in the early 1990's following allograft reconstruction [1], but is also seen with different graft techniques and fixation methods [1–3]. Although no significant correlation between tunnel enlargement and clinical outcomes has currently been reported [4–9], tunnel widening may have serious implications for patients requiring ACL revision surgery. Revision ACL rates range from 10-25% [10], and a reliable assessment of the tunnel width and position is crucial to surgical planning [11].

Different methods for measuring tunnel width have been described in the literature using two dimensional (2D) radiography, computed tomography (CT) and magnetic resonance imaging (MRI) [12–16]. The 2D CT has been

* Correspondence: cwijdicks@sprivail.org
[5]Department of Biomedical Engineering, Steadman Philippon Research Institute, 181 W. Meadow Dr. Suite 1000, Vail 81657 CO, USA
Full list of author information is available at the end of the article

reported to be the best method for identifying the tunnels, especially immediately after surgery [12,17]. Other advantages of CT scans are that they eliminate the scaling issues present in plain radiographs and that they appear to be less affected by geometric factors that may influence the tunnel measurements due to knee positioning during image acquisition. Although providing the most accurate measurements, CT scans also have limitations. Interobserver and intraobserver reliability have been reported to be inconsistent [12,17].

Three dimensional (3D) CT models have been developed to create an accurate 3D model of the bones using imaging software. These models have been largely used to investigate tunnel position following cruciate ligament reconstruction and reportedly have increased intraobserver reliability [18–20]. Additionally, 3D CT models were reported to be the most reliable imaging method of showing conflict between pre-existing and desired femoral tunnel locations prior to ACL revision surgery [21]. However, to the authors' knowledge, 3D CT methods for evaluating tunnel width have not been studied to date.

The purpose of this study was to evaluate the accuracy of three novel methods for measuring tunnel width based on the 3D CT bone model of ACL reconstructed knees. The novel methods were compared to the current clinical method of measuring tunnel width using 2D CT images. We hypothesized that the novel CT bone model methods would be more accurate for measuring tunnel width than the current standard methods.

Methods

Sample selection

Prior to initiation, the study protocol was approved by the Institutional Review Board of the (Regional Committee for Medical Research Ethics) and a signed informed consent for release of scans was received from all participants. The patients' selection criteria were: age between 18 and 40 years, 3 months of rehabilitation prior to the surgical procedure and a complete ACL tear verified by history, physical examination and confirmed by an arthroscopic procedure. Patients were excluded from the study if they presented with ACL revision reconstruction, ACL lesion of the contralateral knee, concomitant PCL, lateral or medial instability at the time of the surgery, established osteoarthritis with Kellgren-Lawrence classification grades 3 or 4 or hamstring grafts unable to have a minimum diameter of 5 mm for each bundle. The 24 patients enrolled into the study were randomized to single-bundle (SB) or double-bundle (DB) ACL reconstruction, with 12 patients in each group.

Imaging protocol and 3D modeling

The CT scanner used was a Philips Brilliance 16-slice scanner, and the imaging specifications used for all patients included 1.5 mm slice thickness, 0.75 mm slice increment, 120 kV, 250 mAs, 500 mm field of view, 512 × 512 resolution. All patients had CT scans performed during the initial two days following surgery with their knee positioned in full extension. The high resolution images were evaluated by an independent investigator who was not involved in the surgical procedure or patient care.

The CT images were exported to an image analysis software (Mimics v1.6, Materialise, Leuven, Belgium) and a manual segmentation of the bone structures, bone tunnels and cortical buttons was performed. The segmentation process relies on using bone-soft tissue density variation on CT images, adjusting a density range to highlight bone anatomy on CT scan images. Manual revision of the CT images was performed to correct errors, and assure that the outline of the bone and tunnels were appropriately filled. This allowed for the creation of a patient-specific 3D bone model of the knee joint, with the tunnels appearing as empty spaces (Figures 1 and 2). This process has previously been validated, and has demonstrated high intraobserver and interobserver reliability and accuracy [22,23].

Measurement methods

Using the 3D model of each patient's knee, three different techniques for measuring tunnel width were evaluated: best fit cylinder, overall wall thickness and transverse section diameter. The best fit cylinder method consisted of creating an analytical best fit cylinder to the entire tunnel length (Figure 3). The wall thickness method consisted of an internal software function (Mimics, Materialise, Leuven, Belgium) that measured the perpendicular distance from each triangle that formed the 3D model to the opposite side of the model (Figure 4). The best fit transverse section method was performed by fitting a center axis to the entire tunnel length and then fitting a circle to the tunnel walls at its mid-length (Figure 5).

The traditional method for measuring tunnel width in a 2D CT scan was also evaluated. The tunnel diameter was measured at the tunnel mid-point in all three image planes (axial, sagittal, and coronal) using a straight line drawing tool (Figure 6). The mean value of the measurements from the three image planes was used for comparison.

The 2D CT measurements and the best fit transverse section method measurements were repeated after one month to determine the intra-observer reliability of the method. The best fit cylinder and wall thickness methods were entirely automated by the software, having a complete agreement between the two consecutive measurements. An orthopedic surgeon (B.C.) trained by a musculoskeletal radiologist performed all measurements.

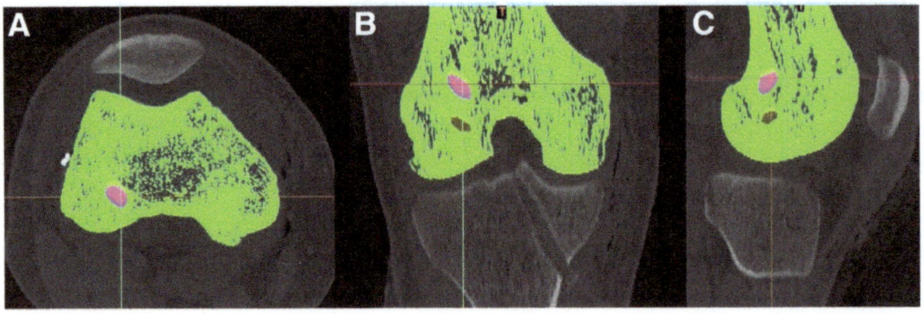

Figure 1 Segmentation process of 2D CT images. Segmentation process performed on the original 2D CT images viewed in axial **(A)**, coronal **(B)** and sagittal **(C)** CT images.

Surgical technique

All procedures were performed by one surgeon (S.J.). The reconstructions relied on ACL anatomical landmarks, with the SB reconstruction targeting to have the tunnel in a central position of the ACL footprint, and the DB reconstruction aimed to place the tunnels in the center of each ACL bundle, as previously described by Muller et al. [24]. The drilling was performed through an accessory anteromedial portal with the knee in hyperflexion for both techniques, following a technique as described by Brown et al. [25]. The gracilis and semitendinosus tendons were harvested and doubled or tripled according to their size and length. The tunnel sizes were defined based on the graft diameters in a 0.5 mm increase graft ruler scale (Smith and Nephew, Andover, MA, USA), and the drill size was selected to match the graft diameter. A suspension device was used for femoral fixation (EndoButton - Smith and Nephew, Andover, MA, USA) and an interference screw (Biosure PK - Smith and Nephew, Andover, MA, USA), was used for tibial fixation.

Statistical analysis

Because the tibia interference screw fixation method produced an intra-operative tunnel widening, and the tunnel size could be significantly different from the original drill size, the tibial tunnels were not used for comparison of methods. The measurements of the femoral ACL reconstruction tunnels were obtained by using the different techniques and were compared to the drill size used to prepare the respective tunnel. Mean (±SD) differences between measurement and drill size are reported. Intra- and inter-method agreement were assessed using the two-way random, single measures, absolute agreement form of the intra-class correlation coefficient (ICC). ICC values were classified as excellent (>0.75), fair to good (0.40 - 0.75) or poor (<0.40) [26–28]. All statistical calculations were performed using IBM SPSS Statistics, Version 20 (Armonk, NY, USA). Histograms of all measurements and differences from drill size were inspected and found to be reasonably normally distributed, prompting the use of parametric statistical tools.

Results

Tunnel size

The drill size range used for the ACL reconstructions in this study was from 5.0 to 9.0 mm and the difference between the average of the drill sizes and the measurements means and respective standard deviation were 0.29 ± 0.4 mm for the 2D CT method, 0.02 ± 0.6 mm for the best fit transverse section method, 0.01 ± 0.8 mm for the best fit cylinder diameter method and 3.34 ± 2.1 mm for the wall thickness method (Figure 7).

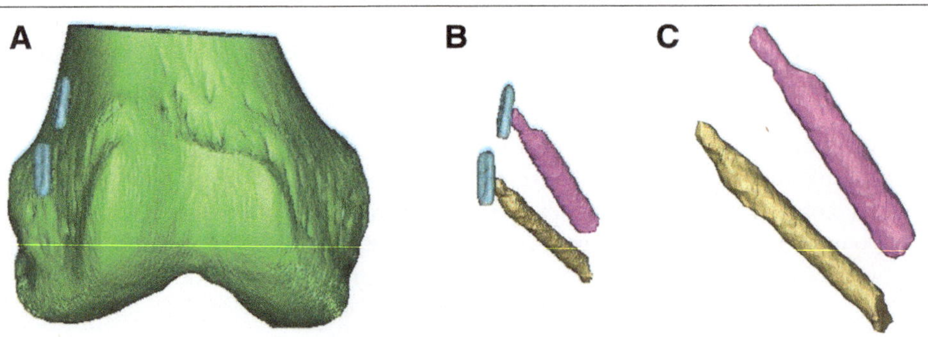

Figure 2 3D model acquisition. CT based 3D model showing all bone structures segmented **(A)**. Same image with the femur hidden **(B)**, and a closer view of the segmented femoral tunnels **(C)**.

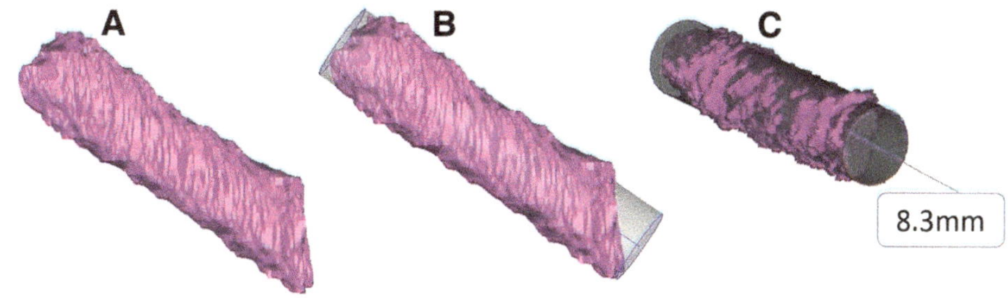

Figure 3 Best fit cylinder method. The original tunnel 3D model was exported to the 3D-matic® software **(A)**. An analytical cylinder was generated **(B)** and, a surface cylinder was created guided by the analytical cylinder. The cylinder diameter was measured **(C)**.

The intraclass correlation coefficient and respective 95% confidence interval range (ICC [95% CI]) comparing the measurements to the drill sizes was 0.922 [0.713-0.97] for the 2D CT method, 0.899 [0.811-0.947] for the best fit transverse section method, 0.745 [0.553-0.862] for the best fit cylinder method and −0.004 [−0.081-0.12] for the wall thickness (Table 1).

Evaluating the measurements obtained on the original 2D CT scans, and comparing the measurements on each image plane (coronal, axial and sagittal) with the average of the drill sizes, there was an ICC [95% CI] of 0.922 [0.713-0.97] for the mean and 0.876 [0.711-0.942] for the measurements obtained on the coronal view, 0.907 [0.548-0.968] for the axial view and 0.876 [0.759-0.936] for the sagittal view (Table 2).

Intra-rater ICCs

The intra-rater agreement (ICC [95% CI]) was excellent for the best-fit circle 0.999 [0.998-0.999] and the 2D CT method 0.969 [0.941-0.984]. The best fit cylinder and the wall thickness methods were totally automated, with total agreement (ICC of 1.00) between measurements.

Discussion

The most important finding of our study was that the 3D best fit transverse section method presented excellent accuracy for measuring tunnel width and excellent intraobserver reliability. Of all the 3D model methods, the best fit cylinder method was the closest to the mean drill size. However, it had a higher standard deviation and lower accuracy, evaluated by the ICC, compared to the transverse section method. The wall thickness method produced significant smaller values than the mean drill size. Additionally, the 2D CT measurement method presented a high correlation to the drill sizes used to ream the tunnels and a high intraobserver reliability.

Several studies evaluated enlargement by comparing late post-operative CT images and the drill sizes used during the procedure. Comparing immediate postoperative images to the drill size diameters, we could access the accuracy of CT based methods. As expected, we obtained a high correlation between the drill diameter and the 2D CT measurements, validating the use of the drill size as the immediate postoperative diameter for the ACL femoral tunnels.

Although the 2D CT method for tunnel enlargement evaluation is commonly used, its limitations regarding

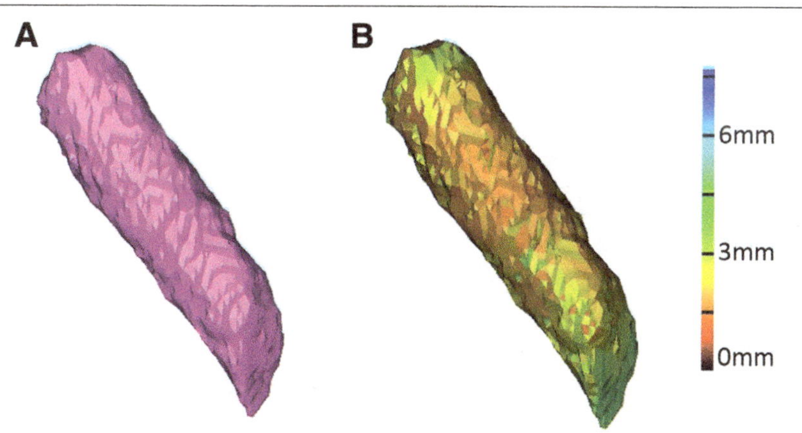

Figure 4 Wall thickness method. The original tunnel 3D model exported to the 3D-matic® software **(A)** and the Wall Thickness function was applied. A color scale showed the distance between the triangles and the opposite wall **(B)**.

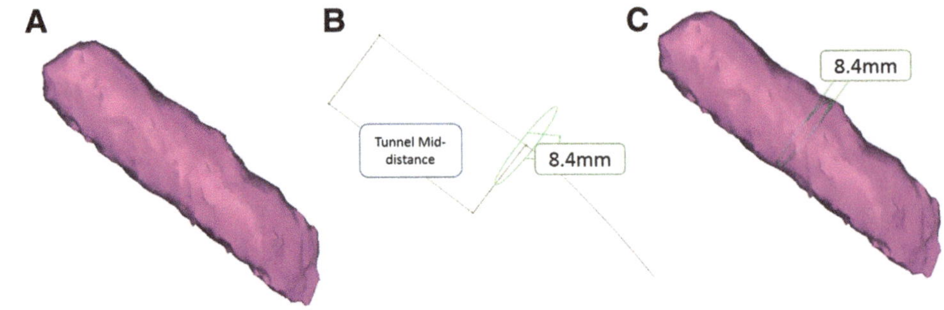

Figure 5 Best transverse section method. The segmented tunnel **(A)** was used as a guide for the automated centerline drawing made by the Mimics® software. Centerline half-way distances were measured and the best fit diameter on this points was evaluated **(B)**. Image of the tunnel model with the measurements on its surface **(C)**.

alignment between CT plane cuts and limb/tunnel orientation have been previously described [17]. The ACL reconstruction technique has lately changed to a more anatomic graft placement with more oblique tunnels related to the femoral axis [29], and this technique change can theoretically increase the tunnel-CT axis orientation mismatch [14] attempted to minimize this factor by reorienting the images to align the tunnel axis, a step that has to be done for every tunnel and can be susceptible to error, especially in the presence of major enlargements, when the tunnel axis is less clear. In this study, the use of the average of all three 2D CT plane measurements improved the 2D method agreement when compared to the measurement in one single image plane (Table 2). However this strategy was time consuming compared to the 3D methods, once the 3D model is available, and hence not commonly used in clinical practice. Additionally, the tunnel enlargement does not seem to be an organized symmetric expansion of the tunnel, and Fink et al. [9] described that the tunnel enlargement differed according to the CT views used for the measurement, a 30.6% enlargement of the tibial tunnel, in the sagittal plane, against a 16.4% coronal plane enlargement was reported 2 years after surgery. All these issues can be potentially eliminated by the use of 3D model methods, because they portray the entire shape of the tunnel and thereby address the 3D geometry of the tunnel.

The best fit transverse section method presented an excellent agreement to the drill sizes (0.899 of ICC) and a mean difference of 0.07 mm to the drill sizes, comparable to 2D CT method with a 0.9222 ICC and 0.33 mm mean difference to the drill size. The intra-rater agreement was excellent (0.999 of ICC) because of the semi-automated nature of the measurement that only varied according to the position of the measurement. The ability of using the 3D image avoids the possible bias of the image cut selection and the tunnel-images mismatch present on 2D measurements. This method preserves the 2D CT method ability of evaluating the enlargement in different portions of the tunnel length. The best fit cylinder method presented a good agreement to the drill size (0.745 of ICC), and the closest mean difference to the drill size 0.04 mm. It has the advantage of evaluating the entire tunnel at once and was automated. The wall thickness method presented a poor agreement to the drill size and had a mean difference compared to the drill sizes of 3.38 mm due to variability in orientation of the triangles that composed the 3D model shape, downsizing the overall measurement.

A high intraobserver agreement value was obtained for the 2D CT method in our study. Previous papers reported much lower intraobserver agreement rates when using

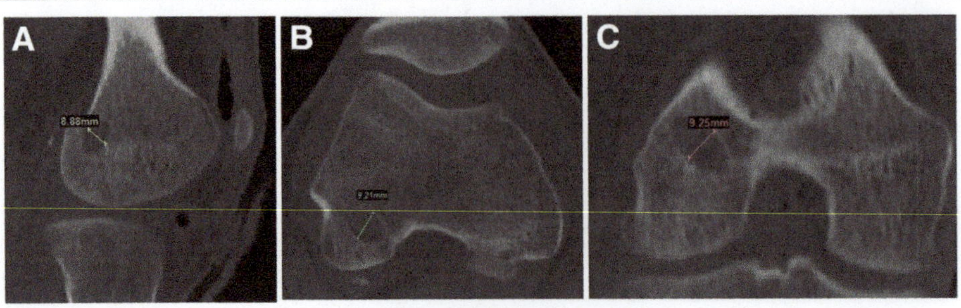

Figure 6 2D CT method. The measurements were made based on the original CT images, and the tunnels were assessed in all three CT planes: coronal **(A)**, sagittal **(B)**, and axial **(C)**.

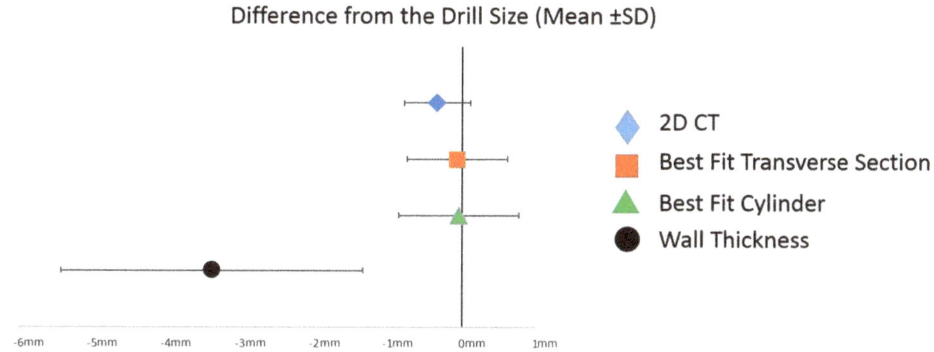

Figure 7 Difference from Drill Size Mean. Shows the difference between the average of the drill size and the mean of the measurements for each method with respective standard deviations.

this method with ICC rates from 0.44 to 0.74 [5,17,30] This difference may be because our patients were evaluated immediately after surgery, when the tunnel remains cylindrical and has not enlarged. Measurement of an enlarged and misshaped tunnel on the 2D CT method would be more difficult, because it would greatly depend on how the enlargement was positioned within the CT field of view, if it was visible in the image planes and in which image the observer choose to perform the measurement. This could lead to a reduced reliability of the method.

3D CT scan is an important adjuvant in a clinical setting, and it has been validated to be the best method for tunnel placement evaluation and for planning a revision cruciate ligament surgery [18–20]. Many CT scanners currently have internal capacity of creating a 3D reconstruction of the bones and software to perform 3D measurements. Additionally this study demonstrated that with simple measurement tools an accurate measurement that addresses the 3D architecture of the tunnels was easily obtained.

This study has some limitations related to a small sample size, and the fact that one investigator performed all the measurements and an inter-observer evaluation was therefore not performed. The images were obtained in the immediate post operative and the effects of an asymmetrical enlargement in methods accuracy could not be evaluated. Additionally, the 2D CT measurements were collected in the original scan images, and the tunnels were not always well aligned to the images axis. However, this is the most usual measurement method on clinical practice, and no standardization for tunnel measurement is available in the literature.

Conclusions

The 3D CT based best-fit transverse section measurement method demonstrated excellent accuracy and reliability for the ACL reconstruction tunnel measurement in immediate post-operative patients. This method was found to be the method of choice for tunnel measurement in 3D models. The best fit cylinder method also presented a high correlation to the drill size, and could be very helpful in revision ACL surgery planning by optimizing the new tunnel size to fit the previous tunnel. The wall thickness method presented poor results in evaluating the tunnels in the 3D model, and would not be recommended.

Table 1 Methods agreement to the drill size

Absolute agreement with drill size			
		ICC[α]	95% CI[β]
2D CT	Mean	0.922	[0.713 to 0.97]
	Coronal	0.876	[0.711 to 0.942]
	Axial	0.907	[0.548 to 0.968]
	Sagittal	0.876	[0.759 to 0.936]
3D Model	Best fit transverse section	0.899	[0.784 to 0.938]
	Best fit cylinder	0.745	[0.553 to 0.862]
	Wall Thickness	−0.004	[−0.081 to 0.12]

Shows the intraclass correlation coefficient (ICC) and respective confidence intervals range ([95%CI]) for the CT and 3D model first measurements compared to the drill sizes.
[α]ICC (intraclass correlation coefficient).
[β]95% CI (95% confidence intervals range).

Table 2 Intra-rater agreement on CT and 3D measurements

Intra-rater absolute agreement			
		ICC[α]	95% CI[β]
2D CT	Mean	0.969	[0.941 to 0.984]
	Coronal	0.949	[0.903 to 0.974]
	Axial	0.947	[0.899 to 0.973]
	Sagittal	0.949	[0.903 to 0.974]
3D Model	Best fit Transverse Section	0.999	[0.998 to 0.999]

Shows the intraclass correlation coefficient (ICC) and respective confidence intervals range ([95%CI]) between the first and second measurements performed with the CT and 3D best fit circle methods.
[α]ICC (intraclass correlation coefficient).
[β]95% CI (95% confidence intervals range).

Abbreviations

ACL: Anterior cruciate ligament; 2D: Two dimensional; CT: Computed tomography; 3D: Three dimensional; SB: Single-bundle; DB: Double-bundle; SD: Standard deviation; ICC: Intraclass correlation coefficient; CI: Confidence interval.

Competing interests

One or more authors receive scientific support from Smith and Nephew, which provided donation of surgical supplies for this study.

Authors' contributions

BC, CA, KJW, SP, RFL, LE and CAW have made significant contributions to the conception, design, and were involved in acquisition, analysis and interpretation of the data. BC, CA, KJW, SP, RFL, LE and CAW have worked on drafting the manuscript and approved the final version of the manuscript to be published.

Acknowledgements

We thank Grant Dornan, MSc, for his contribution of statistical expertise to the analysis of this study. We also thank Steinar Johansen (S.J.), M.D. for performing the surgical procedure and allowing the evaluation of his patients. The orthopedic department of the Oslo University Hospital is gratefully acknowledged for providing the imaging resources. The project was supported by Oslo Sports Trauma Research Center and Steadman Philippon Research Institute.

Author details

[1]Steadman Philippon Research Institute, 181 W. Meadow Dr. Suite 1000, Vail 81657 CO, USA. [2]Department of Orthopaedic Surgery, Oslo University Hospital and Faculty of Medicine, University of Oslo, Oslo, Norway. [3]The Steadman Clinic, Vail, CO, USA. [4]Oslo Sports Trauma Research Center, Oslo, Norway. [5]Department of Biomedical Engineering, Steadman Philippon Research Institute, 181 W. Meadow Dr. Suite 1000, Vail 81657 CO, USA.

References

1. Roberts TS, Drez D, Jr, McCarthy W, Paine R (1991) Anterior cruciate ligament reconstruction using freeze-dried, ethylene oxide-sterilized, bone-patellar tendon-bone allografts Two year results in thirty-six patients. Am J Sports Med 19(1):35–41
2. Peyrache MD, Djian P, Christel P, Witvoet J (1996) Tibial tunnel enlargement after anterior cruciate ligament reconstruction by autogenous bone-patellar tendon-bone graft. Knee Surg Sports Traumatol Arthrosc 4(1):2–8
3. Webster KE, Feller JA, Hameister KA (2001) Bone tunnel enlargement following anterior cruciate ligament reconstruction: a randomised comparison of hamstring and patellar tendon grafts with 2-year follow-up. Knee Surg Sports Traumatol Arthrosc 9(2):86–91
4. Klein JP, Lintner DM, Downs D, Vavrenka K (2003) The incidence and significance of femoral tunnel widening after quadrupled hamstring anterior cruciate ligament reconstruction using femoral cross Pin fixation. Arthroscopy 19(5):470–476
5. Webster KE, Chiu JJ, Feller JA (2005) Impact of measurement error in the analysis of bone tunnel enlargement after anterior cruciate ligament reconstruction. Am J Sports Med 33(11):1680–1687
6. Clatworthy MG, Annear P, Bulow JU, Bartlett RJ (1999) Tunnel widening in anterior cruciate ligament reconstruction: a prospective evaluation of hamstring and patella tendon grafts. Knee Surg Sports Traumatol Arthrosc 7(3):138–145
7. Dyer CR, Elrod BF (1995) Tibial and femoral bone tunnel enlargement following allograft replacement of the anterior cruciate ligament. Arthroscopy 11:353–354
8. Fahey M, Indelicato PA (1994) Bone tunnel enlargement after anterior cruciate ligament replacement. Am J Sports Med 22(3):410–414
9. Fink C, Zapp M, Benedetto KP, Hackl W, Hoser C, Rieger M (2001) Tibial tunnel enlargement following anterior cruciate ligament reconstruction with patellar tendon autograft. Arthroscopy 17(2):138–143
10. Höher J, Möller HD, Fu FH (1998) Bone tunnel enlargement after anterior cruciate ligament reconstruction: fact or fiction? Knee Surg Sports Traumatol Arthrosc 6(4):231–240
11. Hofbauer M, Muller B, Murawski CD, Baraga M, van Eck CF, Fu FH (2013) Strategies for revision surgery after primary double-bundle Anterior Cruciate Ligament (ACL) reconstruction. Knee Surg Sports Traumatol Arthrosc 21(9):2072–2080
12. Webster KE, Feller JA, Elliott J, Hutchison A, Payne R (2004) A comparison of bone tunnel measurements made using computed tomography and digital plain radiography after anterior cruciate ligament reconstruction. Arthroscopy 20(9):946–950
13. Kawaguchi Y, Kondo E, Kitamura N, Kai S, Inoue M, Yasuda K (2011) Comparisons of femoral tunnel enlargement in 169 patients between single-bundle and anatomic double-bundle anterior cruciate ligament reconstructions with hamstring tendon grafts. Knee Surg Sports Traumatol Arthrosc 19(8):1249–1257
14. Siebold R, Cafaltzis K (2010) Differentiation between intraoperative and postoperative bone tunnel widening and communication in double-bundle anterior cruciate ligament reconstruction: a prospective study. Arthroscopy 26(8):1066–1073
15. Choi NH, Oh JS, Jung SH, Victoroff BN (2013) Tibial tunnel widening after hamstring anterior cruciate ligament reconstructions: comparison between rigidfix and Bio- TransFix. The Knee 20(1):31–35
16. Vadalà A, Iorio R, De Carli A, Argento G, Di Sanzo V, Conteduca F, Ferretti A (2007) The effect of accelerated, brace free, rehabilitation on bone tunnel enlargement after ACL reconstruction using hamstring tendons: a CT study. Knee Surg Sports Traumatol Arthrosc 15(4):365–371
17. Marchant MH, Jr, Willimon SC, Vinson E, Pietrobon R, Garrett WE, Higgins LD (2010) Comparison of plain radiography, computed tomography, and magnetic resonance imaging in the evaluation of bone tunnel widening after anterior cruciate ligament reconstruction. Knee Surg Sports Traumatol Arthrosc 18(8):1059–1064
18. Kopf S, Forsythe B, Wong AK, Tashman S, Irrgang JJ, Fu FH (2012) Transtibial ACL reconstruction technique fails to position drill tunnels anatomically in vivo 3D CT study. Knee Surg Sports Traumatol Arthrosc 20(11):2200–2227
19. Meuffels DE, Potters JW, Koning AH, Brown CH, Jr, Verhaar JA, Reijman M (2011) Visualization of postoperative anterior cruciate ligament reconstruction bone tunnels: reliability of standard radiographs, CT scans, and 3D virtual reality images. Acta Orthop 82(6):699–703
20. Youm YS, Cho SD, Eo J, Lee KJ, Jung KH, Cha JR (2012) 3D CT analysis of femoral and tibial tunnel positions after modified transtibial single bundle ACL reconstruction with varus and internal rotation of the Tibia. Knee 20(4):272–276
21. Tscholl PM, Biedert RM, Gal I (2013) Radiological evaluation for conflict of the femoral tunnel entrance area prior to anterior cruciate ligament revision surgery. Int Orthop. doi:10.1007/s00264-013-2126-8. ahead of printl
22. Bryce CD, Pennypacker JL, Kulkarni N, Paul EM, Hollenbeak CS, Mosher TJ, Armstrong AD (2008) Validation of three-dimensional models of in situ scapulae. J Shoulder Elbow Surg 17(5):825–832
23. Moro-oka TA, Hamai S, Miura H, Shimoto T, Higaki H, Fregly BJ, Iwamoto Y, Banks SA (2007) Can magnetic resonance imaging-derived bone models Be used for accurate motion measurement with single-plane three-dimensional shape registration? J Orthop Res 25(7):867–872
24. Muller B, Hofbauer M, Wongcharoenwatana J, Fu F (2012) Indications and contraindications for double-bundle ACL reconstruction. International Orthopaedics (SICOT) 37:239–246
25. Brown CH, Jr, Spalding T, Robb C (2013) Medial portal technique for single-bundle anatomical anterior cruciate ligament reconstruction. International Orthopaedics (SICOT) 37:253–269
26. Chicchetti D, Bronen R, Spencer S, Haut S, Berg A, Oliver P, Tyrer P (2006) Rating scales, scales of measurement, issues of reliability. J Nerv Ment Dis 194(8):557–564
27. Shrout PE, Fleiss JL (1979) Intraclass correlations: uses in assessing rater reliab. Psychol Bulletin 86:420–428
28. Landis JR, Koch GC (1977) The measurement of observer agreement for categorical data. Biometrics 33:159–174
29. Illingworth KD, Hensler D, Working ZM, Macalena JA, Tashman S, Fu FH (2011) A simple evaluation of anterior cruciate ligament femoral tunnel position: the inclination angle and femoral tunnel angle. Am J Sports Med 39(12):2611–2618
30. Järvelä T (2007) Double-bundle versus single-bundle anterior cruciate ligament reconstruction: a prospective, randomize clinical study. Knee Surg Sports Traumatol Arthrosc 15(5):500–507

12

Histological characteristics of ligament healing after bio-enhanced repair of the transected goat ACL

D Tan Nguyen[1*], Sietske Dellbrügge[1], Paul P Tak[2,3], Savio L-Y Woo[4], Leendert Blankevoort[1] and Niek C van Dijk[1]

Abstract

Background: Recently, healing of a ruptured anterior cruciate ligament (ACL) is reconsidered. In a previous study, we have shown that the transected ACL can heal after treatment with the triple X locking suture alone or combined with small intestine submucosa (SIS). The first research question of this study was whether the healing ACLs in both groups show histological characteristics that are typical for ligament healing. Secondly, did the combined treatment with SIS lead to improved histological healing, in terms of the morphology of the fibrous synovial layer, the extracellular matrix (ECM), collagen fiber orientation, cellularity, ratio of myofibroblasts, and collagen type 3 staining. The hypothesis was that SIS enhances the healing by the scaffolding effect, endogenous growth factors, and chemoattractants.

Methods: In the Suture group, the left ACL was transected and sutured with the triple X locking suture repair technique. In the Suture-SIS group, the left ACL underwent the same procedure with the addition of SIS. The right ACL served as internal control. Standard histology and immunostaining of α-smooth muscle actin (SMA) and collagen type 3 were used.

Results: Microscopy showed that the fibrous synovial layer around the ACL was reestablished in both groups. The collagen fibers in the Suture-SIS group stained denser, were more compactly arranged, and the ECM contained fewer voids and fat vacuoles. Neovasculature running between the collagen fibers was observed in both experimental groups. Collagen type 3 stained less in the Suture-SIS group. The cellularity in the Suture group, Suture-SIS group and Control was 1265 ± 1034 per mm^2, 954 ± 378 per mm^2, 254 ± 92, respectively; 49%, 26% and 20% of the cells stain positive for α-SMA, respectively.

Conclusion: The healing ACL in both treated groups showed histological characteristics which are comparable to the spontaneously healing medial collateral ligament and showed that the ACL has a similar intrinsic healing response. Though, no definitive conclusions on the beneficial effects of the SIS scaffold on the healing process can be made.

Keywords: Anterior cruciate ligament; Healing; Bio-enhanced ACL repair; Primary repair; Small intestine submucosa

Background

The anterior cruciate ligament (ACL) of the knee joint is frequently ruptured and may often require reconstruction with autologous tendon grafts to treat chronic knee instability (Beynnon et al. 2005; Woo et al. 2006). The clinical and functional outcome of ACL reconstruction is generally satisfactory, allowing the majority of the patient population to return to work and a part to return to pre-injury level sports activity. However, ACL reconstruction does not fully restore the function of the intact ACL. Additionally, there are several drawbacks (Busam et al. 2008; Drogset et al. 2010; von Porat et al. 2004). Though, it is commonly believed that the ACL does not have a healing response and cannot heal, some researchers are re-exploring methods to repair the ACL in the acute phase (Fisher et al. 2012; Fleming et al. 2009; Murray et al. 2007; Nguyen et al. 2013; Kohl et al. 2013). In a previous study, our research group reported that

* Correspondence: nguyen.ortho.research@live.nl
[1]Department of Orthopedic Surgery, Orthopaedic Research Center Amsterdam, Academic Medical Center, University of Amsterdam, P.O. Box 22660, 1100 DD Amsterdam, The Netherlands
Full list of author information is available at the end of the article

the treatment of the transected ACL with a new suture repair technique in combination with the small intestinal submucosa (SIS) bioscaffold lead to healing in a goat model (Nguyen et al. 2013). The ACLs in both experimental groups were healing and continuous. Biomechanical testing showed that the repaired ACLs contributed to the knee function (Nguyen et al. 2013). The total AP translation of the repaired ACL was 290% to 440% of the intact control under 67 N anterior and posterior tibial load (AP load). The normalized stiffness of the healing ACLs was about half of the control ACLs. The ACLs were retained for this study with the aim to histologically investigate whether the healing ACL has histologically characteristics as the healing medial collateral ligament (MCL). The comparison with the MCL was made as the MCL is regarded as the knee ligament that has a healing response and that can heal spontaneously. As such, the first research question of this study was whether the ACLs treated with the triple X suture alone or combined with small intestine submucosa (SIS) resemble the histological healing characteristics as observed in the healing MCL. Secondly, does the combined treatment with SIS leads to improved histological healing characteristics, in terms of the morphology of the fibrous synovial layer, the extracellular matrix (ECM), collagen fiber orientation, cellularity, ratio of myofibroblasts over total cell count, and collagen type 3 staining. These parameters provide a general evaluation of the healing process in ligaments. Myofibroblasts have shown to play an important role in the healing and remodeling of MCL, with an initial increase in density after injury and steadily normalization during the remodeling phase. Myofibroblasts have also been shown in the injured but non-healing ACL, though the density remained low (<1.5%) (Menetrey et al. 2011). SIS bioscaffold is mainly composed of collagen type 1 and contains endogenous growth factors such as fibroblast growth factors (FGF) and TGF-β, as well as other chemoattractants which enhances the healing (Hodde et al. 1996; Hodde et al. 2005; Voytik-Harbin et al. 1997). Several studies have shown that SIS can act as a provisional scaffold to promote cell migration and to enhance revascularization and repair (Gilbert et al. 2007; Liang et al. 2008; Zantop et al. 2006; Liang et al. 2011; Raeder et al. 2002). It was thus hypothesized that SIS enhances the healing of the ACL and that the SIS-treated ACL is closer to the normal ACL histologically, i.c. compacter ECM, less voids, more cells, less myofibroblasts and less collagen type 3 staining.

Methods

The goat ACLs from the Suture group (n = 4), Suture-SIS group (n = 4), and their respective intact control group (n = 8) were retained from a previous study (Nguyen et al. 2013). Initially, there were five samples in the Suture group; however due to an embedding error and consequently cutting errors one sample was lost for histological analysis. For a detailed description of the animal protocol and surgery, which was approved by the institutional Animal Ethics Committee at the University of Amsterdam, see Nguyen et al., (Nguyen et al. 2013). Briefly, in the left goat knee, a medial parapatellar incision was made to expose the ACL. The ACL was hooked and transected in its midsubstance. In the Suture repair group, the suture repair was performed using absorbable Vicryl 2–0 sutures, using a previously described triple X locking suture technique. Due to its locking configuration, the suture tightens around the collagen fibers when tensile forces are applied, thus providing approximation under tension, greater ultimate tensile strength, and resistance to gapping (Becker and Davidoff 1977; Hatanaka et al. 2000). Subsequently, the medial arthrotomy was closed in separate layers. In the Suture-SIS group, the same procedures were performed as in the Suture group with the addition of porcine derived SIS (Cook Biotech Inc., West Lafayette, IN, USA). Six small pieces of SIS (2 mm x 2 mm x 200 μm) were loosely placed within the midsubstance of the injury site. A hydrated sheet of SIS (5 cm x 2,5 cm x 200 μm) was wrapped around the injury site and affixed with Vicryl 6–0 to the ACL. The ACL in the right hind limb was unoperated in both groups and served as internal intact control. Postoperatively, the animals were allowed full weight bearing immediately after the operation without any external bracing of the operated limb. Free cage activity and later a pasture, food and water was *ad libitum*. At twelve weeks post-surgery, all animals were euthanized and the hind limbs were immediately stored at −20°C until biomechanical testing. The ACLs were kept intact during biomechanical testing and were not tested to failure. The whole ACL was removed from the femur-ACL-tibia complex by cutting the whole ACL from its tibial and femoral bone insertion. The whole ACL was embedded in Tissue-Tek O.C.T. compound (Sakura Finetek, Japan), frozen, and stored at −80°C.

Histology

Five-micrometer thick sections were cut in a cryostat microtome and mounted on glass slides (Star Frost adhesive slides, Knittelgläser, Germany), and stored at −80° C until staining. The cryosections was made by SD and number coded. The staining and analyses were done by DTN and MdB. Standard Haematoxylin & Eosin (H&E) was performed to grossly evaluate the fibrous synovial membrane, the ECM, and cell morphology. Lendrum Masson's trichrome staining was performed to specifically stain the collagen and to evaluate the collagen fiber orientation. The sections were stained sequentially in celestine blue, haematoxiline, Ponceau de Xylidine and tartrazine. The collagen was stained in yellow, the cytoplasm in red and the nuclei in blue. The slides were observed under a light microscope and pictures were taken from the midsubstance at the healing areas with a low magnification (10X) to show the whole ACL and with higher magnifications (100X, 200X and 400X).

Immunohistochemical staining

An AEC (3-Amino-9-ethylcarbazole) labeling immunohistochemical methodology was used with the following antibodies: goat monoclonal mouse anti-human alpha-smooth muscle actin (α-SMA) antibody (Sigma-Aldrich, St. Louis, MO) as a marker for myofibroblasts and monoclonal mouse anti-human collagen type 3 antibody (Abcam, Cambridge, UK) to identify collagen type 3. Briefly, the sections were fixed in 100% acetone for 10 min at room temperature and washed with phosphate-buffered saline (PBS), three times for 5 minutes. Endogenous peroxidase activity was blocked using peroxidase 3% for 30 minutes at room temperature. The sections were rinsed once in PBS and 10% normal goat serum, 1% Bovine Serum Albumin (BSA) in PBS was applied for 1 hour at room temperature as a blocking agent. The monoclonal α-SMA antibody in 5% normal goat serum, 1% BSA in PBS (5 μg/ml) was applied and incubated overnight at 4°C on a shaker. Collagen type 3 was stained with monoclonal mouse collagen type 3 antibody in 5% normal goat serum, 1% BSA in PBS (0.5 μg/ml). Subsequently the sections were washed in PBS three times for 5 minutes each. The secondary antibody, a rabbit anti-mouse immunoglobulin (IgG) horseradish conjugate (HRP) (Abcam, Cambridge, UK), was applied to the sections 1 μg/ml for 60 minutes at room temperature. After a final rinse with PBS, HRP activity was visualized as a brown-red color by incubation with AEC (Sigma-Aldrich). Sections were counterstained with Mayer's haematoxylin and mounted in Kaiser's glycerol gelatin (Merck). Appropriate isotype controls were assessed in all experimental series. Positive controls for α-SMA and collagen type 3 were goat artery vessels and goat skin, respectively.

Digital image analysis

Quantification of α-SMA expressing cells in the healing tissue was performed with digital image analysis (DIA), as previously described (van der Hall et al. 2007). In brief, for each acquisition session the microscope, camera, and computer were calibrated according to a standardized procedure. Settings are recorded and stored and used for the entire session. After immunohistochemical staining, three representative regions of 1.45 x 1.45 mm in each section are identified at low power magnification (without capillaries, fat voids and artifacts) and separated in 18 consecutive high power fields (HPF). The18 HPF images are analyzed by computer-assisted image analysis using a Syndia algorithm on a Qwin-based analysis system (Leica, Cambridge, UK) (Haringman et al. 2005). The software identified positive cells by combining two masks where areas of a nucleus surrounded by a red-brown staining are identified as positive cells, and isolated blue (nuclei without staining) or red are ignored. Positive staining of α-smooth muscle actin was expressed as number of positive cells/mm^2.

Two sections per sample stained for collagen type 3 ($n = 16$) are semi-quantitatively analyzed by DTN and MdB with a standard binocular light microscope (Olympus) at 200X magnification. The expression of collagen type 3 was scored on a 5-point scale (range 0–4), as previously described (Tak et al. 1995). A score of 0 represented no expression, while a score of 4 represented abundant expression of collagen type 3 within the healing tissue. Differences between the two observers are resolved by consensus.

Statistical test

A paired or unpaired Student's t-test was used for statistical analysis, where appropriate. A probability of $p < 0.05$ was considered statistically significant.

Results

Gross morphology

The ACLs in both experimental groups are healing and continuous. The transection site cannot be recognized. The Vicryl sutures and SIS are fully resorbed. In the Suture-SIS group, the ACL appears more opaque and denser than the Suture group (Figure 1). The cross-sectional areas of the healed ACLs in the Suture group and Suture-SIS group as reported previously are 35% and 50% of the intact control (Nguyen et al. 2013).

Fibrous synovial layer

Microscopy shows that the surface of the ACL in both the two experimental groups and the intact control ACLs were covered by a layer of cells and formed the fibrous synovial layer (Figure 2). The sub-intimal synovial layer can be observed along the whole length of the ACL without any disruption.

Extracellular matrix

H&E and Lendrum's Masson's trichrome shows that the ECM in the normal ACL was densely packed with aligned collagen fibers and a crimp pattern. No apparent capillaries, voids or lipid vacuoles can be observed (Figures 3A and 4A). Immunostaining of collagen type 3 shows that there was limited staining, scoring 1 (Figure 5A). In the Suture group the collagen fibers are aligned but loosely packed and with patches of more

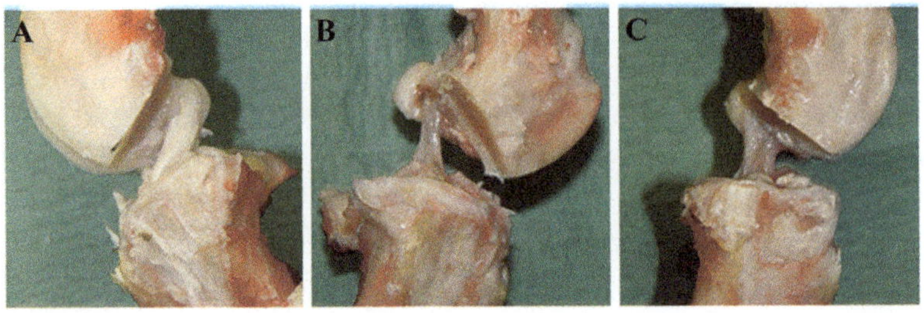

Figure 1 Gross morphology. A) Medial side view of a normal ACL. **B)** A healing ACL after suture repair only. **C)** A healing ACL after suture repair and SIS.

compact fibers but with no crimp pattern at the midsubstance (Figures 3B and 4B). Voids and lipid vacuoles can be observed. Many capillaries can be observed between the fibers, and in some slides the capillaries can be traced through the ACL. Collagen type 3 was present with a score of 2 (Figure 5B). In the Suture-SIS group the collagen fibers were aligned and more compact organized than the Suture group, but with no crimp pattern at the midsubstance (Figures 3C and 4C). Voids and lipid vacuoles can also be observed but was less present than in the Suture group. Many capillaries can be observed between the fibers, and in some slides the capillaries can also be traced through the ACL. Collagen type 3 is present with a score of 2 (Figure 5C). In all groups, the ACLs were vital and there were no necrotic areas.

Fibroblast morphology, cell and myofibroblast density

In the control groups, normal nucleus morphology and cell distribution can be observed within the ACL. Generally, ovoid fibroblast nuclei were located at the proximal ACL, rod-like fibroblast nuclei were located in the midsubstance (Figures 4A and 6A). Round to ovoid shaped nuclei were located at the distal part. Some "chrondroblasts" were observed at the distal part of the ACL. Quantification of the cells with the DIA shows that the cell density in the midsubstance of the Suture control group and Suture-SIS control group was 254 ± 92 cells/mm^2 and 204 ± 93 cells/mm^2, respectively. The ratio of α-SMA positive cells in the control groups was 19% and 20%, respectively (Table 1).

In the Suture group, nucleus morphology and cell distribution were different than in the control group. Limited variation in nucleus morphology was observed. Generally, the nuclei were elongated with more of a spindle shape and were scattered over the whole ACL. The cell density was 1265 ± 1034 and the ratio of α-SMA positive cells over total cell count was 49% (Table 1). The difference in cellularity and the difference in the ratio of the number of α-SMA positive cells over the total number of cells between the Suture group and its control group was statistically not significant ($p > 0.05$).

In the Suture-SIS group, nucleus morphology and cell distribution also differ from the control group and were

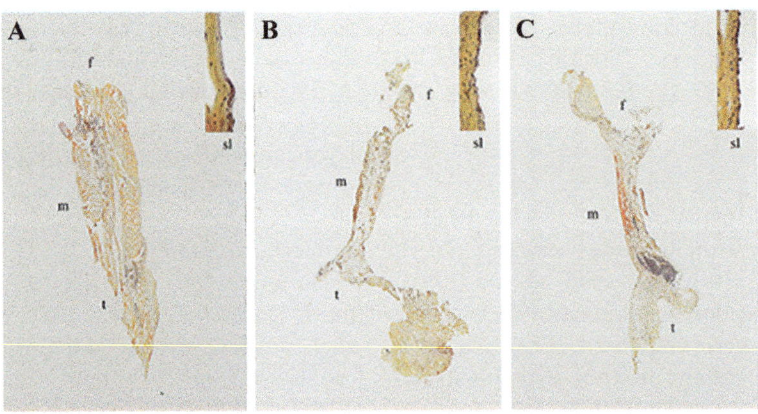

Figure 2 Histologic sections of a normal ACL (A), sutured ACL (B) and sutured ACL with SIS (C) with magnification of subintimal synovial layer at the top right (×100). The sections are stained with Lendrum Masson's trichrome; the collagen fibers are stained in yellow, the cytoplasm in red and the nuclei in blue.

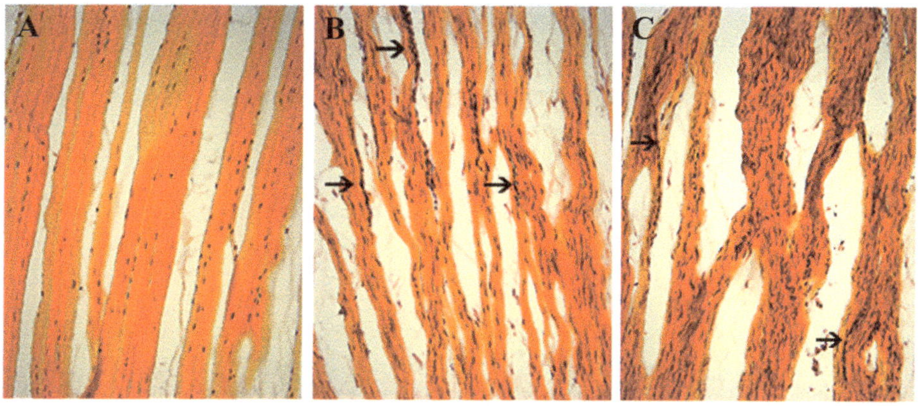

Figure 3 Histologic sections of a normal ACL (A), sutured ACL (B) and sutured ACL with SIS (C). The sections are stained with Lendrum Masson's trichrome; the collagen fibers are stained in yellow, the cytoplasm in red and the nuclei in blue. The ECM of both the Suture and Suture-SIS group have aligned collagen fibers, the collagen fibers in the Suture-SIS group stained denser, more compact arranged and contained less voids and less fat vacuoles. Neovasculature running parallel between the collagen fibers could be observed in both experimental groups. ×100.

comparable to the Suture group (Figures 4C and 6C). The healing ACLs in the Suture-SIS group were hypercellular with a cell density of 954 ± 378 cells/mm^2. The difference in cellularity between the Suture-SIS group and its control group was statistically significant ($p = 0.048$) (Table 1). The ratio of α-SMA positive cells of the Suture-SIS group was 26% and neared the control group (Table 1). Comparing the cellularity and the ratio of α-SMA positive between the Suture group and the Suture-SIS group, shows that there were no statistically significant differences.

Discussion

Previously, our research group has shown that a new suture technique alone or combined with SIS bioscaffold resulted in healing of the transected goat ACL (Nguyen et al. 2013). Knee laxity and ligament stiffness did not return to normal values. The difference between the Suture, Suture-SIS and intact control group was 53% and 51% respectively. However, the outcome was close to previously reported results of bone-patellar tendon-bone ACL reconstructions in goats (Spindler et al. 2009; Abramowitch et al. 2003). The results of this study shows that the healing ACL in the Suture group displayed typical histological characteristics like those observed in spontaneously-healing ligaments, such as the medial collateral ligament (MCL). The MCL's histological characteristics include, for example, disorganized and less compact organized collagen fibers, increased neovascularization, voids (e.g. lipid vacuoles), increased number of myofibroblasts and elevated content of collagen type 3 (Frank et al. 1983; Faryniarz et al. 1996; Amiel et al. 1987; Menetrey et al. 2011). Therefore, it can be concluded that the ACL has a healing response. Adding SIS to the Suture repair seems to biologically enhance

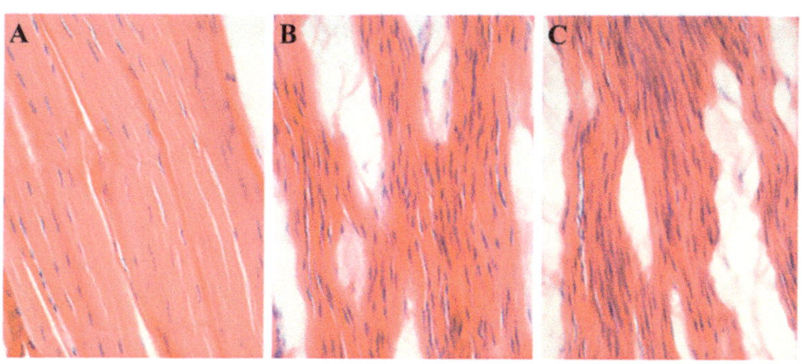

Figure 4 Histologic sections of a normal ACL (A), sutured ACL (B) and sutured ACL with SIS (C). The sections are stained with H&E. Note that the tissue is hypercellular in both the sutured and Suture & SIS ACL and that the nuclei are elongated while in the intact ACL the nuclei are rod-like shaped. ×200.

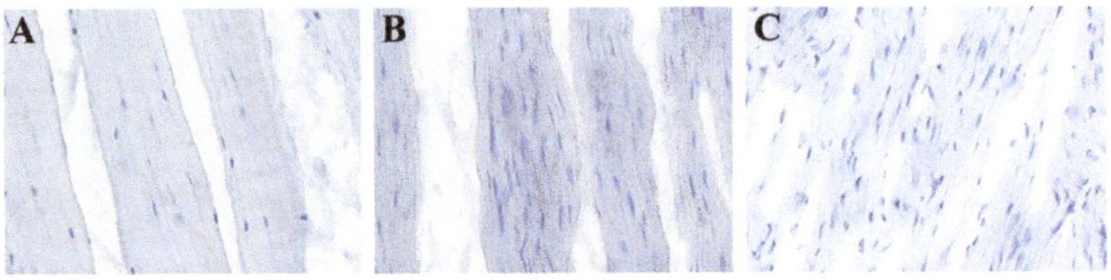

Figure 5 Immunohistologic sections of a normal ACL (A), sutured ACL (B) and sutured ACL with SIS (C). B and C show moderate red-brown staining of collagen type 3. (×400).

the healing as the collagen fibers were more compactly arranged, contain less collagen type 3, and fewer voids and fat vacuoles. The ratio of myofibroblasts to total cell count was more normal. Although this study was not designed to elucidate the mechanism behind the effects of SIS on the healing of the ACL, it was likely that the same mechanisms were involved as previously reported. In previous MCL healing studies, it was also shown that SIS acted as a provisional scaffold to promote cell migration and to enhance revascularization and repair (Gilbert et al. 2007; Liang et al. 2008; Zantop et al. 2006; Liang et al. 2011; Raeder et al. 2002). SIS treatment resulted in a greater alignment of collagen fibers and cells. Ultrastructurally, the SIS-treated group had larger collagen fibrils, and the gene expression of collagen type V, decorin, biglycan, and lumican in the SIS-treated group were significantly down-regulated, correlating with the improved morphological characteristics and mechanical properties (Liang et al. 2008). Other studies have indicated that the hypocellularity of the normal ACL might be a limiting factor leading to the failure of healing of the ACL. However, in this study it was shown that the ACL in the Suture-SIS group can become hypercellular. Thus, hypercellularity may be a positive indicator of ACL healing. Additionally, the fibroblasts in the healing ACLs were not rodlike-shaped but elongated and arranged in an aligned network. This reticular arrangement, hypercellularity, and phenotype may facilitate cell-to-cell communication and aligned deposition of newly formed collagen (Nguyen et al. 2009; Wang et al. 2003; Birk and Zycband 1994). The cells that contribute to the healing may originate from the proliferating internal ligament fibroblasts or may be bone marrow-derived or a combination of these (Zantop et al. 2006; Badylak et al. 2001; Beattie et al. 2009). The ratio of myofibroblasts in the SIS treated ACLs neared that of the normal ACL. Whether this normalization represents a good healing response cannot be answered by this study. It may be a positive indicator, as a decrease in myofibroblasts may indicate that the fibroblasts within the SIS-treated ACLs did not need to maintain the contractile phenotype as they experienced less strain within a larger cross-sectional area. Regarding the vasculature, in both experimental groups, neovasculature through the healing ACL was clearly present. In summary, all these histological observations indicate that the whole ACL was involved in the healing of the injury site.

While this study provides some new insights into the histological morphology of the healing ACLs after Suture and Suture-SIS treatment, there were several limitations. The ACLs were not directly frozen into −80°C which may have influenced and reduced the immunohistological stainings of collagen type 3. Furthermore, the evaluation of the H&E and Lendrum's Masson's trichrome was qualitative, though standard histology is commonly used as it provides a representative impression. Finally, the healing ACLs were examined at one time point which does not allow the evaluation of the

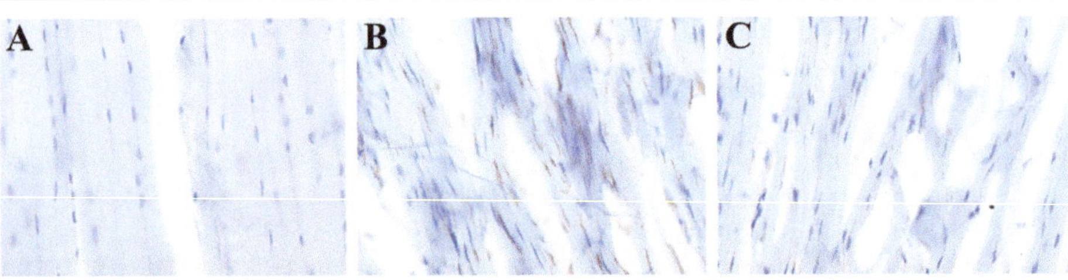

Figure 6 Immunohistologic sections of a normal ACL (A), sutured ACL (B) and sutured ACL with SIS (C). Example of a digital image analysis of α-smooth muscle actin expressing cells. Nuclei stained in blue and α-smooth muscle actin stained in red-brown, identifying α- smooth muscle actin expressing cells. (×400).

Table 1 Total cell density and myofibroblast cell density in the samples of healing ACL tissue (mean ± sd)

	Suture		Suture-SIS	
	Healing	Control	Healing	Control
Number of cells per mm^2	1265 ± 1034	254 ± 92	954 ± 378*	204 ± 93*
Number of myofibroblast per mm^2	642 ± 564	52 ± 22	266 ± 229	36 ± 15
Ratio myofibroblast/total cell density	49%	20%	26%	19%

The difference between Suture-SIS and Control was statistically significant (*paired Student t-test, $p < 0.05$). There was no statistical difference between the Suture and Suture-SIS group.

healing process over time and there was a limited sample size.

Comparing the histological observations of the healing ACL to the ligamentization of tendon grafts in ACL reconstruction, it was shown that the healing ACLs were vital, while it has been reported that necrotic areas within the core of tendon grafts can still be observed during the ligamentization process at 12 weeks (Kondo et al. 2012).

Future studies will include rehabilitation protocols in order to prevent excessive loads on the ACL for potentially a better healing, by e.g. (short-term) casting or internal augmentation devices (Kohl et al. 2013; Fisher et al. 2012).

Conclusions

In conclusion, the healing ACL in both treated groups showed histological characteristics which are comparable to the spontaneously healing medial collateral ligament and shows that the ACL has a similar intrinsic healing response. The addition of SIS appears to biologically enhance the healing process as shown by a continuous fibrous synovial layer, more compact ECM, fewer voids, more aligned collagen fibers, less collagen type 3, and a decreased ratio of myofibroblasts. Though, no definitive conclusions on the beneficial effects of the SIS scaffold on the healing process can be made.

Competing interests

The authors declare that they have no competing interests.

Authors' contributions

DTN contributed to study conception and design, performed surgeries, performed data acquisition, data analysis and interpretation, and drafted the manuscript; SD contributed assisted with surgeries, performed the cryosections, and critically revised the manuscript for important intellectual content; LB contributed to study conception and design, data interpretation, drafted the manuscript and critically revised the manuscript for important intellectual content; PPT, SLYW, CvD contributed to study conception and design, and critically revised the manuscript for important intellectual content. MdB not listed on the author list performed data acquisition, data analysis and interpretation. All authors approved the final manuscript prior to submission.

Acknowledgement

The authors are grateful for the technical assistance of Maarten de Boer and advice of Tamara Ramwadhdoebe with the immunohistochemistry experiments. The study was sponsored by Mozaïek PhD training grant 017.004.076 from the Netherlands Organization for Scientific Research (NWO) and the Marti-Keuning Eckhart foundation.

Author disclosure statement

The SIS material was provided by Cook Biotech Inc., West Lafayette, IN, USA, under a Material Use Agreement, without any monetary compensation and without any condition.
None of the authors had any relation with any other third parties, commercial or otherwise, that has interest in the study or could have influenced the study.

Author details

[1]Department of Orthopedic Surgery, Orthopaedic Research Center Amsterdam, Academic Medical Center, University of Amsterdam, P.O. Box 22660, 1100 DD Amsterdam, The Netherlands. [2]Division of Clinical Immunology and Rheumatology, Academic Medical Center, University of Amsterdam, Amsterdam, The Netherlands. [3]GlaxoSmithKline, Stevenage, U.K. and University of Cambridge, Cambridge, UK. [4]Department of Bioengineering, Musculoskeletal Research Center, University of Pittsburgh, Pittsburgh, USA.

References

Abramowitch SD, Papageorgiou CD, Withrow JD, Gilbert TW, Woo SL (2003) The effect of initial graft tension on the biomechanical properties of a healing ACL replacement graft: a study in goats. J Orthop Res 21(4):708–715, doi: 10.1016/S0736-0266(02)00265-6

Amiel D, Frank CB, Harwood FL, Akeson WH, Kleiner JB (1987) Collagen alteration in medial collateral ligament healing in a rabbit model. Connect Tissue Res 16(4):357–366

Badylak SF, Park K, Peppas N, McCabe G, Yoder M (2001) Marrow-derived cells populate scaffolds composed of xenogeneic extracellular matrix. Exp Hematol 29(11):1310–1318

Beattie AJ, Gilbert TW, Guyot JP, Yates AJ, Badylak SF (2009) Chemoattraction of progenitor cells by remodeling extracellular matrix scaffolds. Tissue Eng A 15(5):1119–1125, doi: 10.1089/ten.tea.2008.0162

Becker H, Davidoff M (1977) Eliminating the gap in flexor tendon surgery. A new method of suture. Hand 9(3):306–311

Beynnon BD, Johnson RJ, Abate JA, Fleming BC, Nichols CE (2005) Treatment of anterior cruciate ligament injuries, part 2. Am J Sports Med 33(11):1751–1767, doi: 10.1177/0363546505279922

Birk DE, Zycband E (1994) Assembly of the tendon extracellular matrix during development. J Anat 184(Pt 3):457–463

Busam ML, Provencher MT, Bach BR Jr (2008) Complications of anterior cruciate ligament reconstruction with bone-patellar tendon-bone constructs: care and prevention. Am J Sports Med 36(2):379–394, doi: 10.1177/0363546507313498

Drogset JO, Strand T, Uppheim G, Odegard B, Boe A, Grontvedt T (2010) Autologous patellar tendon and quadrupled hamstring grafts in anterior cruciate ligament reconstruction: a prospective randomized multicenter review of different fixation methods. Knee Surg Sports Traumatol Arthrosc 18 (8):1085–1093, doi: 10.1007/s00167-009-0996-5

Faryniarz DA, Chaponnier C, Gabbiani G, Yannas IV, Spector M (1996) Myofibroblasts in the healing lapine medial collateral ligament: possible mechanisms of contraction. J Orthop Res 14(2):228–237, doi: 10.1002/jor.1100140210

Fisher MB, Liang R, Jung HJ, Kim KE, Zamarra G, Almarza AJ, McMahon PJ, Woo SL (2012) Potential of healing a transected anterior cruciate ligament with genetically modified extracellular matrix bioscaffolds in a goat model. Knee Surg Sports Traumatol Arthrosc 20(7):1357–1365, doi: 10.1007/s00167-011-1800-x

Fleming BC, Spindler KP, Palmer MP, Magarian EM, Murray MM (2009) Collagen-platelet composites improve the biomechanical properties of healing anterior cruciate ligament grafts in a porcine model. Am J Sports Med 37(8):1554–1563, doi: 10.1177/0363546509332257

Frank C, Woo SL, Amiel D, Harwood F, Gomez M, Akeson W (1983) Medial collateral ligament healing. A multidisciplinary assessment in rabbits. Am J Sports Med 11(6):379–389

Gilbert TW, Stewart-Akers AM, Simmons-Byrd A, Badylak SF (2007) Degradation and remodeling of small intestinal submucosa in canine Achilles tendon repair. J Bone Joint Surg Am 89(3):621–630, doi: 10.2106/JBJS.E.00742

Haringman JJ, Vinkenoog M, Gerlag DM, Smeets TJ, Zwinderman AH, Tak PP (2005) Reliability of computerized image analysis for the evaluation of serial synovial biopsies in randomized controlled trials in rheumatoid arthritis. Arthritis Res Ther 7(4):R862–R867, doi: 10.1186/ar1757

Hatanaka H, Zhang J, Manske PR (2000) An in vivo study of locking and grasping techniques using a passive mobilization protocol in experimental animals. J Hand Surg [Am] 25(2):260–269, doi: 10.1053/jhsu.2000.jhsu25a0260

Hodde JP, Badylak SF, Brightman AO, Voytik-Harbin SL (1996) Glycosaminoglycan content of small intestinal submucosa: a bioscaffold for tissue replacement. Tissue Eng 2(3):209–217, doi: 10.1089/ten.1996.2.209

Hodde JP, Ernst DM, Hiles MC (2005) An investigation of the long-term bioactivity of endogenous growth factor in OASIS Wound Matrix. J Wound Care 14(1):23–25

Kohl S, Evangelopoulos DS, Kohlhof H, Hartel M, Bonel H, Henle P, von Rechenberg B, Eggli S (2013) Anterior crucial ligament rupture: self-healing through dynamic intraligamentary stabilization technique. Knee Surg Sports Traumatol Arthrosc 21(3):599–605, doi: 10.1007/s00167-012-1958-x

Kondo E, Yasuda K, Katsura T, Hayashi R, Kotani Y, Tohyama H (2012) Biomechanical and histological evaluations of the doubled semitendinosus tendon autograft after anterior cruciate ligament reconstruction in sheep. Am J Sports Med 40(2):315–324, doi: 10.1177/0363546511426417

Liang R, Woo SL, Nguyen TD, Liu PC, Almarza A (2008) Effects of a bioscaffold on collagen fibrillogenesis in healing medial collateral ligament in rabbits. J Orthop Res 26(8):1098–1104, doi: 10.1002/jor.20616

Liang R, Fisher M, Yang G, Hall C, Woo SL (2011) Alpha1,3-galactosyltransferase knockout does not alter the properties of porcine extracellular matrix bioscaffolds. Acta Biomater 7(4):1719–1727, doi: 10.1016/j.actbio.2011.01.001

Menetrey J, Laumonier T, Garavaglia G, Hoffmeyer P, Fritschy D, Gabbiani G, Bochaton-Piallat ML (2011) alpha-Smooth muscle actin and TGF-beta receptor I expression in the healing rabbit medial collateral and anterior cruciate ligaments. Injury 42(8):735–741, doi: 10.1016/j.injury.2010.07.246

Murray MM, Spindler KP, Abreu E, Muller JA, Nedder A, Kelly M, Frino J, Zurakowski D, Valenza M, Snyder BD, Connolly SA (2007) Collagen-platelet rich plasma hydrogel enhances primary repair of the porcine anterior cruciate ligament. J Orthop Res 25(1):81–91, doi: 10.1002/jor.20282

Nguyen TD, Liang R, Woo SL, Burton SD, Wu C, Almarza A, Sacks MS, Abramowitch S (2009) Effects of cell seeding and cyclic stretch on the fiber remodeling in an extracellular matrix-derived bioscaffold. Tissue Eng A 15(4):957–963, doi: 10.1089/ten.tea.2007.0384

Nguyen DT, Geel J, Schulze M, Raschke MJ, Woo SL, van Dijk CN, Blankevoort L (2013) Healing of the goat anterior cruciate ligament after a new suture repair technique and bioscaffold treatment. Tissue Eng A 19(19–20):2292–2299, doi: 10.1089/ten.TEA.2012.0535

Raeder RH, Badylak SF, Sheehan C, Kallakury B, Metzger DW (2002) Natural anti-galactose alpha1,3 galactose antibodies delay, but do not prevent the acceptance of extracellular matrix xenografts. Transpl Immunol 10(1):15–24

Spindler KP, Murray MM, Carey JL, Zurakowski D, Fleming BC (2009) The use of platelets to affect functional healing of an anterior cruciate ligament (ACL) autograft in a caprine ACL reconstruction model. J Orthop Res 27(5):631–638, doi: 10.1002/jor.20785

Tak PP, Thurkow EW, Daha MR, Kluin PM, Smeets TJ, Meinders AE, Breedveld FC (1995) Expression of adhesion molecules in early rheumatoid synovial tissue. Clin Immunol Immunopathol 77(3):236–242

van der Hall PO, Kraan MC, Tak PP (2007) Quantitative image analysis of synovial tissue. Method Mol Med 135:121–143

von Porat A, Roos EM, Roos H (2004) High prevalence of osteoarthritis 14 years after an anterior cruciate ligament tear in male soccer players: a study of radiographic and patient relevant outcomes. Ann Rheum Dis 63(3):269–273

Voytik-Harbin SL, Brightman AO, Kraine MR, Waisner B, Badylak SF (1997) Identification of extractable growth factors from small intestinal submucosa. J Cell Biochem 67(4):478–491, doi: 10.1002/(SICI)1097-4644(19971215)67::4<478:AID-JCB6>3.0.CO;2-P

Wang JH, Jia F, Gilbert TW, Woo SL (2003) Cell orientation determines the alignment of cell-produced collagenous matrix. J Biomech 36(1):97–102

Woo SL, Abramowitch SD, Kilger R, Liang R (2006) Biomechanics of knee ligaments: injury, healing, and repair. J Biomech 39(1):1–20, doi: 10.1016/j.jbiomech.2004.10.025

Zantop T, Gilbert TW, Yoder MC, Badylak SF (2006) Extracellular matrix scaffolds are repopulated by bone marrow-derived cells in a mouse model of achilles tendon reconstruction. J Orthop Res 24(6):1299–1309, doi: 10.1002/jor.20071

Osteochondral tissue engineering using a biphasic collagen/GAG scaffold containing rhFGF18 or BMP-7 in an ovine model

Alan Getgood[1*], Frances Henson[2], Carrie Skelton[3], Roger Brooks[3], Hans Guehring[4], Lisa A Fortier[5] and Neil Rushton[3]

Abstract

Background: The aim of this study was to investigate the effect of combining rhFGF18 or BMP-7 with a biphasic collagen/GAG osteochondral scaffold (Chondromimetic) on the repair of osteochondral defects in sheep.

Methods: Osteochondral defects (5.8x6mm) were created in the medial femoral condyle (MFC) and the lateral trochlea sulcus (LTS) of the stifle joint of 24 female sheep. Sheep were randomly assigned to four groups (n = 6); 1) empty defect, 2) scaffold only, 3) scaffold + rhFGF-18 (30 μg) and 4) scaffold + BMP-7 (100 μg). At 6 months the defects underwent non-destructive mechanical testing, gross assessment of repair tissue (ICRS score) and histological analysis (Modified O'Driscoll score).

Results: *ICRS repair score:* Defects treated with scaffold + rhFGF18 (mean 9.83, 95% CI 8.43-11.23) and scaffold + BMP-7 (10, 9.06-10.94) in the MFC had significantly improved ICRS scores compared to empty defects (4.2, 0–8.80) ($p = 0.002$). *Mechanical properties:* BMP-7 treated defects (mean 64.35, 95% CI 56.88-71.82) were significantly less stiff than both the rhFGF18 (mean 84.1, 95% CI 76.8-91.4) and empty defects in the LTS, compared to both contralateral limb ($p = 0.003$), and the perilesional articular cartilage ($p < 0.001$). ***Histology:*** A statistically significant improvement in the modified O'Driscoll score was observed in the rhFGF18 treated group (mean 16.83, 95% CI 13.65-20.61) compared to the empty defects (mean 9, 95% CI 4.88-13.12) ($p = 0.039$) in the MFC. Excellent tissue fill, lateral integration and proteoglycan staining was observed. Only the rhFGF18 defects showed pericellular type VI collagen staining with positive type II collagen and reduced positive type I collagen staining. The majority of defects in the control and BMP-7 groups demonstrated fibrocartilagenous repair tissue.

Conclusion: Statistically significant improvements in gross repair, mechanical properties and histological score were found over empty defects when Chondromimetic was combined with rhFGF18. These results suggest that rhFGF18 may play a significant role in articular cartilage repair applications.

Keywords: Osteochondral repair; Sheep; Biphasic scaffold; rhFGF18

Background

There have been many technological advances in articular cartilage repair techniques over the past decade but the ability to regenerate hyaline cartilage continues to elude us. Procedures such as autologous chondrocyte transplantation and microfracture have, at best, been able to produce a repair tissue with hyaline like features [1]. More recently, a greater focus has been placed on the influence of subchondral bone in the disease process, with articular cartilage now being properly recognised as a composite structure [2]. As a result, tissue engineering principals are now starting to be applied to regenerate the osteochondral unit.

It has been demonstrated that osteochondral defects show improved repair parameters when a scaffold is used within the lesion [3]. Of the scaffolds used, a novel biphasic osteochondral scaffold (Chondromimetic, Orthomimetics/TiGenix, Cambridge, UK) has shown promise in early studies [4]. This collagen/chondroitin sulphate/calcium phosphate scaffold was demonstrated to

* Correspondence: alan.getgood@uwo.ca
[1]The Fowler Kennedy Sport Medicine Clinic 3M Centre, The University of Western Ontario, London, Ontario N6A 3K7, Canada
Full list of author information is available at the end of the article

induce healing with a repair tissue with features of hyaline cartilage at a 6 month end point in the caprine knee [4]. Whilst these results are encouraging, it is likely that a combination of a scaffold and bioactive molecules, such as chondrogenic growth factors, will enhance the healing process [3].

A number of growth factors have been tested both *in-vitro* and *in-vivo* for their chondrogenic properties, including insulin like growth factor 1 (IGF-1) [5] and bone morphogenetic protein 7 (BMP-7) [6,7]. More recently, fibroblast growth factor 18 (FGF18) has also been reported to promote chondrogenesis [8,9]. FGF-18 is a member of the FGF family, in which there are 23 members that bind to 4 structurally related high affinity FGF receptor (FGFR1-4) tyrosine kinases. The essential role of FGF's in signalling in bone and cartilage metabolism is evident from genetic diseases, such as achondroplasia, which are associated with mutations in the FGFR gene.

Studies have shown that FGF18 acts as a ligand for the FGFR3 receptor, expressed on proliferating and prehypertrophic chondrocytes. Liu et al. [10] demonstrated that, in FGF18 knockout mice, the growth plate phenotype was similar to that of mice lacking FGFR3 – there was a delay in ossification and a reduced expression of osteogenic markers. They also showed that in FGF18/FGFR3 knockout mice, expanded zones of proliferating and hypertrophic chondrocytes were formed, with increased chondrocyte proliferation and differentiation. These negative effects in the growth plate are in contrast to the positive effect on mature chondrocytes. Ellsworth et al. have shown a significant direct effect of FGF18 on the growth and proteoglycan synthesis of mature murine and human chondrocytes [11]. An in-vivo study by Power et al. [12] demonstrated that the addition of recombinant human FGF18 (rhFGF18) to microfracture defects in sheep resulted in improved fill and quality of repair tissue with characteristics of hyaline cartilage.

It is therefore possible that FGF18 may play a role in the control of both chondrocyte and bone cell behaviour in tissue repair and warrants an investigation for its use in osteochondral regeneration.

This study was designed to investigate the effect of adding either rhFGF18 (Merck Serono, Darmstadt, Germany) or BMP-7 to a biphasic collagen-glycosaminoglycan (collagen-GAG) scaffold in an ovine osteochondral defect model. The null hypothesis was that neither the addition of rhFGF18 nor BMP-7 would improve the quality of osteochondral repair tissue when compared to a defect filled with scaffold alone.

Methods

This study received approval from both local research ethics committee (University of Cambridge Biomedical Support Services) and the Home Office (United Kingdom Home Office).

Animals: A total of 24 skeletally mature female Welsh Mountain sheep between the ages of 3 and 5 years old were included in the study. Each treatment group contained six sheep (n = 6).

Experimental design: For all animals, full thickness osteochondral defects 5.8 mm wide by 6 mm deep were created in the proximal lateral trochlea sulcus (LTS) and in the medial femoral condyle (MFC) of the right stifle joint using custom made instrumentation. Four treatment groups were used; A - no scaffold in defect ('empty defect'), B - scaffold alone ('scaffold'), C - scaffold plus rhFGF18 (Merck Serono, Darmstadt, Germany, ('scaffold + rhFGF18') and D - scaffold plus BMP-7 (R&D systems, Abingdon, UK) ('scaffold + BMP-7').

Animal anaesthesia, preparation and surgical technique: Prior to surgery animals were selected at random and identification ear tags applied. All animals had food and water removed 24 hours before surgery. General anaesthesia was induced with an injection of thiopentone (3 mg/kg) into the external jugular vein. Maintenance was achieved via inhalational anaesthetic of a mixture of isofluorane, nitrous oxide and oxygen. Perioperative analgesia was provided by pre-operative intramuscular Carprofen (1.5 mg/ml) and antibiotic prophylaxis was given via intramuscular procaine penicillin (10 mg/ml).

The basic surgical procedure was identical for all subjects and performed under strict asepsis by a single surgeon. Each stifle was physically examined for any abnormalities whilst anaesthetised. No gross instability or pathology was found, therefore no animal was excluded from participation within the study.

The animal was placed in a dorsal recumbency position and, following surgical preparation, the right stifle joint opened via a lateral parapatellar approach. Following patella subluxation, the LTS defect was made 10 mm distal to the top of the lateral trochlear ridge aligned with the middle of the lateral trochlear groove. The MFC defect was made 10 mm distal to the condyle groove junction and aligned with the medial crest of the trochlear groove. A 5.8 mm wide × 6 mm deep cylindrical defect was created and a 6mm×6mm collagen-GAG scaffold plus appropriate test substance placed into the defect.

Test substances were reconstituted and added to the scaffold prior to commencing the skin incision. This allowed at least 10 minutes for the growth factor to adsorb on to the scaffold, prior to insertion into the defect. rhFGF-8 was reconstituted via the directions of the supplier with 0.9% saline and added to the scaffolds in a concentration of 150 μg/ml, providing 30 μg per scaffold. Lyophilised BMP-7 was reconstituted with 4 millimolar HCL and applied to the scaffold in a concentration of 500 μg/ml, providing 100 μg per scaffold. This concentration was chosen due to previous studies and following personal communication [6].

The joint was then cycled through a range of motion to ensure a satisfactory rim fixation of the plug, following which the joint was closed in a standard fashion. Postoperatively, animals were allowed to fully weight bear, but kept in small pens for 48 hours to reduce ambulation. All animals were housed indoors for the remaining study period in large pens, which allowed a moderate degree of ambulation. Regular checks were made for any animal displaying signs of postoperative discomfort with additional postoperative analgesia given if required. All further treatments were recorded as appropriate.

Necropsy: Animals were humanely sacrificed at 26 weeks postoperatively using a lethal dose of sodium pentobarbital.

Outcome measures:

1) **Gross Morphology** - The joints were opened and the surface of the osteochondral defect sites blindly scored by 2 observers using the International Cartilage Repair Society score (Table 1). The presence of degenerative change was noted as per the Outerbridge score (Table 2).
2) **Mechanical testing** - Each implant site underwent non-destructive mechanical testing to determine changes to the cartilage surface surrounding the implant or empty defect. Measurements were taken in duplicate from the centre of the osteochondral defect, and at a distance of 1 mm from the original edge of the created osteochondral defect at the 12, 3, 6, and 9 o'clock positions, using a handheld digital durometer (Shore S1, M scale, Instron Ltd, UK). A number between 0–100 (arbitrary unit) would be given (with an inbuilt calibrated error of +/−5) at each site and a mean calculated. These measurements were then repeated in the contralateral limb in the same anatomic sites. The stiffness of the reparative tissue was then expressed as percentage stiffness relative to the control cartilage in the contralateral limb. This therefore allowed a surrogate measure of stiffness to be made, as previously published [4].
3) **Histology** - Specimens were decalcified in formic acid/sodium citrate over two weeks and then processed for routine paraffin embedding. Sections of 7 μm thickness were made through the central portion of the defect. Sections were stained with Safranin O/Fast Green. One slide from the centre of each defect was blindly scored by two investigators using a modified O'Driscoll score (Table 3) [13].
4) **Immunohistochemistry** - Immunohistochemistry was performed as described previously [14]. The following primary antibodies were used in this study; monoclonal mouse anti human type I collagen (MP Biomedicals, US, 1 in 200 dilution), monoclonal mouse anti human type II collagen (MP Biomedicals, US, 1 in 100 dilution) and monoclonal mouse anti-rabbit type VI collagen (Abcam, UK, 1 in 500 dilution). Horseradish peroxidase-conjugated secondary anti-rabbit and mouse immunoglobulin were used as appropriate, and the colour reaction developed with 0.1% 3′, 3-diaminobenzidine tetrachloride (DAB)/0.01% hydrogen peroxide. Normal species-specific serum was used as a control in all experiments. The degree of positive staining for types I, II and VI collagens was evaluated by semi quantitative scoring on a scale of 1 to 4 for intensity i.e. inconspicuous (1), mild (2), moderate (3), and strong (4) [15]. In addition the location of type VI immunoreactivity was noted i.e. pericellular or territorial.

Table 1 ICRS repair score [16]

Characteristic	Grading	Score
Degree of defect repair	Level with surrounding cartilage	4
	75% repair of defect depth	3
	50% repair of defect depth	2
	25% repair of defect depth	1
	0% repair of defect depth	0
Integration to border zone	Complete integration with border zone	4
	Demarcating border <1 mm	3
	¾ of graft integrated, ¼ with notable border >1 mm	2
	½ of graft integrated with surrounding cartilage, ½ with a notable border >1 mm	1
	From no contact to 1/4th of graft integrated with surrounding cartilage	0
Macroscopic appearance	Intact smooth surface	4
	Fibrillated surface	3
	Small, scattered fissures or cracks	2
	Several, small or few but large fissures	1
	Total degeneration of grafted area	0
	Total	**12**

Table 2 Outerbridge score for macroscopic degenerative change [17]

Outerbridge score	Explanation
Grade 0	Normal
Grade I	Mild softening of the articular cartilage
Grade II	Fibrillation and fissuring of chondral surface
Grade III	Cracks in articular cartilage, no subchondral bone exposed
Grade IV	Full thickness chondral defects down to bone

Statistical analysis: Statistical significance between groups for each end point was determined using a one-way analysis

Table 3 Modified O'Driscoll Histology Score [13]

	Characteristic		Grading	Score
I	% Hyaline Cartilage:		80-100	8
			60-80	6
			40-60	4
			20-40	2
			0-20	0
II	Structural Characteristics:	A. Surface irregularity:	Smooth and intact	2
			Fissures	1
			Severe disruption, fibrillation	0
		B. Structural integrity:	Normal	2
			Slight disruption, including cysts	1
			Severe lack of integration	0
		C. Thickness:	100% of normal adjacent cartilage	2
			50-100% or thicker than normal	1
			0-50%	0
		D. Bonding to adjacent cartilage:	Bonded at both ends of graft	2
			Bonded at one end/partially both ends	1
			Not bonded	0
III	Freedom from cellular changes of degeneration:		Normal cellularity, no clusters	2
			Slight hypocellularity, <25% chondrocyte clusters	1
			Moderate hypocellularity, >25% clusters	0
IV	Freedom from degenerate changes in adjacent cartilage:		Normal cellularity, no clusters, normal staining	3
			Normal cellularity, mild clusters, moderate staining	2
			Mild or mod hypocellularity, slight staining	1
			Severe hypocellularity, slight staining	0
V	Reconstitution of subchondral bone:		complete reconstitution	2
			greater than 50% reconstitution	1
			50% or less reconstitution	0
VI	Bonding of repair cartilage to denovo subchondral bone:		complete and uninterrupted	2
			<100% but >50% recon	1
			<50% complete	0
VII	Safranin O staining:		> 80% homogenous positive stain	2
			40-80% homogenous positive stain	1
			<40% homogenous positive stain	0
			TOTAL SCORE	**Max 27**

of variance (ANOVA) and Bonferroni's post hoc test. Where data sets within groups were not found to be normally distributed, a non-parametric Kruskal-Wallis test was instead used, with a post hoc Dunns multiple comparisons test. A level of $p < 0.05$ was accepted as significant in all analyses. GraphPad Prism 5 statistical software package (Graphpad Software Inc., La Jolla, CA) was used for graph production and data analysis.

Results

Gross morphology (Figure 1): At post-mortem two animals in the empty defect group were shown to have sustained

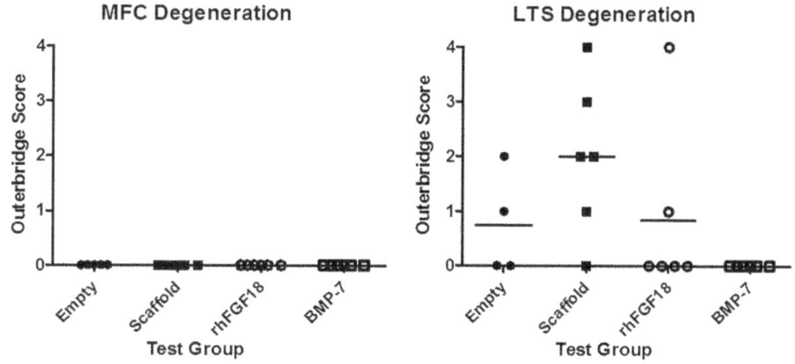

Figure 1 Macroscopic observation of degenerative change in the MFC and LTS at necropsy. The horizontal bars represent the mean value. Non-parametric analysis shows a statistically significant difference between the degeneration in the BMP-7 group compared with the scaffold only ($p = 0.038$).

joint damage and were excluded from the study; one with an undisplaced fracture of the lateral trochlea sulcus which was deemed to affect healing, and the second a subluxated patella which would have influenced its weight bearing properties. Degenerative change was seen in many animals in the LTS, particularly in the empty defect and scaffold only groups. Non-parametric analysis showed a statistically significant difference between the degeneration in the BMP-7 group compared with the scaffold only ($p = 0.038$). Two animals in the BMP-7 group were noted to have osteophyte formation on the MFC.

ICRS repair score (Table 4 *and Figure* 2*)*: Both rhFGF18 (mean 9.83, 95% CI 8.43-11.23) and BMP-7 (10, 9.06-10.94) had significantly improved ICRS repair scores in the MFC compared to empty defects (4.2, 0–8.80) ($p = 0.002$). A trend towards improved repair was seen with both growth factors in comparison to the scaffold only but no statistically significant difference existed between groups ($p > 0.05$). No differences were noted in the LTS.

Mechanical indentation (Table 5*)*: In the MFC, no differences existed between the treatment groups in the mean percentage stiffness of the contralateral limb ($p = 0.31$). In the LTS, BMP-7 was significantly less stiff than both rhFGF18 and the empty defect when compared to the cartilage of contralateral limb ($p = 0.003$). However, the empty defects in the MFC were noted to have higher mean stiffness measurements than normal.

Histology (Table 6 *and Figure* 3*)*: A significantly higher modified O'Driscoll score was seen in the rhFGF18 group (mean16.83, 95% CI 13.65-20.61) in the MFC when compared to the empty defect (9, 4.88-13.12) ($p = 0.039$) (Figure 3). A similar trend was observed in the LTS, with both the rhFGF18 and scaffold only groups scoring higher than the empty defect, however no statistical significance was reached. The BMP-7 group showed the worst results of all in the LTS with a wide variability (7.83, 3.46-12.21) **Tissue repair:** Tissue was seen to have filled the entire original defect in the majority of animals (Figure 4). Good tissue fill was noted in both the cartilaginous and osseous parts of the repair in the empty, scaffold only and rhFGF18 treated groups. In the BMP-7 treated group, poor defect fill was seen in four of the six LTS defects with very poor Safranin O staining in the other two defects. In the MFC, the proteoglycan deposition was improved as seen by increased Safranin O staining; however the thickness of the cartilage layer was mostly reduced in comparison to the native cartilage. In addition, two of the six BMP-7 treated MFC defects contained large subchondral cysts (Figure 4D). In the empty defect and scaffold only groups, moderately positive Safranin O staining was seen in MFC defects, with relatively poor staining in the LTS in scaffold only groups. In the rhFGF18 group excellent Safranin O staining was present throughout the chondral portion of all defects indicating good proteoglycan

Table 4 Mean ICRS Repair Score for each category

	Empty defect		Scaffold only		rhFGF18		BMP-7	
	MFC	LTS	MFC	LTS	MFC	LTS	MFC	LTS
I. Degree of defect repair	2.00	2.60	2.83	2.20	3.83	1.60	4.00	6.40
II. Integration to border zone	1.20	2.50	2.17	2.67	3.67	1.33	3.50	6.50
III. Macroscopic appearance	1.00	3.17	1.33	2.33	2.33	1.83	2.50	7.33
MEAN TOTAL SCORE	**4.20**	**2.67**	**6.33**	**2.50**	**9.83**	**1.00**	**10.00**	**6.50**
p < 0.05	* #				*		#	

* and # indicate significant differences between specific groups $p = 0.002$. All other group comparisons $p > 0.05$.

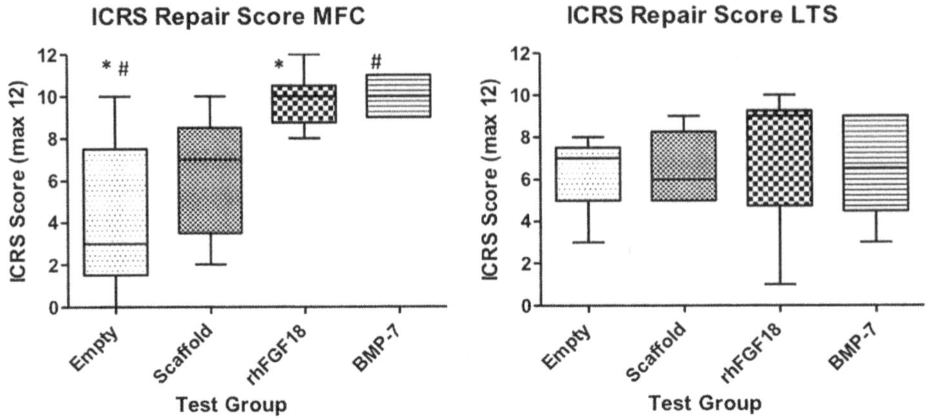

* and # indicate significant differences between specific groups (p=0.002). All other group comparisons p>0.05.

Figure 2 International Cartilage Repair Society gross repair score of MFC and LTS. Box and whisker plots represent the maximum and minimum values, the interquartile range with the horizontal bar representing the median value. Statistically significant differences were noted between the empty defects and rhFGF18 and BMP-7 in the MFC ($p = 0.002$) while no difference was found between groups in the LTS ($p > 0.05$).

production. Good integration of the repair tissue to the parent cartilage was seen in the scaffold only and rhFGF18 groups, however in the BMP-7 group there was poor lateral integration (Figure 5). **Histology:** In empty defects there was disorganised cartilage tissue within the defect, consistent with a fibrocartilagenous repair (Figure 6A). In the scaffold only and BMP-7 groups there was more organisation of the repair cartilage, albeit in defects with poor tissue fill as noted above. In the lateral margins of the repair tissue a more hyaline cartilage structure was noted, with chondrocytes in lacunae arranged in columns in the deep zone, with more flattened chondrocytes in the superficial zone. A similar histological picture was noted in the rhFGF18 group although the organised hyaline like cartilage (Figure 6B) was present over a larger region of the repair tissue with only a central zone showing fibrocartilagenous characteristics. **Immunohistochemistry:** In all empty defects there was strong type I collagen staining throughout the repair tissue. In the scaffold only and BMP-7 groups both type I and type II collagen staining was detected. In the rhFGF18 group there was negative type I collagen staining and strong type II collagen. No empty or BMP-7 treated defects stained positive for pericellular type VI collagen, pericellular type VI collagen was only noted in the lateral margins of the repair tissue in the scaffold only group while there was strong pericellular type VI collagen throughout the majority of the rhFGF-18 defects (Figure 7).

The histology and immunohistochemistry results indicated that, in the empty group there was a fibrocartilage repair, in the scaffold only and BMP-7 defect groups there was a predominately fibrocartilage repair with some evidence of hyaline cartilage at the lateral margins of the defect. In the rhFGF-18 treated group there was a predominately hyaline cartilage repair with fibrocartilage in the centre of the repair.

Discussion

This study has shown that the addition of rhFGF18 to a collagen-GAG osteochondral scaffold can produce objective improvements in osteochondral repair tissue in sheep, when compared to defects either left empty, treated with scaffold alone or when the scaffold is combined with BMP-7. The addition of rhFGF18 resulted in statistically significant improvements in gross appearance and histological score over empty defects in the MFC. The combination of

Table 5 Mechanical testing data

	Empty defect		Scaffold only		rhFGF18		BMP-7	
	MFC	LTS	MFC	LTS	MFC	LTS	MFC	LTS
Mean	126.4	85.4	97.2	79.35	99.42	84.1	90.5	64.35
Std. Deviation	66.78	13.79	13.8	8.072	7.348	6.958	9.479	7.118
Std. Error	29.86	6.167	5.633	3.296	3	2.841	3.87	2.906
Lower 95% CI	43.46	68.28	82.72	70.88	91.71	76.8	80.55	56.88
Upper 95% CI	209.3	102.5	111.7	87.82	107.1	91.4	100.4	71.82
p < 0.05		*				#		* #

* and # indicate significant differences between specific groups $p = 0.003$. All other group comparisons $p > 0.05$.

Table 6 Mean Modified O'Driscoll score for each category

		Empty defect		Scaffold only		rhFGF18		BMP-7	
		MFC	LTS	MFC	LTS	MFC	LTS	MFC	LTS
I	% Hyaline Cartilage:	0.80	1.00	1.00	1.67	3.00	2.00	1.33	0.00
II	Structural Characteristics:								
	A. Surface Irregularity:	0.20	0.75	1.17	1.83	1.83	1.33	0.67	0.83
	B. Structural integrity:	0.40	0.50	0.67	1.00	1.17	0.50	0.83	0.50
	C. Thickness:	0.80	0.75	0.83	0.83	1.33	0.67	1.00	0.33
	D. Bonding to adjacent cartilage:	1.20	1.00	2.00	1.50	1.83	1.67	2.00	1.17
III	Freedom from cellular changes of degeneration:	0.60	0.25	0.67	1.00	0.83	0.83	1.00	0.50
IV	Freedom from degenerate changes in adjacent cartilage:	1.80	1.75	2.17	1.50	2.33	2.33	2.50	2.33
V	Reconstitution of subchondral bone:	1.00	0.75	0.33	0.67	0.67	0.83	1.17	0.50
VI	Bonding of repair cartilage to denovo subchondral bone:	1.60	1.00	1.33	1.67	1.83	1.67	2.00	1.33
VII	Safranin O:	0.60	0.50	1.00	1.00	2.00	1.33	1.50	0.33
	MEAN TOTAL SCORE	**9.00**	**8.25**	**11.17**	**12.70**	**16.83**	**13.20**	**14.00**	**7.83**
	$p < 0.05$	*				*			

* indicates significant differences between specific groups $p = 0.039$. All other group comparisons $p > 0.05$.

scaffold plus rhFGF18 was found to produce similar mechanical properties to native articular cartilage, in contrast to the BMP-7, which was found to be statistically less stiff than both the empty defect and rhFGF18 in the LTS. Histologically, excellent tissue fill of the defects, lateral integration, integrity of neocartilage, and expression of hyaline cartilage markers, such as proteoglycan, type II collagen and pericellular type VI collagen was also observed to a greater degree with rhFGF18. Furthermore, along with BMP-7, rhFGF18 may provide a protective role against perilesional degeneration following osteochondral defect production in the patellofemoral joint and warrants further investigation.

These findings support those of previous studies investigating the role of FGF18 in chondrogenesis. Ellsworth et al. [11] have shown that local delivery of adenovirus expressing FGF18 into the pinnae of nude mice increased the formation of auricular cartilage with high levels of collagen type II and proteoglycan being expressed. Further evidence of its chondrogenic effect were demonstrated by the same group when rhFGF18 was injected intravenously into rats, stimulating expansion of a number of cartilaginous sites including trachea, spine and articular cartilage [18]. In an osteoarthritis small animal model, three injections of rhFGF18 were administered biweekly into rat joints 21 days following meniscus transection [9]. Hyaluronic acid was used both as a carrier vehicle for rhFGF18, and as the control injection. At 6 weeks histological sections representative of the treatment groups showed areas of chondrogenesis with increased proteoglycan deposition and integration of the repair tissue with the native cartilage matrix. Although the repair tissue was not hyaline cartilage, it did show cellular organisation and

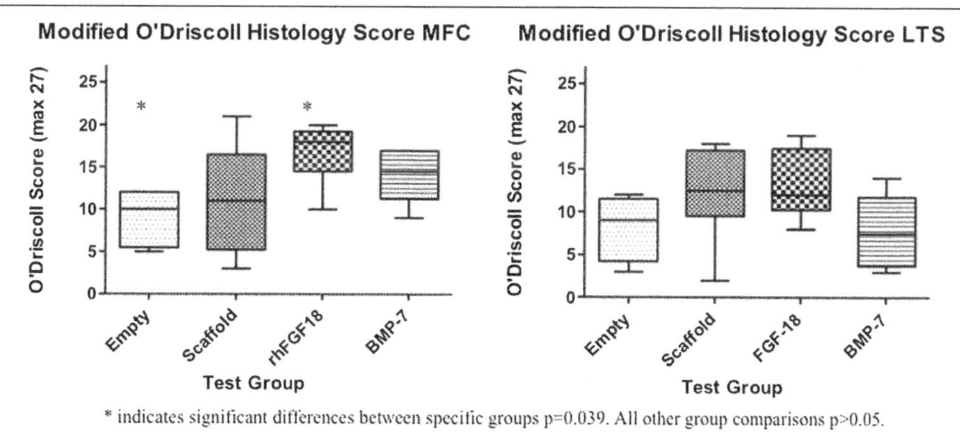

Figure 3 The modified O'Driscoll score for both MFC and LTS ($p > 0.05$) showing comparison between groups. Statistically significant differences were observed between the rhFGF18 and empty defects in the MFC ($p = 0.039$) with no differences observed in the LTS between groups. Box and whisker plots represent the maximum and minimum values, the interquartile range with the horizontal bar representing the median value.

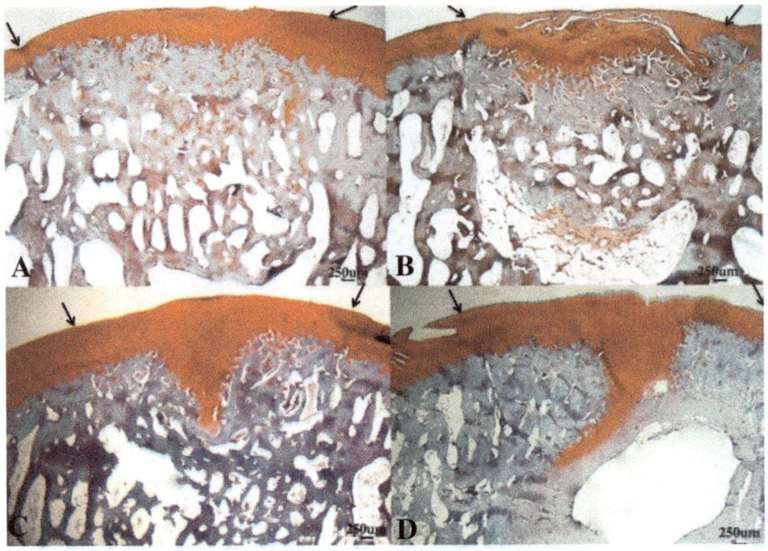

Figure 4 Histological sections stained with Safranin O. A) Empty defect, **B)** Scaffold alone, **C)** Scaffold + rhFGF-18, **D)** Scaffold + BMP-7. In A, B and C there is good tissue fill. Differences in subchondral bone formation can be observed. The empty defect A shows subchondral hypertrophy, whilst in C and D there appears to be a cartilage cleft, with significant proteoglycan staining extending down into the subchondral bone. In D there is a large subchondral cyst. The arrows denote the margins of the defect.

proteoglycan deposition similar to hyaline cartilage without any evidence of angiogenesis. A repair tissue, originating from the joint margins was also noted, migrating over the cartilage surface. These responses were not seen within the normal rat knee joints (i.e. those which were not subjected to meniscus transection), indicating that rhFGF18 may exert its anabolic effects only on damaged cartilage. A more recent study by Lohmander et al. [19] studied the effects of intra-articular rhFGF18 injected into osteoarthritic joints in a double blind, placebo controlled randomised controlled trial. A statistically significant reduction in joint space narrowing was noted in the lateral tibiofemoral compartment, yet no changes were noted in the medial compartment, nor were changes noted in the

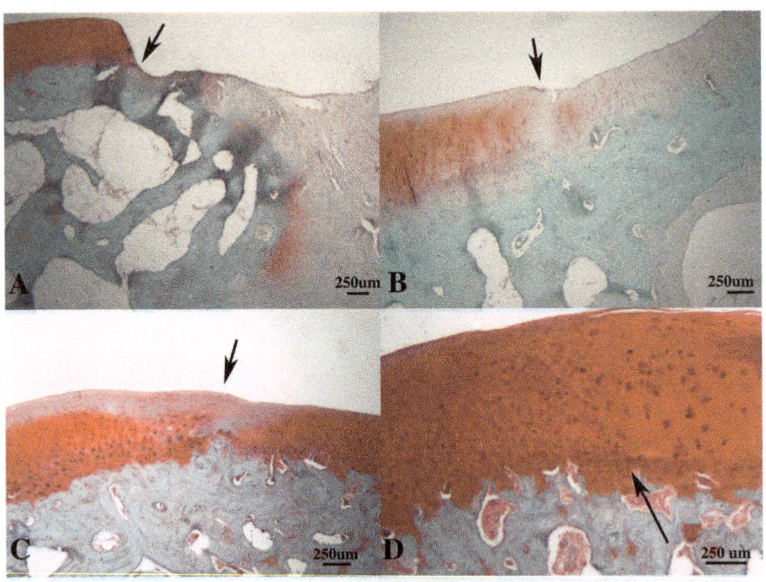

Figure 5 Representative sections showing different grades of integration of repair tissue to parent cartilage. Sections stained with Safranin O. Black arrows indicate the junction between repair tissue and parent cartilage. **A)** Poor repair tissue in the defect and no integration between this tissue and the parent cartilage. **B)** There is integration in this section but a hypocellularity at the junction with a small area of fissuring on the articular surface. **C)** Improved integration but hypocellularity at junction. **D)** Excellent integration between repair tissue (left hand side of arrow) and parent tissue (right hand side of arrow).

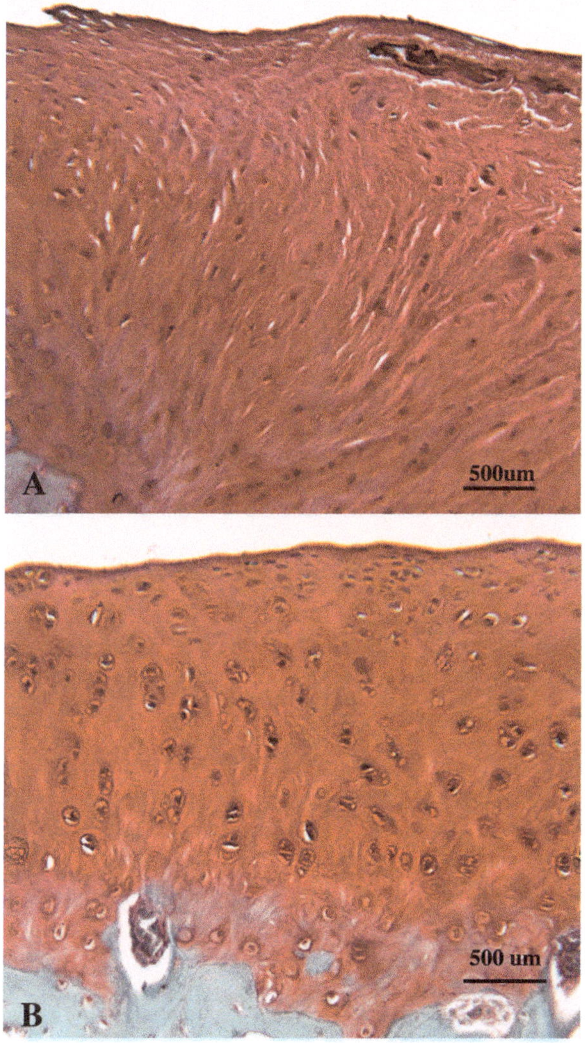

Figure 6 Histological sections stained with Safranin O. A) Fibrocartilagenous repair tissue typical of that seen in empty defects, scaffold alone and BMP-7, **B)** Hyaline cartilage-like repair tissue typical of that seen in scaffold + rhFGF-18 treated defects.

patient reported outcome scores. This may indicate that the mechanism of action of rhFGF18 is in some way determined by the mechanical environment, as medial OA is most often associated with varus alignment and relative offloading of the lateral compartment of the knee. The above findings may have particular value in articular cartilage repair, as in the clinical scenario a mixed picture of acute injury on a background of degenerative disease can often be seen. During articular cartilage repair surgery, it is often the case that the perilesional cartilage is diseased, yet the de novo repair tissue is expected to integrate with it forming functional tissue. Furthermore, it is common practice to 'offload' the repair tissue with a realignment osteotomy to improve the mechanical environment. The possibility of a using a growth factor to promote healing and repair within both the defect and perilesional tissue is therefore appealing.

Surprisingly, BMP-7 performed relatively poorly in this experimental study. BMP-7 is considered to be one of the major anabolic growth factors of articular cartilage [20]. Although the gross repair scores were statistically superior to the empty defect, two animals showed osteophyte formation, a factor, which has been noted in a number of other studies incorporating BMPs [21,22]. The histology in the BMP-7 group, particularly the LTS, was very poor. The majority of defects had poor tissue fill which stained poorly for proteoglycan with architecture mostly resembling fibrous tissue. In the MFC, two of the animals were observed to have large cysts present within the subchondral bone, which would likely provide sub-optimal clinical results. As a result of this tissue repair, the mechanical results were significantly inferior to both the rhFGF18 and empty defect groups.

Most of the literature on BMP-7 suggests that it has a acts as an anabolic growth factor, particularly for chondrocyte homeostasis and repair [6]. However, in this model, the main cell type driving the repair process may not be the chondrocyte *per se*, but is perhaps a mesenchymal stem cell population, resident within the subchondral bone or invading blood vessels, which may not be as responsive to BMP-7 treatment. Knippenberg et al. [23] have shown a preference of BMP-7 to direct chondrogenic differentiation of adipose derived MSC's, compared to an osteogenic lineage by BMP-2. It therefore may not be as potent a growth factor in osteochondral repair as rhFGF18. Alternatively, the dose of BMP-7 used in this model may not have been optimal. The dose of 100 μg per scaffold was chosen based upon personal communication with experts in the field who have previously studied OP-1 (BMP-7) in in-vivo models of cartilage repair [6]. Ideally, further studies should be performed to study different concentrations of growth factor within this model to identify the optimal dose. It should also be noted that the BMP-7 used in this study was not what has been used in other studies provided by Stryker Biotech (Stryker, Kalamazoo, MI), which may have an influence on its biological efficacy.

The positive effects of combining rhFGF18 with a biphasic collagen-GAG scaffold to enhance osteochondral repair is potentially very interesting. rhFGF18 is known to exert an effect on chondrogenesis, as well as osteogenesis [24], so clearly has potential to influence healing across the osteochondral niche. One of the drawbacks of synthetic polymer scaffolds has been reported to be delayed bone formation [25], therefore the addition of a growth factor into the construct, which may speed up the bone regeneration process would be helpful. The ability to control the simultaneous repair of osteochondral tissue is yet to be determined [26]. With increasing time there is a

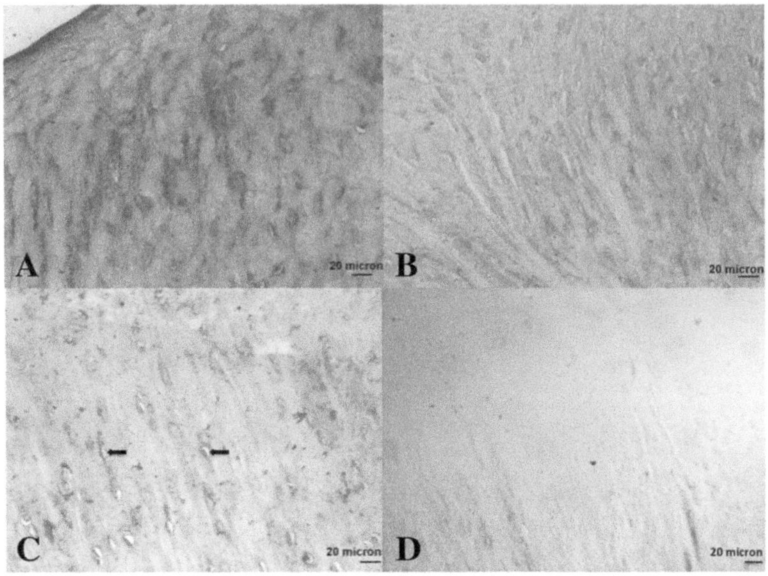

Figure 7 Histological sections following immunohistochemistry to detect type VI collagen. A) Empty defect, **B)** Scaffold alone, **C)** Scaffold + rhFGF-18, **D)** Scaffold + BMP-7. In A, where there is a fibrocartilagenous repair, there is little pericellular matrix staining with marked inter-territorial matrix staining. In C there is marked pericellular staining (black rings around the cells) indicating a more hyaline cartilage like repair tissue.

concern that a process of endochondral bone formation is underway, which could result in an advancing tidemark, chondrocyte hypertrophy and calcification of the articular cartilage component of the osteochondral unit. The fact that FGF18 seems to inhibit growth plate chondrocytes may be somewhat protective of that process, however further studies with longer time points until sacrifice would be required to examine this further.

Limitations of this study include that the dosing schedule may not have been optimal, with further injections of rhFGF18 possibly providing greater benefit. The study time also was only 6 months duration. A number of studies have shown that articular cartilage repair can take upwards of one year for maturation [27], therefore having animals out to 12 months to see if these changes observed become more pronounced or equilibrate, would be of interest. The outcome measures used included a surrogate measure of stiffness and semi quantitative histological analysis. Obtaining objective measurements of stiffness and a biochemical analysis of repair tissue would be advantageous, however would have required a greater numbers of animals. As this was a pilot study, the number of animals included was deliberately reduced and therefore this extra analysis was not possible. Furthermore, it is not clear if the findings, which did not show statistical significance, could be secondary to type II error. Further studies are therefore warranted with larger numbers to ascertain the full potential of the drug.

Conclusion

This study has demonstrated that the combination of rhFGF18 and a collagen-GAG osteochondral scaffold can produce objective improvements in osteochondral repair when incorporated in an acute osteochondral defect model in sheep, although topographic variation may exist between the MFC and LTS. The use of rhFGF18 as a target molecule for articular cartilage repair and osteoarthritis treatment warrants further investigation.

Competing interests

This work was funded via a research grant from the UK Technology Strategy Board, TiGenix Ltd (Cambridge, UK) and Merck Serono (Darmstadt, Germany). Merck Serono have also provided funding to cover the journal processing fee. NR and AG have acted as paid consultants in the past five years for Tigenix and Merck Serono respectively.

Acknowledgements

Dr Brooks acknowledges funding support from the National Institute for Health Research (NIHR).

Author details

[1]The Fowler Kennedy Sport Medicine Clinic 3M Centre, The University of Western Ontario, London, Ontario N6A 3K7, Canada. [2]Department of Veterinary Medicine, University of Cambridge, Cambridge, UK. [3]The University of Cambridge Orthopaedic Research Unit, Cambridge, UK. [4]Merck Serono GmbH, Darmstadt, Germany. [5]Department of Clinical Sciences, Cornell University, Ithaca, USA.

References

1. Saris DB, Vanlauwe J, Victor J, Haspl M, Bohnsack M, Fortems Y, Vandekerckhove B, Almqvist KF, Claes T, Handelberg F, Lagae K, van der Bauwhede J, Vandenneucker H, Yang KG, Jelic M, Verdonk R, Veulemans N, Bellemans J, Luyten FP (2008) Characterized chondrocyte implantation results in better structural repair when treating symptomatic cartilage defects of the knee in a randomized controlled trial versus microfracture. Am J Sports Med 36(2):235–246, 10.1177/0363546507311095
2. Gomoll AH, Madry H, Knutsen G, van Dijk N, Seil R, Brittberg M, Kon E (2010) The subchondral bone in articular cartilage repair: current problems in the

surgical management. Knee Surg, Sports Traumatol, Arthroscopy: Off J of the ESSKA 18(4):434–447, 10.1007/s00167-010-1072-x
3. Henson F, Getgood A (2011) The use of scaffolds in musculoskeletal tissue engineering. Open Orthop J 5(Suppl 2):261–266, 10.2174/1874325001105010261
4. Getgood AM, Kew SJ, Brooks R, Aberman H, Simon T, Lynn AK, Rushton N (2012) Evaluation of early-stage osteochondral defect repair using a biphasic scaffold based on a collagen-glycosaminoglycan biopolymer in a caprine model. Knee 19(4):422–430, 10.1016/j.knee.2011.03.011
5. Fortier LA, Mohammed HO, Lust G, Nixon AJ (2002) Insulin-like growth factor-I enhances cell-based repair of articular cartilage. J Bone Joint Surg 84(2):276–288
6. Chubinskaya S, Hurtig M, Rueger DC (2007) OP-1/BMP-7 in cartilage repair. Int Orthop 31(6):773–781, 10.1007/s00264-007-0423-9
7. Hurtig M, Chubinskaya S, Dickey J, Rueger D (2009) BMP-7 protects against progression of cartilage degeneration after impact injury. J Orthop Res: Off Publ Orthop Res Soc 27(5):602–611, 10.1002/jor.20787
8. Davidson D, Blanc A, Filion D, Wang H, Plut P, Pfeffer G, Buschmann MD, Henderson JE (2005) Fibroblast growth factor (FGF) 18 signals through FGF receptor 3 to promote chondrogenesis. J Biol Chem 280(21):20509–20515, 10.1074/jbc.M410148200
9. Moore EE, Bendele AM, Thompson DL, Littau A, Waggie KS, Reardon B, Ellsworth JL (2005) Fibroblast growth factor-18 stimulates chondrogenesis and cartilage repair in a rat model of injury-induced osteoarthritis. Osteoarthritis and cartilage / OARS, Osteoarthritis Res Soc 13(7):623–631, 10.1016/j.joca.2005.03.003
10. Liu Z, Xu J, Colvin JS, Ornitz DM (2002) Coordination of chondrogenesis and osteogenesis by fibroblast growth factor 18. Genes Dev 16(7):859–869, 10.1101/gad.965602
11. Ellsworth JL, Berry J, Bukowski T, Claus J, Feldhaus A, Holderman S, Holdren MS, Lum KD, Moore EE, Raymond F, Ren H, Shea P, Sprecher C, Storey H, Thompson DL, Waggie K, Yao L, Fernandes RJ, Eyre DR, Hughes SD (2002) Fibroblast growth factor-18 is a trophic factor for mature chondrocytes and their progenitors. Osteoarthritis and Cartilage / OARS, Osteoarthritis Res Soc 10(4):308–320, 10.1053/joca.2002.0514
12. Power J, Hernandez P, Guehring H, Getgood A, Henson F (2014) Intra-articular injection of rhFGF-18 improves the healing in microfracture treated chondral defects in an ovine model. J Orthop Res: Off Pub Orthop Res Soc 32(5):669–676, 10.1002/jor.22580
13. Frenkel SR, Bradica G, Brekke JH, Goldman SM, Ieska K, Issack P, Bong MR, Tian H, Gokhale J, Coutts RD, Kronengold RT (2005) Regeneration of articular cartilage–evaluation of osteochondral defect repair in the rabbit using multiphasic implants. Osteoarthritis and Cartilage / OARS, Osteoarthritis Res Soc 13(9):798–807, 10.1016/j.joca.2005.04.018
14. Henson FM, Davies ME, Jeffcott LB (1997) Equine dyschondroplasia (osteochondrosis)–histological findings and type VI collagen localization. Veterinary J 154(1):53–62
15. Hosgor M, Karaca I, Ozer E, Suzek D, Ulukus C, Ozdamar A (2004) Do alterations in collagen synthesis play an etiologic role in childhood inguinoscrotal pathologies: an immunohistochemical study. J Pediatr Surg 39(7):1024–1029
16. Smith GD, Taylor J, Almqvist KF, Erggelet C, Knutsen G, Garcia Portabella M, Smith T, Richardson JB (2005) Arthroscopic assessment of cartilage repair: a validation study of 2 scoring systems. Arthroscopy: Journal of Arthroscopic & Related Surgery: official publication of the Arthroscopy Association of North America and the International Arthroscopy Association 21(12):1462–1467, 10.1016/j.arthro.2005.09.007
17. Fitzpatrick N, Smith TJ, Evans RB, Yeadon R (2009) Radiographic and arthroscopic findings in the elbow joints of 263 dogs with medial coronoid disease. Veterinary Surg: VS 38(2):213–223, 10.1111/j.1532-950X.2008.00489.x
18. Ellsworth JL, Garcia R, Yu J, Kindy MS (2003) Fibroblast growth factor-18 reduced infarct volumes and behavioral deficits after transient occlusion of the middle cerebral artery in rats. Stroke; J Cerebral Circ 34(6):1507–1512, 10.1161/01.STR.0000071760.66720.5F
19. Lohmander LS, Hellot S, Dreher D, Krantz EF, Kruger DS, Guermazi A, Eckstein F (2014) Intraarticular sprifermin (recombinant human fibroblast growth factor 18) in knee osteoarthritis: a randomized, double-blind, placebo-controlled trial. Arthritis Rheumatol 66(7):1820–1831, 10.1002/art.38614
20. Chubinskaya S, Hakimiyan A, Pacione C, Yanke A, Rappoport L, Aigner T, Rueger DC, Loeser RF (2007) Synergistic effect of IGF-1 and OP-1 on matrix formation by normal and OA chondrocytes cultured in alginate beads. Osteoarthritis and Cartilage / OARS, Osteoarthritis Res Soc 15(4):421–430, 10.1016/j.joca.2006.10.004
21. Gelse K, von der Mark K, Aigner T, Park J, Schneider H (2003) Articular cartilage repair by gene therapy using growth factor-producing mesenchymal cells. Arthritis Rheum 48(2):430–441, 10.1002/art.10759
22. van Beuningen HM, Glansbeek HL, van der Kraan PM, van den Berg WB (1998) Differential effects of local application of BMP-2 or TGF-beta 1 on both articular cartilage composition and osteophyte formation. Osteoarthritis and cartilage / OARS, Osteoarthritis Res Soc 6(5):306–317, 10.1053/joca.1998.0129
23. Knippenberg M, Helder MN, Zandieh Doulabi B, Wuisman PI, Klein-Nulend J (2006) Osteogenesis versus chondrogenesis by BMP-2 and BMP-7 in adipose stem cells. Biochem Biophys Res Commun 342(3):902–908, 10.1016/j.bbrc.2006.02.052
24. Behr B, Sorkin M, Manu A, Lehnhardt M, Longaker MT, Quarto N (2011) Fgf-18 is required for osteogenesis but not angiogenesis during long bone repair. Tissue Eng A 17(15–16):2061–2069, 10.1089/ten.TEA.2010.0719
25. Carmont MR, Carey-Smith R, Saithna A, Dhillon M, Thompson P, Spalding T (2009) Delayed incorporation of a TruFit plug: perseverance is recommended. Arthroscopy: J Arthroscopic & Related Surg: Off Pub Arthroscopy Assoc North Am and the Int Arthroscopy Assoc 25(7):810–814, 10.1016/j.arthro.2009.01.023
26. Getgood A, Brooks R, Fortier L, Rushton N (2009) Articular cartilage tissue engineering: today's research, tomorrow's practice? J Bone Joint Surg 91 (5):565–576, 10.1302/0301-620X.91B5.21832
27. Gikas PD, Morris T, Carrington R, Skinner J, Bentley G, Briggs T (2009) A correlation between the timing of biopsy after autologous chondrocyte implantation and the histological appearance. J Bone Joint Surg 91(9):1172–1177, 10.1302/0301-620X.91B9.22490

Strength of the porcine proximal femoral epiphyseal plate: the effect of different loading directions and the role of the perichondrial fibrocartilaginous complex and epiphyseal tubercle – an experimental biomechanical study

Páll Sigurgeir Jónasson[1*], Lars Ekström[1], Anna Swärd[3], Mikael Sansone[2], Mattias Ahldén[2], Jón Karlsson[1] and Adad Baranto[1]

Abstract

Background: The high loads on adolescent athletes' musculoskeletal system are known to cause morphological and degenerative changes in bone, intervertebral discs and joints. It has been suggested that the cam deformity of the proximal femoral head originates from a subclinical slipped capital femoral epiphysis (SCFE) as a result of non-physiological loading. The perichondrial fibrocartilaginous complex (PFC) and the epiphyseal tubercle are believed to stabilise the proximal femoral epiphysis, but their role is still unclear. The aim of the present study was to develop an experimental, biomechanical model to evaluate the strength of the porcine proximal femoral epiphysis in different loading directions and, furthermore, to investigate the stabilising role of the PFC and the epiphyseal tubercle.

Methods: A descriptive laboratory study. An *in-vitro* model was developed and nine young (5 months) porcine proximal femoral epiphyses were loaded to failure; three in the anterior-posterior direction, three in the lateral-medial direction and three in the vertical direction. The injured proximal femoral epiphyses were then examined both macroscopically and histologically.

Results: Anterior and lateral loading of the proximal femoral epiphysis resulted in failure of the epiphyseal plate, while vertical loading resulted in a fracture epiphyseolysis. The epiphysis was weakest when exposed to a lateral load and strongest when exposed to a vertical load. Despite histological epiphyseolysis, the PFC was intact in 15 of 27 (56%) slices. In histological examinations, the epiphyseal tubercle appears to halt the slide of the epiphysis.

Conclusions: We have developed an experimental, biomechanical model to measure the strength of the proximal femoral epiphyseal plate in different loading directions. The strength of the proximal femur was weakest through the epiphyseal plate. The epiphysis was weakest when exposed to a lateral load and strongest when exposed to a vertical load. The epiphyseal tubercle and the PFC stabilise the epiphysis when the epiphyseal plate is damaged. The findings in the present study indicate that overloading the hips in growing individuals can disrupt the epiphyseal plate. These findings may have implications when it comes to understanding the pathogenesis of cam deformity of the hip.

Keywords: Hip; Load; Epiphysiolysis; Epiphyseal plate; Porcine; Epiphyseal tubercle; Perichondrial fibrocartilaginous complex

* Correspondence: pallsj@gmail.com
[1]Department of Orthopaedics, Institute of Clinical Sciences at Sahlgrenska Academy, University of Gothenburg and Sahlgrenska University Hospital, Gothenburg, Sweden
Full list of author information is available at the end of the article

Background

The skeleton of the growing individual is susceptible to mechanical injuries, but the growing bone is also capable of adapting to varying stresses [1]. Some physiological load is needed for normal bone growth, [2] but exceeding this physiological load can lead to unwanted morphological changes and different pathologies of the bone and joints [3,4].

Adolescent athletes in sports where high demands are imposed on the back have been shown to have a high frequency of abnormalities in the vertebral endplates, apophyseal ring and intervertebral discs [5,6]. A systematic review of sports-related growth plate injuries reported similar results for the upper and lower extremities [3].

The cam deformity is a non-spherical extension of the femoral head at the antero-superior head-neck junction of the proximal femur. It is more common in adolescent athletes, participating in high-load sports, compared with an age-matched control group [7] and it is thought to be a frequent cause of hip pain in athletes [8]. The etiology of the cam deformity is not known. One suggested explanation is that it is caused by a subclinical epiphysiolysis of the proximal femoral epiphysis [9-11].

In 1976, Chung et al. reported that the perichondrial fibrocartilaginous complex (PFC) was an important stabiliser of the human epiphyseal plate. When the PFC was excised, the shear strength of the plate decreased significantly [12]. Other researchers have proposed that a defect in the PFC or thinning of the periosteum may precipitate subclinical slipped capital femoral epiphysis (SCFE) [13,14]. The epiphyseal tubercle is also believed to stabilise the proximal femoral epiphyseal plate. It is a tuberosity, eccentrically and inferiorly placed on the capital epiphysis, projecting into an appropriately shaped socket in the metaphysis. The tubercle is believed to hold the epiphysis in place in a chronic SCFE [15-17].

During routine daily activities, the hip joint is mainly loaded vertically [18-21]. The way the load is distributed in the hip joint in deep flexion or during sport is largely unknown.

The purpose of the present study was to create a porcine model in order to estimate the difference in strength of the proximal femoral epiphysis in relation to different loading directions. Furthermore, the aim was to explore the stabilising roles of the PFC and epiphyseal tubercle, utilising a histological analysis.

The hypothesis was that the epiphyseal plate would be the weakest link in the proximal femur and that its strength would be greatest during vertical loading.

Methods

Experimental animals and procedures

The proximal femur from nine young (5 months) porcine hips were dissected and cleaned of soft tissue, muscle and capsular attachments. The porcine subjects were male domestic pigs, obtained from the local abattoir, with a median weight of 90 kg (range 85–95). The diameter of the femoral heads was measured in the coronal and sagittal planes with a measurement error of less than 1 mm using a slide caliper [22].

Mechanical test procedures

Nine femurs were used in pilot tests of the model in order to establish a correct fixation method; the remaining nine femurs were used for the study.

The prepared proximal femurs were fixed with cement in a metal fixture and attached to the actuator of a servo hydraulic universal testing machine (MTS Test Star, Minneapolis, MN, USA). A custom-made aluminium rod with a small plastic cup (25 mm in diameter), contoured to the shape of the femoral head, was attached to the upper crosshead of the testing machine. The deformation control mode was set at a rate of 0.05 mm/sec. Force and deformation were recorded continuously and failure was defined as a sudden decrease in force, which could be seen on the force/deformation diagram on the computer. Furthermore the failure was visual and audible to the researchers (the first and second authors) in all test cases. Loading was stopped immediately after the first sign of failure.

The physeal line was clearly visible on the surface of the femoral head and was used as a guide for the placement of the plastic cup, which was proximally to the line. The proximal epiphysis was then loaded to failure in one of three directions. Three femurs were loaded from the lateral side in the coronal plane, three femurs were loaded from the anterior side in the sagittal plane and three femurs were loaded vertically (Figures 1, 2 and 3). On those loaded from the lateral side, the major trochanter was removed to facilitate access for the loading rod with the

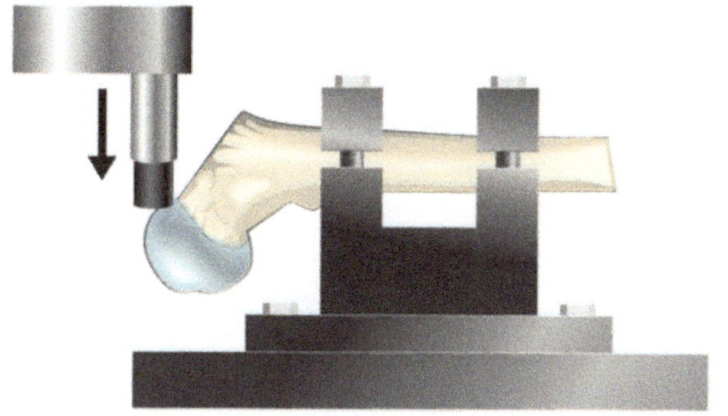

Figure 1 Set-up for lateral loading of the specimens. The major trochanter was removed to facilitate access for the loading rod.

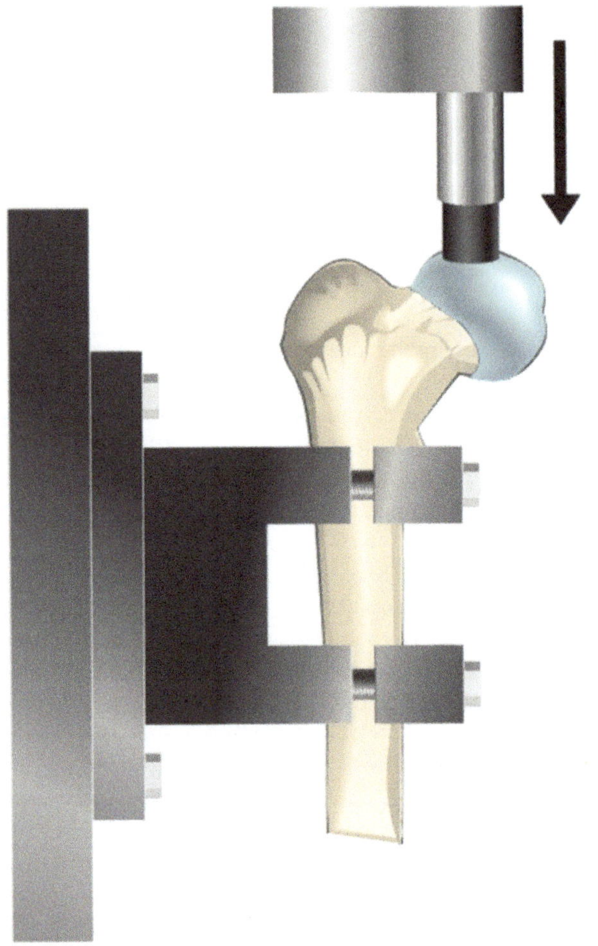

Figure 2 Set-up for vertical loading of the specimens.

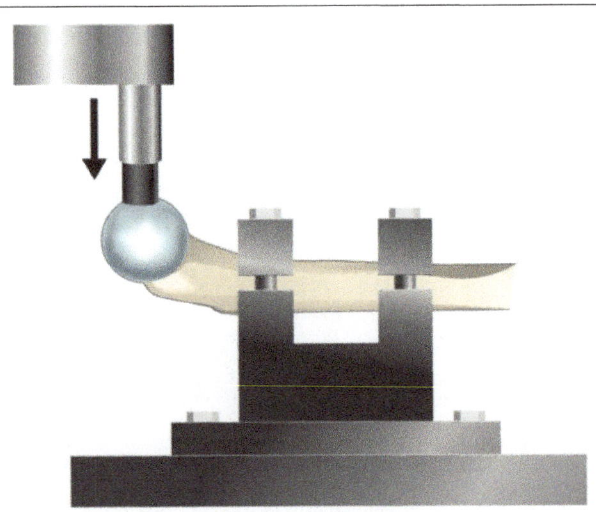

Figure 3 Set-up for anterior loading of the specimens.

plastic cup. After failure, the size of the footprint left by the plastic cup on the femoral head and its distance from the physeal line were measured. Any signs of epiphyseolysis or fracture, visual or palpable, were registered if present.

Macroscopic and histological examinations

The specimens were then stored in a –20°C freezer until completely frozen. When frozen, they were sawn into four equally thick primary slices in the loading plane using a bandsaw. The slices were decalcified, dehydrated, fixed in paraffin and cut in 4 μm slices using a microtome. Four slices from each specimen were then stained with hematoxylin-eosin and alcian blue solution. The histological slices were examined microscopically for injuries by the first and the second author (an orthopedic surgeon and a research engineer respectively).

The histological presence of epiphyseolysis, the percentage of the epiphyseal plate that was damaged, the epiphyseal zone that was damaged and a Salter-Harris classification were registered for each slice. The integrity of the PFC and the presence of the epiphyseal tubercle were also noted and registered.

Results

Anterior load

Imposing an anterior load on all three specimens resulted in failure at a median load of 1,750 N (range 1,679-1,756). On histological examination, subtotal epiphyseolysis was present in two specimens and total epiphyseolysis was present in one specimen. The damage wandered erratically between the resting and the ossifying zones of the epiphyseal line (Figure 4). PFC damage could not be assessed in one slice and was seen on only

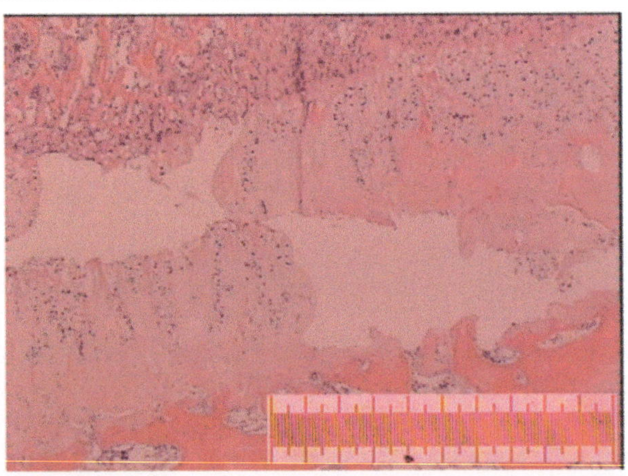

Figure 4 Photomicrograph showing damaged epiphyseal plate. In the anterior and lateral loaded specimens, the damage wandered between the resting and ossifying zones. Sample stained with hematoxylin-eosin solution. Magnification X25. Scale bar equals 1 mm.

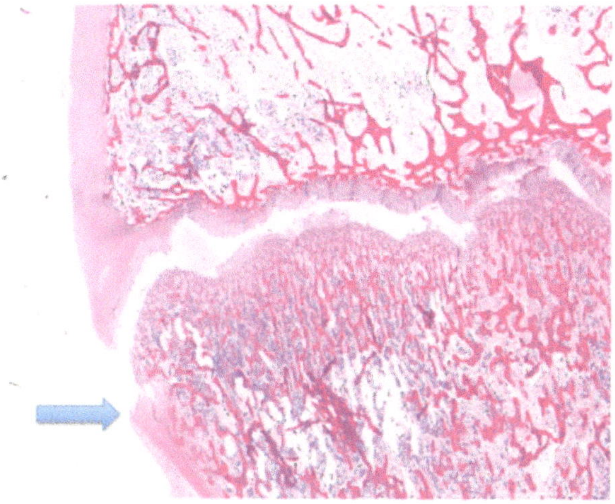

Figure 5 Epiphysiolysis with a damaged PFC (arrow). Sample stained with hematoxylin-eosin solution. Scanned slide, no magnification.

one slice of the remaining eleven (Figure 5). Macroscopically, a small cleavage was seen proximal to the footprint over the epiphyseal line (Figure 6). On palpation, no movement could be detected between the epiphysis and metaphysis after failure.

Lateral load

Imposing a lateral load on all three specimens resulted in failure at a median load of 920 N (range 918–1,148). On histological examination, subtotal epiphysiolysis was found in all specimens, with the damage wandering erratically between the resting and ossifying zones (Figure 4). On those slices in which the epiphyseal tubercle was present, it appeared as though it was partially dislodged and was pressing against the medial wall of the metaphyseal socket (Figure 7). PFC integrity could not be assessed in two slices and the PFC was damaged on eight of the remaining ten slices. Macroscopically, a small cleavage was seen proximal to the footprint, over the epiphyseal line. On palpation, no movement could be detected between the epiphysis and metaphysis.

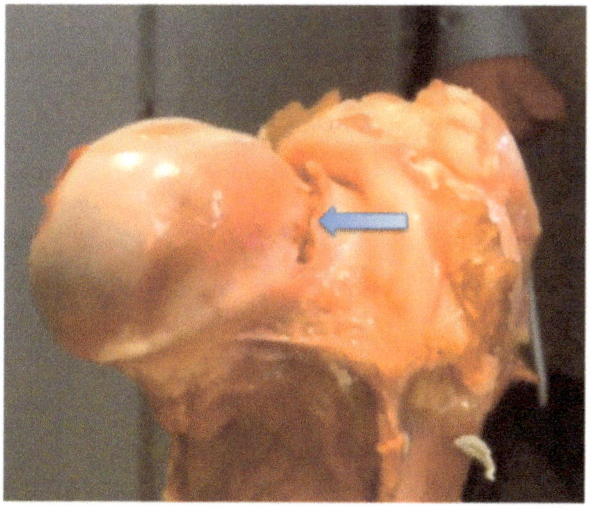

Figure 6 A small cleavage (arrow) over the epiphyseal line can be seen after failure.

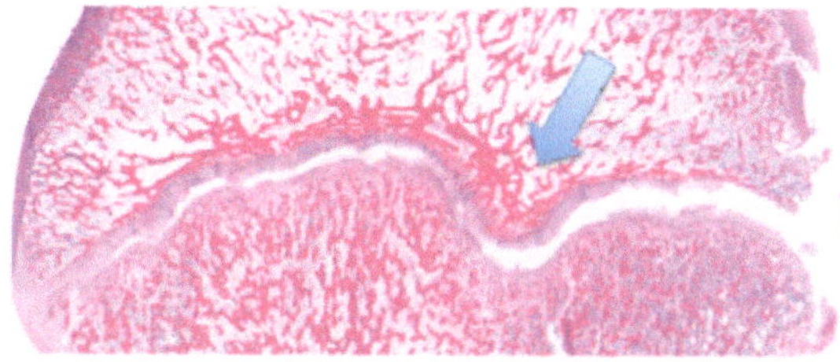

Figure 7 The epiphyseal tubercle (arrow) pressing against the medial wall of the metaphyseal socket. The PFC is damaged. Sample stained with hematoxylin-eosin solution. Scanned slide, no magnification.

Vertical load

Imposing a vertical load on all three specimens resulted in failure at a median load of 7,397 N (range 7,008-7,413). On histological examination, all specimens showed signs, to a varying degree, of epiphyseolysis and fracture epiphyseolysis Salter Harris type 2. The epiphyseolysis was primarily in the ossifying zone. The epiphyseal tubercle was present in one slice in every specimen and the fractures tended to originate laterally to the epiphyseal tubercle and extend through the medial cortex of the femoral neck. The integrity of the PFC could not be assessed in six slices, but the PFC was damaged in three of the remaining six slices. Macroscopically, a cleavage was seen laterally over the epiphyseal line and an obvious fracture, medially on the femoral neck, was seen. On palpation, movement over the fracture could easily be detected.

General

Loading of all the specimens (9 of 9) resulted in an epiphyseolysis (anterior load and lateral load) or a fracture epiphyseolysis. The epiphyseal plate showed the greatest strength in response to vertical loading (mean 7,273 N (SD 229)) and the least strength in response to lateral loading (mean 995 N (SD 132)), with the strength in response to anterior loading falling in between (mean 1,728 N (SD 43)).

The femoral heads were of similar size and the plastic cup on the rod left a shallow footprint on the femoral head after loading. The size of the

Table 1 Macroscopic characteristics with load and deformation at failure for all specimens

Direction of load	Specimen	AP diameter (mm)	ML diameter (mm)	Load at failure (N)	Deformation at failure (mm)	Footprint (mm)	Footprint distance from epiphyseal line (mm)	Macroscopic epiphyseolysis
Anterior load								
	1	35	36	1756	7.4	22 × 8	6	Yes
	2	35	37	1750	7.5	21 × 7	5	Yes
	3	35	36	1679	8.7	20 × 8	5	Yes
	Mean (SD)	35	36	1728 (43)	7.9			
Lateral load								
	1	34	36	1148	7.1	14 × 8	4	Yes
	2	34	36	918	7.0	15 × 4	3	Yes
	3	37	38	920	7.1	17 × 4	4	Yes
	Mean (SD)	35	37	995 (132)	7.1			
Vertical load								
	1	38	39	7397	5.0	25 × 25	5	Yes
	2	37	39	7413	6.6	25 × 25	9	Yes
	3	38	38	7008	6.4	25 × 25	4	Yes
	Mean (SD)	38	39	7273 (229)	6.0			

indentation from the plastic cup was clearly detectable on the femoral head and the size of the footprint was related to the load – larger footprints at higher load failures. The macroscopic characteristics of the porcine hips, the footprint size and distance from the physeal line and the load and deformation at failure are presented in Table 1. A sample loading/deformation curve is presented in Figure 8.

On nine of thirty-six slices, PFC integrity could not be estimated. During preparation of the slices, the metaphyseal part of the PFC disappeared, making judgement of its integrity impossible. The PFC was damaged on 12 of the remaining 27 slices. All specimens loaded laterally showed some damage to the PFC. The epiphyseal tubercle was identified on 12 of 36 slices. Its presence was confirmed in all specimens apart from one loaded anteriorly. The microscopic characteristics are presented in Table 2.

The force/deformation graphs for lateral, anterior and vertical loads are presented in Figures 2, 3 and 4 respectively.

Discussion

The main finding in the present study is that the epiphyseal plate is the weakest point in the young porcine proximal femur. Loading to failure resulted in epiphyseolysis or fracture epiphyseolysis in all the specimens. The model was consistent and easy to set up.

Load at failure was lowest for the laterally loaded specimens (995 N) and highest for the vertically loaded specimens (7,273 N). The load set-up in the present model resulted primarily in a tensile load over the epiphyseal plate in the laterally loaded specimens, a shear load in the anteriorly loaded specimens and a compressive load in those loaded vertically. The highest strength was

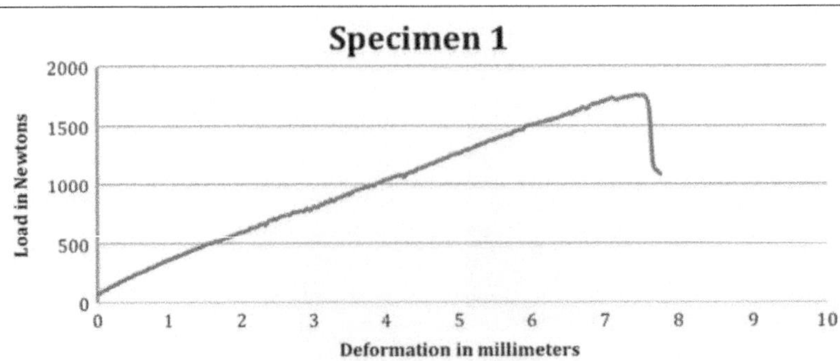

Figure 8 Anterior loaded specimen sample load/deformation curve.

Table 2 Microscopic characteristics of the specimens

Specimen	Slide	Microscopic epiphyseolysis present	Percentage of epiphysis damaged	Epiphyseal zone damaged	Salter Harris classification	Perichondral fibrocartilaginous complex damaged	Epiphyseal tubercle present
Anterior specimen 1							
	1	Yes	100	Resting/ ossifying	1	No	No
	2	Yes	68	Resting	1	No	No
	3	Yes	77	Resting/ ossifying	1	No	No
	4	Yes	100	Resting/ ossifying	2	Yes	Yes
Anterior specimen 2							
	1	Yes	89	Resting/ ossifying	2	No	No
	2	Yes	63	Ossifying	1	No	No
	3	Yes	80	Resting/ ossifying	1	N/A	No
	4	Yes	81	Resting/ ossifying	1	No	No
Anterior specimen 3							
	1	Yes	100	Resting/ ossifying	1	No	No
	2	Yes	100	Resting/ ossifying	1	No	No
	3	Yes	100	Resting/ ossifying	1	No	Yes
	4	Yes	100	Resting/ ossifying	1	No	Yes
Lateral specimen 1							
	1	Yes	83	Resting/ ossifying	1	Yes	No
	2	Yes	84	Ossifying	1	No	No
	3	Yes	87	Resting/ ossifying	1	N/A	Yes
	4	Yes	100	Resting/ ossifying	2	No	Yes
Lateral specimen 2							
	1	Yes	100	Resting/ ossifying	2	Yes	No
	2	Yes	55	Resting/ ossifying	1	Yes	No
	3	Yes	75	Resting/ ossifying	1	Yes	Yes
	4	Yes	75	Resting/ ossifying	1	Yes	Yes
Lateral specimen 3							
	1	Yes	64	Resting/ ossifying	1	Yes	No
	2	Yes	100	Resting/ ossifying	2	N/A	No
	3	Yes	78	Resting/ ossifying	1	Yes	Yes

Table 2 Microscopic characteristics of the specimens *(Continued)*

4	Yes	72	Resting/ ossifying	1	Yes	Yes
Vertical specimen 1						
1	Yes	100	Ossifying	1	No	No
2	Yes	50	Ossifying	1	No	No
3	Yes	30	Ossifying	1	N/A	Yes
4	Yes fracture	30	Resting	2	N/A	No
Vertical specimen 2						
1	Yes fracture	70	Ossifying	2	Yes	No
2	Yes fracture	80	Ossifying	2	Yes	No
3	Yes fracture	100	Ossifying	2	N/A	Yes
4	Yes fracture	50	Ossifying	2	Yes	No
Vertical specimen 3						
1	Yes fracture	80	Ossifying	2	No	No
2	Yes fracture	100	Ossifying	2	N/A	No
3	Yes fracture	100	Ossifying	2	N/A	Yes
4	Yes fracture	100	Ossifying	2	N/A	No

therefore to be expected in the vertically loaded specimens, where the loading direction is comparable to the loading direction *in vivo* [18-21].

The vertical load mainly caused failure in the ossifying zone of the epiphyseal plate, while a more random pattern of failure between different epiphyseal zones was seen in the other groups. In a study of cattle, Moen et al. reported that compressive forces tended to cause failure in the ossifying zone [23].

Chung et al. [12] reported a significant decrease in shear strength when the PFC was excised. They loaded their specimens anteriorly. In the present study, all but one slice from the anteriorly loaded specimens showed an undamaged PFC (figure 9), while some PFC damage was seen in all laterally loaded specimens. This indicates that the PFC performs a stabilising function, at least when the epiphysis is loaded anteriorly. In the vertically loaded specimens, the integrity of the PFC could not be assessed in six of 12 slices. The disappearance of the metaphyseal part during the preparation of the slices might indicate that the PFC was damaged.

The epiphyseal tubercle was identified in all specimens apart from one of the anteriorly loaded specimens. On the slices from the laterally loaded specimens where the tubercle was identified, the tubercle can be seen pressing against the metaphyseal socket, stopping the slide of the epiphysis (Figure 7). The same finding was seen on the slices from the vertically loaded specimens, where the tubercle appears to stop the epiphysis in its slide. Due to the compressive forces applied in the vertically loaded specimens, the tubercle compresses the medial wall of the socket, resulting in a fracture of the metaphysis through the medial cortex instead of dislodging the tubercle from the socket. This implies that the tubercle performs a stabilising function during vertical and lateral loading.

On microscopic examination of the vertically loaded specimens, the epiphyseal plate was damaged laterally to the epiphyseal tubercle. The cam deformity is usually located antero-superiorly on the femoral head [24] and therefore laterally to the epiphyseal tubercle. It is possible to speculate that the cam deformity

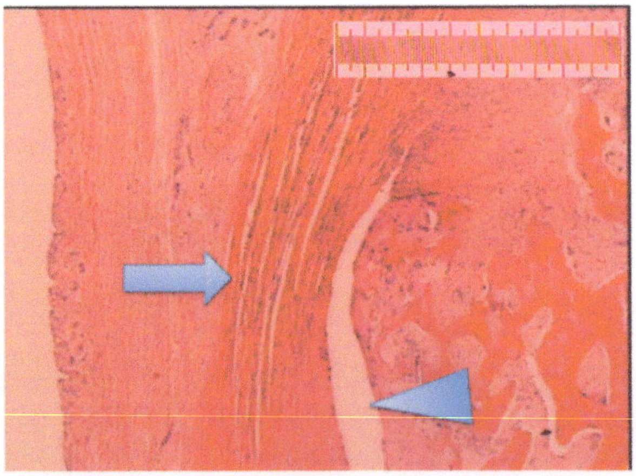

Figure 9 Photomicrograph showing microscopic epiphyseolysis (arrowhead) with the PFC (arrow) intact. Sample stained with hematoxylin-eosin solution. Magnification X20. Scale bar equals 1 mm.

develops from a partial epiphyseolysis, where the epiphyseal tubercle prevents total epiphyseolysis or dislodges partially in total epiphyseolysis. Rotation of the epiphysis around the eccentric epiphyseal tubercle has also been suggested as a possible cause of chronic SCFE [16,17].

Anterior and lateral loading forces around the femoral head are small during routine activities [18-21]. The way loading occurs during sports and in deep flexion is unknown. Muscle action and ligament constraints around the hip joint most probably prevent the joint being loaded from an anterior direction *in vivo*. In reality, the hip joint is probably loaded somewhere between the vertical and anterior loading directions in deep flexion. A posterior slope of the femoral epiphysis increases the anterior load on the epiphyseal plate and is a known predictor of SCFE [25] and anterior load also appears to increase in deep flexion [26]. It is possible to speculate that the strength of the epiphyseal plate is therefore lower when the hip is in flexion.

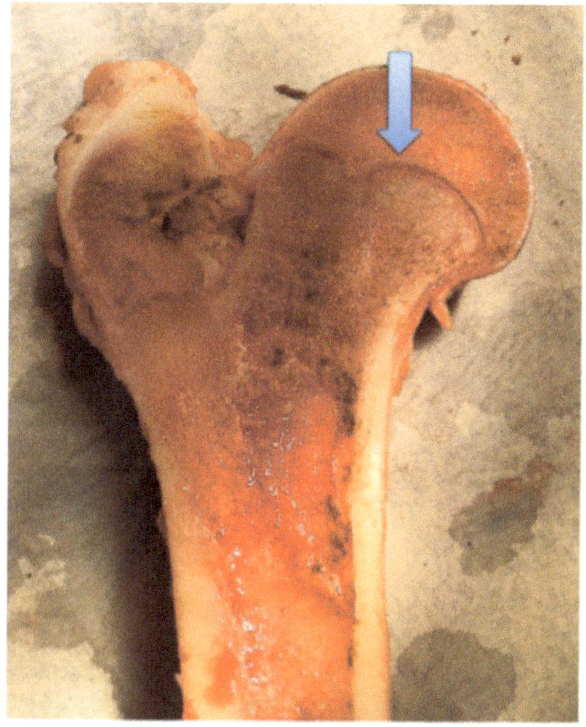

Figure 10 Porcine proximal femur split coronally. The major trochanter is relatively larger than in a human and the femoral neck shorter. The growth plate and the epiphyseal tubercle are clearly visible in this specimen (arrow).

Limitations

Using an *in-vitro* porcine model can be regarded as a limitation when it comes to understanding human hip joint diseases, but many studies of hip biomechanics and hip conditions use a porcine model, especially in pediatric orthopedics, [27-34] and, in a phenomenological study like the present one, it is thought to be appropriate.

During the preparation of the specimens, all the soft tissues were removed. The muscles and ligaments of the hip most certainly play a major role in dynamic hip biomechanics. Our conclusions are not affected by this fact, as we are only investigating semi-static strength.

Macroscopically, the porcine hip is comparable to the human hip, the main difference being a more prominent major trochanter and a shorter femoral neck (Figure 10). Ipsen et al. reported that, in one-year-old pigs, the proximal femoral epiphysis is similar in size to that in adolescent humans and its shear strength is comparable to that reported by Chung et al. [12,35]. The specimens in the present study are of comparable size to those in a 10-year-old child and the shear strength of the anteriorly loaded specimens was comparable to the values reported by Chung et al. [12]. The microscopic characteristics of the porcine epiphyseal plate are identical to those of the human epiphyseal plate, with the different epiphyseal growth zones clearly visible (Figure 11).

Conclusion

This model is consistent and simple. The weakest part in the young porcine proximal femur was the epiphyseal plate. This location of weakness may explain the cam deformity found in young athletes. The epiphyseal plate is strongest when exposed to vertical load, weaker when exposed to anterior load and weakest when exposed to lateral load. The epiphyseal tubercle and the PFC are important stabilisers of the epiphysis.

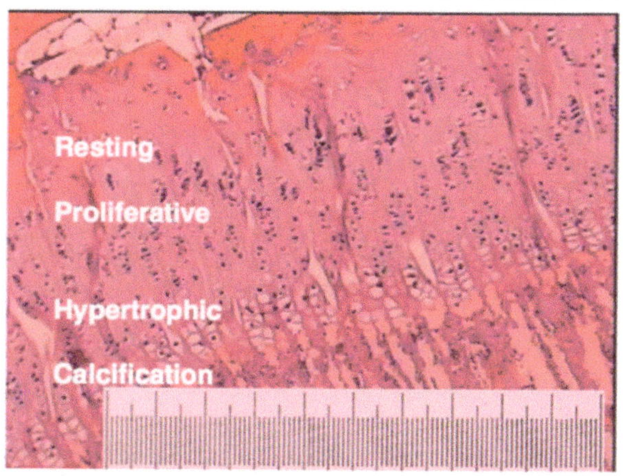

Figure 11 The different zones of the porcine epiphyseal plate. Sample stained with hematoxylin-eosin solution. Magnification X40. Scale bar equals 1 mm.

Competing interests

The authors have no financial or non-financial competing interests.

Authors' contribution

PJ and LE participated in designing the study, performing the experiments and writing the article. AS, MS and MA participated in writing the article. JK and AB participated in designing the study and writing the article. All authors read and approved the final manuscript.

Author details

[1]Department of Orthopaedics, Institute of Clinical Sciences at Sahlgrenska Academy, University of Gothenburg and Sahlgrenska University Hospital, Gothenburg, Sweden. [2]Orthocenter/IFK-KLINIKEN, Sports Medicine Clinic, Gothenburg, Sweden. [3]Östersund Hospital, Östersund, Sweden.

References

1. Arkin AM, Katz JF (1956) The effects of pressure on epiphyseal growth; the mechanism of plasticity of growing bone. J Bone Joint Surg Am 38-A (5):1056–1076
2. Malina RM (1969) Exercise as an influence upon growth. Review and critique of current concepts Clinical pediatrics 8(1):16–26
3. Caine D, DiFiori J, Maffulli N (2006) Physeal injuries in children's and youth sports: reasons for concern? Br J Sports Med 40(9):749–760
4. Strobino LJ, French GO, Colonna PC (1952) The effect of increasing tensions on the growth of epiphyseal bone. Surgery, gynecology & obstetrics 95(6):694–700
5. Lundin O, Hellstrom M, Nilsson I, Sward L (2001) Back pain and radiological changes in the thoraco-lumbar spine of athletes. A long-term follow-up Scand J Med Sci Sports 11(2):103–109
6. Sward L, Hellstrom M, Jacobsson B, Nyman R, Peterson L (1991) Disc degeneration and associated abnormalities of the spine in elite gymnasts. A magnetic resonance imaging study. Spine (Phila Pa 1976) 16(4):437–443
7. Siebenrock KA, Ferner F, Noble PC, Santore RF, Werlen S, Mamisch TC (2011) The cam-type deformity of the proximal femur arises in childhood in response to vigorous sporting activity. Clin Orthop Relat Res 469 (11):3229–3240
8. Murray RO, Duncan C (1971) Athletic activity in adolescence as an etiological factor in degenerative hip disease. J Bone Joint Surg Br 53(3):406–419
9. Murray RO (1965) The aetiology of primary osteoarthritis of the hip. The British journal of radiology 38(455):810–824
10. Harris WH (1986) Etiology of osteoarthritis of the hip. Clin Orthop Relat Res 213:20–33
11. Goodman DA, Feighan JE, Smith AD, Latimer B, Buly RL, Cooperman DR (1997) Subclinical slipped capital femoral epiphysis. Relationship to osteoarthrosis of the hip J Bone Joint Surg Am 79(10):1489–1497
12. Chung SM, Batterman SC, Brighton CT (1976) Shear strength of the human femoral capital epiphyseal plate. J Bone Joint Surg Am 58(1):94–103
13. Pritchett JW, Perdue KD (1988) Mechanical factors in slipped capital femoral epiphysis. J Pediatr Orthop 8(4):385–388
14. Billing L, Bogren HG, Henrikson B, Wallin J (2004) Slipped capital femoral epiphysis. The mechanical function of the periosteum: new aspects and theory including bilaterality. Acta radiologica Supplement 431:1–27
15. Liu RW, Armstrong DG, Levine AD, Gilmore A, Thompson GH, Cooperman DR (2013) An anatomic study of the epiphyseal tubercle and its importance in the pathogenesis of slipped capital femoral epiphysis. J Bone Joint Surg Am 95(6):e341–348
16. Tayton K (2007) Does the upper femoral epiphysis slip or rotate? J Bone Joint Surg Br 89(10):1402–1406
17. Tayton K (2009) The epiphyseal tubercle in adolescent hips. Acta Orthop 80(4):416–419
18. Correa TA, Crossley KM, Kim HJ, Pandy MG (2010) Contributions of individual muscles to hip joint contact force in normal walking. J Biomech 43(8):1618–1622
19. Bergmann G, Deuretzbacher G, Heller M, Graichen F, Rohlmann A, Strauss J, Duda GN (2001) Hip contact forces and gait patterns from routine activities. J Biomech 34(7):859–871
20. Bergmann G, Graichen F, Rohlmann A (2004) Hip joint contact forces during stumbling. Langenbeck's archives of surgery/Deutsche Gesellschaft fur Chirurgie 389(1):53–59
21. Brand R (1982) Forces on the femoral head during activities of daily living. Iowa Orthop J 2:43–49
22. Kosashvili Y, Backstein D, Safir O, Ran Y, Loebenberg MI, Ziv YB (2008) Hemiarthroplasty of the hip for fracture-what is the appropriate sized femoral head? Injury 39(2):232–237
23. Moen CT, Pelker RR (1984) Biomechanical and histological correlations in growth plate failure. J Pediatr Orthop 4(2):180–184
24. Rakhra KS, Sheikh AM, Allen D, Beaule PE (2009) Comparison of MRI alpha angle measurement planes in femoroacetabular impingement. Clin Orthop Relat Res 467(3):660–665
25. Barrios C, Blasco MA, Blasco MC, Gasco J (2005) Posterior sloping angle of the capital femoral physis: a predictor of bilaterality in slipped capital femoral epiphysis. J Pediatr Orthop 25(4):445–449
26. Sparks DR, Beason DP, Etheridge BS, Alonso JE, Eberhardt AW (2005) Contact pressures in the flexed hip joint during lateral trochanteric loading. J Orthop Res 23(2):359–366
27. Baranto A, Ekstrom L, Hellstrom M, Lundin O, Holm S, Sward L (2005) Fracture patterns of the adolescent porcine spine: an experimental loading study in bending-compression. Spine (Phila Pa 1976) 30(1):75–82
28. Baranto A, Ekstrom L, Holm S, Hellstrom M, Hansson HA, Sward L (2005) Vertebral fractures and separations of endplates after traumatic loading of adolescent porcine spines with experimentally-induced disc degeneration. Clin Biomech (Bristol, Avon) 20(10):1046–1054
29. Dodds MK, Lee J, McCormack D (2008) Transarticular stabilization of the immature femoral head: assessment of a novel surgical approach to the dislocating pediatric hip in a porcine model. J Pediatr Orthop 28(1):36–42
30. Hosalkar HS, Varley ES, Glaser DA, Farnsworth CL, Wenger DR (2011) Intracapsular hip pressures in a porcine model: does position and volume matter? J Pediatr Orthop B 20(5):278–283
31. Kishan S, Upasani V, Mahar A, Oka R, Odell T, Rohmiller M, Newton P, Wenger D (2006) Biomechanical stability of single-screw versus two-screw fixation of an unstable slipped capital femoral epiphysis model: effect of screw position in the femoral neck. J Pediatr Orthop 26(5):601–605
32. Pawaskar SS, Grosland NM, Ingham E, Fisher J, Jin Z (2011) Hemiarthroplasty of hip joint: An experimental validation using porcine acetabulum. J Biomech 44(8):1536–1542
33. Upasani V, Kishan S, Oka R, Mahar A, Rohmiller M, Pring M, Wenger D (2006) Biomechanical analysis of single screw fixation for slipped capital femoral epiphysis: are more threads across the physis necessary for stability? J Pediatr Orthop 26(4):474–478
34. Wenger D, Miyanji F, Mahar A, Oka R (2007) The mechanical properties of the ligamentum teres: a pilot study to assess its potential for improving stability in children's hip surgery. J Pediatr Orthop 27(4):408–410
35. Ipsen BJ, Williams JL, Harris MJ, Schmidt TL (2002) Shear Strength of the Pig Capital Femoral Epiphyseal Plate. An Experimental Model for Human Slipped Capital Femoral Epiphysis Fixation Studies. Paper presented at the ASME 2002 International Mechanical Engineering Congress and Exposition, New Orleans, Louisiana, USA, November 17-22, 2002

Immune modulation as a therapeutic strategy in bone regeneration

Claudia Schlundt[1,2], Hanna Schell[1], Stuart B Goodman[3], Gordana Vunjak-Novakovic[4], Georg N Duda[1,2*] and Katharina Schmidt-Bleek[1,2]

Abstract

We summarize research approaches and findings on bone healing and regeneration that were presented at a workshop at the 60th annual meeting of the Orthopedic Research Society (ORS) in New Orleans in 2014. The workshop was designed to discuss the role of inflammation in bone regeneration in the context of fundamental biology, and to develop therapeutic strategies that involve immune modulation. Delayed or non-healing of bone is a major clinical problem, with around 10% of fracture patients suffering from unsatisfying healing outcomes. Inflammation is traditionally seen as a defense mechanism, but was recently found essential in supporting and modulating regenerative cascades. In bone healing, macrophages and T- and B-cells interact with progenitor cells, bone forming osteoblasts and remodeling osteoclasts. Among the cells of the innate immunity, macrophages are promising candidates for targets in immune-modulatory interventions that would overcome complications in bone healing and bone-related diseases. Among the cells of the adaptive immune system, CD8+ T cells have been shown to have a negative impact on bone fracture healing outcome, whereas regulatory T cells could be promising candidates that have a positive, modulating effect on bone fracture healing. This workshop addressed recent advances and key challenges in this exciting interdisciplinary research field.

Keywords: Osteoimmunology; Regeneration; Macrophages; Immune modulation; Bone healing; Revascularization

Introduction

Bone healing

Vertebrates have a bony skeleton that acts as a scaffold for the body. Healthy bone has a remarkable capacity for self-repair (Figure 1). Although bone healing is for the most part an efficient process, around 10% of patients suffer from delayed healing or non-union, leading to the application of complex, expensive, and often invasive, treatment strategies [1].

Fracture healing is a highly complex process that includes the participation of different cell types (immune cells, progenitor cells, mesenchymal cells) [2] and their signalling molecules (cytokines, growth factors, chemokines) [3]. The healing process, which is initiated after injury, results in effective reconstitution of the initial structure of bone tissue, without scar formation. The regenerative reconstitution can be divided into several consecutive steps: inflammation, soft callus formation, hard callus formation, and remodelling (Figure 2).

The inflammatory phase starts with the formation of a hematoma caused by the influx of blood following tissue injury and vascular disruption. Because of its angiogenetic and osteogenetic potential, the formation of fracture hematoma in the early healing phase is an indispensable step for successful healing [4,5]. Removal of the early fracture hematoma was shown to impair bone healing in animal studies, whereas transplantation of the hematoma leads to ectopic bone formation [6,7], demonstrating its osteogenic potential. During the inflammatory phase, the fracture area is characterized by hypoxia (low pH, high lactate) that induces expression of the transcription factor *Hypoxia inducible factor 1α* (Hif1α) that further triggers the expression of angiogenic factors such as *Vascular Endothelial Growth Factor* (VEGF). Revascularization is a prerequisite for the repair phase, including the formation of new cartilage and finally new bone (Figure 3). Immune cells, located in the fracture area, release cytokines as a

* Correspondence: georg.duda@charite.de
[1]Julius Wolff Institut and Center for Musculoskeletal Surgery, Charité - Universitätsmedizin Berlin, Augustenburger Platz 1, 13353 Berlin, Germany
[2]Berlin-Brandenburg Center for Regenerative Therapies, Charité – Universitätsmedizin Berlin, Augustenburger Platz 1, 13353 Berlin, Germany
Full list of author information is available at the end of the article

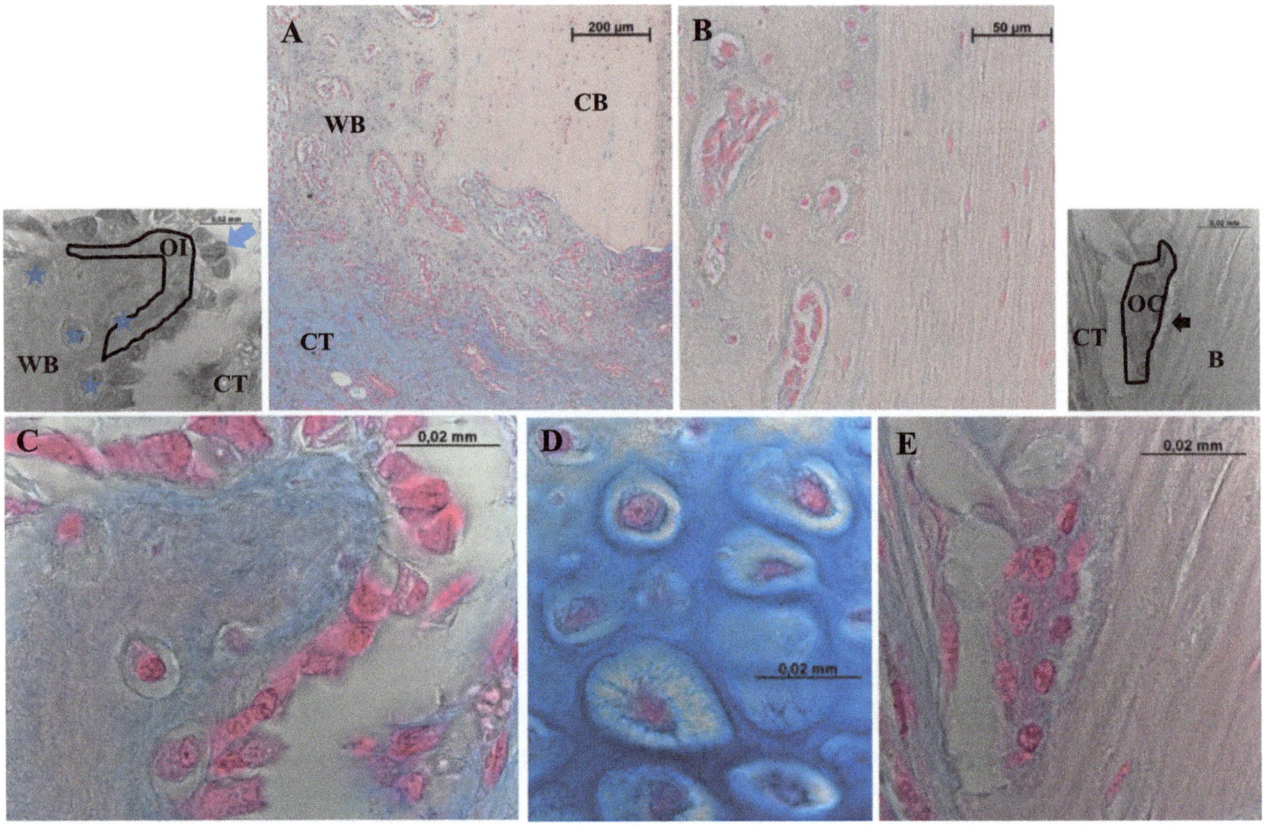

Figure 1 Bone healing. A regenerative process leading to bone formation with restored form/ function if successful. **A**: Intramembranous bone formation along osteomized cortical bone (CB) clearly shows the newly formed woven bone (WB) on the left. Further from the bone edge connective tissue is visible, that remains in the osteotomy gap at this healing stage. **B**: The difference between lamellar bone (CB) on the right is clearly visible when compared to the heterogeneous newly formed woven bone (WB) on the left. Important cells in bone formation: **C**: Cells depositing new bone are osteoblasts. The small black and white image explains this image. The arrow indicates an osteoblast in typical palisade form sitting in a row with other osteoblasts on the surface of newly synthesized bone. The region marked with a line and stained blue in "C" shows osteoid (OI), the extracellular matrix, yet unmineralized, synthesized by the osteoblasts. Freshly embedded in the newly formed woven bone at least 4 osteocytes can be seen, surrounded by mineralized matrix (★). **D**: Endochondral bone formation is initiated by a cartilaginous phase, with chondrocytes becoming hypertrophic and then being replaced by osteoblasts and woven bone. **E**: Osteoclasts (OC) are multinuclear bone resorbing cells, sitting on the bone surface. Clearly visible is the ruffled border, which is the actual bone resorbing area of the active osteoclast. (Images are taken from a large animal bone healing model in sheep, 3 mm osteotomy gap, stable external fixation, staining: Alcian blue).

consequence of an injury [8]. This leads to a recruitment of mesenchymal stromal cells (MSC) to the site of injury where they further proliferate and differentiate thus promoting revascularization.

Osteoimmunology

The immune and skeletal systems share a number of regulatory and signaling molecules. This cross-linkage of the immune and skeleton systems has led to new directions in research and the emergence of "osteoimmunology" [9]. Bone is constantly remodelled due to the action of osteoblast and osteoclast. Osteoblasts are bone-producing cells which are derived from MSCs. Osteoclasts are the bone resorbing counterparts to bone forming osteoblasts. They differentiate from hematopoietic stem cells (HSC) and thus share the same progenitor as cells of the immune system (Figure 4).

In numerous autoimmune diseases, disorders of the skeletal system are commonly found. This has highlighted the fact that there is little known concerning the direct and indirect interactions between bone and the immune system [10-12]. However, recent research clearly showed the influence of the immune system on the bone healing success [13], thus identifying the immune system as a possible tool for new therapeutic approaches. The interconnectivity and complexity of cellular and molecular interactions between the immune system and bone tissue creates a major challenge to develop therapeutic approaches that can specifically target one system without detrimentally affecting the other. With aging of the

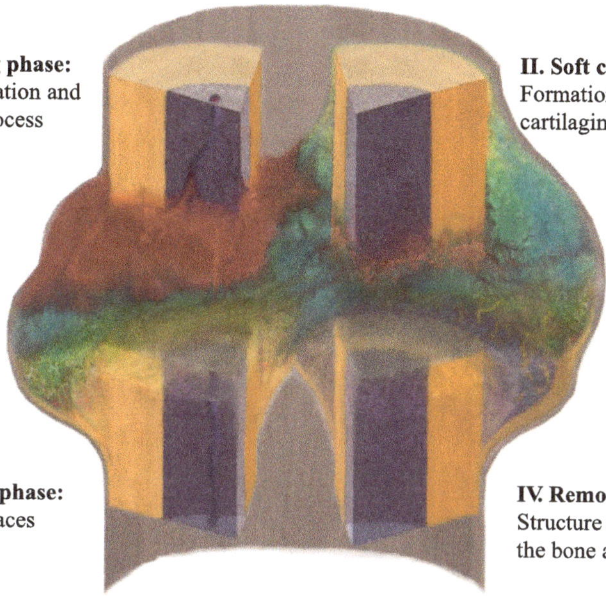

Figure 2 Different phase of the bone healing process. This scheme shows the consecutive/partly overlapping bone healing phases (I-IV) occurring in secondary bone healing. The illustration follows the tissue coloring of the histological Movat's Pentachrome staining, where bone appears yellow, cartilage appears green, bone marrow is purple, vessels are depicted in red.

population in industrialized countries, understanding of this interplay appears to be crucial.

Review

Impact of the immune system on bone fracture healing

Innate immunity

Macrophage Innate immunity is the first line of defense to recognize and attack pathogens entering the body. This includes physiological barriers (epithelial and mucosa) but also cellular defense mechanisms accomplished by macrophages, mast cells and natural killer cells [14].

The innate immune system plays an important role in tissue repair and in maintaining tissue homeostasis. Among the cells of the innate immunity, tissue resident macrophages are recognized as key elements for the orchestration of the recovery processes to re-establish tissue integrity and function after damage [15]. Macrophages, originally believed to be solely pro-inflammatory and destructive phagocytes, were found in 1992 to have ability to convert to a pro-healing phenotype [16]. Since then, it has been shown that macrophages are necessary for angiogenesis, wound healing, tumor growth, and limb regeneration [17-20]. To distinguish this new phenotype from their familiar "classically activated" counterparts, these macrophages were referred to as "alternatively activated". Since then, these "M2" macrophages, named following the helper T cell nomenclature (Th1/Th2) and in contrast to pro-inflammatory "M1" macrophages, have been associated with the resolution of wound healing *in vivo* in chronic leg ulcers [21], atherosclerotic lesions [22], traumatic spinal cord injury [23], and inflammatory renal disease [24]. For research studies and therapeutic applications, monocytes isolated from peripheral human blood can be differentiated into macrophages through the addition of the monocyte colony stimulating factor MCSF, and polarized to different macrophage phenotypes via the addition of specific cytokines [25] (Figure 5).

Depending on the micro-environment, macrophages display distinct activation (also called polarization) states. They are divided into the "classical activated" pro-inflammatory M1 type macrophages and into the "alternatively activated" anti-inflammatory, pro-tissue regeneration and repair M2 type macrophages. Within the M2 population, there are different subtypes, characterized by their surface receptor expression and cytokine secretory profile, as: M2a (anti-inflammatory), M2b (immune-regulatory) and M2c (remodelling) [26] (Figure 6).

Role of macrophages in joint replacement-induced osteolysis: an example of osteoimmunology

Total joint replacement (TJR) is a successful orthopaedic intervention for end stage arthritis. Wear particles are an unwanted by-product of all TJRs and are the cause for the development of chronic inflammation at the implant site [27]. A consistent inflammatory reaction leads to delayed osseointegration of the implant and finally to osteolysis (periprosthetic bone loss) and implant loosening. So far, there are no nonsurgical treatment strategies to overcome wear particle-induced osteolysis. Macrophages are one of the first cells infiltrating the inflammatory reaction

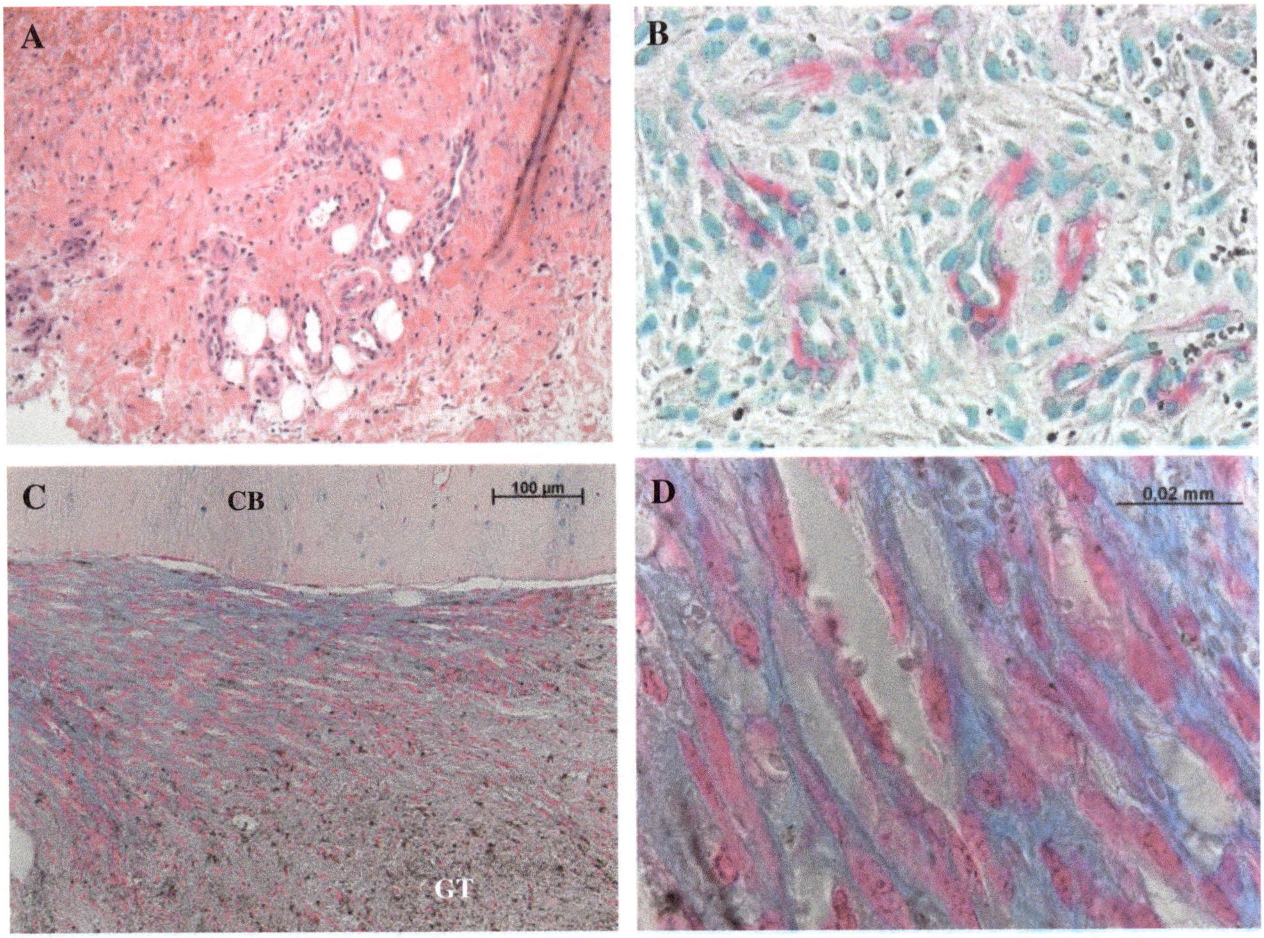

Figure 3 Onset of revascularization in bone healing. Seven days after performing a standardized osteotomy in a sheep's tibia, the maturating granulation tissue clearly shows newly formed vessels (**A**: hematoxilin-eosin staining; 20 × magnification, **B**: α-SMA, methylgreen counterstaining, vessels depicted in red, 40 × magnification). For these vessels to be this highly developed, revascularization in the hematoma must have started earlier. **C** and **D** (Alcian blue staining): The importance of the revascularization becomes evident when observing the cutting edge of cortical bone (CB) where a high number of vessels developed between bone and granulation tissue remnants (GT). The density of this capillary formation is illustrated in D, where endothelial cells, indicating vessel borders, lie nearly wall to wall.

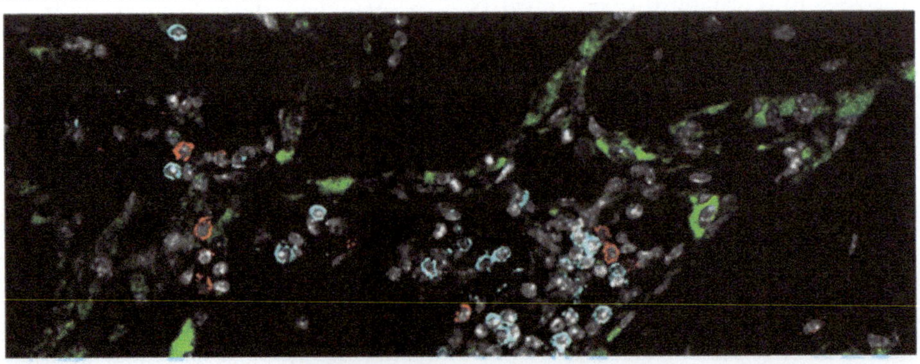

Figure 4 Interactions between osteoclasts and immune cells in a mouse osteotomy model. In areas of newly formed woven bone (14 days after fracture, mouse model) the tight interaction between osteoclasts (green (katepsin K)) and immune cells (T cells = red (CD3); B cells = blue (B220)) is eminent. Osteoclasts line the dark areas of newly formed bone in this image.

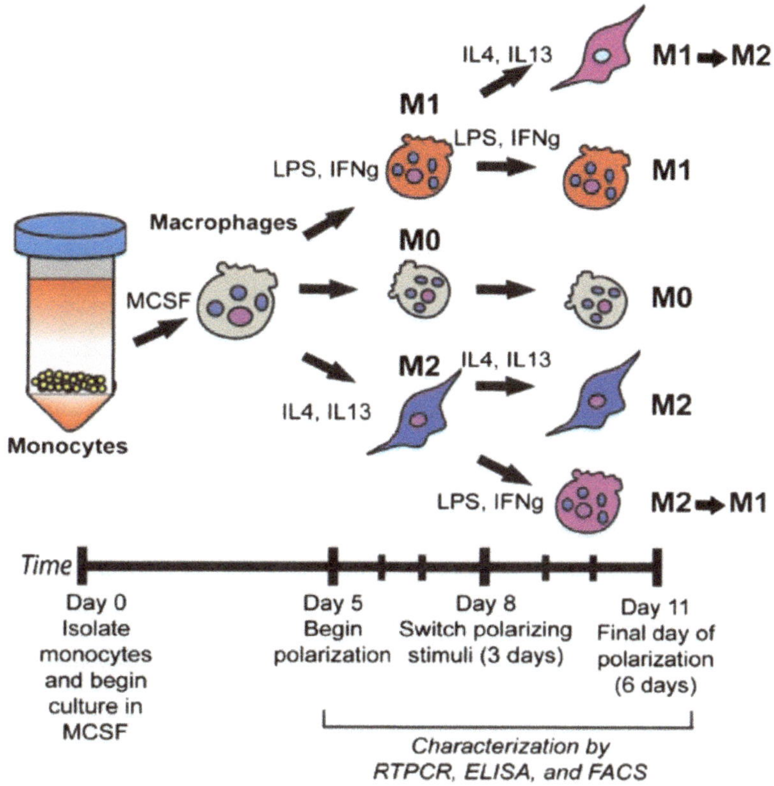

Figure 5 Derivation of subsets of human macrophages from monocytes. Monocyte-derived macrophages were exposed to M1- or M2-polarizing stimuli for 3 days followed by polarizing stimuli of the other phenotype for an additional 3 days (M1- > M2 and M2- > M1). Unstimulated macrophages (M0) or macrophages cultured under M1- or M2-polarizing stimuli for 6 days (M1 and M2), with a media change at day 3, served as controls. Reproduced with permission from [8].

induced by wear particles in TJRs [28]. Because of their plasticity, macrophages could be a promising therapeutic target, in the special case of wear particle-induced osteolysis to enhance osseointegration of the implant, and in general to enhance bone healing.

One main key regulator for the migration and infiltration of monocytes and macrophages is the monocyte chemoattractant protein-1 (MCP-1) [29]. Gibon et al. showed in 2012 that a systemic therapeutic intervention in the MCP-1-CCR2 chemokine-receptor axis (CCR2 is the receptor for MCP-1) leads to less systemic migration of macrophages to the site of particle infusion and further, to decreased osteolysis [30,31]. The reverse effect was observed after local administration of MCP-1. This study gave the first hint that the MCP-1-CCR2 axis plays an important role in the recruitment of macrophages to the localization of wear particles. It also showed that bone injury is not only a local event but rather a systemic process affecting further tissues and organs. Blocking of the MCP1-CCR-2 axis by addition of a mutant MCP-1 protein, 7ND, which competes with MCP-1 for the binding to CCR-2 on macrophages, leads also to a decreased migration of macrophages *in vitro. In vivo* studies using 7ND are currently in progress. In the presence of 7ND, a diminished secretion of pro- as well as anti-inflammatory cytokines by macrophages was observed ([32,33]). The simultaneous decrease of pro- and anti-inflammatory cytokine secretion could be explained by a re-establishment of the homeostatic status. Both studies illustrate the crucial role that macrophages play in regulating inflammatory processes in bone probably due to their secreted cytokine profile. An investigation of the responsible macrophage subset would be an interesting and indispensable question to answer with regard to the development of nonsurgical treatment approaches for wear particle-induced osteolysis in humans. Recent *in vitro* and vivo studies have demonstrated that polarization of macrophages from an M1 to an M2 phenotype using local delivery of IL-4 mitigates wear particle-induced bone loss [34].

Modulation of macrophages in tissue engineering approaches: revascularization of bone grafts

In tissue engineering, revascularization of the transplanted tissue is a crucial prerequisite for a complete integration and functionality of the transplant in the host. Living, functional bone grafts, customized to the patient´s need, are of great clinical need e.g. in the case of congenital abnormalities, cancer resections and trauma [35].

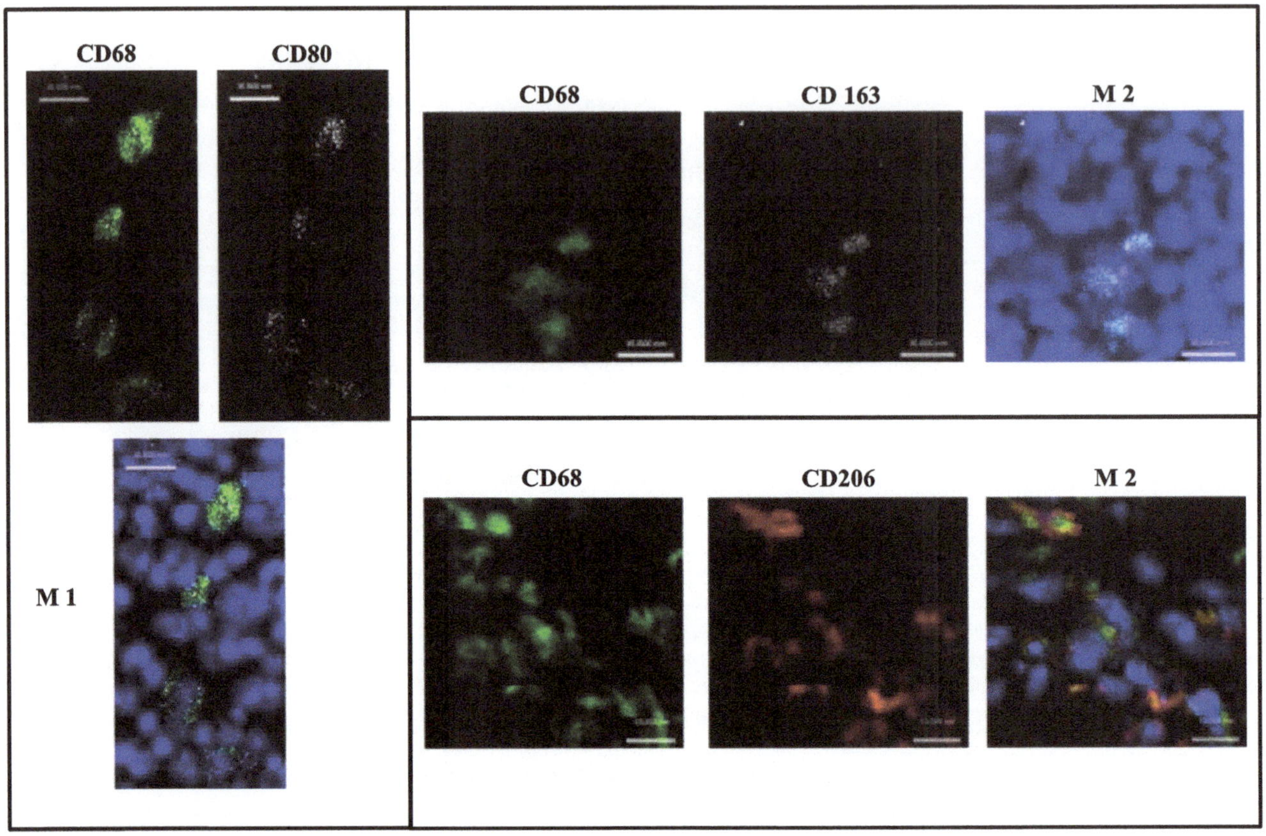

Figure 6 During bone regeneration different types of macrophages are found in a mouse osteotomy model. M1 macrophages positive for the CD68 macrophage marker and the M1 marker CD80 are found, for the M2 macrophages we detected cells positive for CD68 and CD163 and other M2 macrophages positive for CD68 and CD 206.

The tissue engineering paradigm involves the use of the patient's own stem cells capable of osteogenesis and vasculogenesis, biomaterial scaffolds that act as a template for bone formation, and a bioreactor providing nutrition, oxygen supply and regulatory signals. In an ideal case, the missing or defective bone should be repaired using a living, functional bone graft that corresponds to the exact shape of the bone being replaced or regenerated. Current studies are achieving this goal through the use of the patient's own stem cells and image-based and guided scaffold and bioreactor design. One of the main challenges is to ensure the revascularization with blood perfusion of the bone graft, to maintain its viability and function. The developing vasculature guaranties the needed supply of nutrients and, during normal development, serves as a template for the forming bone. Therefore, for successful bone tissue engineering strategies a synergistic formation of the new bone and new blood vessels is an indispensable condition [36].

Because of their early appearance in inflammatory processes, the action of macrophages and their polarization state could be important for vascularization of implanted bone in humans [24].

It is still unclear what are the exact roles of various macrophage subsets in vascularization of biomaterials. To answer this question, Spiller et al. analysed the expression profiles of M1, M2a and M2c polarized macrophages *in vitro* with focus on the expression of genes and proteins important for angiogenesis. They also analysed the pro-angiogenetic potential of conditioned media from these polarized macrophage subsets in an *in vitro* sprouting assay with human endothelial cells. Interestingly, it was not one single subset of macrophages acting as the key regulator of vasculogenesis. Instead, an interplay between the M1 and M2 subset gave the best pro-angiogenic stimuli.

In order to confirm the findings from the *in vitro* studies, the vascularization process and the macrophage phenotype were evaluated *in vivo*. The following collagen scaffold types were subcutaneously implanted in a mouse model: glutaraldehyde-crosslinked (initiation of a moderate inflammatory response expected), soaked in LPS (M1 polarization expected) and unmodified (control). Ten days post-implantation, the scaffolds and the surrounding tissue were analysed with regards to the appearance of blood vessels (histological staining for CD31) and macrophage subsets in and around the scaffold (discrimination between M1 and M2). The unmodified scaffold showed no vascularization and was surrounded by a fibrous capsule in which was detected a strong signal for M2 macrophages. As expected, in the LPS soaked scaffold there were large numbers of inflammatory cells but no blood vessels, and were strongly stained for the M1 subset. In the third scaffold type, which was well vascularized, a staining for both, M1 and M2 macrophages was observed [24].

Taken together the findings of this study suggest that coordinated involvement of both subsets of macrophages guides new blood vessel formation (Figure 7). A model was proposed in which M1 macrophages promote sprouting of blood vessels via secretion of VEGF, bFGF, IL8, RANTES, and TNFalpha; M2c macrophages support angiogenesis, by increasing vascular remodeling via production of MMP9; M2a macrophages promote fusion of blood vessels through currently unidentified secreted factors. M2a macrophages may also regulate the actions of M1 macrophages via production of TIMP3, and may recruit pericytes via secretion of PDGF-BB. The interplay between M1 and M2 macrophages in regulating angiogenesis, and particularly the effects of timing requires much more work [24].

Adaptive immunity

The adaptive (acquired) immune system is characterized by high antigen specificity. Main cell types of the adaptive immunity are B and T cells that recognize non self-proteins by their highly specified antigen receptors. The uniqueness of the adaptive immune system is the enormously high variety of these antigen receptors whereby a vast number of different antigens can be detected. Another important characteristic of the adaptive immune system is its memory. The memory enables a much faster reaction of this part of the immune system during a renewed contact with an already known antigen. Besides activation of the cells of the adaptive immune system via their receptors, another possible activation occurs via signals released by the innate immune system demonstrating the high interconnectivity between both parts of the vertebrate immune system.

In addition to its obvious crucial role in the fight against pathogens, the adaptive immunity also plays an important role during the healing process of a fractured bone, illustrating the interdependency between the bone and the immune system [37].

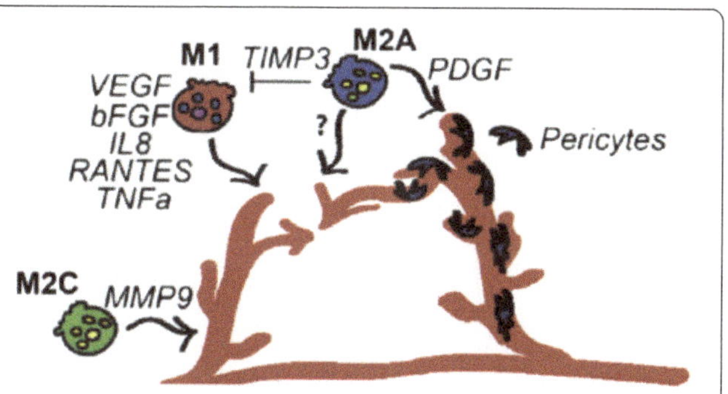

Figure 7 Proposed model for macrophage-mediated angiogenesis. M1 macrophages promote sprouting of blood vessels via secretion of VEGF, bFGF, IL8, RANTES, and TNFa. M2a macrophages promote fusion of blood vessels through as-yet unidentified secreted factors. M2a macrophages may also regulate the actions of M1 macrophages via production of TIMP3, and may recruit pericytes via secretion of PDGF-BB, although this was not directly assessed in this study. M2c macrophages may function in vascular remodeling, given their high levels of production of MMP9. Reproduced with permission from [28].

Negative impact of the immune system in the regenerative processes After an injury, the disruption of the blood vessels leads to hematoma formation that is accompanied by inflammation. This immediate body reaction is a phylogenetically ancient, adaptive response [38]. In the context of wound healing, it is an indispensable step for the initiation of the healing cascade [4]. Wound healing is a multistage and complex process including a multitude of different regulatory mechanisms and molecules, especially in the inflammatory reaction, determining the course of regeneration versus scar formation.

One of the key factors could be the age of the adaptive immune system. Whitby and Ferguson [39] showed that wounds in early mammalian embryos heal without scar formation [39]. At these early stages, the immune system is not yet fully developed. This leads to the assumption, that a fully developed immune system thought to be perfectly adapted to act against the invasion of pathogens, could have a negative impact in the course of wound healing (Figure 8). This raises the question whether the evolutionary development of such a highly efficient immune response takes into account drawbacks for the body's regenerative capacity. The immune system ages throughout the life of an individual. Therefore, the cellular composition is different between a young and an older organism that has been exposed to a multitude of antigens and developed an immune memory. This aging process could be the reason for the diminished regenerative capacity of bone in the aged. This assumption is confirmed by the finding of an enhanced healing after rejuvenation of the immune system [40]. Furthermore, mice with a blunted immune system (germ free housing) develop a significant higher bone density compared to control animals [41].

The question is: Do certain cells of the adaptive immunity have a negative impact on wound healing? The answer is yes: $CD8^{+}$ T cells as part of the adaptive immune response were found to negatively influence wound healing [42,43]. They could therefore be a promising therapeutic target in wound healing treatment strategies in general and especially in bone healing because the bone marrow

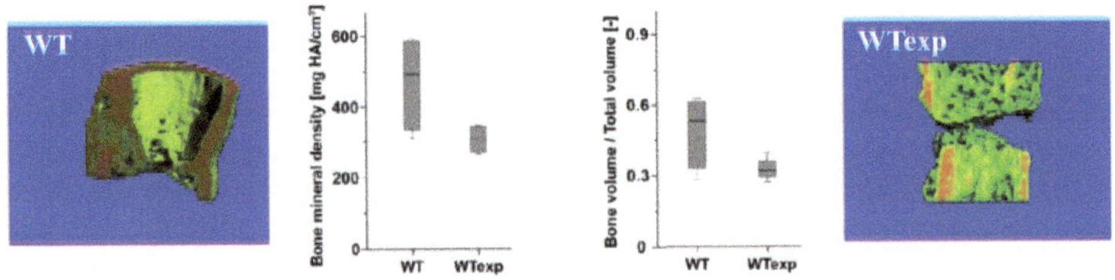

Figure 8 Bone healing in mice under different housing conditions. Analyzing bone healing in a mouse, which has been raised in a SPF (specific pathogen free) surrounding (WT) and a mouse, that had contact with pathogens and thus the possibility to develop its adaptive immune system (higher effector/ memory T cell count) (Wtexp): it became apparent, that the exposed animals showed a diminished healing capacity when compared with animals of SPF raising. This was documented through µCT evaluation showing lower bone mineral density and a lower bone volume/total volume in exposed animals. This data has been earlier published in the context of the negative influence of terminally differentiated CD8+ T cells in bone healing [13].

microenvironment harbors, contrary to other tissues, a higher percentage of $CD8^+$ T cells than $CD4^+$ T cells under physiological conditions [44]. Reinke et al. has shown in humans that an enhanced level of terminally differentiated effector memory CD8 + T cells correlates with delayed fracture healing. This was further confirmed in a mouse osteotomy model where a specific depletion of CD8+ T cells led to an improved bone healing [13]. Whether the cells themselves or their secreted cytokines have to be finally targeted has still to be evaluated.

Positive impact of the adaptive immune system in regenerative processes The T cell population is highly diverse. These cells secrete different inflammatory cytokines and proteins (like Wnt ligands) and thereby promote bone resorption and bone formation, respectively. Furthermore, bone homeostasis is regulated by T cells via their crosstalk with bone marrow stromal cells. Among the T cell population, CD4+ and CD8+ T cell subsets seem to play different roles in bone formation. *In vitro* studies showed that the osteogenetic differentiation in human MSC cultures significantly increases with conditioned media of unstimulated CD4+ T cells. This was further confirmed by the up-regulation of the expression of osteogenic markers such as runt-related transcription factor 2 (Runx2), osteocalcin (OC), bone sialoprotein (BSP), and alkaline phosphatase (ALP) [45]. In contrast, no such effect was seen with the conditioned medium from $CD8^+$ cells. A positive role of CD4+ T cells was further evaluated in wound healing without identifying the responsible subset [42]. Regulatory T cells, a subpopulation of CD4+ T cells, are a promising candidate for a positive regulator in wound and bone healing. Several studies cement this assumption.

A correlation between high bone mass and decreased bone resorption was observed in mice with an increased amount of regulatory T cells [44,46]. In addition, regulatory T cells counteract transplant rejection due to their tolerogenic capacity [47], have a negative impact on osteoclasts [48] and were shown to enhance bone healing of a skull defect in mice when integrated in autologous bone graft [49] (Figure 9).

Conclusion

The current therapies for the treatment of non-healing bone fractures and bone disease are still unsatisfactory. Fracture healing is a highly complex process involving

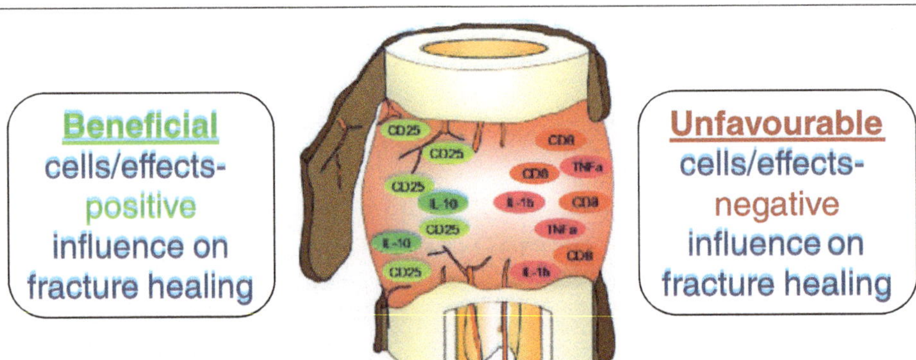

Figure 9 Beneficial and unfavourable immune cells in bone healing. The cellular composition of the bone hematoma that forms upon vessel disruption during injury, is an important criterion towards successful healing. To date certain cells of the adaptive immune system and their influence on regenerative processes have been determined which are depicted in this figure.

different cells and released factors, tissue matrix and the inflammatory and immune system. For a successful healing outcome, the spatial and temporal interplay of these different components has to be well orchestrated. Therefore, in-depth understanding of bone regeneration on the molecular, cellular and tissue level is indispensable for the development of new therapeutic approaches.

Both the innate and adaptive immunity play a crucial role by initiating and regulating the healing cascades. The impact of immune cells in musculoskeletal diseases illustrates how crucial it is to better understand the signaling processes during the inflammatory phase of healing. This importance is further supported by the growing needs of our aging population, where the risk of fracture and poor recovery become more frequent. The aging population presents new challenges to both clinicians and researchers.

To develop new treatment strategies, the challenges we need to address include: (*i*) An early assessment of poor healing so that advanced treatment options can be implemented as soon as possible, for best outcomes, and (*ii*) Timely coordination of the therapeutic intervention with the progression of healing. There are already several approaches developed to address each of these aspects. Based on a better understanding of the signaling cascades and the types, roles and timing of presentation of the participating molecules and cells, a biomarker to "predict" the healing outcome of a patient would be most useful. In this context, the finding that a special subset of CD8+ T cells has a negative impact on fracture healing is already an important step in the early clinical evaluation of fractured patients.

The use of biomaterials to support the healing process is another important aspect in treating musculoskeletal disease. Biomaterials are used as a structural template for the regenerating tissues, including bone, and at the same time they can function as a source of biological factors. A biomaterial can be designed to optimize the regenerative mechanisms by delivering the right amounts of factors at the right time and to the right location within the bone healing area. The new generation of biomaterial scaffolds is being designed to recapitulate the local cytokine and/or growth factor milieu of development and remodeling, and to stimulate specific cell subsets to proliferate and differentiate in the desired and patient-specific way. One example discussed at the workshop was the incorporation of factors recruiting M1 macrophages over an initial period of time (to initiate vascularization) along with the factors (immobilized for sustained action) to recruit M2 macrophages (to mature and stabilize vasculature). So far, little is known about the specific role of the M1 and M2 types in the different musculoskeletal diseases and healing phases (e.g. revascularization of a fractured bone or a bone transplant) and further research is needed to evaluate their potential. This ORS workshop from 2014 with its topics of osteoimmunology in fracture healing, joint replacement loosening, and *in vitro* model systems demonstrates the wide spectrum of bone-immuno-interplay. Future research should pay attention to this relevant field.

Competing interests

The authors declare that they have no competing interest.

Authors' contributions

CS, HS, GND and KSB participated equally in drafting the manuscript in particular the osteoimmunological section. SBG participated equally in drafting the manuscript in particular the wear particle induced osteolysis section. GVN participated equally in drafting the manuscript in particular the section about the revascularization of bone grafts. All of the authors read and approved the final manuscript.

Acknowledgements

The studies reported in this review have been supported by the German research Foundation (DFG SCHE 1594/1, DU 298/21, SCHM 2977/3), the Berlin Brandenburg Center for Regenerative Therapies, the NIH (grants DE016525, EB002520 and AR061988 to GVN) and NIH grants 2R01AR055650, 1R01AR063717 and the Ellenburg Chair in Surgery at Stanford University (SBG). We thank Tobias Thiele for designing Figure 2.

Author details

[1]Julius Wolff Institut and Center for Musculoskeletal Surgery, Charité - Universitätsmedizin Berlin, Augustenburger Platz 1, 13353 Berlin, Germany. [2]Berlin-Brandenburg Center for Regenerative Therapies, Charité – Universitätsmedizin Berlin, Augustenburger Platz 1, 13353 Berlin, Germany. [3]Department of Orthopaedic Surgery and (by courtesy) Bioengineering, Stanford University Medical Center Outpatient Center, 450 Broadway St., M/C 6342, 94063 Redwood City, CA, USA. [4]Department of Biomedical Engineering and Department of Medicine, Columbia University, 622 west 168th Street, VC12-234, 10032 New York, NY, USA.

References

1. Einhorn TA, Lane JM (1998) Significant advances have been made in the way surgeons treat fractures. Clin Orthop Relat Res (355 Suppl.):S2–3
2. Schmidt-Bleek K, Petersen A, Dienelt A, Schwarz C, Duda GN (2014) Initiation and early control of tissue regeneration - bone healing as a model system for tissue regeneration. Expert Opin Biol Ther 14:247–259
3. Ai-Aql ZS, Alagl AS, Graves DT, Gerstenfeld LC, Einhorn TA (2008) Molecular mechanisms controlling bone formation during fracture healing and distraction osteogenesis. J Dent Res 87:107–118
4. Kolar P, Schmidt-Bleek K, Schell H, Gaber T, Toben D, Schmidmaier G, Perka C, Buttgereit F, Duda GN (2010) The early fracture hematoma and its potential role in fracture healing. Tissue Eng Part B Rev 16:427–434
5. Lienau J, Schmidt-Bleek K, Peters A, Haschke F, Duda GN, Perka C, Bail HJ, Schutze N, Jakob F, Schell H (2009) Differential regulation of blood vessel formation between standard and delayed bone healing. J Orthop Res 27:1133–1140
6. Mizuno K, Mineo K, Tachibana T, Sumi M, Matsubara T, Hirohata K (1990) The osteogenetic potential of fracture haematoma. Subperiosteal and intramuscular transplantation of the haematoma. J Bone Joint Surg (Br) 72:822–829
7. Park SH, Silva M, Bahk WJ, McKellop H, Lieberman JR (2002) Effect of repeated irrigation and debridement on fracture healing in an animal model. J Orthop Res 20:1197–1204
8. Einhorn TA, Majeska RJ, Rush EB, Levine PM, Horowitz MC (1995) The expression of cytokine activity by fracture callus. J Bone Miner Res 10:1272–1281
9. Arron JR, Choi Y (2000) Bone versus immune system. Nature 408:535–536
10. Bultink IE, Lems WF, Kostense PJ, Dijkmans BA, Voskuyl AE (2005) Prevalence of and risk factors for low bone mineral density and vertebral fractures in patients with systemic lupus erythematosus. Arthritis Rheum 52:2044–2050

11. Schoon EJ, Blok BM, Geerling BJ, Russel MG, Stockbrugger RW, Brummer RJ (2000) Bone mineral density in patients with recently diagnosed inflammatory bowel disease. Gastroenterology 119:1203–1208
12. Spector TD, Hall GM, McCloskey EV, Kanis JA (1993) Risk of vertebral fracture in women with rheumatoid arthritis. BMJ 306:558
13. Reinke S, Geissler S, Taylor WR, Schmidt-Bleek K, Juelke K, Schwachmeyer V, Dahne M, Hartwig T, Akyuz L, Meisel C, Unterwalder N, Singh NB, Reinke P, Haas NP, Volk HD, Duda GN (2013) Terminally Differentiated CD8+ T Cells Negatively Affect Bone Regeneration in Humans. Sci Transl Med 5:177ra136
14. Janeway CA Jr, Medzhitov R (2002) Innate immune recognition. Annu Rev Immunol 20:197–216
15. Chazaud B (2014) Macrophages: supportive cells for tissue repair and regeneration. Immunobiology 219:172–178
16. Stein M, Keshav S, Harris N, Gordon S (1992) Interleukin 4 potently enhances murine macrophage mannose receptor activity: a marker of alternative immunologic macrophage activation. J Exp Med 176:287–292
17. Chung ES, Chauhan SK, Jin Y, Nakao S, Hafezi-Moghadam A, van Rooijen N, Zhang Q, Chen L, Dana R (2009) Contribution of macrophages to angiogenesis induced by vascular endothelial growth factor receptor-3-specific ligands. Am J Pathol 175:1984–1992
18. Condeelis J, Pollard JW (2006) Macrophages: obligate partners for tumor cell migration, invasion, and metastasis. Cell 124:263–266
19. Godwin JW, Pinto AR, Rosenthal NA (2013) Macrophages are required for adult salamander limb regeneration. Proc Natl Acad Sci U S A 110:9415–9420
20. van Amerongen MJ, Harmsen MC, van Rooijen N, Petersen AH, van Luyn MJ (2007) Macrophage depletion impairs wound healing and increases left ventricular remodeling after myocardial injury in mice. Am J Pathol 170:818–829
21. Krishnamoorthy L (2006) The role of macrophages in human wound healing and their response to a tissue engineered dermal replacement in human chrinic wounds
22. Khallou-Laschet J, Varthaman A, Fornasa G, Compain C, Gaston AT, Clement M, Dussiot M, Levillain O, Graff-Dubois S, Nicoletti A, Caligiuri G (2010) Macrophage plasticity in experimental atherosclerosis. PLoS One 5:e8852
23. Kigerl KA, Gensel JC, Ankeny DP, Alexander JK, Donnelly DJ, Popovich PG (2009) Identification of two distinct macrophage subsets with divergent effects causing either neurotoxicity or regeneration in the injured mouse spinal cord. J Neurosci 29:13435–13444
24. Spiller K, Nassiri S, Witherel CE, Anfang RR, Ng J, Nakazawa KR, Vunjak-Novakovic G (2014) Sequential delivery of immunomodulatory cytokines to facilitate the M1-to-M2 transition of macrophages and enhance vascularization of bone scaffolds. Biomaterials in press
25. Spiller KL, Freytes DO, Vunjak-Novakovic G (2014) Macrophages Modulate Engineered Human Tissues for Enhanced Vascularization and Healing. Annals of biomedical engineering. [Epub ahead of print]
26. Mantovani A, Sica A, Sozzani S, Allavena P, Vecchi A, Locati M (2004) The chemokine system in diverse forms of macrophage activation and polarization. Trends Immunol 25:677–686
27. Rao AJ, Gibon E, Ma T, Yao Z, Smith RL, Goodman SB (2012) Revision joint replacement, wear particles, and macrophage polarization. Acta Biomater 8:2815–2823
28. Nich C, Takakubo Y, Pajarinen J, Ainola M, Salem A, Sillat T, Rao AJ, Raska M, Tamaki Y, Takagi M, Konttinen YT, Goodman SB, Gallo J (2013) Macrophages-Key cells in the response to wear debris from joint replacements. Journal of biomedical materials research. Part A 101:3033–3045
29. Deshmane SL, Kremlev S, Amini S, Sawaya BE (2009) Monocyte chemoattractant protein-1 (MCP-1): an overview. J Interferon Cytokine Res 29:313–326
30. Gibon E, Ma T, Ren PG, Fritton K, Biswal S, Yao Z, Smith L, Goodman SB (2012) Selective inhibition of the MCP-1-CCR2 ligand-receptor axis decreases systemic trafficking of macrophages in the presence of UHMWPE particles. J Orthop Res 30:547–553
31. Gibon E, Yao Z, Rao AJ, Zwingenberger S, Batke B, Valladares R, Smith RL, Biswal S, Gambhir SS, Goodman SB (2012) Effect of a CCR1 receptor antagonist on systemic trafficking of MSCs and polyethylene particle-associated bone loss. Biomaterials 33:3632–3638
32. Keeney M, Waters H, Barcay K, Jiang X, Yao Z, Pajarinen J, Egashira K, Goodman SB, Yang F (2013) Mutant MCP-1 protein delivery from layer-by-layer coatings on orthopedic implants to modulate inflammatory response. Biomaterials 34:10287–10295
33. Yao Z, Keeney M, Lin TH, Pajarinen J, Barcay K, Waters H, Egashira K, Yang F, Goodman S (2013) Mutant monocyte chemoattractant protein 1 protein attenuates migration of and inflammatory cytokine release by macrophages exposed to orthopedic implant wear particles. J Biomed Mater Res Part A 102:3291–3297
34. Roa A, Nich C, Dhulipale LS, Gibon E, Valladeras R, Zwingenberger S, Smith RL, Goodman SB (2013) Local effect of IL-4 delivery on polyethylene particle induced osteolysis in the murine calvarium. J Biomed Mater Res 101:1926–1934
35. Spiller KL, Anfang RR, Spiller KJ, Ng J, Nakazawa KR, Daulton JW, Vunjak-Novakovic G (2014) The role of macrophage phenotype in vascularization of tissue engineering scaffolds. Biomaterials 35:4477–4488
36. de Peppo GM, Vunjak-Novakovic G, Marolt D (2014) Cultivation of human bone-like tissue from pluripotent stem cell-derived osteogenic progenitors in perfusion bioreactors. Methods Mol Biol 1202:173–184
37. Konnecke I, Serra A, El Khassawna T, Schlundt C, Schell H, Hauser A, Ellinghaus A, Volk HD, Radbruch A, Duda GN, Schmidt-Bleek K (2014) T and B cells participate in bone repair by infiltrating the fracture callus in a two-wave fashion. Bone 64:155–165
38. Opal SM (2000) Phylogenetic and functional relationships between coagulation and the innate immune response. Crit Care Med 28:S77–80
39. Whitby DJ, Ferguson MW (1991) Immunohistochemical localization of growth factors in fetal wound healing. Dev Biol 147:207–215
40. Xing Z, Lu C, Hu D, Miclau T 3rd, Marcucio RS (2010) Rejuvenation of the inflammatory system stimulates fracture repair in aged mice. J Orthop Res 28:1000–1006
41. Sjogren K, Engdahl C, Henning P, Lerner UH, Tremaroli V, Lagerquist MK, Backhed F, Ohlsson C (2012) The gut microbiota regulates bone mass in mice. J Bone Miner Res 27:1357–1367
42. Park JE, Barbul A (2004) Understanding the role of immune regulation in wound healing. Am J Surg 187:11S–16S
43. Schaffer M, Barbul A (1998) Lymphocyte function in wound healing and following injury. Br J Surg 85:444–460
44. Pacifici R (2013) Osteoimmunology and its implications for transplantation. Am J Transplant 13:2245–2254
45. Grassi F, Cattini L, Gambari L, Manferdini C, Piacentini A, Gabusi E, Facchini A, Lisignoli G (2013) T cell subsets differently regulate osteogenic differentiation of human mesenchymal stromal cells in vitro. J Tissue Eng Regen Med. [Epub ahead of print]
46. Zaiss MM, Frey B, Hess A, Zwerina J, Luther J, Nimmerjahn F, Engelke K, Kollias G, Hunig T, Schett G, David JP (2010) Regulatory T cells protect from local and systemic bone destruction in arthritis. J Immunol 184:7238–7246
47. van Maurik A, Herber M, Wood KJ, Jones ND (2002) Cutting edge: CD4+ CD25+ alloantigen-specific immunoregulatory cells that can prevent CD8+ T cell-mediated graft rejection: implications for anti-CD154 immunotherapy. J Immunol 169:5401–5404
48. Zaiss MM, Axmann R, Zwerina J, Polzer K, Guckel E, Skapenko A, Schulze-Koops H, Horwood N, Cope A, Schett G (2007) Treg cells suppress osteoclast formation: a new link between the immune system and bone. Arthritis Rheum 56:4104–4112
49. Liu Y, Wang L, Kikuiri T, Akiyama K, Chen C, Xu X, Yang R, Chen W, Wang S, Shi S (2011) Mesenchymal stem cell-based tissue regeneration is governed by recipient T lymphocytes via IFN-gamma and TNF-alpha. Nat Med 17:1594–1601

Clinical results of multilayered biomaterials for osteochondral regeneration

Elizaveta Kon[1*], Giuseppe Filardo[1], Francesco Perdisa[2], Giulia Venieri[2] and Maurilio Marcacci[2]

Abstract

Several techniques have been used during the years to treat chondral and osteochondral lesions. Among them, the emerging trend in the field of osteochondral regeneration is to treat the entire osteochondral unit by implanting cell-free scaffolds, which provide a three-dimensional support for the cell growth and may act themselves as stimuli for an "in situ" tissue regeneration. Various multi-layered products have been proposed that mimic both the subchondral bone and the cartilaginous layer. Among these, three have currently been reported in the literature. One has been widely investigated: it is a nanocomposite three-layered collagen-hydroxyapatite scaffold, which is showing promising results clinically and by MRI even at mid-term follow-up. The second is a PLGA-calcium-sulfate bilayer scaffold: however, the literature findings are still controversial and only short-term outcomes of limited case-series have been published. The most recent one is a solid aragonite-based scaffold, which seems to give promising clinical and MRI outcomes, even if the literature is still lacking more in-depth evaluations.
Even though the Literature related to this topic is quickly increasing in number, the clinical evidence it is still limited to some case series, and high-level studies are needed to better demonstrate their real effectiveness.

Introduction

Different techniques have been proposed over the years for chondral disease, but treating osteochondral disease is still an arduous challenge for the orthopedic surgeon. Among the currently available surgical approaches, bone marrow stimulation procedures aim at favoring the healing process in the lesion site, taking advantage of the migration of stem cells from the subchondral bone with minimal invasiveness and limited costs, even though paired with well-known limitations (Orth et al. 2012; Kon et al. 2011b). The surgical alternative traditionally consists of more aggressive techniques based on autologous or allogenic tissue transplantation that provides an immediate viable tissue in the lesion site (Gomoll et al. 2012a; Filardo et al. 2014c). The complexity of cartilage-bone interface and the differences between cartilage and subchondral bone layers, including both composition and biomechanical properties, particularly impede successful regenerative treatment (Pape et al. 2010; Madry et al. 2010; Orth et al. 2013). However, progress in the field of biomaterials has led to a new strategy for the treatment of such defects of joint articular surface. Based on the rationale of providing a temporary three-dimensional structure for the growth of living cells and guide for tissue formation, various biopolymers assembled in the form of a scaffold have been developed (Kon et al. 2012a). An ideal scaffold should mimic the biology, architecture, and functional properties of the native tissue, thus promoting cell attachment, proliferation, and differentiation. Other key requirements are biocompatibility and biodegradability: the scaffold should support the early phases of tissue formation and then be gradually replaced by the regenerating tissue. Following this rationale, such constructs were first applied in combination with cultured cells (chondrocytes) such as a 3D support for a better tissue regeneration, thus producing good results even at mid-long term follow-up (Filardo et al. 2014b; Brix et al. 2014). Subsequently, this kind of matrix was applied as "one-step" surgical augmentation to marrow-stimulating techniques, by implanting into the defect alone, thus avoiding any cell addition (Anders et al. 2013; Gille et al. 2013), or in combination with mesenchymal stem cells, harvested and seeded during the same surgical procedure (Gobbi et al. 2014).

In fact, from a clinical point of view, an ideal graft should be an off-the-shelf product, thus allowing easy

* Correspondence: e.kon@biomec.ior.it
[1]Nano-Biotechnology Laboratory, Rizzoli Orthopaedic Institute, Via di Barbiano n. 1/10, 40136 Bologna, Italy
Full list of author information is available at the end of the article

handling and less expensive one-step procedures, and avoiding problems due to cell manipulation and culture.

With this in mind and an increasing awareness of the crucial role of the subchondral bone in the pathogenesis of articular degeneration, new bi-layered constructs have been developed to reproduce the different biological and functional requirements for the growth of both bone and cartilage tissues, with the aim of providing a treatment to the entire osteochondral unit. In fact, the above-mentioned regenerative techniques showed several limitations when applied to primary osteochondral defects (i.e. OCDs) (Filardo et al. 2012a) or articular lesions in a degenerative context, where the subchondral bone is more frequently involved (Filardo et al. 2013c; Filardo et al. 2012b). As previously reported, some scaffolds displayed a potential to act by themselves as stimuli for the differentiation of resident bone marrow stem cells, by inducing an "in situ" tissue regeneration that allows an orderly and durable osteochondral tissue without the need for any cell augmentation (Kon et al. 2012b; O'Shea and Miao 2008; Keeney and Pandit 2009; Lopa and Madry 2014).

Among the many different multi-layered scaffolds specifically developed to reproduce both bone and cartilage either with or without the addition of cells (Shimomura et al. 2014b), only a few acellular ones have currently been investigated with clinical trials (Table 1). The aim of the present review is to illustrate the available literature evidence, by focusing on the clinical results obtained with these osteochondral scaffolds.

Review

Collagen-hydroxyapatite based three-layer scaffold: MaioRegen™

The most widely studied multi-layered scaffold is MaioRegen™ (Fin-ceramica, Faenza, Italy), a nanostructured implant consisting of different ratios of collagen (coll) and hydroxyapatite (HA) organized in three-layers (Figure 1; Table 1). The composition of the graft resembles that of the extracellular matrixes of cartilage and bone tissue, and is based on nucleation of HA nanocrystals onto self-assembled coll fibers (Tampieri et al. 2008) to generate a chemically and morphologically-graded biomimetic material. Equine type I coll acts as an organic matrix for the mineralization process, due to its good physicochemical stability, processability, high safety and biocompatibility profile, due to the removal of all potentially immunogenic telopeptides. The mineral phase is represented by magnesium–hydroxyapatite (Mg-HA). Magnesium ions have been introduced to increase the physicochemical, structural, and morphological affinities of the composite with natural bone (Serre et al. 1998). The final design of the scaffold mimics the natural structure of both cartilage and subchondral bone layers: the cartilaginous upper layer is smooth on the surface and consists entirely of Type I coll; the intermediate layer is made of a combination of Type I coll (60%) and Mg-HA (40%); and the lower one consists of a mineralized blend of Type I coll (30%) and Mg-HA (70%). Safety and efficacy of the product have been shown through preclinical studies (Kon et al. 2010a; Kon et al. 2010b), where similar results were obtained with or without loading the implant with cultured autologous chondrocytes. The scaffold appeared to be able to induce an ordered *in situ* regeneration, possibly through progenitor cells from the bone marrow surrounding the implantation site, thus allowing the regeneration of a good quality and well-integrated tissue in the animal model. Moreover, both histological and immunohistochemical evaluations showed type II coll in the cartilage region down to the subchondral bone, and the uniform presence of type I coll in the subchondral layer, even if aspects of ongoing remodeling were still present at 6 months (Kon et al. 2010a). These preclinical findings prompted researchers to bring this method to the clinical practice as a "cell-free" technique.

The preliminary results of this biomimetic graft were reported in the first clinical trial in 2010 in 13 patients (15 lesions): a high-resolution magnetic resonance imaging (MRI) evaluation was performed at 5–8 weeks and 6 months after surgery (Kon et al. 2010b), which showed a complete integration of the implant in 13 of 15 lesions at 5-8 weeks of follow-up, whereas a partial detachment was found in 2 patients. The 6-month evaluation made with MOCART (Magnetic Resonance Observation of Cartilage Repair Tissue) score, showed the ongoing maturation process, with good filling of the lesion and integration of

Table 1 Specifics of the osteochondral scaffolds

Name	Trufit CB™	Maioregen™	Agili-C™
Number of layers	2	3	2
Bone phase	Ca-sulfate	70% HA – 30% Coll I 40% HA – 60% Coll I	Aragonite
Cartilage phase	Hydrophilic polimer (PGA, PLGA, surfactant)	100% Coll I	Hyaluronate-impregnated aragonite
Plug size	Ø 5 - 11 mm cylinders	Square 35 x 35 mm (manual sizing)	Ø 6 - 18 mm cylinders
Plug depth	Max 18 mm (to be cut)	6 ± 2 mm (swelling)	15 or 20 mm

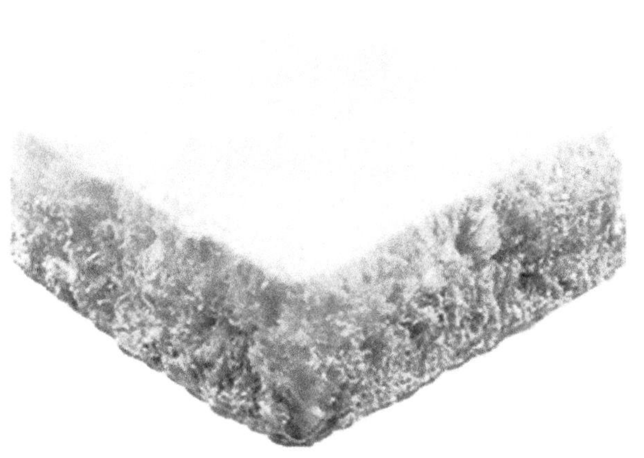

Figure 1 HA-Collagene type I three-layer scaffold (Maioregen™, Finceramica, Italy).

the graft. Subsequently, the same group reported the results of a pilot clinical study at 24 months of follow-up (Kon et al. 2011a). Twenty-eight consecutive patients (9 women, 21 men; mean age, 29.3 years) treated for knee chondral or osteochondral lesions (size 1.5 - 6.0 cm^2) improved significantly from baseline to the different follow-up times in both the International Knee Documentation Committee (IKDC) and Tegner scores. Further analysis highlighted a faster recovery for patients with higher pre-injury activity level, whereas a slower one was found in patients who presented adverse events, in older ones or those who had undergone previous surgery, and for lesions located at the patella. Finally, most of the MRIs showed complete filling of the cartilage layer and complete integration of the graft. Twenty-seven patients of the same series (Kon et al. 2014a) were then evaluated for up to 5 years' follow-up, where the clinical results recorded at 24 months were confirmed as stable over time up to the mid-term follow-up. In detail, the IKDC subjective score improved from 40.0 ± 15.0 to 76.5 ± 14.5 and 77.1 ± 18.0, and the Tegner score from 1.6 ± 1.1 to 4.0 ± 1.8 and 4.1 ± 1.9 at 2 and 5 years, respectively. MRI evaluation of 23 lesions was also performed at 2 years and at final follow-up, revealing significant improvements in both mean MOCART score and subchondral bone status over time, although some abnormalities persisted. However, no correlation was found between imaging and clinical outcomes. This biomaterial has also been tested for the treatment of OCD (osteochondritis dissecans) lesions. Twenty-seven consecutive patients affected by symptomatic femoral condyle OCD (average defect size 3.4 ± 2.2 cm^2) were treated and prospectively evaluated by subjective and objective IKDC and Tegner scores at 2 years' follow-up. A statistically significant improvement in all clinical scores was present at 1 year, and a further improvement was obtained the following year, with no correlation between size and outcome. The MRI evaluations showed good defect filling and implant integration, although most of the scans presented inhomogeneity of the regenerating tissue and the presence of subchondral bone alterations. However, even in this case, no correlation between the MOCART score and clinical outcome was found (Filardo et al. 2013a). These positive results suggest that an osteochondral approach is key for this pathologic entity, which primarily involves the subchondral bone, and shows good results also for the treatment of large lesions.

Analogously, Delcogliano et al. obtained an encouraging outcome at 24 months' follow-up on 19 patients affected by large-sized articular defects treated with the same scaffold (Delcogliano et al. 2013), and subsequently demonstrated positive findings in 49 patients of a multicenter study, thus supporting the potential of this product also for the treatment of large osteochondral lesions (Berruto et al. 2014). Similar results were also reported in a bigger series of 79 patients affected by femoral condyles or trochlea lesions (size 3.2 ± 2.0 cm^2) and evaluated prospectively both clinically and with MRI at 12 and 24 months of follow-up, where a significantly better outcome was recorded in traumatic lesions compared to degenerative ones (Kon et al. 2014b).

Some encouraging findings have been also documented by applying this biomimetic approach in cases of "complex" lesions involving the subchondral bone. A 46-year-old former athlete (Kon et al. 2009) was successfully treated by implanting the scaffold in multifocal osteochondral defects of the medial femoral condyle, trochlea and patella, and concurrently by restoring the correct alignment of a varus knee through a closing-wedge high tibial osteotomy. Good clinical outcome and positive MRI results were recorded at 12 months' follow-up. Favourable findings were reported also in a 50-year-old woman affected by a tibial plateau osteochondral defect following a Schatzker type II fracture (Filardo et al. 2009). Due to the complexity of the lesion, an integrated mechanical and biological approach was applied to restore the previous anatomic features. Besides filling the bone and cartilage defect with this three-layered implant, the tibial plateau was elevated by an opening-wedge osteotomy and filled with homologous bone graft, and finally a dynamic external distractor was applied to allow early mobilization while protecting the implant. Twelve months later the patient was pain free and returned to a satisfactory activity level, stable until the 4 years' follow-up. A further case report dealt with an Olympic-level female athlete affected by multifocal degenerative knee lesions. The patient underwent a complex combined treatment: implantation of the scaffold, autologous osteochondral grafting, patellar realignment, and meniscal allograft transplantation to address both joint surface lesions and associated comorbidities. The patient was able to return to high-level competitions within

24 months after surgery (Perdisa et al. 2014). Following these promising outcomes, obtained through a combined mechanical and biological approach as a salvage procedure, a more extensive application was experimented for complex osteochondral lesions. Thirty-three patients affected by "complex" knee lesions, according to defined criteria (Filardo et al. 2013b), were treated by implanting this multi-layered scaffold and combining concurrent procedures to address axial misalignment and meniscal resection sequelae. A good clinical outcome was recorded at 24 months' follow-up. The clinical results were then compared with those of a homogeneous group of 23 patients previously treated with a similar protocol but with the implantation of a chondral scaffold. A better outcome was found in the osteochondral scaffold group. Finally, the biomimetic scaffold was also tested for the treatment of unicompartmental OA in young patients (Marcacci et al. 2013), to attempt an alternative solution to metal resurfacing. Currently, the main surgical indication in a young and active population affected by unicompartmental OA consists of unloading osteotomies or unicompartmental metal resurfacing (Gomoll et al. 2012b), but the high functional demands and the young age of this kind of patient increase the risk of prosthetic revision. In this challenging population, characterized by a combination of high functional demands and great expectations regarding their recovery on one hand, and a limited choice of treatment options on the other, a solution to delay or even avoid metal resurfacing is highly desirable. The osteochondral scaffold was then implanted in a group of 43 patients affected by unicompartmental OA (Kellegren-Lawrence < =3), with full-thickness focal cartilage lesions in stable knees. Concurrent procedures were performed when required (15 osteotomies, 11 meniscal scaffolds and 9 meniscal allograft implantations). The clinical outcome showed a significant clinical improvement from pre-op to the 3 years' follow-up. The best benefits were obtained in patients under 40 years old; thus, the authors recommended this surgical approach as a new treatment option for young OA patients.

A recent study tried to define the best fixation method for this scaffold, by performing a comparative mechanical test on a cadaver human knee model (24 scaffolds fixed only by press-fit, 24 scaffolds by fibrin glue) exposed to continuous passive motion (CPM). A statistically significant difference was obtained between press-fit and fibrin glue implants with each score used. Whereas scaffolds implanted only by a press-fit technique are exposed to deformation, delamination, and dislodgement, scaffolds fixed by fibrin glue showed better layer cohesiveness. Furthermore, implant stability and integrity were maintained even when load was applied to simulate early weight bearing. Following these results the authors recommended the use of fibrin glue in the clinical practice, to improve early post-operative stability and integrity of the implant, and thus allowing a safer and faster recovery (Filardo et al. 2014a).

Poli-lactic (PLGA), poli-glycolic acid (PGA), calcium sulfate biphasic polimer: TruFit™

TruFit™ (Smith & Nephew, Andover, MA) is a bilayer scaffold made of a semiporous 75:25 PLGA-PGA calcium-sulfate biopolymer, shaped into form by different size cylinders (Figure 2; Table 1).

The design should allow a complete resorption over time, which aims to provide a complete filling of the defect with regenerating tissue (Slivka et al. 2001). Promising preclinical results showed an *in vivo* good quality of the regenerating tissue, with similar gross and histological findings either with or without the addition of cells (Niederauer et al. 2000). The scaffold was then introduced into the clinical practice with the indication to backfill autologous grafts donor sites, anyway it has been mainly used off-label,

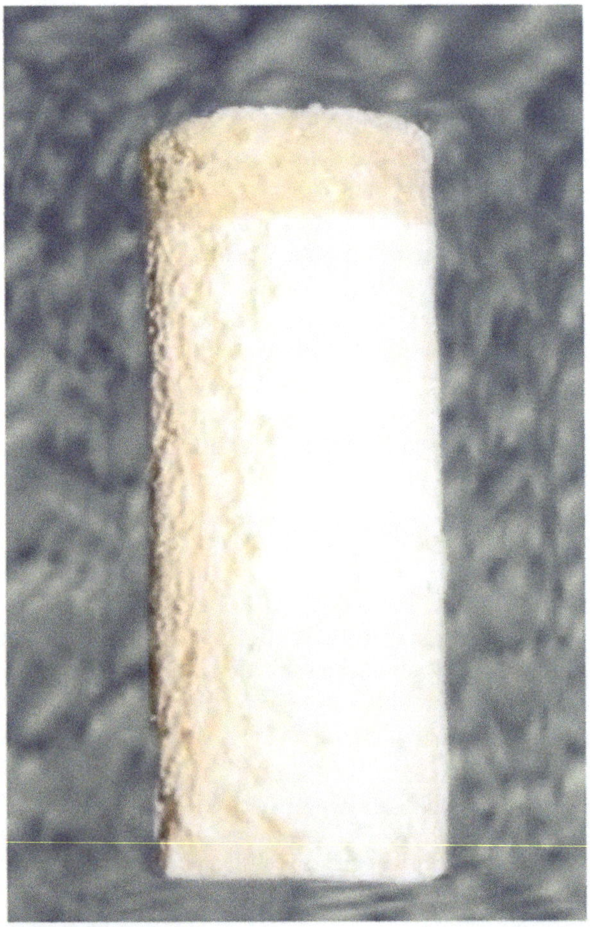

Figure 2 Polimeric PLGA-PGA and Calciun sulfate bi-layer scaffold (Trufit CB™, Smith & Nephew, USA).

by direct implantation for the treatment of focal articular surface defects, where it showed some controversial results, although long-term durability evaluations are still lacking (Melton et al. 2010; Williams and Gamradt 2008).

The first reports described using this scaffold to fill the donor site during OAT procedures: Bedi et al. (Bedi et al. 2010) found a slow improvement in MRI appearance of the implant site, whereas Barber et al. documented no signs of maturation, osteoconduction, or ossification of the scaffold in any of the 9 patients evaluated with CT scans (Barber and Dockery 2011). Moreover, Quarch et al. (Quarch et al. 2014) showed that filling donor site defects with TruFit™ in patients who underwent OAT, did not produce clinical improvements since the donor site morbidity was already low anyway.

Other studies reported the application of this bone graft substitute for the treatment of articular cartilage knee defects. Also in this case the controversial effectiveness of this implant was shown. Positive findings were documented by Carmont et al. in a case report of a symptomatic 18-year-old patient treated with this scaffold for a large chondral lesion on the lateral femoral condyle. The patient had complete relief of symptoms and was able to return to sports; moreover, the authors suggested that, although an intermediate post-operative interval can be associated with unfavorable MRI findings, the plug appearance may significantly improve at further follow-up (Carmont et al. 2009). With quantitative MRI, using delayed Gadolinium-enhanced technique, Bekkers et al. evaluated the results of 13 patients at a mean of 12 months after the implantation of this plug in their femoral condyles. These findings were positive both in terms of clinical outcome and cartilage-like signal of the graft in its superficial layer (Bekkers et al. 2013).

Conversely, other authors documented poor results. Dhollander et al. (Dhollander et al. 2012) recorded a failure rate of 20% (3 out of 15 patients) at 1-year follow-up and biopsies showing fibrous vascularized repair tissue. An even higher number of failures have been reported when applying this scaffold to patellar defects: 70% of 10 patients treated needed a reoperation due to implant failure within the first 24 months after surgery (Joshi et al. 2012); thus, the authors advised against the use of this scaffold for this kind of lesion. Finally, the comparison of a group of 35 patients treated with this scaffold implantation and 31 patients using mosaicplasty for similar defects, showed significantly higher outcomes for the latter ones (Hindle et al. 2013).

Crystalline coral aragonite-hyaluronic acid bilayer scaffold: Agili-C™

The most recent literature describes a novel aragonite-based osteochondral scaffold applied into clinical practice (Agili-C™, CartiHeal (2009) Ltd, Israel), developed in shape of cylinders, with a similar surgical rationale than the mosaic-like osteochondral autograft transplantation. It is a rigid cell-free implant consisting of two layers: a bone phase made of calcium carbonate in the aragonite crystalline form, and a superficial cartilage phase composed of modified aragonite and hyaluronic acid (Figure 3; Table 1). Preclinical analysis (Kon et al. 2013b) revealed the safety and potential of this scaffold, thus showing its biodegradability and intrinsic restorative potential. Particularly, its ability to recruit cells from the surrounding tissues, allowed a good regeneration of the entire osteochondral unit to be produced: histological and immunohistochemical stainings showed the presence of collagen type I only in the bone phase and type II in the cartilage layer. This led to the translation of this scaffold as a one-step implantation without any cell augmentation into the clinical setting. Only one case report (Kon et al. 2013a) describing the clinical use of this construct is currently available in the literature: a 47-year-old non-professional sportsman affected by a post-traumatic osteochondral lesion around 2 cm^2 on the medial femoral condyle was treated successfully and resumed his pre-injury sport activity after 18 months. The MRI evaluation performed at 24 months of follow-up showed promising findings with the restoration of the articular surface.

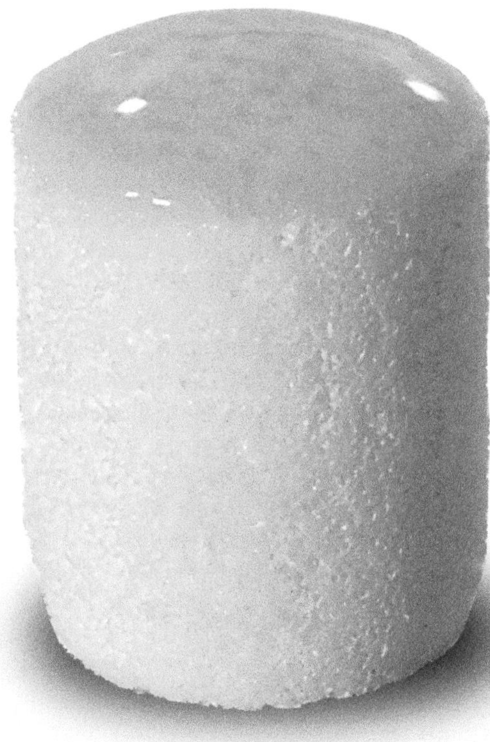

Figure 3 Aragonite-based osteochondral scaffold (Agili-C™, CartiHeal (2009) Ltd, Israel).

Conclusion

The subchondral bone is often involved when the articular surface is damaged and needs to be treated to have a correct and durable restoration of the most superficial layers of the joint. In this context, tissue engineering research has led to the development of several osteochondral substitutes. Even though the association of several biomaterials with different cell strategies is being tested preclinically, these techniques mainly require cell isolation and culture, as well as two different surgical procedures (Zhang et al. 2013b; Shimomura et al. 2014a; Schleicher et al. 2013b; Zhang et al. 2013a; Schleicher et al. 2013a; Duan et al. 2013). This is probably one of the reasons why, despite the favorable results, none of them has already been reported for the clinical use. In fact, the advantages of these new biomaterials include also the possibility to perform a one-step surgical procedure, off-the-shelf availability, a simpler and faster surgical technique, and lower costs. Among commercialized scaffolds, three have been documented in the literature to date. Concerning the polymeric PLGA-calcium-sulfate bilayer scaffold, the reported results are quite controversial, both from clinical and imaging points of view. Conversely, the three-layered scaffold is showing promising results. Also in this case controversial findings have been reported from the imaging point of view, but significant improvements have been repeatedly documented in the mid-term follow-up, with encouraging outcomes even for the treatment of complex osteochondral lesions (including OCDs, large size lesions, unicompartmental OA and combined knee injuries), with the possibility to address also larger articular defects. Thus, this procedure may be a valid treatment option for osteochondral lesions and a possible solution to delay the need for more aggressive approaches in "complex" patients. On the other hand the persistence of an altered signal and a slow maturation process of the osteochondral unit suggest that further improvements are still possible to obtain a better tissue regeneration and an optimal and durable clinical outcome. Finally, a novel aragonite-based product is showing promising preliminary results, but the literature on this new product is still limited and it isn't still available for the clinical use.

Despite the clinical improvement highlighted by most of the reported studies for a wide range of indications, some common controversial findings seem to emerge with regard to the quality of the regenerative tissue, as testified by alterations in the MRI appearance of the grafts. Experimental studies are ongoing to test new and different multi-layered biomaterials and their interaction with cells and the environment in an in vivo setting. On the other hand further clinical studies are needed to assess the real effectiveness of the available grafts with high level trials, and to better identify the target of patients which would get most benefit from these procedures for osteochondral regeneration.

Competing interests

F. Perdisa and G. Venieri have no conflict of interests.

Authors' contribution

EK and MM made the senior editing. GF, FP and GV performed the Literature analysis and manuscript writing. All authors read and approved the final manuscript.

Authors' information

E. Kon is consultant for CartiHeal (2009) Ltd (Israel) and has stocks of CartiHeal (2009) Ltd (Israel). She is consultant and receives institutional support from Finceramica Faenza Spa (Italy). She receives institutional support from Fidia Farmaceutici Spa (Italy), IGEA Clinical Biophysics (Italy), BIOMET (USA) and Kensey Nash (USA).

G. Filardo is consultant and receives institutional support from: Finceramica Faenza Spa (Italy), Fidia Farmaceutici Spa (Italy), CartiHeal (2009) Ltd (Israel). He is consultant for: EON Medica SRL (Italy). He receives Institutional Support from: IGEA Clinical Biophysics (Italy), BIOMET (USA) and Kensey Nash (USA).

M. Marcacci receives royalties and research institutional support from Fin-Ceramica Faenza SpA (Italy). He receives institutional support from: Fidia Farmaceutici Spa (Italy), CartiHeal (2009) Ltd (Israel), IGEA Clinical Biophysics (Italy), BIOMET (USA) and Kensey Nash (USA).

Acknowledgements

The present study was partially supported by OPHIS European Project: COMPOSITE PHENOTYPIC TRIGGERS FOR BONE AND CARTILAGE REPAIR (FP7-NMP-2009-SMALL 3-246373).

Author details

[1]Nano-Biotechnology Laboratory, Rizzoli Orthopaedic Institute, Via di Barbiano n. 1/10, 40136 Bologna, Italy. [2]Biomechanics Laboratory, Rizzoli Orthopaedic Institute, Via di Barbiano n. 1/10, 40136 Bologna, Italy.

References

Anders S, Volz M, Frick H, Gellissen J (2013) A Randomized, controlled trial comparing Autologous Matrix-Induced Chondrogenesis (AMIC(R)) to microfracture: analysis of 1- and 2-year follow-up data of 2 centers. Open Orthop J 7:133–143

Barber FA, Dockery WD (2011) A computed tomography scan assessment of synthetic multiphase polymer scaffolds used for osteochondral defect repair. Arthroscopy 27(1):60–64

Bedi A, Foo L, Williams RI, Potter H, Cartilage Study Group (2010) The maturation of synthetic scaffolds for osteochondral donor sites of the knee: An MRI and T2-mapping analysis. Cartilage 1(1):20–28

Bekkers JE, Bartels LW, Vincken KL, Dhert WJ, Creemers LB, Saris DB (2013) Articular cartilage evaluation after TruFit plug implantation analyzed by delayed gadolinium-enhanced MRI of cartilage (dGEMRIC). Am J Sports Med 41(6):1290–1295

Berruto M, Delcogliano M, de Caro F, Carimati G, Ferrua P, Uboldi F, Ziveri G, De Biase C (2014) Treatment of large knee osteochondral lesions with a biomimetic scaffold: results from 49 patients at 2-years' minimum follow-up in a multicenter study. Am J Sports Med 42(7):1607–1617

Brix MO, Stelzeneder D, Chiari C, Koller U, Nehrer S, Dorotka R, Windhager R, Domayer SE (2014) Treatment of Full-Thickness Chondral Defects With Hyalograft C in the Knee: Long-term Results. Am J Sports Med

Carmont MR, Carey-Smith R, Saithna A, Dhillon M, Thompson P, Spalding T (2009) Delayed incorporation of a TruFit plug: perseverance is recommended. Arthroscopy 25(7):810–814

Delcogliano M, de Caro F, Scaravella E, Ziveri G, De Biase CF, Marotta D, Marenghi P, Delcogliano A (2013) Use of innovative biomimetic scaffold in the treatment for large osteochondral lesions of the knee. Knee Surg Sports Traumatol Arthrosc 22(6):1260–9

Dhollander AA, Liekens K, Almqvist KF, Verdonk R, Lambrecht S, Elewaut D, Verbruggen G, Verdonk PC (2012) A pilot study of the use of an osteochondral scaffold plug for cartilage repair in the knee and how to deal with early clinical failures. Arthroscopy 28(2):225–233

Duan P, Pan Z, Cao L, He Y, Wang H, Qu Z, Dong J, Ding J (2013) The effects of pore size in bilayered poly(lactide-co-glycolide) scaffolds on restoring osteochondral defects in rabbits. J Biomed Mater Res A May 2. [Epub ahead of print]

Filardo G, Di Martino A, Kon E, Delcogliano M, Marcacci M (2009) Midterm results of a combined biological and mechanical approach for the treatment of a complex knee lesion. Cartilage 3(3):288–292

Filardo G, Kon E, Berruto M, Di Martino A, Patella S, Marcheggiani Muccioli GM, Zaffagnini S, Marcacci M (2012a) Arthroscopic second generation autologous chondrocytes implantation associated with bone grafting for the treatment of knee osteochondritis dissecans: Results at 6 years. Knee 19(5):658–663

Filardo G, Kon E, Di Martino A, Patella S, Altadonna G, Balboni F, Bragonzoni L, Visani A, Marcacci M (2012b) Second-generation arthroscopic autologous chondrocyte implantation for the treatment of degenerative cartilage lesions. Knee Surg Sports Traumatol Arthrosc 20(9):1704–1713

Filardo G, Kon E, Di Martino A, Busacca M, Altadonna G, Marcacci M (2013a) Treatment of knee osteochondritis dissecans with a cell-free biomimetic osteochondral scaffold: clinical and imaging evaluation at 2-year follow-up. Am J Sports Med 41(8):1786–1793

Filardo G, Kon E, Perdisa F, Di Matteo B, Di Martino A, Iacono F, Zaffagnini S, Balboni F, Vaccari V, Marcacci M (2013b) Osteochondral scaffold reconstruction for complex knee lesions: a comparative evaluation. Knee 20(6):570–576

Filardo G, Vannini F, Marcacci M, Andriolo L, Ferruzzi A, Giannini S, Kon E (2013c) Matrix-assisted autologous chondrocyte transplantation for cartilage regeneration in osteoarthritic knees: results and failures at midterm follow-up. Am J Sports Med 41(1):95–100

Filardo G, Drobnic M, Perdisa F, Kon E, Hribernik M, Marcacci M (2014a) Fibrin glue improves osteochondral scaffold fixation: study on the human cadaveric knee exposed to continuous passive motion. Osteoarthritis Cartilage 22(4):557–565

Filardo G, Kon E, Andriolo L, Di Matteo B, Balboni F, Marcacci M (2014b) Clinical profiling in cartilage regeneration: prognostic factors for midterm results of matrix-assisted autologous chondrocyte transplantation. Am J Sports Med 42(4):898–905

Filardo G, Kon E, Perdisa F, Balboni F, Marcacci M (2014c) Autologous osteochondral transplantation for the treatment of knee lesions: results and limitations at two years' follow-up. Int Orthop Mar 25. [Epub ahead of print]

Gille J, Behrens P, Volpi P, de Girolamo L, Reiss E, Zoch W, Anders S (2013) Outcome of Autologous Matrix Induced Chondrogenesis (AMIC) in cartilage knee surgery: data of the AMIC Registry. Arch Orthop Trauma Surg 133(1):87–93

Gobbi A, Karnatzikos G, Sankineani SR (2014) One-step surgery with multipotent stem cells for the treatment of large full-thickness chondral defects of the knee. Am J Sports Med 42(3):648–657

Gomoll AH, Filardo G, Almqvist FK, Bugbee WD, Jelic M, Monllau JC, Puddu G, Rodkey WG, Verdonk P, Verdonk R, Zaffagnini S, Marcacci M (2012a) Surgical treatment for early osteoarthritis. Part II: allografts and concurrent procedures. Knee Surg Sports Traumatol Arthrosc 20(3):468–486

Gomoll AH, Filardo G, de Girolamo L, Espregueira-Mendes J, Marcacci M, Rodkey WG, Steadman JR, Zaffagnini S, Kon E (2012b) Surgical treatment for early osteoarthritis. Part I: cartilage repair procedures. Knee Surg Sports Traumatol Arthrosc 20(3):450–466

Hindle P, Hendry JL, Keating JF, Biant LC (2013) Autologous osteochondral mosaicplasty or TruFit plugs for cartilage repair. Knee Surg Sports Traumatol Arthrosc 22(6):1235–40

Joshi N, Reverte-Vinaixa M, Diaz-Ferreiro EW, Dominguez-Oronoz R (2012) Synthetic resorbable scaffolds for the treatment of isolated patellofemoral cartilage defects in young patients: magnetic resonance imaging and clinical evaluation. Am J Sports Med 40(6):1289–1295

Keeney M, Pandit A (2009) The osteochondral junction and its repair via bi-phasic tissue engineering scaffolds. Tissue Eng Part B Rev 15(1):55–73

Kon E, Delcogliano M, Filardo G, Altadonna G, Marcacci M (2009) Novel nano-composite multi-layered biomaterial for the treatment of multifocal degenerative cartilage lesions. Knee Surg Sports Traumatol Arthrosc 17(11):1312–1315

Kon E, Delcogliano M, Filardo G, Fini M, Giavaresi G, Francioli S, Martin I, Pressato D, Arcangeli E, Quarto R, Sandri M, Marcacci M (2010a) Orderly osteochondral regeneration in a sheep model using a novel nano-composite multilayered biomaterial. J Orthop Res 28(1):116–124

Kon E, Mutini A, Arcangeli E, Delcogliano M, Filardo G, Nicoli Aldini N, Pressato D, Quarto R, Zaffagnini S, Marcacci M (2010b) Novel nanostructured scaffold for osteochondral regeneration: pilot study in horses. J Tissue Eng Regen Med 4(4):300–308

Kon E, Delcogliano M, Filardo G, Busacca M, Di Martino A, Marcacci M (2011a) Novel nano-composite multilayered biomaterial for osteochondral regeneration: a pilot clinical trial. Am J Sports Med 39(6):1180–1190

Kon E, Filardo G, Berruto M, Benazzo F, Zanon G, Della Villa S, Marcacci M (2011b) Articular cartilage treatment in high-level male soccer players: a prospective comparative study of arthroscopic second-generation autologous chondrocyte implantation versus microfracture. Am J Sports Med 39(12):2549–2557

Kon E, Filardo G, Di Martino A, Marcacci M (2012a) ACI and MACI. J Knee Surg 25(1):17–22

Kon E, Filardo G, Roffi A, Andriolo L, Marcacci M (2012b) New trends for knee cartilage regeneration: from cell-free scaffolds to mesenchymal stem cells. Curr Rev Musculoskelet Med 5(3):236–243

Kon E, Drobnic M, Davidson PA, Levy A, Zaslav KR, Robinson D (2013a) Chronic post-traumatic cartilage lesion of the knee treated with an acellular osteochondral regenerating implant - case history with rehabilitation guidelines. J Sport Rehabil Nov 14. [Epub ahead of print]

Kon E, Filardo G, Robinson D, Eisman JA, Levy A, Zaslav K, Shani J, Altschuler N (2013b) Osteochondral regeneration using a novel aragonite-hyaluronate bi-phasic scaffold in a goat model. Knee Surg Sports Traumatol Arthrosc 22(6):1452–64

Kon E, Filardo G, Di Martino A, Busacca M, Moio A, Perdisa F, Marcacci M (2014a) Clinical results and MRI evolution of a nano-composite multilayered biomaterial for osteochondral regeneration at 5 years. Am J Sports Med 42(1):158–165

Kon E, Filardo G, Perdisa F, Di Martino A, Busacca M, Balboni F, Sessa A, Marcacci M (2014b) A one-step treatment for chondral and osteochondral knee defects: clinical results of a biomimetic scaffold implantation at 2 years of follow-up. J Mater Sci Mater Med Mar 6. [Epub ahead of print]

Lopa S, Madry H (2014) Bioinspired scaffolds for osteochondral regeneration. Tissue Eng Part A Jan 29. [Epub ahead of print]

Madry H, van Dijk CN, Mueller-Gerbl M (2010) The basic science of the subchondral bone. Knee Surg Sports Traumatol Arthrosc 18(4):419–433

Marcacci M, Zaffagnini S, Kon E, Marcheggiani Muccioli GM, Di Martino A, Di Matteo B, Bonanzinga T, Iacono F, Filardo G (2013) Unicompartmental osteoarthritis: an integrated biomechanical and biological approach as alternative to metal resurfacing. Knee Surg Sports Traumatol Arthrosc 21(11):2509–2517

Melton JT, Wilson AJ, Chapman-Sheath P, Cossey AJ (2010) TruFit CB bone plug: chondral repair, scaffold design, surgical technique and early experiences. Expert Rev Med Devices 7(3):333–341

Niederauer GG, Slivka MA, Leatherbury NC, Korvick DL, Harroff HH, Ehler WC, Dunn CJ, Kieswetter K (2000) Evaluation of multiphase implants for repair of focal osteochondral defects in goats. Biomaterials 21(24):2561–2574

Orth P, Goebel L, Wolfram U, Ong MF, Graber S, Kohn D, Cucchiarini M, Ignatius A, Pape D, Madry H (2012) Effect of subchondral drilling on the microarchitecture of subchondral bone: analysis in a large animal model at 6 months. Am J Sports Med 40(4):828–836

Orth P, Cucchiarini M, Kohn D, Madry H (2013) Alterations of the subchondral bone in osteochondral repair–translational data and clinical evidence. Eur Cell Mater 25:299–316. discussion 314-296

O'Shea TM, Miao X (2008) Bilayered scaffolds for osteochondral tissue engineering. Tissue Eng Part B Rev 14(4):447–464

Pape D, Filardo G, Kon E, van Dijk CN, Madry H (2010) Disease-specific clinical problems associated with the subchondral bone. Knee Surg Sports Traumatol Arthrosc 18(4):448–462

Perdisa F, Filardo G, Di Matteo B, Di Martino A, Marcacci M (2014) Biological knee reconstruction: a case report of an Olympic athlete. Eur Rev Pharmacol Sci 18(suppl 1):76–80

Quarch VM, Enderle E, Lotz J, Frosch KH (2014) Fate of large donor site defects in osteochondral transfer procedures in the knee joint with and without TruFit Plugs. Arch Orthop Trauma Surg 134(5):657–66

Schleicher I, Lips KS, Sommer U, Schappat I, Martin AP, Szalay G, Hartmann S, Schnettler R (2013a) Biphasic scaffolds for repair of deep osteochondral defects in a sheep model. J Surg Res 183(1):184–192

Schleicher I, Lips KS, Sommer U, Schappat I, Martin AP, Szalay G, Schnettler R (2013b) Allogenous bone with collagen for repair of deep osteochondral defects. J Surg Res 185(2):667–675

Serre CM, Papillard M, Chavassieux P, Voegel JC, Boivin G (1998) Influence of magnesium substitution on a collagen-apatite biomaterial on the production of a calcifying matrix by human osteoblasts. J Biomed Mater Res 42(4):626–633

Shimomura K, Moriguchi Y, Ando W, Nansai R, Fujie H, Hart DA, Gobbi A, Kita K, Horibe S, Shino K, Yoshikawa H, Nakamura N (2014a) Osteochondral repair using a scaffold-free tissue-engineered construct derived from synovial mesenchymal stem cells and a hydroxyapatite-based artificial bone. Tissue Eng Part A Mar 21. [Epub ahead of print]

Shimomura K, Moriguchi Y, Murawski CD, Yoshikawa H, Nakamura N (2014b) Osteochondral tissue engineering with biphasic scaffold: current strategies and techniques. Tissue Eng Part B Rev Feb 26. [Epub ahead of print]

Slivka MA, Leatherbury NC, Kieswetter K, Niederauer GG (2001) Porous, resorbable, fiber-reinforced scaffolds tailored for articular cartilage repair. Tissue Eng 7(6):767–780

Tampieri A, Sandri M, Landi E, Pressato D, Francioli S, Quarto R, Martin I (2008) Design of graded biomimetic osteochondral composite scaffolds. Biomaterials 29(26):3539–3546

Williams RJ, Gamradt SC (2008) Articular cartilage repair using a resorbable matrix scaffold. Instr Course Lect 57:563–571

Zhang S, Chen L, Jiang Y, Cai Y, Xu G, Tong T, Zhang W, Wang L, Ji J, Shi P, Ouyang HW (2013a) Bi-layer collagen/microporous electrospun nanofiber scaffold improves the osteochondral regeneration. Acta Biomater 9(7):7236–7247

Zhang W, Chen J, Tao J, Hu C, Chen L, Zhao H, Xu G, Heng BC, Ouyang HW (2013b) The promotion of osteochondral repair by combined intra-articular injection of parathyroid hormone-related protein and implantation of a bi-layer collagen-silk scaffold. Biomaterials 34(25):6046–6057

17

Cyclical loading causes injury in and around the porcine proximal femoral physeal plate: proposed cause of the development of cam deformity in young athletes

Páll Sigurgeir Jónasson[3*], Lars Ekström[1], Hans-Arne Hansson[4], Mikael Sansone[2], Jón Karlsson[1], Leif Swärd[2] and Adad Baranto[1]

Abstract

Background: The repetitive load to which the adolescent athlete's body is exposed during training and competition affects bone growth. In previous studies, abnormalities of the spine and extremities of adolescent athletes have been described on radiographs and this also applies to the hip. The cam deformity of the hip is an extension of the physeal plate and develops during the adolescent athlete's growth. Studies of the porcine spine have shown that the vertebral endplates, apophyseal rings and intervertebral discs are susceptible to both static and repetitive loads. The proximal physeal plate of the porcine femur is susceptible to static loads, but no studies have been performed on its susceptibility to repetitive loads. The purpose of this study was to investigate the susceptibility of the proximal porcine femur to repetitive loads.

Methods: Descriptive laboratory study. Seven proximal femurs from four young (5 months) pigs were loaded repetitively (50,000 cycles) using a previously developed model. Three were loaded vertically, three antero-superiorly and one was used as a control. All femurs were examined macroscopically, histologically and with MRI after loading.

Results: No macroscopic injuries were detected on any of the femurs after loading. Fluid redistribution was seen in all femurs on MRI compared with the unloaded control. Injuries were seen in all loaded femurs on microscopic examination of histological samples. Injuries, perpendicularly to the physeal plate and fractures adjacent to the plate, were seen in the vertically loaded specimens. In the antero-superiorly loaded specimen, the injury in the growth plate was parallel to the plate.

Conclusion: Repeated loading of the young porcine hip leads to histological injuries in and adjacent to the physeal plate. These injuries are likely to cause growth disturbances in the proximal femur. We propose that such injuries may be induced in adolescent athletes and offer a plausible explanation for the development of the cam deformity.

Keywords: Hip; Adolescent; Athlete; Physeal plate; Porcine; Biomechanics; Cam; Femoroacetabular impingement

* Correspondence: pallsj@gmail.com
[3]SportsMed, Gothenburg, Sweden
Full list of author information is available at the end of the article

Background

For normal bone growth, physiological load is required (Malina 1969). Exceeding the normal physiological load may result in growth disturbances and unwanted morphological changes in the bone and joints (Caine et al. 2006; Strobino et al. 1952).

Abnormalities in the vertebral endplates, apophyseal rings and intervertebral discs have been demonstrated in the adolescent athlete participating in sports exposing the spine to high loads (Lundin et al. 2001; Sward et al. 1991). Abnormalities in the upper and lower extremities have also been reported in adolescent athletes (Caine et al. 2006). The etiology of the cam deformity of the femoral head-neck junction is multifactorial (Siebenrock and Schwab 2013). There is increasing evidence that the cam deformity can develop during growth periods in adolescent athletes (Siebenrock et al. 2011; Agricola et al. 2014).

Repetitive loading during the performance of sports may lead to injuries to the physeal plate and growth interruption in young athletes. The microtrauma and occasional macrotrauma to which the adolescent athlete's growing body is exposed affect the growing bone and joints. There are two ways this growth interruption can possibly occur; either directly, because of damage to the growth plate, or indirectly, because of interruptions to the growth plate blood supply. The growth plate blood supply is mainly derived from the epiphyseal side, through the epiphyseal artery, or the metaphyseal side, through the metaphyseal artery (Figure 1). Interruption of the epiphyseal blood supply causes narrowing of the growth plate and eventually growth cessation. Interruption of the metaphyseal blood supply causes widening of the physeal plate and may weaken it, but it does not cause growth cessation (Trueta and Amato 1960).

In a previous study, Jónasson et al. created an *in-vitro*, porcine model in which the effect of different loads and loading directions on the porcine proximal femur was investigated (Jonasson et al. 2014). The physeal plate was shown to be the weakest link in the proximal femur and especially susceptible to shearing forces. High loads to failure on the proximal femur resulted in physeolysis or fracture combined with physeolysis in all specimens.

The growth zone and, to a lesser extent, the endplate, is the weakest part of the young porcine lumbar spine when loaded in flexion, extension or axially (Baranto et al. 2005a; Baranto et al. 2005b). Biomechanical studies investigating the effect of cyclical loading and then axial compression to failure of the porcine spine have disclosed that the endplate and the growth zone are the weakest part of the cyclically loaded functional spinal units (Thoreson et al. 2010). There are no previous biomechanical studies investigating the effect of cyclical loading on the porcine proximal femur.

The purpose of the present study was to use the previously established model to investigate the effect of

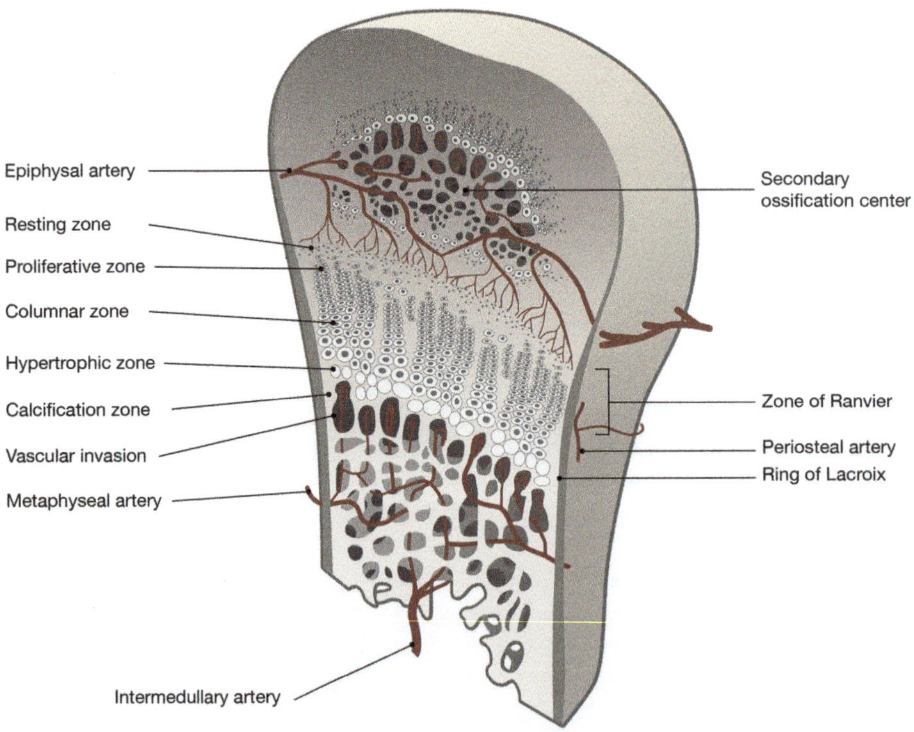

Figure 1 Anatomy and blood supply of the physis. The physis has been expanded to visualize the different cellular zones.

cyclical, sub-maximum loading on the porcine proximal femur. The hypothesis was that sub-maximum repetitive loading of the young porcine proximal femur would cause injuries in the physeal plate or in the epiphyseal or metaphyseal bone, adjacent to the physeal plate.

Methods

Experimental animals and procedures

Seven proximal femurs from four young (5 months) porcine hips were dissected and carefully cleaned of soft tissue, muscle and capsular attachments. The subjects were male domestic pigs, retrieved from the local abattoir, with a median weight of 90 kg (range 85–95). The diameter of the femoral heads was measured in the coronal and sagittal planes with a measurement error of less than 1 mm using a slide calliper (Kosashvili et al. 2008).

Mechanical test procedures

One femur was used as a control. Six femurs were used for the mechanical testing procedures. The control was treated in exactly the same way as the other specimens bar the loading procedure.

The prepared proximal femurs were fixed with Plastic Padding™ (Loctite Technology) in a metal fixture and attached to the actuator of a servo hydraulic universal testing machine (MTS Test Star, Minneapolis, MN, USA). A custom-made aluminium rod with a small plastic cup (25 mm in diameter), contoured to the shape of the femoral head, was attached to the upper crosshead of the testing machine. The femurs were then loaded repetitively at 2 Hz for 50,000 cycles. Two Hz represents a good compromise between strain rate and exposure time in order to minimise the impact of dehydration. It is also closer to a normal running (1.5 Hz) cadence as opposed to a faster loading set-up. Fifty thousand cycles is equal to running four marathons (Thoreson et al. 2010). The number of cycles was used to correspond to a weekly cumulative load exposure during sport activities, e.g. long-distance runner and football players training between 11 and 16 hours a week. Three femurs (labelled 1–3) were loaded vertically with 2,500 N (Figure 2) and three femurs (labelled 4–6) were loaded with 2,000 N antero-superiorly (Figure 3), simulating 45° of hip flexion.

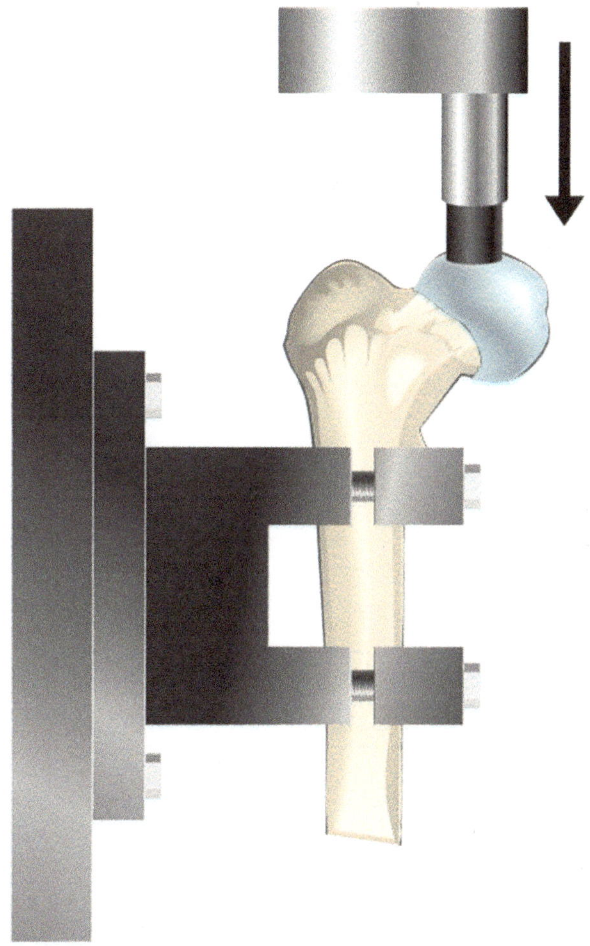

Figure 2 Setup for vertical loading of the specimens.

Macroscopic examination

The physeal plate was clearly visible on the surface of the femoral head and was used as a guide for the placement of the plastic cup, proximally to the physeal plate. After loading, the sizes of the footprint left by the plastic cup on the femoral head and its distance from the physeal plate were measured. Any signs of epiphyseolysis or fracture, visual or palpable, were registered, if present.

Magnetic resonance imaging

Directly after loading, Magnetic Resonance Imaging (MRI) was performed on all specimens, including the control femur, in a Philips Achieva 3.0™ (Philips Healthcare Inc.) using a wrist protocol, an extremity coil and SPAIR sequences. The MRI from each specimen was compared with the control and the difference in signal intensity was registered in eight different zones (Figure 4), medially and laterally to the epiphyseal tubercle in the epiphysis and the metaphysis and adjacent to the physeal plate, above and below.

Microscopic and histological examinations

The specimens were then stored in a –20°C freezer until completely frozen. When frozen, they were sawn into four equally thick primary slices in the coronal plane using a band saw. The slices were numbered from one to four, with slice number one as the most anterior and slice 4 the most posterior. The slices were decalcified, dehydrated, fixed in paraffin and cut in 4 μm slices using a microtome. Four slices from each specimen were then

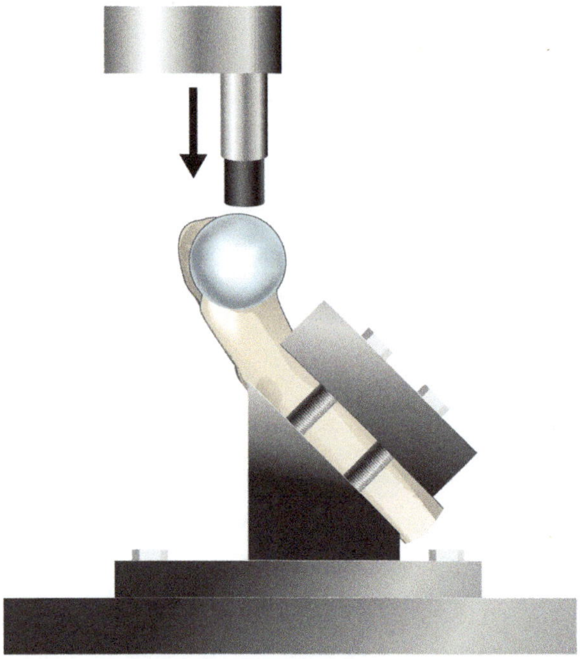

Figure 3 Setup for antero-superior loading of the specimens, simulating 45° of flexion.

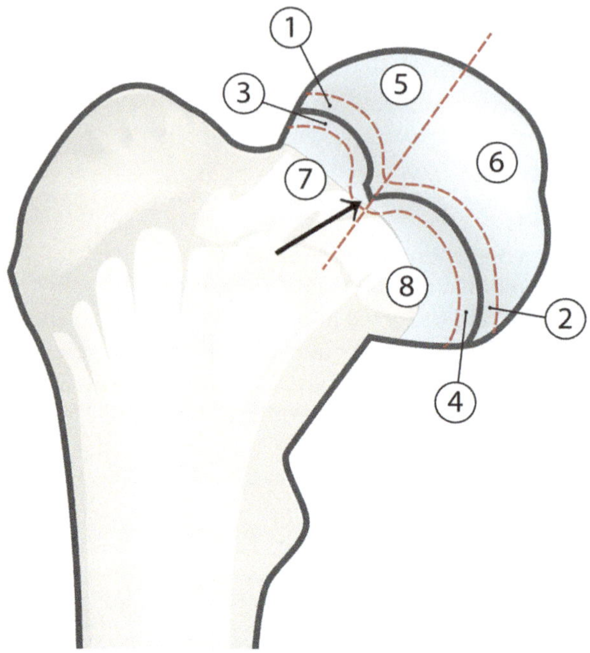

Figure 4 The different zones compared on the MRI of the control to the MRI of the loaded specimens. **1** = Superior and adjacent to the physeal line, laterally to the epiphyseal tubercle (Black arrow). **2** = Superior and adjacent to the physeal line, medially to the epiphyseal tubercle. **3** = Inferior and adjacent to the physeal line, laterally to the epiphyseal tubercle. **4** = Inferior and adjacent to the physeal line, medially to the epiphyseal tubercle. **5** = Epiphysis, laterally to the epiphyseal tubercle. **6** = Epiphysis, medially to the epiphyseal tubercle. **7** = Metaphysis, laterally to the epiphyseal tubercle. **8** = Metaphysis, medially to the epiphyseal tubercle.

stained with hematoxylin-eosin and alcian blue solution and the histological slices were examined microscopically for injuries by one of the co-authors, an experienced histologist.

The histological presence of damage to the physeal plate or adjacent bone was registered for each slice.

The procedure for the preparation of the sections planned for microscopy has previously been shown not to induce any structural changes (Baranto et al. 2005a; Baranto et al. 2005b), as was further confirmed for the control specimen.

Results

Macroscopic features

The macroscopic features of the specimens are shown in Table 1.

Caput diameters ranged from 35 × 35 mm to 38 × 39 mm (average 37 × 37.3 mm). In the specimens loaded vertically, the footprint was 7 mm from the physeal plate. In the specimens loaded in 45° of flexion, the distance of the footprint from the physeal plate varied between 5 and 14 mm.

No macroscopic damage was visible or palpable on any of the specimens after loading.

Histological findings

Damage to the physeal plate was seen in all specimens. No injuries were seen in the control. In the vertically loaded specimens, the damage tended to run parallel to the cellular columns of the physeal plate and perpendicularly to the physeal plate (Figure 5). In contrast, in the antero-superiorly loaded specimens, the damage ran parallel to the physeal plate (Figure 6). Microscopic fractures of the adjacent bone were seen in all vertically loaded specimens and in one of those loaded antero-

Table 1 Macroscopic features of the specimens

Specimen	A-P diameter (mm)	M-L diameter (mm)	Footprint distance from epiphyseal line (mm)	Macroscopic damage present
1	35	35	7	No
2	38	39	7	No
3	37	38	7	No
4	38	38	14	No
5	38	38	9	No
6	36	36	5	No
Control	37	38	NA	No
Average	37	37.4		

A-P; anterior-posterior.
M-L; medial-lateral.

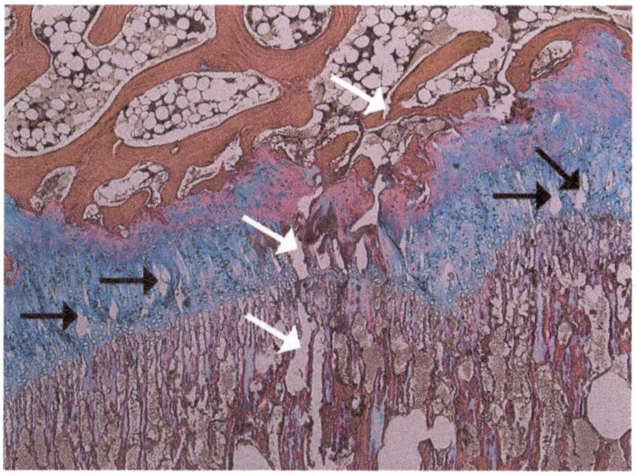

Figure 5 In the vertically loaded specimens the injuries of the physeal line (black arrows) lay perpendicular to the physeal line, parallel to the cellular columns of the physeal line. On this microscopic picture, a fracture (white arrows) extending from the epiphyseal bone (above) through the physeal line and into metaphyseal bone (below) is seen.

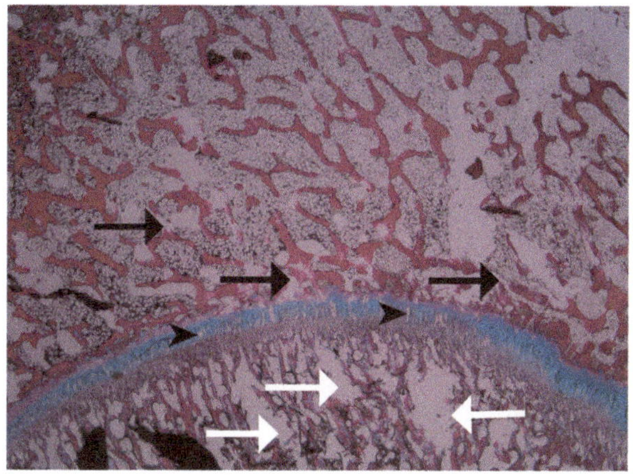

Figure 7 A microscopic photograph of a vertically loaded specimen. Fractures of the epiphyseal bone (above, black arrows) and metaphyseal bone (below, white arrows) are seen and the injuries in the physeal line (black arrowheads) are aligned parallel with the cellular columns of the physeal line.

superiorly (Figure 7). Generally, more damage was seen in the slides from the vertically loaded specimens compared with those loaded antero-superiorly. Microscopic fractures, whether in the epiphyseal bone or metaphyseal bone, tended to concentrate laterally in the epiphyseal tubercle, where the bone density was higher than peripherally (Figure 8). The bone density was evaluated based on the light microscopic inspection of stained sections, disclosing a distinct difference in bone structure on either side of the epiphyseal tubercle.

Vertically loaded specimens

In specimen 1, three of four slides showed physeal plate injury and microscopic fractures of both the epiphyseal and metaphyseal bone. No damage was seen on the fourth slide.

In specimen 2, two of four slides showed physeal plate injury and microscopic fractures of the metaphyseal bone. On the remaining two slides, no damage was seen.

In specimen 3, two slides showed injuries to the physeal plate and, in one of them, microscopic fractures were also seen in the epiphyseal bone. One slide showed no injuries, while, in one, artefacts made assessment difficult.

Antero-superiorly loaded specimens

In specimen 4, three of four slides showed injuries to the physeal plate. No damage was seen on the remaining slide.

In specimen 5, microscopic fractures in the epiphyseal bone and physeal plate injury were seen on one slide.

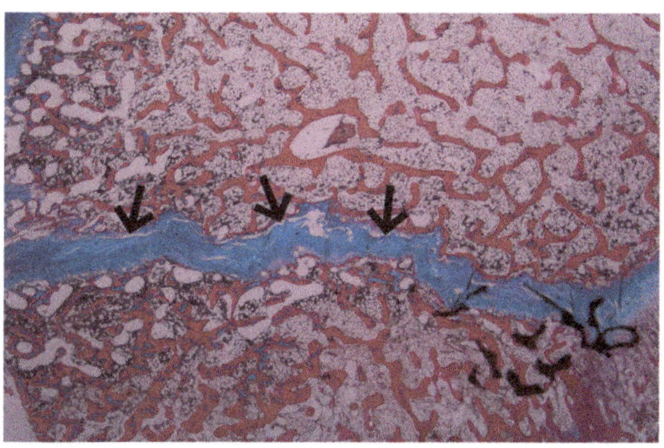

Figure 6 Microscopic photograph of an antero-superiorly loaded specimen. In the antero-superiorly loaded specimens the injuries lay parallel to the physeal line (black arrows).

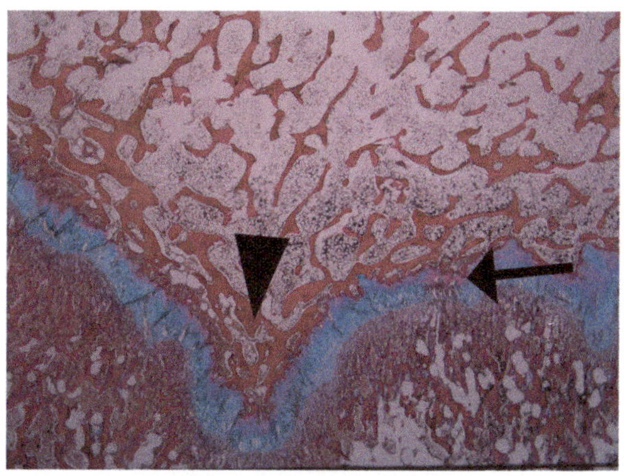

Figure 8 A microscopic picture of the epiphyseal tubercle (black arrowhead) in a vertically loaded specimen. The bone density is higher around the tubercle and injuries (black arrow) were often seen in the zone were the bone becomes less dense.

No damage was seen on two slides and, in one, artefacts made assessment difficult.

In specimen 6, physeal plate damage was seen on one slide, while no injuries were seen on the remaining three slides.

MRI findings

A summary of the MRI findings in the specimens is presented in Table 2.

As compared with the control specimen, differences were seen adjacent to the physeal plate, medially to the tubercle, in the majority of specimens (5 of 6). A reduced signal was demonstrated above the line and an increased signal below the physeal plate (Figure 9). In specimen 4, an increased signal was seen in the metaphysis and a reduced signal was seen laterally in the epiphysis of specimen 6.

No fractures or separations/avulsions were found in any specimen on MRI.

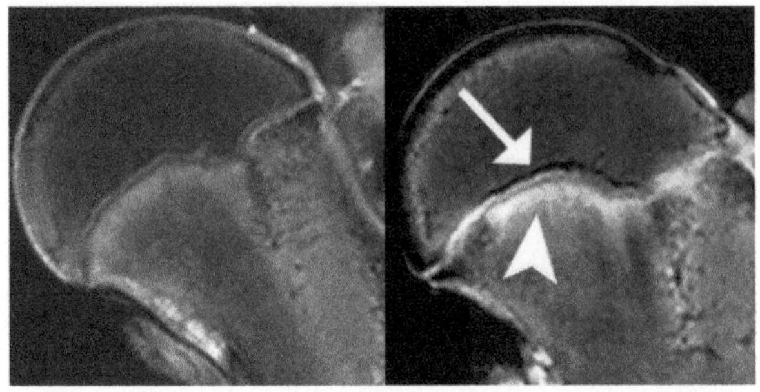

Figure 9 MRI image of the control hip (left) and a vertically loaded hip (right). After loading, difference in signal intensity was seen medially to the epiphyseal tubercle. A lower signal was seen above the epiphyseal line (white arrow) and higher signal below the epiphyseal line (white arrowhead).

Discussion

The main finding in the present study was that, after repetitive sub-maximum loading of the young porcine proximal femur, microscopic injuries to the physeal plate and adjacent bone were demonstrable. All specimens showed histological physeal plate injuries and fractures in the adjacent bone were seen in four of six specimens. On MRI, a reduced fluid signal was seen adjacent to the physeal plate in all cases.

The age and size of the samples were comparable to those in a previous study in which the proximal femora were loaded to failure (Jonasson et al. 2014). Hip-joint loading has been shown to reach levels of up to nine times body weight during different daily activities (Bergmann et al. 2001; Bergmann et al. 1993, 2004; Cleather et al. 2013). In this study, we decided to apply about 35-40% of the failure load reported in the static strength study (Jonasson et al. 2014). As no static failure load data were available, the failure load of the antero-superiorly loaded specimens was estimated to be between the vertical failure load (7,273 N) and the anterior failure load (1,728 N). This resulted in 2,500 N (equivalent to 255 kg) for the vertically loaded specimens (35% failure load) and 2,000 N (equivalent to 204 kg) for the antero-superiorly loaded specimens (40% estimated failure load). The specimens used in this study came from animals weighing about 90 kg. The load levels that were chosen are more than twice the body weight (2.2-2.7). Weight distribution in a pig is approximately 60% front and 40% rear limbs (Meijer et al. 2014). This results in a load that is 5.5 to 6.75 times the rear limb weight distribution. However, it is important to recognise that the stance load is not equivalent to the hip-joint load. To our knowledge, no data that quantify the load and movement in the porcine hip joint during daily activity have been presented. Based on estimations of the load to which a human hip joint is subjected during activity, it is believed that the load levels chosen in the present study are reasonable

Table 2 MRI findings of the different zones of femoral head in the specimens

Specimen	Zones							
	1	2	3	4	5	6	7	8
		Adjacent to the physeal plate			Epiphysis		Metaphysis	
	Superior		Inferior					
	Medially	Laterally	Medially	Laterally	Medially	Laterally	Medially	Laterally
1	-	-	+	+	0	0	0	0
2	-	+	+	0	0	0	0	0
3	-	0	+	+	0	0	0	0
4	0	0	+	0	0	0	+	+
5	-	0	+	-	0	0	0	0
6	-	0	0	0	0	-	0	0
Control	0	0	0	0	0	0	0	0

+ and − indicate a higher and a lower signal respectively, compared with the control.

and perhaps even under-estimated. The size and shear strength of the specimens are comparable to those of a 10- to 12-year-old child (Chung et al. 1976; Ipsen et al. 2002). In a previous study in which cyclical loading was applied for 20,000 cycles to the porcine spine, no differences were seen in failure load compared with non-cyclically loaded spines (Thoreson et al. 2010). In the present study, 50,000 cycles were applied; this is approximately comparable to running four marathons for a person of average height or cumulative exposure during one week of top athletic activity. Although comparisons between the porcine model used in the present study and the conditions in the human hip are open to debate, we conclude that the load applied in this study is well within the physiological range possible during sporting activities.

It is not known how loading forces vary in the hip joint during hip movements. Biomechanical studies have shown that, during routine activities, vertical load dominates (Bergmann et al. 2004). What happens in deep flexion of the hip is so far not known. The joint capsule, ligaments and muscles around the hip joint probably prevent changes in loading directions to a certain degree. The extreme range of motion performed during sporting activities and the load applied simultaneously may create unfavourable forces over the physeal plate, creating microscopic injuries that could lead to growth disturbance.

MRI of dead tissue has certain limitations and interpreting the findings is therefore difficult. A difference in fluid distribution was noted within the tissue. Mechanical loading of the tissue probably alters the distribution of fluid. With heavier loads, more redistribution of fluid can occur. Differences in signal intensity between loaded specimens and controls were predominantly observed adjacent to the physeal plate, medially to the epiphyseal tubercle. No separations or injuries could be seen in the cartilage and no fractures were observed, probably due to the poor ability of MRI to detect microfractures. Perhaps micro-CT analysis of the whole specimen could show fracture injuries in the skeletal part of the femur.

Although no macroscopic injuries to the specimens were detected on examination after loading, all specimens showed signs of microscopic injuries. The signs were often subtle and might produce only a few symptoms or even be asymptomatic in an individual (Kaeding and Miller 2013). In the vertically loaded specimens, injuries were seen both in and adjacent to the physeal plate, while physeal plate injuries predominated in the antero-superiorly loaded specimens. The physeal plate has previously been shown to be sensitive to shearing forces (Jonasson et al. 2014). It is possible to speculate that more shearing forces are applied to the physeal plate in the antero-superiorly loaded specimens and this explains the difference in injury patterns between loading directions.

Differences on MRI were predominantly medial to the epiphyseal tubercle, while microscopic injuries were predominantly found laterally to the epiphyseal tubercle. This could be explained by the stabilising function of the epiphyseal tubercle (Jonasson et al. 2014; Tayton 2009), causing the majority of the load to be distributed laterally to the tubercle, thereby causing fractures, while the minority of the load is evenly distributed medially, causing only fluid redistribution.

The cam deformity is located laterally to the epiphyseal tubercle. It is believed to develop during growth in adolescents and appears to be an extension of the physis (Siebenrock et al. 2011; Siebenrock et al. 2004; Agricola et al. 2014). The findings in the present study support the hypothesis that repeated high loads on the adolescent hip can lead to growth disturbance, due to physeal injury and microfractures in the trabecular bone, and consequently the development of cam deformity.

The present study has certain limitations. Relating results from an *in-vitro*, animal model, to the *in-vivo*, human condition is and always will be debatable. Porcine models are commonly used in studies of the hip and spine and in paediatric orthopaedics (Baranto et al. 2005a; Baranto et al. 2005b; Dodds et al. 2008; Hosalkar et al. 2011; Jonasson et al. 2014; Kishan et al. 2006; Pawaskar et al. 2011; Thoreson et al. 2010; Upasani et al. 2006; Wenger et al. 2007; Lundin et al. 2000; Karlsson et al. 1998; Kaigle et al. 1998) and are accepted in the literature as appropriate models (Pearce et al. 2007).

We conclude that the loads applied were within physiological limits. The number of cycles can be regarded as high, but the amount of training performed by many elite athletes is fairly severe, with more than 20 hours' training every week. Further research is needed to investigate the effect of load level and the number of load cycles on the fatigue properties of the femoral head.

Conclusion

In-vitro cyclical, physiological loading of the young porcine hip leads to histological injuries in and adjacent to the physeal plate. We propose that these injuries are likely to cause growth disturbances seen in adolescent athletes. These injures are also seen on MRI and offer a plausible explanation for the development of the cam deformity of the hip.

Competing interests

The authors declare that they have no competing interests.

Authors' contributions

PSJ and LE performed the mechanical procedures. PSJ and AB investigated the MRI's. PSJ, LE, JK, LS and AB developed the study setup. HAH performed the histological examination. All authors participated in the writing and proofreading of the manuscript. All authors read and approved the final manuscript.

Author details

[1]Department of Orthopaedics, Institute of Clinical Sciences at Sahlgrenska Academy, University of Gothenburg, and Sahlgrenska University Hospital, Gothenburg, Sweden. [2]Orthocenter/IFK-Kliniken, Gothenburg, Sweden. [3]SportsMed, Gothenburg, Sweden. [4]Institute of Biomedicine, Sahlgrenska Academy, University of Gothenburg, Gothenburg, Sweden.

References

Agricola R, Heijboer MP, Ginai AZ, Roels P, Zadpoor AA, Verhaar JA, Weinans H, Waarsing JH (2014) A cam deformity is gradually acquired during skeletal maturation in adolescent and young male soccer players: a prospective study with minimum 2-year follow-up. Am J Sports Med 42(4):798–806

Baranto A, Ekstrom L, Hellstrom M, Lundin O, Holm S, Sward L (2005a) Fracture patterns of the adolescent porcine spine: an experimental loading study in bending-compression. Spine (Phila Pa 1976) 30(1):75–82

Baranto A, Ekstrom L, Holm S, Hellstrom M, Hansson HA, Sward L (2005b) Vertebral fractures and separations of endplates after traumatic loading of adolescent porcine spines with experimentally-induced disc degeneration. Clin Biomech (Bristol, Avon) 20(10):1046–1054

Bergmann G, Deuretzbacher G, Heller M, Graichen F, Rohlmann A, Strauss J, Duda GN (2001) Hip contact forces and gait patterns from routine activities. J Biomech 34(7):859–871

Bergmann G, Graichen F, Rohlmann A (1993) Hip joint loading during walking and running, measured in two patients. J Biomech 26(8):969–990

Bergmann G, Graichen F, Rohlmann A (2004) Hip joint contact forces during stumbling. Langenbecks Arch Surg 389(1):53–59

Caine D, DiFiori J, Maffulli N (2006) Physeal injuries in children's and youth sports: reasons for concern? Br J Sports Med 40(9):749–760

Chung SM, Batterman SC, Brighton CT (1976) Shear strength of the human femoral capital epiphyseal plate. J Bone Joint Surg Am 58(1):94–103

Cleather DJ, Goodwin JE, Bull AM (2013) Hip and knee joint loading during vertical jumping and push jerking. Clin Biomech (Bristol, Avon) 28(1):98–103

Dodds MK, Lee J, McCormack D (2008) Transarticular stabilization of the immature femoral head: assessment of a novel surgical approach to the dislocating pediatric hip in a porcine model. J Pediatr Orthop 28(1):36–42

Hosalkar HS, Varley ES, Glaser DA, Farnsworth CL, Wenger DR (2011) Intracapsular hip pressures in a porcine model: does position and volume matter? J Pediatr Orthop B 20(5):278–283

Ipsen BJ, Williams JL, Harris MJ, Schmidt TL (2002) Shear Strength of the Pig Capital Femoral Epiphyseal Plate: An Experimental Model for Human Slipped Capital Femoral Epiphysis Fixation Studies. Paper presented at the ASME 2002 International Mechanical Engineering Congress and Exposition, New Orleans, Louisiana, USA

Jonasson P, Ekstrom L, Sward A, Sansone M, Ahlden M, Karlsson J, Baranto A (2014) Strength of the porcine proximal femoral epiphyseal plate: the effect of different loading directions and the role of the perichondrial fibrocartilaginous complex and epiphyseal tubercle - an experimental biomechanical study. J Exp Orthop 1(1):4

Kaeding CC, Miller T (2013) The comprehensive description of stress fractures: a new classification system. J Bone Joint Surg Am 95(13):1214–1220

Kaigle A, Ekstrom L, Holm S, Rostedt M, Hansson T (1998) In vivo dynamic stiffness of the porcine lumbar spine exposed to cyclic loading: influence of load and degeneration. J Spinal Disord 11(1):65–70

Karlsson L, Lundin O, Ekstrom L, Hansson T, Sward L (1998) Injuries in adolescent spine exposed to compressive loads: an experimental cadaveric study. J Spinal Disord 11(6):501–507

Kishan S, Upasani V, Mahar A, Oka R, Odell T, Rohmiller M, Newton P, Wenger D (2006) Biomechanical stability of single-screw versus two-screw fixation of an unstable slipped capital femoral epiphysis model: effect of screw position in the femoral neck. J Pediatr Orthop 26(5):601–605

Kosashvili Y, Backstein D, Safir O, Ran Y, Loebenberg MI, Ziv YB (2008) Hemiarthroplasty of the hip for fracture-what is the appropriate sized femoral head? Injury 39(2):232–237

Lundin O, Ekstrom L, Hellstrom M, Holm S, Sward L (2000) Exposure of the porcine spine to mechanical compression: differences in injury pattern between adolescents and adults. Eur Spine J 9(6):466–471

Lundin O, Hellstrom M, Nilsson I, Sward L (2001) Back pain and radiological changes in the thoraco-lumbar spine of athletes. A long-term follow-up. Scand J Med Sci Sports 11(2):103–109

Malina RM (1969) Exercise as an influence upon growth. Review and critique of current concepts. Clin Pediatr 8(1):16–26

Meijer E, Bertholle CP, Oosterlinck M, van der Staay FJ, Back W, van Nes A (2014) Pressure mat analysis of the longitudinal development of pig locomotion in growing pigs after weaning. BMC Vet Res 10:37

Pawaskar SS, Grosland NM, Ingham E, Fisher J, Jin Z (2011) Hemiarthroplasty of hip joint: An experimental validation using porcine acetabulum. J Biomech 44(8):1536–1542

Pearce AI, Richards RG, Milz S, Schneider E, Pearce SG (2007) Animal models for implant biomaterial research in bone: a review. Eur Cell Mater 13:1–10

Siebenrock KA, Ferner F, Noble PC, Santore RF, Werlen S, Mamisch TC (2011) The cam-type deformity of the proximal femur arises in childhood in response to vigorous sporting activity. Clin Orthop Relat Res 469(11):3229–3240

Siebenrock KA, Schwab JM (2013) The cam-type deformity-what is it: SCFE, osteophyte, or a new disease? J Pediatr Orthop 33(Suppl 1):S121–125

Siebenrock KA, Wahab KHA, Werlen S, Kalhor M, Leunig M, Ganz R (2004) Abnormal extension of the femoral head epiphysis as a cause of cam impingement. Clin Orthop Relat Res 418:54–60

Strobino LJ, French GO, Colonna PC (1952) The effect of increasing tensions on the growth of epiphyseal bone. Surg Gynecol Obstet 95(6):694–700

Sward L, Hellstrom M, Jacobsson B, Nyman R, Peterson L (1991) Disc degeneration and associated abnormalities of the spine in elite gymnasts. A magnetic resonance imaging study. Spine (Phila Pa 1976) 16(4):437–443

Tayton K (2009) The epiphyseal tubercle in adolescent hips. Acta Orthop 80 (4):416–419

Thoreson O, Baranto A, Ekstrom L, Holm S, Hellstrom M, Sward L (2010) The immediate effect of repeated loading on the compressive strength of young porcine lumbar spine. Knee Surg Sports Traumatol Arthrosc 18(5):694–701

Trueta J, Amato VP (1960) The vascular contribution to osteogenesis. III changes in the growth cartilage caused by experimentally induced ischaemia. J Bone Joint Surg Br 42-B:571–587

Upasani V, Kishan S, Oka R, Mahar A, Rohmiller M, Pring M, Wenger D (2006) Biomechanical analysis of single screw fixation for slipped capital femoral epiphysis: are more threads across the physis necessary for stability? J Pediatr Orthop 26(4):474–478

Wenger D, Miyanji F, Mahar A, Oka R (2007) The mechanical properties of the ligamentum teres: a pilot study to assess its potential for improving stability in children's hip surgery. J Pediatr Orthop 27(4):408–410

18

Histological changes of semitendinosus autograft after anterior cruciate ligament reconstruction in an immature rabbit model

Marco Giordano[1*], Francesco Falciglia[1], Alessia Poggiaroni[1], Angelo Gabriele Aulisa[1], Pietro Savignoni[1] and Vincenzo Guzzanti[1,2]

Abstract

Introduction: The anterior cruciate ligament (ACL) injury is one of the most common in the knee. Tendons can be used as alternative grafts for ACL repair, with tendon "ligamentization" often reported in literature. The purpose of this study was to evaluate the morphological and histological changes occurring in a semitendinosus tendon (ST) during ACL reconstruction in growing rabbits.

Materials and methods: Twenty-one 8-week-old New Zealand white rabbits, weighing about 1500 g underwent reconstructive surgery on the right knee. In two cases the left knee was used to verify the normal microstructure of the ACL and ST in rabbits. The rabbits were then randomly divided into seven groups and sacrificed at 1, 4, 6, 8, 12, 24 and 48 weeks after surgery. The specimens were evaluated under light microscopy to analyze the changes in the intra-articular tract of the graft. The evidence of necrosis, neovascularization and organization of the collagen fibers were investigated.

Results: One month after surgery, numerous disorganized fibroblasts and collagenous fibers were identified. A marked reduction of cellular necrosis was observed in the early phase of the neo-ligament healing process. After 4 weeks, these fusiform-like cells became more rounded. By 8 weeks, the collagen fibers had become aligned in parallel with newly formed capillaries and highly differentiated fibroblasts. At 24 and 48 weeks the transplanted tendon differed histologically from both tendon and ligament.

Conclusions: The data of the present study showed that ligamentization did not occur until at least 24 months post-operatively and, during healing, the grafted tendon assumed a unique micro-architecture that was a middle between a tendon and a ligament.
The ACL reconstruction in pediatric age has become more frequent in these past recent years. The use of semitendinosus graft with preservation of its distal attachment should be the gold standard in skeletally immature patients.

Keywords: Immature animal models; Anterior cruciate ligament; Ligamentization; Intra-articular tract; Semitendinosus tendon

Background

Anterior cruciate ligament (ACL) injuries in the skeletally immature athletes have been reported with increasing frequency, accounting for 31 % of the total knee injuries (Shea et al. 2004). ACL reconstruction in adolescents is still discussed. Non operative management is an appealing option in reason of the risk of physeal damage, however the recent literature uniformly indicates that conservative treatment of ACL tears in children results in a higher rate of instability that may progress to intra-articular damage, including meniscal tears (Fabricant et al. 2013; Henry et al. 2009; Ramsky et al. 2013). For this reason, there has been an increasing interest in the early operative management to restore stability in skeletally immature knees (Falciglia et al. 2014). Several aspects of the biology and biomechanics of the reconstruction of the anterior cruciate ligament have been underlined, but only

* Correspondence: marco.giordano@opbg.net
[1]Orthopaedics and Traumatology Division, Bambino Gesù Children's Hospital, Institute of Scientific Research, Piazza San Onofrio 4, I-00165 Rome, Italy
Full list of author information is available at the end of the article

few studies have been conducted on the process of ligamentization in childhood.

Although tendons have different both biological and histological features compared to ligaments, numerous studies have reported the use of tendons for ligamentous repair.

One of the still debatable questions is to clarify how the so-called “neo-ligament” really progressively loses its tendon specific biological characteristics exhibiting ligamentous histological properties. While there has been a wide number of studies exploring the various aspects of ACL reconstruction in adults only limited data are available regarding the human or animal tendon graft healing process in skeletally immature patients.

In the early twentieth century Roux, Bertocchi-Bianchetti, and Vallone published the first experimental studies on the histological characteristics of tendon grafts (Amiel et al. 1986).

Later, Carnevali indicated that the graft preserved its original features on its intra-articular tract (Claes et al. 2011). Amiel (1986) proposed the concept of graft ligamentization.

In a recent review, Claes examined several animal studies and showed that the implanted tendons indeed seemed to remodel into a ligamentous ACL-like structure (Claes et al. 2011; Scheffler et al. 2008). ACL reconstruction in children and adolescents with open physes requires physeal sparing procedures. Surgery should respect the biology and biomechanics of reconstruction of the anterior cruciate ligament in order to minimize the surgeons fear regarding the possibility of consequences on the growth of the lower limbs.

Different tendons have been proposed for surgical ACL reconstruction in skeletally immature patients but the semitendinosus is certainly the most commonly used. The purpose of this study was to evaluate the morphological and histological changes that occur in the intra-articular tract of a semitendinosus tendon, when used to reconstruct the ACL in growing rabbits, preserving its distal insertion. The study was performed on growing animals to determine the type and the extent of the lesions that develop in the intrarticular tract. Immature animals should have a greater potential for tissue regeneration. The hypothesis was that the so-called graft ligamentization process never completes beyond what was already stated during the maturation phase in other experimental studies in mature animal models.

Methods

This experimental study is an histological qualitative description of the ultrastructural changes of semitendinosus autograft used for the anterior cruciate ligament reconstruction in an immature rabbit model. The experiment was approved by the local ethics committee and followed the guidelines for the care and use of animals at our institution. The principles of laboratory animal care were followed, as well as specific national laws where applied.

All rabbits used for the study were provided by the animal enclosure of the Catholic University of the Sacred Heart of Rome (Rome, Italy). The animals received antibiotic prophylaxis with 10 mg/kg amoxicillin (Amoxysol - Bayer Spa) (preoperative administration and two additional doses at intervals of 72 h) and analgesic therapy with 30 mg ketorolac (Toradol - Recordati Spa) for 2 days postoperatively. All the healthy rabbits were enrolled in the study. Exclusion criteria were limping, pain or other signs of disease as septic arthritis.

They have been observed for 1 week following surgery in adequate cages and then sent back to the farm under veterinarian care.

In 1934 Galeazzi proposed the anterior cruciate ligament reconstruction in humans using the semitendinosus tendon (Galeazzi 1934). Carnevali used this technique in animal models in 1938 (Carnevali 1938). For the study twenty-one 8-week-old New Zeland white rabbits, weighing about 1500 ± 200 g, underwent surgery on the right knee using this last technique (Fig. 1). The left knee was

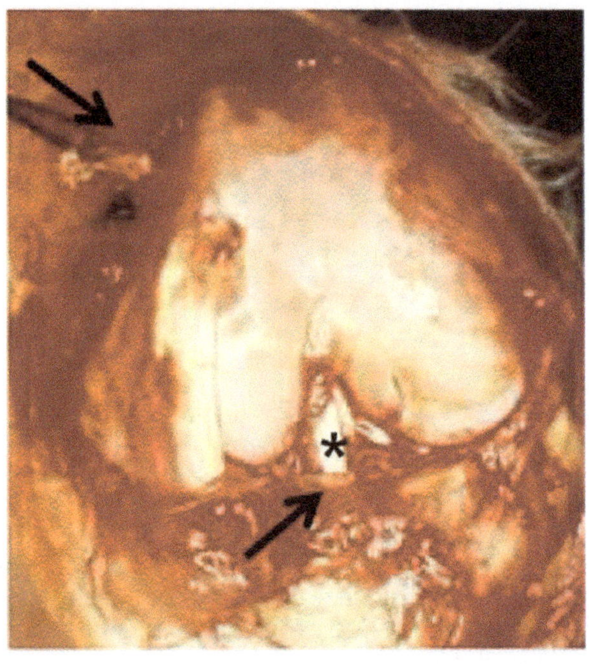

Fig. 1 Carnevali's technique: intraoperative field. The right knees joint was exposed. The ST and G tendons are divided from the musculotendinous junction, preserving the distal insertion site. Once the ACL was accurately removed the oblique 2-mm-diameter tunnels were drilled, mediolaterally in the tibia and anteroposteriorly in the femur (arrows), passing through the original attachments of the ACL and through the growth plates. Then, the semitendinosus tendon (*) was threaded through the tibial and femoral tunnels and then sutured to the periosteum of the lateral part of the femoral metaphysis with 2.0 silk thread

used to compare. The animals were anaesthetized with diazepam (Ziapam – Laboratoire Tvm) (3 to 5 mg/kg) and with intramuscular ketamine (Inoketam – Virbac Srl) (500 mg/kg).

The right knees joints were exposed through a medial parapatellar incision. The ACL was accurately removed and the original footprints were marked using a sterile pencil. Oblique 2-mm-diameter tunnels were drilled, mediolaterally in the tibia and anteroposteriorly in the femur, passing through the original attachments of the ligament and through the growth plates. Then, the semitendinosus tendon was cut at its proximal muscle-tendon junction, but left uninjured at its distal attachment site. The tendon was then threaded through the tibial and femoral tunnels and then sutured to the periosteum of the lateral part of the femoral metaphysis with 2.0 silk thread. The operated knees were immobilized in a cast for seven days, with all efforts made to minimize suffering and to avoid weight bearing. After surgery, the animals returned to their cages and were feeded with water and standard rabbit diet "ad libitum".

The animals were then randomly divided into seven groups of three and sacrificed at 1, 4, 6, 8, 12, 24 and 48 weeks after surgery. The right limb of each animal was dissected, measured with a caliper (DIN 862, Mauser-Messzeug-GMBH, Oberndorf/Neckar, Germany) and radiographed to detect deformity and leg-length discrepancy. In two cases the left knee was used to compare the normal ultrastructure of the ACL in rabbits (Fig. 2).

For the experimental and control limbs, the samples were fixed in 10 % formalin. Later they were decalcified in EDTA and embedded in paraffin. Longitudinal 5 μm-thick sections were stained with hematoxylin and eosin (H&E), Masson's trichrome, Alcian-PAS and Alcian Blue with different $MgCl_2$ concentrations (Quintarelli and Dellovo 1965). The specimens were evaluated under light microscopy (Leica DM RB) to analyze changes in the intra-articular tract of the graft. All specimens were compared with the normal rabbit ACL structure.

Statistic

Quantitative variables were presented as means and SD or proportion where appropriate. The variables that the study had taken in account and qualitatively described were the following: necrosis, neovascularization and organization of the collagen fibers.

Results

Any complication with the animals, throughout the entire period of the study, was observed. All grafts were intact at the time of evaluation and they did not have the pearly appearance of the normal ACL. No failure of the semitendinosus graft was observed at the sacrificed time. At 1 week after surgery, the graft tissue showed focal cell-free areas with poor necrosis. Tissue necrosis was better evaluable at 3–4 weeks, as the intense inflammatory response, but it was no longer detectable after 40 days from surgery. 1 month after surgery, many fibroblasts were present, and numerous disorganized collagenous fibers were observed. The fibrillar collagen, such as type I and III, are the essential building blocks that provide tendon and ligaments with their elasticity and strength. The fibroblastic cells had a central position in the tendon with an initial longitudinal arrangement. The vascularization was still poor and vessels were located on the grafts periphery (Fig. 3a).

In the semitendinosus tendon, the fibroblastic cells appeared fusiform (Fig. 3b), which was different from the ACL rounder fibroblasts. However, after 4 weeks, these fusiform-like cells became more rounded. The collagen fibers became more organized after the first month with areas of disorganized collagen matrix (Fig. 3c). From the fourth to the eighth week after surgery the typical

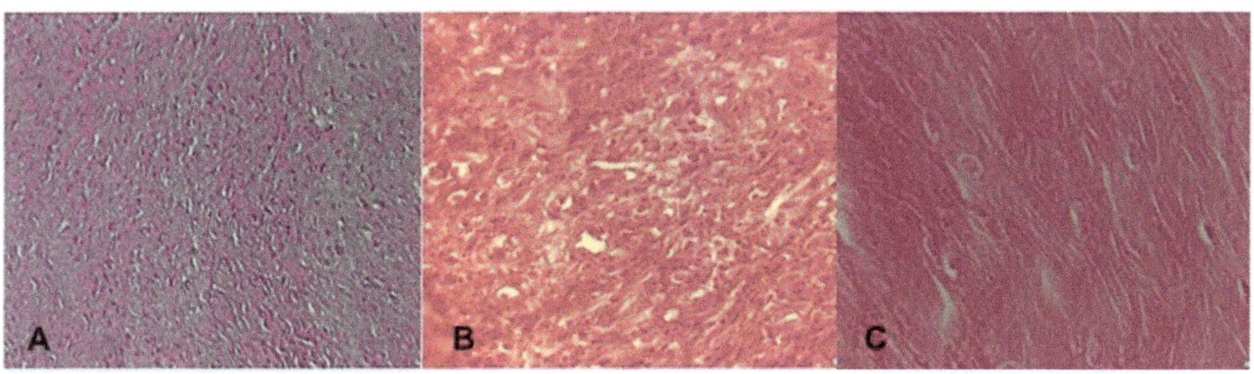

Fig. 2 Normal structure of the anterior cruciate ligament in the growing rabbit. H&E staining (**a**) Original magnification x20; (**b**) Original magnification x60; (**c**) Original magnification x100

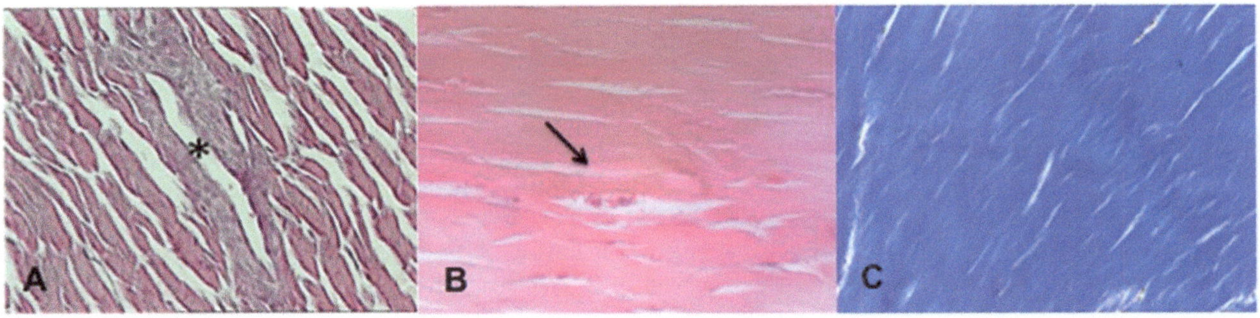

Fig. 3 H&E staining (**a**) (Original magnification x40) One month after surgery the graft tissue showed regions of cell-free areas and necrosis. *Vessel located in the periphery of the graft and runned parallel to the collagen fiber bundles in the septa at forty days; **b** (Original magnification x100) fusiform fibroblast (arrow) in the central portion of the tendon. **c** Masson trichrome staining (Original magnification x40) Disorganized collagenous fibers at 4 weeks

inflammatory cell population gradually disappeared and the small necrosis areas were not detectable.

At 8 weeks after surgery, the collagen fibers aligned in parallel with the new capillaries and with the fibroblastic cells that had become highly differentiated (Fig. 4). The semitendinosus tendon, which initially had no vessels after grafting, gradually became vascularized, expecially after 40 days after surgery. The grafts, however, did not appear to resemble the ACL at this timepoint, with the mean graft cross-sectional area significantly higher in the operated knee as compared with the normal left knee ligament. At the end of the healing process of the neo-ligament (24 weeks) the loss of the regular collagen orientation and crimp pattern was observed with the shift of the diameter of the collagen fibrils, from large to small, the reduction of collagen type I fibrils and an increase of collagen type III synthesis. The histological features observed in the sacrificed animals at 24 weeks (Fig. 5) were not subject to further changes at 48 weeks (Fig. 6). Between 24 and 48 weeks the graft had not yet acquired the characteristics of the normal rabbit ACL in the intra-articular tract of the sections. Table 1 summarizes the major histological characteristics at each time-point.

Discussion

The most noteworthy findings in the current study were: 1) The semitendinosus graft did not undergo full ligamentization and, after 48 weeks, its original appearance at the microstructural level was different; 2) A marked reduction of cellular necrosis was observed in the early phase of the neo-ligament healing process.

The ACL reconstruction in pediatric age has become more frequent in these past recent years. In skeletally immature patients, physeal-sparing procedures are recommended for the reconstruction of the injured ACL. The use of patellar tendon should be avoided for the potential risk of premature physeal closure and subsequent tibial recurvatum (Meller et al. 2008), moreover it may interfere with the delicate changes of the extensor mechanism during growth (progressive reduction of laxity, reduction of Q angle, lower limb torsional changes and gradual patella lowering). For these reasons the semitendinous graft is

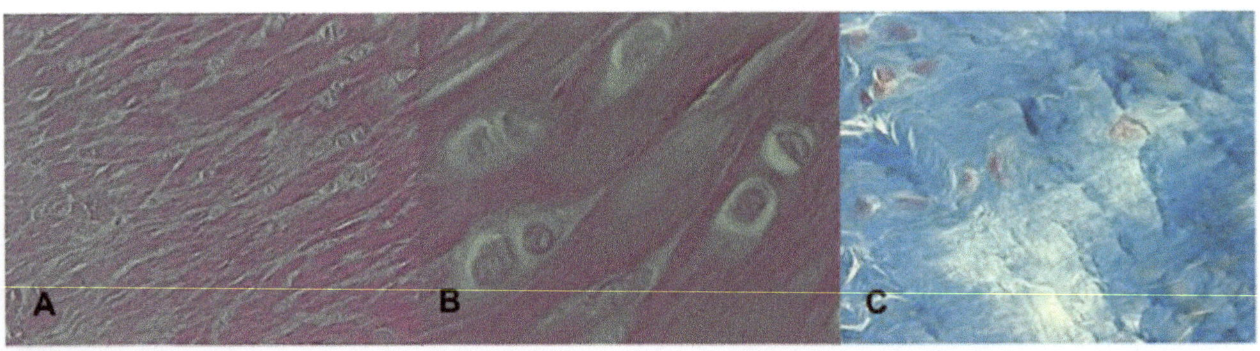

Fig. 4 H&E staining (**a**) (Original magnification x40). Fibroblastic cells of the semitendinosus tendon at 2 months after surgery. **b** (Original magnification x100). Fibroblastic cells with large nuclei and abundant cytoplasm 8 weeks after surgery. **c** Masson trichrome staining (Original magnification x60) Collagenous fibers of the semitendinosus tendon at 8 weeks after surgery

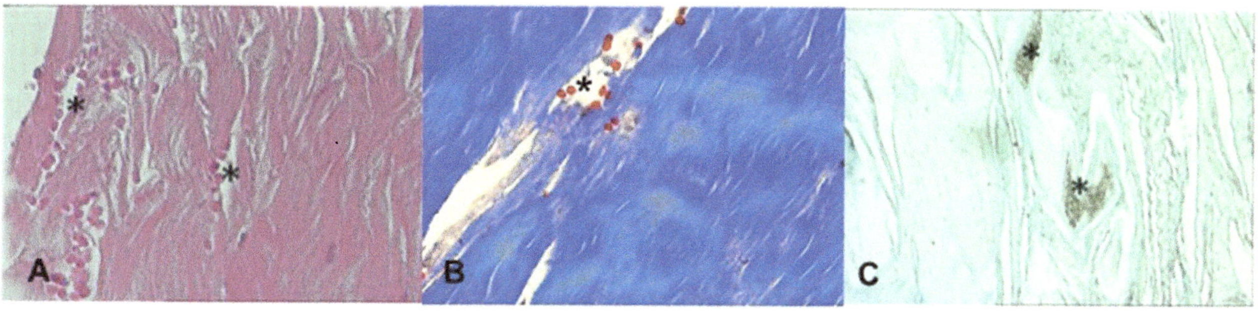

Fig. 5 Peripheral and core vessels(*) in the semitendinosus tendon 24 weeks after surgery. **a** H&E staining (Original magnification x40). **b** Masson trichrome staining (Original magnification x40) (**c**) Alcian Blue (Original magnification x20)

widely used for ACL reconstruction in children and teenage. Carnevali's surgical technique, used in this study, satisfies these requirements.

The ligamentization process was never evaluated on skeletally immature rabbits before. In Literature there were only a few papers on growing animal models, but no studies on growing rabbits has ever been performed before. This last aspect makes the study on skeletally immature patients original. In particular in other studies, the experiments were performed on mature rabbits (Amiel et al 1986; Blickenstaff et al. 1997; Papachristou et al. 2007; Tohyama et al. 2006); in others immature sheep (Meller et al. 2009), mature sheep (Blickenstaff et al. 1997; Mayr et al. 2012) or an immature canine model (Chudik et al. 2007). Besides, while we used the semitendinosus tendon, other studies used the Achilleous tendon (Li et al. 2009) the patellar tendon (Amiel et al. 1986; Falconiero et al. 1998), the superficial flexor digitorum tendon and the gastrocnemius tendon (Li et al. 2009). Few studies considered the remodeling of autografts after anterior cruciate ligament reconstruction in mature human patients (Claes et al. 2011; Scheffler et al. 2008).

Amiel (1986) proposed the concept of graft ligamentization. In his study, he used a rabbit model for ACL reconstruction and transplanted the autogenous patellar tendon in 37 adult rabbits of approximately 6 to 8 months old. He showed that patellar autograft underwent a process of "ligamentization" when placed in the ACL environment and that the cells responsible for this change were of an extragraft origin. He concluded that the ligamentization process was a continuous development of the tendon into a substance similar to a normal ligament. Other studies supported these findings (Falconiero et al. 1998; Marumo et al. 2005; Sanchez et al. 2010).

On the opposite side, Bosch demonstrated that the autograft tissue was different from the original tendon both structurally and mechanically, and that it would never approach the characteristics of a normal ligament (Bosch and Kasperczyk 1992). He also stressed the importance of the four different phases of the autograft healing process: necrosis, revitalization, collagen formation and remodeling. This was supported by Blickenstaff, who concluded that, at the end of the healing period of 52 weeks, the graft was different from the original ligament, but also had different

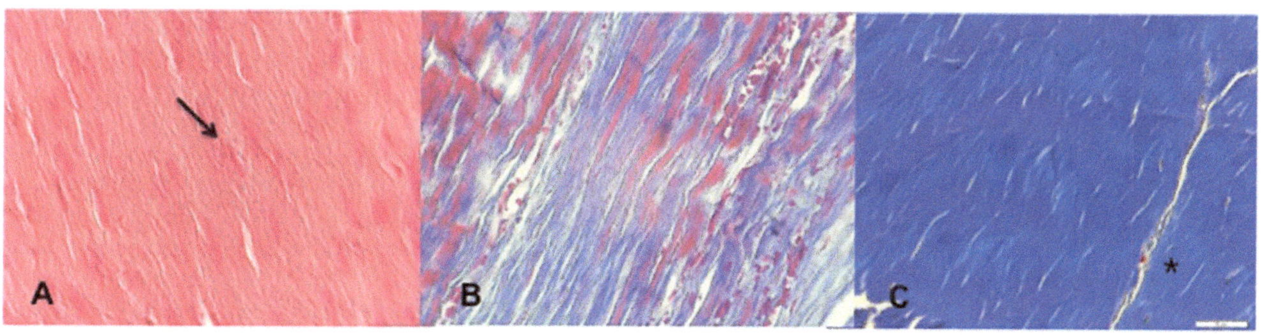

Fig. 6 **a** H&E staining (Original magnification x60). Despite the histological changes the neoligament at 48 weeks after surgery does not assume the characteristics of the normal rabbits ACL. The fibers showed a slight separation with increased waviness. The cellularity and vascularity were graded as normal. The fibrocytes have different characteristics from the fibroblastic cells observed few time after surgery. **b** Masson trichrome staining (Original magnification x20). Semitendinosus tendon 48 weeks after surgery. An increased longitudinal and parallel orientation of the collagen bundles was observed; **c** Masson trichrome staining (Original magnification x40). At 48 weeks the neoligament was viable. Red cells were present in the peripheric portion of the graft

Table 1 Major histological characteristics at each time-point in ST graft

	1 week	4 weeks	6 weeks	8 weeks	12 weeks	24 weeks	48 weeks
Necrosis	Focal cell-free areas with small necrosis	Cell-free areas with poor necrosis	Gradually disappeares		No necrosis sign		
Neovascularization	No vessel	Poor and located on the grafts periphery	Vessel located in the periphery of the graft and runned parallel to the collagen fiber bundles in the septa	Vessel located from periphery to central area	Normal vascularity		
Organization of the collagen fibers	ST tendon characteristics	Disorganized collagenous fibers	Initial longitudinal arrangement	Collagen fibers aligned in parallel with the new capillaries and with the fibroblastic cells	Loss of regular collagen orientation and crimp pattern	Slight separation with increased waviness of fibers	
					Shift of the diameter of the collagen fibrils, from large to small	Unimodal appearance of collagen fibrils	
					Reduction of collagen type I fibrils	Failure restauration of collagen orientation to normality	
					Increase of collagen type III synthesis		
Cellularity	Inflammatory cell population		Aligned longitudinally, more rounded fibroblastic cells with large nuclei and abundant cytoplasm	Highly differentiated fibroblastic cells	Normal cellularity		
	Disorganized and randomly arranged fusiform-like fibroblastic cells with plump nuclei			Gradual disappearance of the typical inflammatory cell population	Fibrocyte have different characteristics from fibroblastic cells		

characteristics from the original tendon (Blickenstaff et al. 1997).

Kennedy analyzed the evolution of intra-articular semitendinosus (ST) transfer in rabbits concluding that the surgical ACL reconstruction was a failure (Kennedy et al. 1980). In accordance with Amiel's paper, Tohyama published a study showing that the patellar tendon graft underwent important changes in its structure that could be divided into the upper mentioned four stages (Tohyama et al. 2006). He concluded that the matrix changes were caused by the adaptation of the patellar tendon to the ACL environment.

In literature only one experimental study on rabbit models used the semitendinosus tendon for ACL reconstruction with preservation of the distal insertion. In this study the specimens were taken up to 12 weeks after surgery, instead in our study they were extended beyond 24 weeks after surgery reaching the rabbits skeletal maturity, which verifies approximately at about 28 weeks. (Masoud et al. 1986 and Kaweblum et al. 1994). Papachristou immobilized rabbits for 2 weeks after surgery, instead in our study we immobilized the animals for only one week to avoid the potential risk of osteonecrosis. Despite the time points of the samples explanted were not completely overlapped, in the first month after surgery the results were similar (absence of avascular necrosis, disorganized collagen fibers). Papachristou described average or intense vascularization with new formed vessels at 3 weeks. This last finding, in our study, was observed between the 4th and the 6th week. The phase of cell differentiation was more markedly observed between the 6th and the 12th week. After this time point we evidenced the maturation phase of the graft which maintained vital up to 48 weeks after surgery.

Our study analyzed the trend and the graft patterns across different timepoints to verify the microscopic changes that occurred during the healing process. After surgery, the space between the graft and the original bone was filled with a fibrovascular tissue. The healing process occurred by the establishment of collagen fibers and neovascularization. The graft showed a fibroblasts number increase during the early postoperative period (about 1 month). The fibroblastic cells appeared disorganized and randomly arranged (Fig. 3). It was believed that the cells were metabolically active because of the presence of plump nuclei. After this timepoint, the fibroblasts aligned longitudinally became rounded and their nuclei less ovoidal (Fig. 4).

The study confirmed, even in growing rabbits, that the findings reported by other authors such as the graft vascularization began only 30–40 days after surgery (Amiel et al. 1986) and the initial focal necrosis areas were no more detectable after 4–6 weeks (Ekdahl et al. 2008; Stener et al. 2012). The new vessels initially appeared on the grafts periphery and later were present within the central zone (Fig. 4). Collagen orientation did not return to normality during the study period (48 weeks). Moreover, at the electron microscopic analysis, the diameter of the collagen fibrils lost their normal bimodality appearance changing in unimodal as described by Abe et al. (1993).

As a collateral finding, although it was not the aim of this study, any necrosis sign in the physis was observed. Therefore, drilling a tunnel through the region of the growth plate did not alter bone growth; although, there was transient hypertrophy in the portion, which disappeared within the first month after surgery (Guzzanti et al. 1994).

The remodeling phase of the healing process of the tendon graft is the most vulnerable phase because of the increased necrosis, revascularization and extra-cellular infiltration (Claes et al. 2011; Papachristou et al. 2007; Pauzenberger et al. 2013). Other animal studies have shown that the patellar tendon, similar to the semitendinosus tendon, underwent more extended avascular necrosis and revascularization after transplantation (Amiel et al. 1986; Bosch and Kasperczyk 1992). These histological observations, compared with human studies, showed that especially in the early phase there was a marked necrosis in the central portion of the graft (Amiel et al. 1986; Bosch and Kasperczyk 1992). Although the preservation of the distal insertion of the semitendinosus tendon did not improve the final graft histological feature, and even the time of the different phases of the remodeling process were not modified, however, this study noted a marked reduction in cellular necrosis, only in focal areas observed. This aspect was due to the increased vascularization of the neoligament directly given by the preservation of the distal attachment of the semitendinosus that improved both revascularization and growth of fibroblasts, as observed by Papachristou. This finding is very important because it reduces the vulnerability of the graft especially during the first weeks after ACL reconstruction.

Even though this study showed a lower percentage of cellular necrosis, it is better to be more cautious and avoid an early and intensive rehabilitation treatment in adolescents, this not for the histological weakness but for the uncertainty on their prudent post-surgical conduct.

A thorough knowledge of the graft healing process is necessary to improve aspects of the surgical technique and in particular for the rehabilitation program.

The understanding of the ligamentization process is still far from definitive answers. However one thing is clear: the neoligament doesn't assume the histological characteristics of the normal anterior cruciate ligament, expressing always an intermediate structure between the tendon and the ligament. However, clinical experience in the use of the semitendinosus for the ACL injured reconstruction shows that the ultrastructural appearance of the graft, viable at any given time point of the studies, at the end of the healing process provides sufficient guarantees such as to justify its use.

The major limitation of our study was the lack of biomechanical analysis and the ability to transfer the findings of this animal model to human tendon transplantation surgeries. The core biopsy of the graft would be appropriate even in childhood. However, the minor surgical cases and the rarity of degenerative disease in this population make second-look arthroscopy extremely rare and conditioned by small percentage of biopsies taken from the center of the graft.

Findings showed in experimental animal models, in their general concept about the progressive biologic changes that develop in the transplanted semitendinosus tendon, could be useful to lead ACL reconstruction in pediatric and adolescent population.

Conclusion

The ligamentization process is not present up to 48 weeks after surgery in growing rabbit models. The grafted ST tendon changes into a new entity during the healing process, assuming a micro-architecture somehow between the tendon and the ligament ones. Semitendinosus graft undergoes a process of adaptation rather than full restoration of the intact ACL's biology properties.

The use of semitendinosus for ACL reconstruction with preservation of its distal insertion should be the gold standard in skeletally immature patients.

Abbreviations

ACL: anterior cruciate ligament; ST: semitendinosus tendon;
H&E: hematoxylin and eosin.

Competing interests

Authors certify that there is no conflict of interest with any financial organization regarding the present manuscript.

Authors' contributions

All authors contributed equally to this work, all authors read and approved the final manuscript.

Author details

[1]Orthopaedics and Traumatology Division, Bambino Gesù Children's Hospital, Institute of Scientific Research, Piazza San Onofrio 4, I-00165 Rome, Italy.
[2]University of Cassino (FR), Cassino, Italy.

References

Abe S, Kurosaka M, Iguchi T, Yoshiya S, Hirohata K (1993) Light and electron microscopic study of remodeling and maturation process in the autogenous graft for anterior cruciate ligament reconstruction. Arthroscopy 9(4):394–405
Amiel D, Kleiner JB, Akeson WH (1986) The natural history of the anterior cruciate ligament autograft of patellar tendon origin. Am J Sports Med 14(6):449–462
Blickenstaff KR, Grana WA, Egle D (1997) Analysis of a semitendinosus autograft in a rabbit model. Am J Sports Med 25(4):554–559

Bosch U, Kasperczyk WJ (1992) Healing of the patellar tendon autograft after posterior cruciate ligament reconstruction-a process of ligamentization? An experimental study in a sheep model. Am J Sports Med 20(5):558–566

Carnevali SL (1938) La ricostruzione dei legamenti crociati del ginocchio (studio clinico e sperimentale). Arch di Ortopedia LIV:718–757

Chudik S, Beasley L, Potter H, Wickiewicz T, Warren R, Rodeo S (2007) The influence of femoral technique for graft placement on anterior cruciate ligament reconstruction using a skeletally immature canine model with a rapidly growing physis. Arthroscopy 23(12):1309–1319

Claes S, Verdonk P, Forsyth R, Bellemans J (2011) The "Ligamentization" process in anterior cruciate ligament reconstruction. What happens to the human graft? A systemic review of the literature. Am J Sports Med 20(5):1–8

Ekdahl M, Wang JH, Ronga M, Fu FH (2008) Graft healing in anterior cruciate ligament reconstruction. Knee Surg Sports Traumatol Arthrosc 16(10):935–947

Fabricant PD, Jones KJ, Delos D, Cordasco FA, Mars RG, Pearle AD, Warren RF, Green DW (2013) Reconstruction of the anterior cruciate ligament in the skeletally immature athlete: a review of current concept. J Bone Joint Surg Am 95(5):e28

Falciglia F, Di Lazzaro A, Guzzanti V (2014) The Knee: ligamentous tears. In: Guzzanti V (ed) Pediatric and Adolescent Sports Traumatology. Springer 12:141–55

Falconiero RP, Di Stefano VJ, Cook TM (1998) Revascularization and ligamentization of autogenous anterior cruciate ligament grafts in humans. Arthroscopy 14(2):197–205

Galeazzi R (1934) La ricostruzione dei legamenti crociati del ginocchio. Atti e memorie della Società Lombarda di Chirurgia

Guzzanti V, Falciglia F, Gigante A, Fabbriciani C (1994) The effect of intra-articular ACL reconstruction on the growth plates of rabbit. J Bone Joint Surg Br 76(6):960–963

Henry J, Chotel F, Chouteau J, Fessy MH, Berard J, Moyen B (2009) Rupture of the anterior cruciate ligament in children: early reconstruction with open physes or delayed reconstruction to skeletal maturity? Knee Surg Sports Traumatol Arthrosc 17:748–755

Kaweblum M, Aguilar MC, Blancas E, Kaweblum J, Lehman WB, Grant AD, Strongwater AM (1994) Histological and radiographic determination of the age of physeal closure of the distal femur, proximal tibia, and proximal fibula of the New Zealand white rabbit. J Orthop Res 12(5):747–749

Kennedy JC, Roth JH, Mendenhall HV, Sanford JB (1980) Presidential address. Intraarticular replacement in the anterior cruciate ligament-deficient knee. Am J Sports Med 8(1):1–8

Li Z, Liu Y, Shi B et al (2009) An experimental study on anterior cruciate ligament reconstruction with remnants and remaining bundle preservation. Zhongguo Xiu Fu Chong Jian Wai Ke Za Zhi 23(3):282–286

Marumo K, Saito M, Yamagishi T, Fujii K (2005) The "Ligamentization"process in human anterior cruciate ligament reconstruction with autogenous patellar and hamstring tendons. A biochemical study. Am J Sports Med 33(8):1166–1173

Masoud I, Shapiro F, Kent R, Moses A (1986) A longitudinal study of the growth of the New Zealand white rabbit: cumulative and biweekly incremental growth rates for body length, body weight, femoral length, and tibial length. J Orthop Res 4(2):221–231

Mayr HO, Stoehr A, Dietrich M, von Eisenhart-Rothe R, Hube R, Senger S, Suedkamp NP, Bernstein A (2012) Graft-dependent differencences in the ligamentization process of anterior cruciate ligament grafts in a sheep trial. Knee Surg Sports Traumatol Arthrosc 20(5):947–956

Meller R, Brandes G, Drögëmuller C, Fritz F, Schiborra F, Fehr M, Hankemeier S, Krettek C, Hurschler C (2009) Graft remodeling during growth following anterior cruciate ligament reconstruction in skeletally immature sheep. Arch Orthop Trauma Surg 129(8):1037–1046

Meller R, Kendoff D, Hankemeier S, Jagodzinski M, Grotz M, Knobloch K, Krettek C (2008) Hindlimb growth after a transphyseal reconstruction of the anterior cruciate ligament: a study in skeletally immature sheep with wide-open physes. Am J Sports Med 36(12):2437–2443

Papachristou G, Nikolaou V, Efstathopoulos N, Sourlas J, Lazarettos J, Frangia K, Papalois A (2007) ACL reconstruction with swmitendinosus tendon autograft without detachment of its tibial insertion: a histologic study in a rabbit model. Knee Surg Sports Traumatol Arthrosc 15(10):1175–1180

Pauzenberger L, Syré S, Schurz M (2013) "Ligamentization" in Hamstring Tendon Grafts After Anterior Cruciate Ligament Reconstruction: A Systematic Review of the Literature and a Glimpse Into the Future. Arthroscopy 29(10):1712–1721

Quintarelli G, Dellovo MC (1965) The chemical and histochemical properties of alcian blue. IV. Further studies on the methods for the identification of acid glycosaminoglycans. Histochemie 5(():196–209

Ramsky DE, Kanj WW, Franklin CC, Baldwin KD, Ganley TJ (2013) Anterior Cruciate Ligament tears in children and adolescent: a meta-analysis of nonoperative versus operative treatment. Am J Sport Med. doi:10.1177/0363546513510889

Sanchez M, Anitua E, Azofra J, Prado R, Maruzabal F, Andia I (2010) Ligamentization of tendon grafts treated with an endogenous preparation rich in growth factors: gross morphology and histology. Arthroscopy 26(4):470–480

Scheffler SU, Unterhauser FN, Weiler A (2008) Graft remodeling and ligamentization after cruciate ligament reconstruction. Knee Surg Sports Traumatol Arthrosc 16(9):834–842

Shea KG, Pfeiffer R, Jo HW, Curtin M, Apel PJ (2004) Anterior cruciate ligament injury in pediatric and adolescent soccer players: an analysis of insurance data. J Pediatr Orthop 24(6):623–628

Stener S, Ejerhed L, Movin T, Sernert N, Papadogiannakis N, Kartus J (2012) The reharvested patellar tendon has the potential for ligamentization when used for anterior cruciate ligament revision surgery. Knee Surg Sports Traumatol Arthros 20(6):1168–1174

Tohyama H, Yasuda K, Uchida H (2006) Is the increase in type III collagen of the patellar tendon graft after ligament reconstruction really caused by "ligamentization" of the graft? Knee Surg Sports Traumatol Arthrosc 14(12):1270–1277

19

New trends in articular cartilage repair

Magali Cucchiarini[1,2*], Christel Henrionnet[2,3], Didier Mainard[2,3], Astrid Pinzano[2,3] and Henning Madry[1,2,4]

Abstract

Damage to the articular cartilage is an important, prevalent, and unsolved clinical issue for the orthopaedic surgeon. This review summarizes innovative basic research approaches that may improve the current understanding of cartilage repair processes and lead to novel therapeutic options. In this regard, new aspects of cartilage tissue engineering with a focus on the choice of the best-suited cell source are presented. The importance of non-destructive cartilage imaging is highlighted with the recent availability of adapted experimental tools such as Second Harmonic Generation (SHG) imaging. Novel insights into cartilage pathophysiology based on the involvement of the infrapatellar fat pad in osteoarthritis are also described. Also, recombinant adeno-associated viral vectors are discussed as clinically adapted, efficient tools for potential gene-based medicines in a variety of articular cartilage disorders. Taken as a whole, such advances in basic research in diverse fields of articular cartilage repair may lead to the development of improved therapies in the clinics for an improved, effective treatment of cartilage lesions in a close future.

Keywords: Cartilage repair; Bioengineering; Non-invasive second harmonic generation imaging; Stem cells; rAAV gene therapy; Osteoarthritis; Infrapatellar fat pad

Introduction

Articular cartilage damage is an important, prevalent, and unsolved clinical issue following joint trauma or during osteoarthritis (OA). In the absence of vascularity, the cartilage does not have access to progenitor cells that may support and participate in regenerative processes. Clinical interventions such as marrow stimulation techniques that support cell invasion from the bone marrow do not restore the original cartilage structure and function in the lesions. Instead, these options lead to the formation of a poorly organized, mechanically inadapted fibrocartilage made of type-I collagen instead of type-II collagen with proteoglycans that are normally found in the hyaline cartilage (Johnstone et al. 2013). Furthermore, such fibrocartilaginous repair tissue may not integrate well with the surrounding, unaffected cartilage (Khan et al. 2008), and may induce the development of osteoarthritis over time (Schinhan et al. 2012).

New, effective treatments are thus needed to enhance the intrinsic repair capacities of injured articular cartilage that might be envisaged based on a better understanding of the pathological events underlying cartilage degradation. In this regard, original findings from active basic and applied experimental research have emerged that may allow to elaborate novel concepts for therapy. They include the identification of new components and tissues involved in the pathological processes of cartilage damage and the development of cell-, gene-, and tissue engineered-based approaches that may positively influence the protective and reparative activities of this highly specialized tissue in sites of injury.

Review

Bioengineering and cartilage

Cartilage tissue engineering is the creation of functional substitutes of native cartilage by attaching cells with a chondrogenic potential to polymer scaffolds. Once generated and tested *in vitro*, such constructs might be directly implanted in sites of cartilage injury in the patient, especially in the case of well circumscribed (focal) lesions. The three-dimensional (3D) environment of a scaffold is crucial in cartilage engineering strategies for cell entrapment, proliferation, and chondrogenic differentiation. A scaffold must display the several, following features: they must be biocompatible, must allow for cell adhesion and proliferation, and preferably be biodegradable. Various biodegradable

* Correspondence: mmcucchiarini@hotmail.com
[1]Center of Experimental Orthopaedics, Saarland University Medical Center and Saarland University, Bldg 37, Kirrbergerstr. 1, D-66421 Homburg, Germany
[2]Cartilage Net of the Greater Region, Homburg, Germany
Full list of author information is available at the end of the article

scaffolds based on natural or synthetic polymers have been developed for cartilage tissue engineering (Madry et al. 2002; Sohier et al. 2007; Henrionnet et al. 2010; Henrionnet et al. 2012; Huot et al. 2013; Tritz-Schiavi et al. 2010; Heiligenstein et al. 2011b; Heiligenstein et al. 2011a; Madry et al. 2013; Madry et al. 2014; Rey-Rico et al. 2014b). The importance of the scaffold microarchitecture has been demonstrated for articular cartilage repair (Matsiko et al. 2014).

Chondrocytes may provide the best source of cells for cartilage engineering. Due to the relatively low cellularity of the cartilage, *in vitro* expansion phases are necessary to obtain a sufficient number of cells. Yet, expansion of chondrocytes leads to rapid cell dedifferentiation and consequently to the loss of the chondrogenic phenotype (Benya et al. 1978). Alternative cell sources include embryonic stem cells (ESCs), inducible pluripotent stem cells (iPSCs), and mesenchymal stem cells (MSCs) (de Isla et al. 2010; Stoltz et al. 2010; Orth et al. 2014). ESCs are pluripotent cells derived from the blastocyst but their use is still limited by the risk of teratoma formation and by ethical concerns. iPSCs are other promising cells for clinical applications but again, a risk of tumorigenicity has been identified with their use (Yamashita et al. 2013). MSCs are an alternative valid source of cells for cartilage regeneration as they can be easily gained and expanded *in vitro* without losing their differentiation potential. MSCs can be obtained from the adult bone marrow (BMSCs), adipose tissue, umbilical cord, Wharton's jelly, and the synovial membrane. BMSCs are currently the most studied and best characterized progenitor cells for cartilage engineering. Recently, a new, promising strategy for cartilage regeneration has been identified by isolating MSCs from the synovial fluid, with expansion over a short period of time, leading to the successful differentiation of the cells in chondrocytes (Matsukura et al. 2014). Notably, higher levels of synovial fluid-derived MSCs have been reported in the knee joint of patients with degenerated cartilage and OA. On the basis of their morphology and gene expression profiles, synovial fluid-derived MSCs are more similar to synovium-derived MSCs than to BMSCs (Sekiya et al. 2012).

Three important parameters apart from the origin of the transplantable cells may be used to maintain the chondrocyte phenotype and/or to promote chondrogenic differentiation: 1) the presence of growth or soluble factors, 2) the effects of mechanical loading, and 3) the stimulation by environmental factors such as hypoxia. The presence of growth or soluble factors (e.g. vitamins) in the culture medium is known to modulate the conditions of chondrocyte culture and chondrogenic differentiation. Members of the transforming growth factor beta (TGF-β) superfamily are good candidates to promote chondrogenesis (Figure 1) (Madry et al. 2014; Henrionnet et al. 2010). Addition of such factors, alone or in combination with others (bone morphogenetic proteins; fibroblast growth factors, i.e. FGFs) during the phase of chondrocyte expansion allows for a better maintenance of the chondrocyte phenotype and for an effective chondrogenic differentiation of MSCs (Perrier et al. 2011). Induction of stem cell differentiation by applying mechanical forces is another innovative concept in artificial tissue generation (Henrionnet et al. 2012). Hydrostatic pressure is a key component of the *in vivo* joint environment and has been shown to enhance the chondrogenesis of stem cells. It can act synergistically with growth factors to upregulate the expression of SOX9 (a key chondrogenic transcription factor) and the synthesis of cartilage-specific matrix molecules (proteoglycans, type-II collagen) while downregulating the expression of genes associated with terminal differentiation (type-X collagen) (Vinardell et al. 2012). *In vivo*, the cartilage and chondrocytes are exposed to low oxygen tension (2-7% saturation), contributing to the maintenance of the chondrocyte phenotype and to a tight control of the chondrogenic commitment and differentiation of various types of MSCs. MSC isolation and expansion under hypoxic conditions (3%) increases the ability of the cells to undergo a more robust chondrogenesis. Studies also suggest that hypoxia, like growth factors, may be a potential tool to control hypertrophic MSC differentiation (Studer et al. 2012). Of note, the majority of the studies available thus far are limited to combining one or two of these modulators while the concomitant effects of factors, loading, and hypoxia have not been documented yet although such a setup clearly represents the "real articular joint condition".

Non-invasive characterization of cartilaginous implants

In cartilage bioengineering, early detection according to the organization of the collagen network is a crucial step in the differentiation process of autologous cells seeded in a collagen biomaterial (matrix). To achieve a purpose-made biofunctionality, engineered cartilage needs to exhibit biochemical and physical properties similar to those of the native, hyaline cartilage. Additionally, early analysis of the amount of type-II collagen produced *versus* resident-matrix type-I collagen is a crucial step for non-destructive, preclinical implantation validation. The goal of our work was to develop a novel, non-invasive procedure that permits to characterize the collagen network in 3D constructs by Second Harmonic Generation (SHG) imaging (Stoltz et al. 2010).

To integrate the notion of multiscale imaging in real "clinical" live (non-sliced samples, sterile, non-invasive) analyses, a two-photon excitation laser was adapted to a macroscope optical way. To combine multidimensional fluorescence data (time and spatial), a new multimodality imaging (SHG-TCSPC) based on the SHG method was considered to detect especially collagen matrix and Time Correlated Single Photon Counting (TCSPC) method to

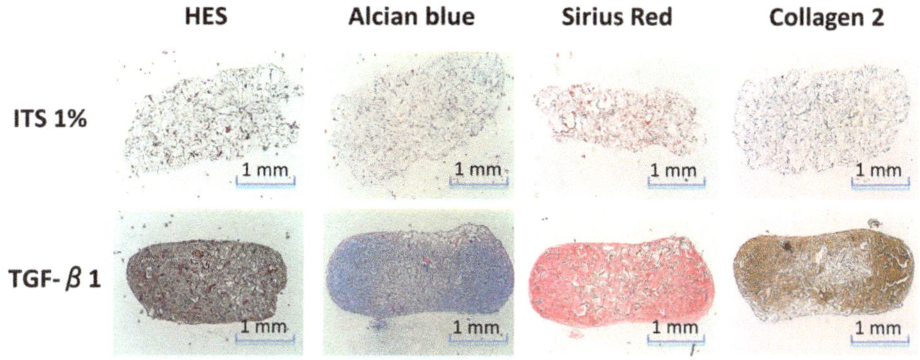

Figure 1 Chondrogenic differentiation of human bone marrow-derived MSCs in collagen sponges after 28 days of culture in presence of TGF-β1 *versus* defined chondrogenic ITS medium. TGF-β1-induced matrix synthesis inside the sponge (HES: Hematoxylin-Eosine-Saffron) rich in proteoglycans (Alcian blue) and collagens (Sirius Red), particularly in type-II collagen.

contrast signal (auto-fluorescence background, SHG and immunolabelling staining) (McCourtie & Poxton 1990; Werkmeister et al. 2009). For both SHG-TCSPC optical systems (microscopy and macroscopy), an index F-SHG based on decay time response measured by TCSPC for respectively fluorescence (F) and SHG values was introduced. This index was previously defined in relation with the behavior of cells (F for proliferation; SHG for collagen synthesis) (Dumas et al. 2010).

The technique was validated using human BMSCs (hBMSCs) as a population of cells capable of chondrogenic differentiation when subjected to appropriate culture conditions (Kuroda & Dezawa 2014). hBMSCs were seeded in a scaffold (collagen sponge) that offers a high level of complexity, recapitulating the 3D organization of chondral tissue, and maintained in culture using the highly chondrogenic TGF-β1 growth factor. hBMSC-seeded 3D collagen sponges were processed to evaluate the effects of TGF-β1 upon type-II collagen expression in the extracellular matrix by macroscopic analysis of entire sponges (7-mm diameter) *versus* microscopic (histological) evaluation (5-μm thick sections). Similar increases in type-II collagen expression produced by the cells seeded in the constructs were noted after 28 days of culture with TGF-β1 using either microscopic or macroscopic tests. The levels achieved were always higher than in the absence of growth factor, regardless of the technique applied (Hematoxylin-Eosine-Saffron and Sirius red staining, immunolabelling, multiphoton imaging, TCSPC-SHG, F-SHG index).

Collagen network SHG imaging simplifies the interaction study between cells and collagen or molecules linked to collagen. Indeed, microscopy multiphoton allows to observe a first fluorescent marker via 2 photon-excitation-fluorescence and to visualize collagen without marking with SHG (Werkmeister et al. 2008). From a general point of view, such findings demonstrate the relevance of SHG microscopy to control the quality of a biomaterial in real time, without sacrifice, and especially to follow this individual evolution according to the patient's cell capacity to differentiate into chondrocytes. Moreover, the possibility of detecting collagen as a harmonophore via TCSPC-SHG, without the need for an exogenous probe, may be advantageous to measure *ex vivo* cartilage degeneration (density and homogeneity of the collagen matrix). This technique may be used for the convenient and rapid screening of a large number of biomaterials simultaneously, noninvasively, and nondestructively, as a means to optimize the implant before grafting in a cartilage lesion (Figure 2). The next step will be to be able to discriminate between type-I and type-II collagens as previously described (Su et al. 2010).

Second Harmonic Generation is thus a sensitive technique for a "live" characterization of fibrillar collagens *versus* more conventional techniques. As it can be applied to many types of samples, SHG is robust, without additional manipulation among the studies using fluorescent markers. Despite its cost, it is so far the only procedure capable of defining the 3D organization of collagen in engineered tissues.

Recombinant adeno-associated viral vectors as efficient tools for musculoskeletal gene therapy

Application of chondroreparative and chondroregenerative factors to sites of cartilage damage is an attractive approach to improve the quality of the healing response of cartilage to injury. Yet, a direct administration of recombinant molecules is impeded by their relatively short pharmacological half-lives (some minutes) due to the rapid clearance from the host. Approaches based on the transfer of genetic coding sequences have the advantage of allowing for the sustained production of a candidate agent in a desired location like in a cartilage lesion (Cucchiarini & Madry 2005).

Recombinant adeno-associated virus (rAAV) vectors are currently the best suited, clinically relevant gene

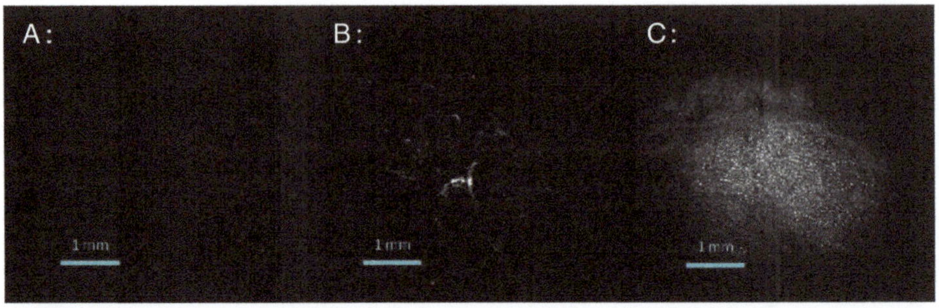

Figure 2 Direct observation of three different scaffolds by TCSPC-SHG macroscopy for the detection of collagen as a harmonophore. **(A)** Sponge without cells; **(B)** MSCs cultured for 28 days in sponges in the presence of ITS; **(C)** MSCs cultured for 28 days in sponges in the presence of TGF-β1.

delivery systems for human gene therapy and regenerative medicine as they are based on the non-pathogenic, replication defective adeno-associated virus (AAV) and have been reported for both their elevated gene transfer efficiencies and higher safety compared with other more classical classes of vectors (nonviral vectors, adenoviral, retro-/lenviral, or herpes simplex virus-derived vectors) (Frisch et al. 2014a; Cucchiarini et al. 2014; Madry & Cucchiarini 2013; Cucchiarini & Madry 2013; Madry et al. 2011; Cucchiarini & Madry 2005; Cucchiarini et al. 2003). This is mostly due to the fact that all AAV coding sequences can be removed from the recombinant vector genome and replaced by a transgene cassette, and that rAAV are mainly kept as highly stable episomal structures that can be expressed over extended periods of time without the need for integration in undesired (oncogenic) sites in the host genome (Figure 3).

Early work demonstrated the ability of rAAV vectors coding for reporter genes (*E. coli* beta-galactosidase gene; *Discosoma sp.* red fluorescent protein) to successfully modify normal and OA human adult articular chondrocytes in primary culture *in vitro*, in cartilage explant tissue *in situ*, and in sites of articular damage *in vivo* (Arai et al. 2000; Madry et al. 2003). In these systems, the transduction efficiencies exceeded 70%, resulting in reporter gene expression within cartilage explant tissue to a depth exceeding 450 μm that remained present for at least 150 days.

The benefits of applying various rAAV vectors to deliver growth (FGF-2; insulin-like growth factor I, i.e. IGF-I; TGF-β) and transcription (SOX9) factors in cartilage lesions in clinically relevant animal models of focal defects and of OA were next documented, allowing to improve the capacities of this tissue for stable repair for at least 4 months *in vivo* without development of a deleterious host immune response to the vectors or the transgene products (Cucchiarini & Madry 2014; Cucchiarini et al. 2013; Cucchiarini et al. 2005). Also of note, all these constructs were successful to transduce various human cells of the musculoskeletal system *in vitro* and *in situ*, including human normal and OA articular chondrocytes (Madry et al. 2003) and bone marrow-derived mesenchymal stem cells (hMSCs) (Cucchiarini et al. 2011; Stender et al. 2007). Such approaches led to the significant and durable remodelling of OA cartilage (at least 3 months) (Venkatesan et al. 2013; Weimer et al. 2012; Cucchiarini et al. 2009; Cucchiarini et al. 2007) and to enhance the chondrogenic differentiation of MSCs (Rey-Rico et al. 2014a; Frisch et al. 2014b;

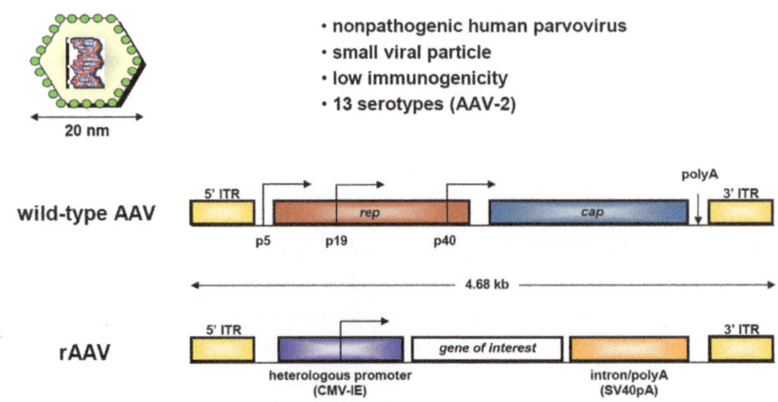

Figure 3 Generation and characteristics of recombinant adeno-associated virus (rAAV) gene therapy vectors.

Frisch et al. 2014c; Venkatesan et al. 2012; Cucchiarini et al. 2011; Pagnotto et al. 2007) while delaying undesirable, premature chondrocyte hypertrophy and terminal differentiation (Cucchiarini et al. 2011; Venkatesan et al. 2012).

Altogether, rAAV vectors appear as particularly advantageous gene vehicles capable of promoting the effective, durable, and safe healing and remodelling of injured articular cartilage. The recent example of the market authorization of Glybera® (alipogene tiparvovec, an rAAV vector engineered to express the lipoprotein lipase in the muscles of patients with lipoprotein lipase deficiency) (Carpentier et al. 2012; Gaudet et al. 2012a; Gaudet et al. 2012b; Rip et al. 2005; Ross et al. 2004), the first commercially-approved gene therapy product in the West by the European Medicines Agency (EMA 2012) is thus a strong, motivating sign to develop clinically grade rAAV-based products for articular cartilage regenerative medicine.

Evidence for an inflammatory and degradative role of the infrapatellar fat pad in OA

While early research in OA focused mostly on the articular cartilage, an innovating hypothesis has been proposed that may take into account 1) the well-established link between OA and obesity and 2) the changes in the whole OA joint, including synovium, bone, muscle, ligaments, joint capsule, and cartilage (Pottie et al. 2006). It is now well recognized that OA develops in the highly metabolic and inflammatory environment of adiposity. The sole role of biomechanical loading can not explain the increased risk for OA in non-weightbearing joints among overweight persons, and recent studies indicated that adiposity (rather than simply excess in body mass) is detrimental to the joint (Ding et al. 2008; Teichtahl et al. 2009; Toda et al. 1998; Wang et al. 2009). In obese subjects, the adipose tissue exhibits an aberrant secretion pattern. The enlarged adipose tissue is infiltrated with activated macrophages and several other types of inflammatory cells, leading to an increased production of proinflammatory adipokines (Lumeng et al. 2007).

As an articular adipose tissue, the infrapatellar fat pad (IFP) is an important candidate to become the focus of investigations that aim at further understanding the pathophysiology of OA (Clockaerts et al. 2010). Until recently, this extrasynovial but intraarticular tissue has been neglected even though it clearly releases growth factors, cytokines, and adipokines (Ushiyama et al. 2003). Work from our laboratory showed that in addition to the synovium, the IFP is an important source of adipokines in the joint, especially leptin and adiponectin (Presle et al. 2006). A crosstalk between adipocytes and other cells in the IFP may then regulate the cellular functions both in the cartilage and the synovium and promote articular changes associated with OA. Such work demonstrated a contribution of the IFP to local inflammation in knee OA and to cartilage degeneration through the release of cytokines and adipokines, in relation to the better characterized subcutaneous adipose tissue (scAT).

In these studies, specimens of cartilage, synovium, IFP, and scAT were obtained from OA patients undergoing total knee replacement surgery. Conditioned media were generated from cultured IFP and scAT explants, and cells (chondrocytes, synoviocytes) were isolated after sequential enzymatic digestion of the corresponding tissues. The data showed that the IFP released elevated amounts of leptin and adiponectin. Interestingly, the IFP from male OA patients exhibited similar secretory activity than the scAT, but the production of both adipokines differed between both adipose tissues for female OA patients. The IFP was the major source of adiponectin while the scAT released elevated levels of leptin. Besides, the conditioned media from IFP strongly induced the expression of microsomal prostaglandin E synthase-1 (mPGES-1) and cyclooxygenase-2 (COX-2) both in chondrocytes and synoviocytes. The mRNA level for inducible nitric oxide (NO) synthase (iNOS) was markedly increased in chondrocytes but not in synoviocytes. The expression of the genes encoding degradative enzymes (metalloproteinase 13, i.e. MMP13; ADAMS with thrombospondin motifs 4, i.e. ADAMTS-4) and to a lesser extent that of IGF-I was upregulated in the chondrocytes. In contrast, the conditioned media from the IFP did not stimulate the expression of TGF-β, aggrecan, or type-II collagen. Conditioned media from the IFP increased the production of PGE2 and NO and the activity of MMP13 in chondrocytes, stimulating also the release of PGE2 in culture supernatants from synoviocytes (Table 1). Similar effects were noted with the scAT but at different extents compared with the patient-matched IFP.

Table 1 Effects of IFP-conditioned media on gene expression in patient-matched chondrocytes and synoviocytes

Genes	Chondrocytes	Synoviocytes
iNOS	427.22 ± 123.76*	2.63 ± 0.45*
COX-2	57.39 ± 12.85*	362.75 ± 145*
mPGES-1	41.25 ± 7.51*	13.64 ± 1.82*
MMP13	18.29 ± 2.96*	ND
ADAMTS-4	86.64 ± 21.13*	ND
IGF-I	8.86 ± 2.04*	4.60 ± 2.64
TGF-β1	1.49 ± 0.28	1.09 ± 0.16
Type-II collagen	1.43 ± 0.19	ND
Aggrecan	1.27 ± 0.18	ND

The expression of inflammatory genes (iNOS, mPGES-1, COX-2) and of genes coding for matrix components (type-II collagen, aggrecan) or for factors involved in cartilage remodelling (MMP13, ADAMTS-4, IGF-I, TGF-β1) was analyzed in patient-matched cells (n = 20) by real-time quantitative PCR after 24 h of culture in paired conditioned medium. Data are expressed as means ± SEM of the mean over control values. *$P \leq 0.05$ between IFP conditioned media-treated and control cells.

The data indicated that IFP is a particularly active organ with a major endocrine function, releasing notably leptin and adiponectin. The IFP and scAT exhibited different secretory patterns for adipokines in female OA patients. More importantly, the IFP may also be an important source of inflammation for chondrocytes and synoviocytes, thus contributing to articular changes associated with OA. Future studies on the identification of IFP-derived inflammatory mediators and on the characterization of infiltrating immune cells will be critical to understand the biology of this tissue.

Discussion

Despite the availability of various options in the clinics, lesions to the articular cartilage remain a major unsolved problem due to the poor healing properties inherent to this avascular tissue. The development of new, effective therapeutic regimens is therefore critical to stimulate the intrinsic repair capacities of the cartilage. The use of basic science tools including cells, genes, and biomaterials that might be implanted in sites of cartilage lesions may open new avenues of clinically adapted research in orthopaedic surgery. Challenges that remain to advance the field of cartilage engineering include the choice of the best suited source of cells to undergo optimal chondrocyte differentiation without undesirable, premature chondrocyte hypertrophy and osseous metaplasia in dedicated scaffolds (Johnstone et al. 2013). Advances in high-resolution cartilage imaging greatly increased the ability to generate information on its 3D structure in a non-destructive fashion (Zehbe et al. 2010; Goebel et al. 2012; Goebel et al. 2014). Especially noteworthy is the recent availability of adapted experimental tools such as Second Harmonic Generation (SHG) imaging to perform a "live" structural characterization of cartilaginous constructs prior to implantation *in vivo*. In the field of gene therapy, the recent example of the market authorization of an rAAV vector-based gene medicine raises strong hopes for a clinical translation of this potent technology for musculoskeletal applications. Finally, the IFP has been identified as another particularly active organ involved in OA. It remains to be seen whether apart from its roles in OA, the IFP and in particular its associated mediators might be of value as targets for therapeutic interventions to enhance cartilage repair. Such advances in basic scientific and translational research in diverse fields of articular cartilage repair may have strong value to further develop improved clinical therapies (Madry 2014).

Conclusion

In light of the new advancements in basic and applied experimental cartilage research, establishing a constant exchange of knowledge between scientists and clinicians appears to be the most adapted method to generate new, effective therapeutic options for an optimal treatment of articular cartilage lesions in patients.

Competing interests

The authors declare that they have no competing interests.

Authors' contributions

MC, CH, DM, AP, and HM participated equally in drafting the manuscript. MC participated equally in drafting the manuscript in particular the Recombinant adeno-associated viral vectors as efficient tools for musculoskeletal gene therapy section. CH participated equally in drafting the manuscript in particular the Non-invasive characterization of cartilaginous implants section. DM participated equally in drafting the manuscript in particular the Evidence for an inflammatory and degradative role of the infrapatellar fat pad in OA section. AP participated equally in drafting the manuscript in particular the Bioengineering and cartilage section. HM participated equally in drafting the manuscript in particular the Discussion section. All of the authors read and approved the final manuscript.

Acknowledgments

This work was presented during the Research Day session of the Annual Congress of the *Société Française d'Arthroscopie*, December 3rd, 2014, Luxembourg. The authors thank the presenters, discussion moderators, and all the participants to the Symposium for their valuable input and contributions. We wish to confirm that there are no known conflicts of interest associated with this publication and there has been no financial support for this work that could have influenced its outcome. The authors are also grateful to P. Gégout-Pottie, P. Gillet, J.-B. Gross, C. Guillaume, and N. Presle (all from the Ingénierie Moléculaire et Physiopathologie Articulaire, UMR 7365 CNRS, Université de Lorraine, Vandoeuvre Lès Nancy, France) for helpful discussions.

Author details

[1]Center of Experimental Orthopaedics, Saarland University Medical Center and Saarland University, Bldg 37, Kirrbergerstr. 1, D-66421 Homburg, Germany. [2]Cartilage Net of the Greater Region, Homburg, Germany. [3]Ingénierie Moléculaire et Physiopathologie Articulaire, Unité Mixte de Recherches 7365 Centre National de la Recherche Scientifique, Université de Lorraine, F-54505 Vandoeuvre Lès Nancy, France. [4]Department of Orthopaedic Surgery, Saarland University Medical Center and Saarland University, D-66421 Homburg/Saar, Germany.

References

Arai Y, Kubo T, Fushiki S, Mazda O, Nakai H, Iwaki Y, Imanishi J, Hirasawa Y (2000) Gene delivery to human chondrocytes by an adeno associated virus vector. J Rheumatol 27(4):979–982

Benya PD, Padilla SR, Nimni ME (1978) Independent regulation of collagen types by chondrocytes during the loss of differentiated function in culture. Cell 15 (4):1313–1321

Carpentier AC, Frisch F, Labbe SM, Gagnon R, de Wal J, Greentree S, Petry H, Twisk J, Brisson D, Gaudet D (2012) Effect of alipogene tiparvovec (AAV1-LPL (S447X)) on postprandial chylomicron metabolism in lipoprotein lipase-deficient patients. J Clin Endocrinol Metab 97(5):1635–1644, doi:10.1210/jc.2011-3002

Clockaerts S, Bastiaansen-Jenniskens YM, Runhaar J, Van Osch GJ, Van Offel JF, Verhaar JA, De Clerck LS, Somville J (2010) The infrapatellar fat pad should be considered as an active osteoarthritic joint tissue: a narrative review. Osteoarthritis Cartilage 18(7):876–882, doi:10.1016/j.joca.2010.03.014

Cucchiarini M, Ekici M, Schetting S, Kohn D, Madry H (2011) Metabolic activities and chondrogenic differentiation of human mesenchymal stem cells following recombinant adeno-associated virus-mediated gene transfer and overexpression of fibroblast growth factor 2. Tissue Eng Part A 17(15–16):1921–1933, doi: 10.1089/ten.TEA.2011.0018

Cucchiarini M, Madry H (2005) Gene therapy for cartilage defects. J Gene Med 7(12):1495–1509

Cucchiarini M, Madry H (2013) The potential of gene transfer for the treatment of osteoarthritis. Regen Med 9(1):5–8, doi: 10.2217/rme.13.70

Cucchiarini M, Madry H (2014) Overexpression of human IGF-I via direct rAAV-mediated gene transfer improves the early repair of articular cartilage defects *in vivo*. Gene Ther 21(9):811–819, doi:10.1038/gt.2014.58

Cucchiarini M, Madry H, Guilak F, Saris DB, Stoddart MJ, Koon Wong M, Roughley P (2014) A vision on the future of articular cartilage repair. Eur Cell Mater 27:12–16

Cucchiarini M, Madry H, Ma C, Thurn T, Zurakowski D, Menger MD, Kohn D, Trippel SB, Terwilliger EF (2005) Improved tissue repair in articular cartilage defects *in vivo* by rAAV-mediated overexpression of human fibroblast growth factor 2. Mol Ther 12(2):229–238

Cucchiarini M, Orth P, Madry H (2013) Direct rAAV SOX9 administration for durable articular cartilage repair with delayed terminal differentiation and hypertrophy *in vivo*. J Mol Med (Berl) 91(5):625–636, doi: 10.1007/s00109-012-0978-9

Cucchiarini M, Terwilliger EF, Kohn D, Madry H (2009) Remodelling of human osteoarthritic cartilage by FGF-2, alone or combined with Sox9 via rAAV gene transfer. J Cell Mol Med 13(8B):2476–2488, doi: 10.1111/j.1582-4934.2008.00474.x

Cucchiarini M, Thurn T, Weimer A, Kohn D, Terwilliger EF, Madry H (2007) Restoration of the extracellular matrix in human osteoarthritic articular cartilage by overexpression of the transcription factor SOX9. Arthritis Rheum 56(1):158–167

Cucchiarini MC, Ren XL, Perides G, Terwilliger EF (2003) Selective gene expression in brain microglia mediated via adeno-associated virus type 2 and type 5 vectors. Gene Ther 10(8):657–667

de Isla N, Huseltein C, Jessel N, Pinzano A, Decot V, Magdalou J, Bensoussan D, Stoltz JF (2010) Introduction to tissue engineering and application for cartilage engineering. Biomed Mater Eng 20(3):127–133, doi: 10.3233/BME-2010-0624

Ding C, Parameswaran V, Cicuttini F, Burgess J, Zhai G, Quinn S, Jones G (2008) Association between leptin, body composition, sex and knee cartilage morphology in older adults: the Tasmanian older adult cohort (TASOAC) study. Ann Rheum Dis 67(9):1256–1261, doi: 10.1136/ard.2007.082651

Dumas D, Henrionnet C, Hupont S, Werkmeister E, Stoltz JF, Pinzano A, Gillet P (2010) Innovative TCSPC-SHG microscopy imaging to monitor matrix collagen neo-synthetized in bioscaffolds. Biomed Mater Eng 20(3):183–188, doi: 10.3233/BME-2010-0630

EMA W (2012) Glybera

Frisch J, Venkatesan JK, Rey-Rico A, Madry H, Cucchiarini M (2014) Current progress in stem cell-based gene therapy for articular cartilage repair. Curr Stem Cell Res Ther. doi:CSCRT-EPUB-62443

Frisch J, Venkatesan JK, Rey-Rico A, Schmitt G, Madry H, Cucchiarini M (2014) Determination of the chondrogenic differentiation processes in human bone marrow-derived mesenchymal stem cells genetically modified to overexpress transforming growth factor-beta via recombinant adeno-associated viral vectors. Hum Gene Ther. doi:10.1089/hum.2014.091

Frisch J, Venkatesan JK, Rey-Rico A, Schmitt G, Madry H, Cucchiarini M (2014c) Influence of insulin-like growth factor I overexpression via recombinant adeno-associated vector gene transfer upon the biological activities and differentiation potential of human bone marrow-derived mesenchymal stem cells. Stem Cell Res Ther 5(4):103, doi: 10.1186/scrt491

Gaudet D, Methot J, Dery S, Brisson D, Essiembre C, Tremblay G, Tremblay K, de Wal J, Twisk J, van den Bulk N, Sier-Ferreira V, van Deventer S (2012a) Efficacy and long-term safety of alipogene tiparvovec (AAV1-LPLS447X) gene therapy for lipoprotein lipase deficiency: an open-label trial. Gene Ther 20(4):361–369, doi: 10.1038/gt.2012.43

Gaudet D, Methot J, Kastelein J (2012b) Gene therapy for lipoprotein lipase deficiency. Curr Opin Lipidol 23(4):310–320, doi: 10.1097/MOL.0b013e3283555a7e

Goebel L, Orth P, Muller A, Zurakowski D, Bucker A, Cucchiarini M, Pape D, Madry H (2012) Experimental scoring systems for macroscopic articular cartilage repair correlate with the MOCART score assessed by a high-field MRI at 9.4 T - comparative evaluation of five macroscopic scoring systems in a large animal cartilage defect model. Osteoarthritis Cartilage 20(9):1046–1055, doi: 10.1016/j.joca.2012.05.010

Goebel L, Zurakowski D, Muller A, Pape D, Cucchiarini M, Madry H (2014) 2D and 3D MOCART scoring systems assessed by 9.4 T high-field MRI correlate with elementary and complex histological scoring systems in a translational model of osteochondral repair. Osteoarthritis Cartilage 22(10):1386–1395, doi: 10.1016/j.joca.2014.05.027

Heiligenstein S, Cucchiarini M, Laschke MW, Bohle RM, Kohn D, Menger MD, Madry H (2011a) Evaluation of nonbiomedical and biomedical grade alginates for the transplantation of genetically modified articular chondrocytes to cartilage defects in a large animal model *in vivo*. J Gene Med 13(4):230–242, doi: 10.1002/jgm.1557

Heiligenstein S, Cucchiarini M, Laschke MW, Bohle RM, Kohn D, Menger MD, Madry H (2011b) *In vitro* and *in vivo* characterization of nonbiomedical- and biomedical-grade alginates for articular chondrocyte transplantation. Tissue Eng Part C Methods 17(8):829–842, doi: 10.1089/ten.tec.2010.0681

Henrionnet C, Roeder E, Gillet R, Galois L, Bensoussan D, Mainard D, Netter P, Gillet P, Pinzano A (2010) Expression of chondrogenic genes by undifferentiated vs. differentiated human mesenchymal stem cells using array technology. Biomed Mater Eng 20(3):175–181, doi: 10.3233/BME-2010-0629

Henrionnet C, Wang Y, Roeder E, Gambier N, Galois L, Mainard D, Bensoussan D, Gillet P, Pinzano A (2012) Effect of dynamic loading on MSCs chondrogenic differentiation in 3-D alginate culture. Biomed Mater Eng 22(4):209–218, doi: 10.3233/BME-2012-0710

Huot S, Rohman G, Riffault M, Pinzano A, Grossin L, Migonney V (2013) Increasing the bioactivity of elastomeric poly(epsilon-caprolactone) scaffolds for use in tissue engineering. Biomed Mater Eng 23(4):281–288, doi: 10.3233/BME-130752

Johnstone B, Alini M, Cucchiarini M, Dodge GR, Eglin D, Guilak F, Madry H, Mata A, Mauck RL, Semino CE, Stoddart MJ (2013) Tissue engineering for articular cartilage repair–the state of the art. Eur Cell Mater 25:248–267

Khan IM, Gilbert SJ, Singhrao SK, Duance VC, Archer CW (2008) Cartilage integration: evaluation of the reasons for failure of integration during cartilage repair. A review. Eur Cell Mater 16:26–39

Kuroda Y, Dezawa M (2014) Mesenchymal stem cells and their subpopulation, pluripotent muse cells, in basic research and regenerative medicine. Anat Rec (Hoboken) 297(1):98–110, doi: 10.1002/ar.22798

Lumeng CN, Deyoung SM, Bodzin JL, Saltiel AR (2007) Increased inflammatory properties of adipose tissue macrophages recruited during diet-induced obesity. Diabetes 56(1):16–23, doi: 10.2337/db06-1076

Madry H (2014) Translating orthopaedic basic science into clinical relevance. J Exp Orthop 1(1):5, doi: 10.1186/s40634-014-0005-x

Madry H, Cucchiarini M (2013) Advances and challenges in gene-based approaches for osteoarthritis. J Gene Med 15(10):343–355, doi: 10.1002/jgm.2741

Madry H, Cucchiarini M, Terwilliger EF, Trippel SB (2003) Efficient and persistent gene transfer into articular cartilage using recombinant adeno-associated virus vectors *in vitro* and *in vivo*. Human Gene Ther 14(4):393–402

Madry H, Kaul G, Zurakowski D, Vunjak-Novakovic G, Cucchiarini M (2013) Cartilage constructs engineered from chondrocytes overexpressing IGF-I improve the repair of osteochondral defects in a rabbit model. Eur Cell Mater 25:229–247

Madry H, Orth P, Cucchiarini M (2011) Gene therapy for cartilage repair. Cartilage 2(3):201–225, doi: 10.1007/s00167-010-1071-y

Madry H, Padera R, Seidel J, Langer R, Freed LE, Trippel SB, Vunjak-Novakovic G (2002) Gene transfer of a human insulin-like growth factor I cDNA enhances tissue engineering of cartilage. Hum Gene Ther 13(13):1621–1630

Madry H, Rey-Rico A, Venkatesan JK, Johnstone B, Cucchiarini M (2014) Transforming growth factor beta-releasing scaffolds for cartilage tissue engineering. Tissue Eng Part B Rev 20(2):106–125, doi: 10.1089/ten.TEB.2013.0271

Matsiko A, Gleeson JP, O'Brien FJ (2014) Scaffold mean pore size influences mesenchymal stem cell chondrogenic differentiation and matrix deposition. Tissue Eng Part A. doi:10.1089/ten.TEA.2013.0545

Matsukura Y, Muneta T, Tsuji K, Koga H, Sekiya I (2014) Mesenchymal stem cells in synovial fluid increase after meniscus injury. Clin Orthop Relat Res 472 (5):1357–1364, doi: 10.1007/s11999-013-3418-4

McCourtie J, Poxton IR (1990) Characterisation of Bacteroides from sheep periodontal disease by SDS-PAGE of outer membrane proteins. FEMS Microbiol Lett 59(1–2):5–9

Orth P, Rey-Rico A, Venkatesan JK, Madry H, Cucchiarini M (2014) Current perspectives in stem cell research for knee cartilage repair. Stem Cells Cloning 7:1–17, doi:10.2147/SCCAA.S42880 sccaa-7-001

Pagnotto MR, Wang Z, Karpie JC, Ferretti M, Xiao X, Chu CR (2007) Adeno-associated viral gene transfer of transforming growth factor-beta1 to human mesenchymal stem cells improves cartilage repair. Gene Ther 14(10):804–813

Perrier E, Ronziere MC, Bareille R, Pinzano A, Mallein-Gerin F, Freyria AM (2011) Analysis of collagen expression during chondrogenic induction of human bone marrow mesenchymal stem cells. Biotechnol Lett 33(10):2091–2101, doi: 10.1007/s10529-011-0653-1

Pottie P, Presle N, Terlain B, Netter P, Mainard D, Berenbaum F (2006) Obesity and osteoarthritis: more complex than predicted. Ann Rheum Dis 65 (11):1403–1405, doi: 10.1136/ard.2006.061994

Presle N, Pottie P, Dumond H, Guillaume C, Lapicque F, Pallu S, Mainard D, Netter P, Terlain B (2006) Differential distribution of adipokines between serum and synovial fluid in patients with osteoarthritis. Contribution of joint tissues to their articular production. Osteoarthritis Cartilage 14(7):690–695, doi: 10.1016/j.joca.2006.01.009

Rey-Rico A, Frisch J, Venkatesan JK, Schmitt G, Madry H, Cucchiarini M (2014) Determination of effective rAAV-mediated gene transfer conditions to support chondrogenic differentiation processes in human primary bone marrow aspirates. Gene Ther. doi: 10.1038/gt.2014.90

Rey-Rico A, Venkatesan JK, Sohier J, Moroni L, Cucchiarini M, Madry H (2014b) Adapted chondrogenic differentiation of human mesenchymal stem cells via controlled release of TGF-beta1 from poly(ethylene oxide)-terephtalate/poly (butylene terepthalate) multiblock scaffolds. J Biomed Mater Res A 103 (1):371–383, doi: 10.1002/jbm.a.35181

Rip J, Nierman MC, Sierts JA, Petersen W, Van den Oever K, Van Raalte D, Ross CJ, Hayden MR, Bakker AC, Dijkhuizen P, Hermens WT, Twisk J, Stroes E, Kastelein JJ, Kuivenhoven JA, Meulenberg JM (2005) Gene therapy for lipoprotein lipase deficiency: working toward clinical application. Hum Gene Ther 16 (11):1276–1286, doi: 10.1089/hum.2005.16.1276

Ross CJ, Twisk J, Meulenberg JM, Liu G, van den Oever K, Moraal E, Hermens WT, Rip J, Kastelein JJ, Kuivenhoven JA, Hayden MR (2004) Long-term correction of murine lipoprotein lipase deficiency with AAV1-mediated gene transfer of the naturally occurring LPL(S447X) beneficial mutation. Hum Gene Ther 15 (9):906–919, doi: 10.1089/hum.2004.15.906

Schinhan M, Gruber M, Vavken P, Dorotka R, Samouh L, Chiari C, Gruebl-Barabas R, Nehrer S (2012) Critical-size defect induces unicompartmental osteoarthritis in a stable ovine knee. J Orthop Res 30(2):214–220, doi: 10.1002/jor.21521

Sekiya I, Ojima M, Suzuki S, Yamaga M, Horie M, Koga H, Tsuji K, Miyaguchi K, Ogishima S, Tanaka H, Muneta T (2012) Human mesenchymal stem cells in synovial fluid increase in the knee with degenerated cartilage and osteoarthritis. J Orthop Res 30(6):943–949, doi: 10.1002/jor.22029

Sohier J, Hamann D, Koenders M, Cucchiarini M, Madry H, van Blitterswijk C, de Groot K, Bezemer JM (2007) Tailored release of TGF-beta1 from porous scaffolds for cartilage tissue engineering. Int J Pharm 332(1–2):80–89, doi: 10.1016/j.ijpharm.2006.09.037

Stender S, Murphy M, O'Brien T, Stengaard C, Ulrich-Vinther M, Soballe K, Barry F (2007) Adeno-associated viral vector transduction of human mesenchymal stem cells. Eur Cell Mater 13:93–99

Stoltz JF, Magdalou J, Netter P, Pinzano A (2010) Papers from the 5th Scientific Meeting on Cartilage Engineering, February 2010, Nancy, France. Foreword. Biomed Mater Eng 20(3):119, doi: 10.3233/BME-2010-0622

Studer D, Millan C, Ozturk E, Maniura-Weber K, Zenobi-Wong M (2012) Molecular and biophysical mechanisms regulating hypertrophic differentiation in chondrocytes and mesenchymal stem cells. Eur Cell Mater 24:118–135

Su PJ, Chen WL, Li TH, Chou CK, Chen TH, Ho YY, Huang CH, Chang SJ, Huang YY, Lee HS, Dong CY (2010) The discrimination of type I and type II collagen and the label-free imaging of engineered cartilage tissue. Biomaterials 31 (36):9415–9421, doi: 10.1016/j.biomaterials.2010.08.055

Teichtahl AJ, Wluka AE, Wang Y, Hanna F, English DR, Giles GG, Cicuttini FM (2009) Obesity and adiposity are associated with the rate of patella cartilage volume loss over 2 years in adults without knee osteoarthritis. Ann Rheum Dis 68(6):909–913, doi:10.1136/ard.2008.093310

Toda Y, Toda T, Takemura S, Wada T, Morimoto T, Ogawa R (1998) Change in body fat, but not body weight or metabolic correlates of obesity, is related to symptomatic relief of obese patients with knee osteoarthritis after a weight control program. J Rheumatol 25(11):2181–2186

Tritz-Schiavi J, Charif N, Henrionnet C, de Isla N, Bensoussan D, Magdalou J, Benkirane-Jessel N, Stoltz JF, Huselstein C (2010) Original approach for cartilage tissue engineering with mesenchymal stem cells. Biomed Mater Eng 20(3):167–174, doi: 10.3233/BME-2010-0628

Ushiyama T, Chano T, Inoue K, Matsusue Y (2003) Cytokine production in the infrapatellar fat pad: another source of cytokines in knee synovial fluids. Ann Rheum Dis 62(2):108–112

Venkatesan JK, Ekici M, Madry H, Schmitt G, Kohn D, Cucchiarini M (2012) SOX9 gene transfer via safe, stable, replication-defective recombinant adeno-associated virus vectors as a novel, powerful tool to enhance the chondrogenic potential of human mesenchymal stem cells. Stem Cell Res Ther 3(3):22, doi: 10.1186/scrt113

Venkatesan JK, Rey-Rico A, Schmitt G, Wezel A, Madry H, Cucchiarini M (2013) rAAV-mediated overexpression of TGF-beta stably restructures human osteoarthritic articular cartilage *in situ*. J Transl Med 11:211, doi: 10.1186/1479-5876-11-211

Vinardell T, Rolfe RA, Buckley CT, Meyer EG, Ahearne M, Murphy P, Kelly DJ (2012) Hydrostatic pressure acts to stabilise a chondrogenic phenotype in porcine joint tissue derived stem cells. Eur Cell Mater 23:121–132

Wang Y, Simpson JA, Wluka AE, Teichtahl AJ, English DR, Giles GG, Graves S, Cicuttini FM (2009) Relationship between body adiposity measures and risk of primary knee and hip replacement for osteoarthritis: a prospective cohort study. Arthritis Res Ther 11(2):R31, doi: 10.1186/ar2636

Weimer A, Madry H, Venkatesan JK, Schmitt G, Frisch J, Wezel A, Jung J, Kohn D, Terwilliger EF, Trippel SB, Cucchiarini M (2012) Benefits of rAAV-mediated IGF-I overexpression for the long-term reconstruction of human osteoarthritic cartilage by modulation of the IGF-I axis. Mol Med 18(1):346–358, doi: 10.2119/molmed.2011.00371

Werkmeister E, de Isla N, Marchal L, Stoltz JF, Dumas D (2008) Interest of second harmonic generation imaging for diagnosis in thick and opaque tissue. Biorheology 45(3–4):375–383

Werkmeister E, de Isla N, Netter P, Stoltz JF, Dumas D (2009) Collagenous extracellular matrix of cartilage submitted to mechanical forces studied by second harmonic generation microscopy. Photochem Photobiol 86(2):302–310, doi: 10.1111/j.1751-1097.2009.00648.x

Yamashita A, Liu S, Woltjen K, Thomas B, Meng G, Hotta A, Takahashi K, Ellis J, Yamanaka S, Rancourt DE (2013) Cartilage tissue engineering identifies abnormal human induced pluripotent stem cells. Sci Rep 3:1978, doi: 10.1038/srep01978

Zehbe R, Haibel A, Riesemeier H, Gross U, Kirkpatrick CJ, Schubert H, Brochhausen C (2010) Going beyond histology. Synchrotron micro-computed tomography as a methodology for biological tissue characterization: from tissue morphology to individual cells. J R Soc Interface 7(42):49–59, doi: 10.1098/rsif.2008.0539

20

What quantitative mechanical loading stimulates *in vitro* cultivation best?

Jerry Natenstedt[1], Aimee C Kok[2], Jenny Dankelman[1] and Gabrielle JM Tuijthof[1,2*]

Abstract

Articular cartilage has limited regeneration capacities. One of the factors that appear to affect the *in vitro* cultivation of articular cartilage is mechanical stimulation. So far, no combination of parameters has been identified that offers the best results. The goal is to review the literature in search of the best available set of quantitative mechanical stimuli that lead to optimal *in vitro* cultivation.

The databases Scopus and PubMed were used to survey the literature, and strict in- and exclusion criteria were applied regarding the presence of quantitative data. The review was performed by studying the type of loading (hydrostatic compression or direct compression), the loading magnitude, the frequency and the loading regime (duration of the loading) in comparison to quantitative evidence of cartilage quality response (cellular, signaling and mechanical).

Thirty-three studies met all criteria of which 8 studied human, 20 bovine, 2 equine, 1 ovine, 1 porcine and 1 canine cells using four different types of cultivated constructs. Six studies investigated loading magnitude within the same setup, three studies the frequency, and seven the loading regime. Nine studies presented mechanical tissue response. The studies suggest that a certain threshold exits for enhanced cartilage *in vitro* cultivation of explants (>20 % strain and 0.5 Hz), and that chondrocyte-seeded cultivated constructs show best results when loaded with physiological mechanical stimuli. That is a loading pressure between 5–10 MPa and a loading frequency of 1 Hz exerted at intermittent intervals for a period of a week or longer. Critical aspects remain to be answered for translation into *in vivo* therapies.

Keywords: Chondrocytes; BMMSC; Compression; Mechanical loading; *in vitro*; Collagen type II; GAG; Cell therapy

Introduction

Articular cartilage is a nonlinearly permeable, viscoelastic multiphasic material containing chondrocytes and proteoglycan aggregates (3-10 % of volume) that are surrounded by an extracellular matrix (ECM), whose primary constituents are water with mobile ions (60-85 % of volume) and collagen type II (10-30 % of volume) (Fig. 1) (Mow et al. 1999; Schulz and Bader 2007; Khan and Scott 2009; Madry et al. 2010). Damaged articular cartilage presents itself as partial chondral, full thickness chondral or osteochondral defects (Fig. 1). Partial or full thickness lesions show limited ability to regenerate due to its avascular and highly structured nature, which prevents progenitor cells and chondrocytes to migrate to the defect-site (Heath and Magari 1996; Zengerink et al. 2006; Khan et al. 2008; Magnussen et al. 2008; Khan and Scott 2009). For osteochondral defects, the subchondral bone plate is breached leading to an inflow of blood containing bone marrow-derived mesenchymal stem cells (BMMSCs) that populate the defect site (Khan and Scott 2009; Madry et al. 2011). These cells may differentiate into chondrocytic cells, which in turn can regenerate the ECM (Angele et al. 2003; Bahuleyan et al. 2009). This repair tissue mostly contains collagen type I and degrades over time (Khan et al. 2008; Madry et al. 2011; Hannon et al. 2014). However, newer tissue engineered techniques are clinically applied in which tissue engineered constructs with or without (autologous) cells are used to enhance cartilage regeneration with more hyaline like cartilage as result (Brittberg 2010; Fortier et al. 2011; Hildner et al. 2011; Spiller et al. 2011). Over the last decade, numerous studies have been

* Correspondence: g.j.m.tuijthof@tudelft.nl
[1]Department of Biomechanical Engineering, Faculty of Mechanical, Materials and Maritime Engineering, Delft University of Technology, Mekelweg 2, Delft 2628 CD, The Netherlands
[2]Department of Orthopedic Surgery, Academic Medical Centre, Meibergdreef 9, Amsterdam, AZ 1105, The Netherlands

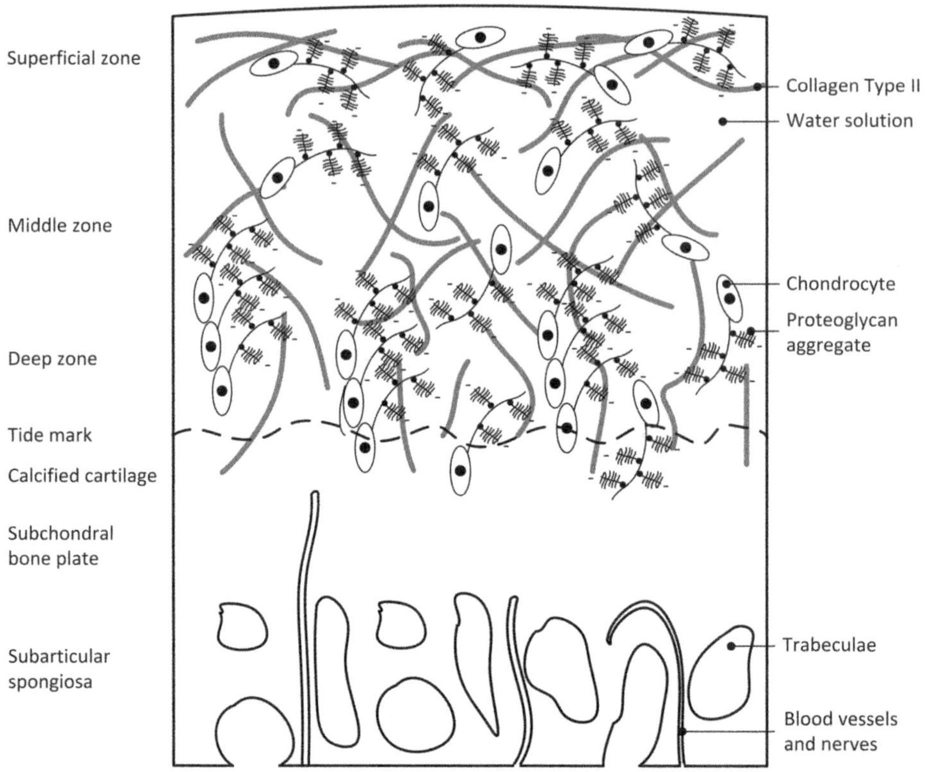

Fig. 1 Cellular structure of cartilage. Defects are sustained in different layers: partial thickness chondral defect (up till the deep zone), full thickness chondral defect (up till the calcified cartilage) and osteochondral defect (crossing the subchondral bone plate) base on (Madry et al. 2010)

published that unravelled important factors influencing the cartilage regeneration process (e.g. (Chung and Burdick 2008; Khan et al. 2008; Brittberg 2010; Fortier et al. 2011; Hildner et al. 2011; Spiller et al. 2011)).

This review will focus on the mechanical loading to promote cartilage cultivation. Mechanical stimuli promote ECM production (Grodzinsky et al. 2000), increase chondrocyte activity, and aid to protect the ECM temporarily from excessive loading (Mow et al. 1999). Due to its unique composition, cartilage can be loaded up to 18 MPa *in vivo*, which is up to 15 times the body weight (Darling and Athanasiou 2003; Elder and Athanasiou 2009; Spiller et al. 2011). If an underdeveloped ECM sustains such high loading, it can collapse; and can further deteriorate eventually leading to a full stop in intrinsic repair (Darling and Athanasiou 2003). A similar mechanism is seen when damaged cartilage (with a disrupted ECM) is loaded during gait with physiological values of around 5 times the body weight (van Dijk et al. 2010a, 2010b).

On the other hand, biomechanical intermittent cyclic loading has shown to stimulate regeneration of cartilage tissue (Arokoski et al. 2000; Bonassar et al. 2001; Waldman et al. 2004; Chung and Burdick 2008; Fan and Waldman 2010; Hess et al. 2010; Potier et al. 2010). Tissue engineering studies show that dynamic compression increases cartilage *in vitro* cultivation rather than static compression (Schulz and Bader 2007; Elder and Athanasiou 2008, 2009; Mizuno and Ogawa 2011). Important loading parameters appear to be the magnitude, frequency and duration (Ikenoue et al. 2003). So far, no combination of parameters has been identified that offers the best result in *in vivo* regeneration. Unfortunately, a first search in the literature indicated that none of the retrieved *in vivo* studies provided quantitative values to identify this combination. Therefore, the goal of this study is to review the literature in search of the best available set of quantitative mechanical stimuli that increase cartilage *in vitro* cultivation; and possibly deduct suggestions for *in vivo* cartilage regeneration.

Review

Methods

The databases Scopus and PubMed where used to survey the literature. The following keywords and synonyms were used to retrieve candidate studies: *(Mechan* OR Biomech*) AND (load* OR loading OR stimulat* OR compress* OR shear OR forces) AND articular cartilage AND (repair OR regeneration OR healing).* Both original and review papers were included from 1980 until April 18th 2015 and the search was limited to English language. The in- and exclusion criteria were formulated based on strict interpretation of the research question.

Inclusion criteria

Studies were included if they:

- Studied dynamic loading.
- Harvested either chondrocyte or BMMSC cultures from larger animal models (canine, bovine, equine, porcine, human). Larger animals provide a closer environment and metabolism to the human cartilage case (Chu et al. 2010).
- Provided quantitative values of the applied mechanical stimuli (loading magnitude, frequency, type and regime).
- Provided quantitative values of the effect on the cartilage quality response (e.g. cellular or mRNA response in terms of increased percentage).

Exclusion criteria

Studies were excluded if they only:

- Used computational methods to simulate the mechanical properties or regenerating capabilities of cartilage.
- Determined the mechanical properties of cartilage (e.g. stiffness or elastic strain limit).
- Presented operative techniques to promote cartilage healing (e.g. grafting and graft-ingrowth, arthroplasty, or microfracturing).
- Studied *in vivo* loading to stimulate cartilage, for example by specific physical therapy protocols, and did not provide quantitative data on the mechanical stimuli and/or effect on the cartilage quality response.
- Studied non-articular cartilage (e.g. cartilage of the ear).
- Examined the effect of non-mechanical factors (e.g. hormonal, chemical, or electrical) that can stimulate cartilage cultivation or regeneration.
- Harvested chondrocytes or stem cells from small animals (e.g. rodent) (Chu et al. 2010).
- Performed continuous static compression as loading regime.

From the included studies, the cell donor and culture, the construct, the additives, the type of loading (hydrostatic compression or direct compression), the loading magnitude, the frequency and the loading regime (duration of the loading) were documented as input parameters, and the quantitative evidence of cartilage quality response (cellular, signaling and mechanical responses) was documented as output parameter. Unfortunately, variety in testing conditions such as cell source, cultivated constructs, and the chosen cartilage quality response parameters only allowed for a qualitative comparison. To enhance comparison, the applied loading regime is presented in one format: the frequency, the total time of loading per day, the total number of days and total loading hours. Additionally, the loads were mostly expressed in pressure (P or σ equals force per area expressed in Pa) (Shepherd and Seedhom 1999; Darling and Athanasiou 2003). However, some studies use the strain (ε), defined as the percentage of cartilage thickness decrease. To enhance uniformity, the strain values were converted into pressure values using the formula for linear elastic materials:

$$\sigma = E \cdot \varepsilon \qquad (1)$$

Where E is the Young's modulus, which is a material property, and σ is the compression load expressed in Pa. Since cartilage is a viscoelastic multiphasic material (Mow et al. 1999), multiple parameters are needed to describe its material behaviour. In this study, an approximation of the Young's modulus was used: the 'instantaneous' compressive modulus of cartilage (E_c) (Shepherd and Seedhom 1999). Substituting E_c and ε in Equation (1) gives the compression load. The value of E_c depends on the joint donor site (Shepherd and Seedhom 1999). To this end, the range of values for the human knee joint (between 6 and 12 MPa) was filled out in Eq. (1) together with the applied strain to calculate E_c for studies that used the human knee, the bovine and canine stifle joint as donor sites (Shepherd and Seedhom 1999). In a similar fashion, the range of values for the human ankle (between 11 and 19 MPa) was filled out for bovine or canine metatarsal donor joints (Shepherd and Seedhom 1999).

Finally, this review presents the changes found in cellular, signaling and mechanical response due to the mechanical stimuli, which were indicated as an increased (+) or decreased (−) response compared to controls or as no change or similar (=) (Tables 1, 2, 3, 4, 5).

Results

After a first title and abstract scan of the 836 hits combined from Scopus and PubMed, 106 papers were left to be reviewed completely, which eventually resulted in 33 studies that were eligible for inclusion. Generally, the tissue engineering studies investigated the effect of mechanical stimuli on cultivated constructs at least in one study arm compared to unstimulated controls (Darling and Athanasiou 2003; Mauck et al. 2003). Tables 1, 2, 3, 4, 5 summarize the results.

Cell sources, cultivated constructs and additives

Two cell sources (chondrocytes and BMMSC) were studied from 6 mammal types: 8 studies used human cells, 20 bovine, 2 equine, 1 ovine, 1 porcine and 1 canine. First, 27 studies used chondrocytes as cell source (Tables 1, 2, 3, 4). Chondrocytes are responsible for the production of the ECM (Meachim and Stockwell 1973; Buckwalter and Mankin 1998; Cohen et al. 1998), since they are likely to synthesize collagen type II and proteoglycans (Schulz and

Table 1 Results on changes in cellular, signaling and/or mechanical response to explants for hydrostatic and direct compression (Fig. 2). PG is proteoglycan; MMP is matrix metalloproteinases; # is number; h is hours; h/day is hours per day; – is decrease or inhibition; = is no change or status quo; + is increase; ++ is highest increase. *-symbol implies pressure converted from strain, which is added in brackets

Study	Cell source, cultivated construct, additive(s)	Magnitude (MPa)	Freq (Hz)	Loading (h/day)	Loading (# days)	Loading (total h)	Culture composition (change -, =, +)	mRNA response (change -, =, +)	Other findings (change -, =, +)
Hydrostatic compression									
Parkinnen 1993 (Parkkinen et al. 1993)	Bovine	5	0.5	1.5	1	1.5	+ PG synthesis		
	Explant		0.25						
	Fetal calf serum		0.05				= PG synthesis		
			0.0167						
Direct compression									
Li 2013 (Li et al. 2013)	Young Bovine Bruised Explant Serum free medium, 20 g/ml ascorbic acid	0.6-1.2* (10 %)	0.5	4	4	16	+ PG synthesis	+ aggrecan + collagen II	Control show better results compared to bruised explants
		1.2-2.4* (20 %)					++ PG synthesis	++ aggrecan ++ collagen II	
		1.8-3.6* (30 %)					+ PG synthesis	+ aggrecan = collagen II	
Okuda 2013 (Okuda et al. 2013)	Young Bovine, Explant 20 % Fetal bovine serum; 50 mg/L L-ascorbic acid	0.6-1.2* (10 %)	1	3.5	5	17.5	+ sGAG + # of cells		+ compressive modulus
Torzilli 1996 (Torzilli et al. 1996)	Bovine, Explant 10 % Fetal bovine serum; 50 μg/mL ascorbic acid	1	1	24	1	24	- PG synthesis		
Torzilli 2011 (Torzilli et al. 2011)	Bovine, Explant 10 % Fetal bovine serum; 50 μg/mL ascorbic acid	0.5 (10 %)	0.5	24	3	72	= PG content	= MMP −3, −13	

Table 2 Results on changes in cellular, signaling and/or mechanical response to chondrocyte-seeded meshes for hydrostatic and direct compression (Fig. 2). PGA is polyglycolic acid; PEGT/PBT is polyethylene glycol terephthalate/polybutylene terephthalate; Sox9 is the gene that regulates chondrogenic differentiation; # is number; h is hours; h/day is hours per day; – is decrease or inhibition; = is no change or status quo; + is increase; ++ is highest increase. *-symbol implies pressure converted from strain, which is added in brackets; **loading was performed every other day for 1 h twice a day with 8 h rest in between

Study	Cell source, cultivated construct, additive(s)	Magnitude (MPa)	Freq (Hz)	Loading (h/day)	Loading (# days)	Loading (total h)	Culture composition (change -, =, +)	mRNA response (change -, =, +)	Other findings (change -, =, +)
Hydrostatic compression									
Carver 1999a (Carver and Heath 1999a)	Young equine Mesh nonwoven PGA 10 % Fetal bovine serum; 50 μg/mL ascorbic acid	3.4	0.25	2	35	70	+ GAG = collagen II = # of chondrocytes		GAG increase strongest at 6.9 MPa for young
		6.9					+ GAG + collagen II = # of chondrocytes		
	Adult equine Mesh nonwoven PGA 10 % Fetal bovine serum; 50 μg/mL ascorbic acid	3.4					+ GAG + collagen II = # of chondrocytes		Collagen II increase strongest at 6.9 MPa for young and adult
		6.9					= GAG + collagen II = # of chondrocytes		
Carver 1999b (Carver and Heath 1999b)	Young equine Mesh nonwoven PGA 10 % Fetal bovine serum; 50 μg/mL ascorbic acid	3.44	0.25	2	35	70	+ GAG + collagen = # of chondrocytes		+ E- modulus
Direct compression									
Démarteau 2003 (Démarteau et al. 2003)	Human Mesh PEGT/PBT Foam 10 % Fetal bovine serum; growth factor TGF-β1, FGF-2, PDGFbb	0.3-0.6* (5 %)	0.1	4	3	12	+ GAG	= Sox9 = aggrecan = collagen II	Measured peak loading 0.018 MPa
Hilz 2014 (Hilz et al. 2014)	Bovine, Mesh Polyurethane 25 % Fetal calf serum;50 μg/mL L-ascorbic acid	1.2-2.4* (20 %)	1	2**	21	16	+ GAG + aggrecan + collagen II	=Sox9 +collagen II	
El-ayoubi 2011 (El-Ayoubi et al. 2011)	Canine, Mesh poly-L-Lactide 10 % Fetal bovine serum	0.6-1.2* (10 %)	1	3	14	42	+ # of cells		

Table 3 Results on changes in cellular, signaling and/or mechanical response to chondrocyte cultivated constructs for hydrostatic compression (Fig. 2). PG is proteoglycan; MMP is matrix metalloproteinases; h is hours; h/day is hours per day;;- is decrease or inhibition; + is increase; ++ is highest increase; = is no change or status quo. *-symbol implies pressure converted from strain, which is added in brackets, **-symbol is increased aggrecan only with 4 h

Study	Cell source, cultivated construct, additive(s)	Magnitude (MPa)	Freq (Hz)	Loading (h/day)	Loading (# days)	Loading (total h)	Culture composition (change -, =, +)	mRNA response (change -, =, +)	Other findings (change -, =, +)
Ikenoue 2003 **(Ikenoue et al. 2003)**	Human Monolayer 10 % Fetal bovine serum	1	1	4	1	4		= aggrecan	Loading of 16h gave better results compared to 4h
								= collagen II	
		5	1					+ aggrecan	
		10						= collagen II	
		1	1	4	4	16		+ aggrecan	
								+ collagen II	
		5	1					+ aggrecan	
								++ collagen II	
		10	1					++ aggrecan	
								++ collagen II	
Elder 2008 **(Elder and Athanasiou 2008)**	Young bovine, Agarose gel, 20 % Fetal bovine serum; 50 µg/mL L-ascorbic acid	1	0.1	1	5	5	+ GAG		= Aggregate modulus
							= collagen II and # of cells		= E-modulus
		5	0.1				= GAG		+ Aggregate modulus
							= collagen II and # of cells		= E-modulus
		10	0.1				+ GAG		= Aggregate modulus
							= collagen II and # of cells		++ E-modulus
		1	1				= GAG		+ Aggregate modulus
							= collagen II and # of cells		+ E-modulus
		5	1				= GAG		= Aggregate modulus
							= collagen II and # of cells		= E-modulus
		10	1				++ GAG		++ Aggregate modulus
							= collagen II and # of cells		++ E-modulus

Table 3 Results on changes in cellular, signaling and/or mechanical response to chondrocyte cultivated constructs for hydrostatic compression (Fig. 2). PG is proteoglycan; MMP is matrix metalloproteinases; h is hours; h/day is hours per day;;- is decrease or inhibition; + is increase; ++ is highest increase; = is no change or status quo. *-symbol implies pressure converted from strain, which is added in brackets, **-symbol is increased aggrecan only with 4 h *(Continued)*

Hu 2006 **(Hu and Athanasiou** 2006**)**	Young bovine, Agarose gel, 10 % Fetal bovine serum; 50 μg/mL L-ascorbic acid	10	1	4	40	160	= GAG (no loss) + collagen II		= Aggregate modulus
Mizuno 2011 **(Mizuno and Ogawa** 2011**)**	Young bovine, Aggregate pellet, Collagen solution, 10 % Fetal bovine serum	0.5	0.5	24	7	168	+ sGAG	+ aggrecan, + collagen II, + MMP-3, −13	
Kawanishi 2007 **(Kawanishi et al.** 2007**)**	Young bovine, Aggregate pellet, 10 % Fetal bovine serum; 50μg/mL ascorbic acid	5	0.5	4	4	16	+ GAG	+ aggrecan	
							+ sGAG	+ collagen II	
Suh 1999 **(Suh et al.** 1999**)**	Bovine, Monolayer, 10 % Fetal bovine serum	−0.08 vacuum	0.14	6	1	6	+ PG synthesis	+ aggrecan	
							= collagen synthesis	= collagen II	
Parkinnen 1993 **(Parkkinen et al.** 1993**)**	Bovine, Monolayer, 10 % Fetal calf serum	5	0.5	1.5	1	1.5	- PG synthesis		
			0.25						
			0.05						
			0.0167				= PG synthesis		
			0.5	20	1	20	+ PG synthesis		
			0.25						
			0.05				= PG synthesis		
			0.0167				- PG synthesis		
			0.0082				= PG synthesis		
			0.0034						
Jortikka 2000 **(Jortikka et al.** 2000**)**	Bovine, Monolayer, 10 % Fetal bovine serum	5	0.5	20	1	20	+ PG synthesis		
Smith 1996 **(Smith et al.** 1996**)**	Bovine, Monolayer Ham's F-12 medium; 3 % Fetal bovine serum	10	1	4	1	4	+ PG synthesis	+ aggrecan	
								+ collagen II	
Smith 2000 **(Smith et al.** 2000**)**	Bovine, Monolayer, Ham's F-12 medium	10	1	2,4,8,12, 24	1	2,4,8,12, 24		+ aggrecan**, + collagen II	Superior increase compared to one loading period
				4	4	16		++ aggrecan, + + collagen II	
Heyland 2006 **(Heyland et al.** 2006**)**	Porcine chondrocytes, Beads alginate, 10 % Fetal bovine serum	0.3	0.0083	6	4	24	+ GAG, = collagen II		
				6	7	42	= GAG, + collagen II		= E-modulus

Table 4 Results on changes in cellular, signaling and/or mechanical response to chondrocyte cultivated constructs for direct compression (Fig. 2). OA is osteoarthritis; MMP is matrix metalloproteinases; PG is proteoglycan; h is hours; h/day is hours per day; – is decrease or inhibition; + is increase; ++ is highest increase; = is no change or status quo. *-symbol implies pressure converted from strain, which is added in brackets,** -symbol is increase only present 12 h post stimulation, ^-symbol is increase only present after 6 h post stimulation

Study	Cell source, cultivated construct, additive(s)	Magnitude (MPa)	Freq (Hz)	Loading (h/day)	Loading (# days)	Loading (total h)	Culture composition (change -, =, +)	mRNA response (change -, =, +)	Other findings (change -, =, +)
Nebelung 2012 (Nebelung et al. 2012)	Human OA Hydrogel collagen type I 10 % Human serum	0.6-1.2* (10 %)	0.3	24	28	672	= proteoglycan	= aggrecan	= E-modulus
							= collagen II	+ collagen II	
								+ MMP-13	
Shelton 2003 (Shelton et al. 2003)	Bovine, Agarose gel Type VII 20 % Fetal calf serum	1.7-2.9* (15 %)	0.3	24	2	48	- GAG		
			1				+ GAG		
			3				= GAG		
Omata 2012 (Omata et al. 2012)	Bovine, Agarose gel Type VII 20 % Fetal bovine serum; 0.85 mM L-ascorbic acid	1.7-2.9* (15 %)	1	6	22	132			+ E-modulus
Hung 2004 (Hung et al. 2004)	Bovine, Agarose gel Type VII 10 % Fetal bovine serum; growth factor: TGF-β1, IGF-1	0.6-1.2* (10 %)	1	3	3	9		+ aggrecan	= aggregate modulus
				3	20	60			+ E-modulus
									+ aggregate modulus
Nicodemus 2010 (Nicodemus and Bryant 2010)	Young bovine, Hydrogel polyethylene glycol, 5 % Fetal bovine serum; 50 mg/L L-ascorbic acid	1.2-2.4* (20 %)	0.3	24	7	168	+ GAG	+ aggrecan	
								- collagen II	
								- MMP-3	
								= MMP-13	
				6	7	42	= GAG	= aggrecan	
								+ collagen II	
								+ MMP-3, –13	
Waldman 2004 (Waldman et al. 2004)	Bovine, Monolayer on top of calcium polyphosphate mesh, 5 % Fetal bovine serum	0.3-0.6* (5 %)	1	.1 (400 cycles)	3.5	0.5	= PG synthesis		
							++ coll. synthesis		
		0.6-1.2* (10 %)					++ PG synthesis		
		1.2-2.4* (20 %)					= coll. synthesis		
		0.3-0.6* (5 %)		0.6 (2000 cycles)	3.5	2	= PG synthesis		
							+ coll. synthesis		
		0.6-1.2* (10 %)					+ PG synthesis		
		1.2-2.4* (20 %)					= coll. synthesis		

Table 4 Results on changes in cellular, signaling and/or mechanical response to chondrocyte cultivated constructs for direct compression (Fig. 2). OA is osteoarthritis; MMP is matrix metalloproteinases; PG is proteoglycan; h is hours; h/day is hours per day; – is decrease or inhibition; + is increase; ++ is highest increase; = is no change or status quo. *-symbol implies pressure converted from strain, which is added in brackets,** -symbol is increase only present 12 h post stimulation, ^-symbol is increase only present after 6 h post stimulation *(Continued)*

		0.3-0.6* (5 %)	1	0.1	7	1	= PG synthesis = coll. synthesis		= E-modulus
				0.1	14	2	+ PG synthesis + coll. synthesis		+ E-modulus
De Croos 2006 (De Croos et al. 2006)	Bovine, Monolayer on top of calcium polyphosphate mesh 5 % Fetal bovine serum	0.001	1	<1 h	1	<1 h	+ PG synthesis ^ + coll. synthesis ^	+ aggrecan ** + collagen II ** + MMP-3, –13	

Table 5 Results on changes in cellular and/or signaling response to BMMSC cultivated constructs under hydrostatic compression (Fig. 2). Sox9 is the gene that regulates chondrogenic differentiation; h is hours; h/day is hours per day; – is decrease or inhibition; and + is increase; ++ is highest increase; = is no change or status quo

Study	Cell source, cultivated construct, additive(s)	Magnitude (MPa)	Freq (Hz)	Loading (h/day)	Loading (# days)	Loading (total h)	Culture composition (change -, =, +)	mRNA response (change -, =, +)
Mesh								
Wagner 2008 (Wagner et al. 2008)	Human BMMSC, Mesh Collagen Type 1 50 mg/mL bovine serum albumin; 50 μg/mL L-ascorbic acid; 10^{-9} M dexamethasone	1	1	4	10	40	+ proteoglycan	+ Sox9 + aggrecan + collagen II
Luo 2007 (Luo and Seedhom 2007)	Ovine BMMSC, Mesh non-woven filamentous plasma-treated polyester 10 % Fetal bovine serum; 50 μg/mL ascorbic acid; 10^{-7} M dexamethasone	0.1	0.25	0.5	7	3.5	+ GAG = collagen	
				0.5	10	5	++ GAG + collagen	
Gel								
Miyanishi 2006a (Miyanishi et al. 2006a)	Human BMMSC, Aggregate pellet 1.25 mg/mL bovine serum albumin; 50 μg/mL ascorbic acid; 10^{-7} M dexamethasone	0.1	1	4	14	56	= sGAG	+ Sox9 + aggrecan = collagen II
		1					+ sGAG	++ Sox9 + aggrecan = collagen II
		10					++ sGAG	++ Sox9 ++ aggrecan + collagen II
Miyanishi 2006b (Miyanishi et al. 2006b)	Human BMMSC, Aggregate pellet 1.25 mg/mL bovine serum albumin; 50 cpg/mL ascorbic acid; 10^{-7} M dexamethasone	10	1	4	14	56		+ Sox9 + aggrecan + collagen II
Angele 2003 (Angele et al. 2003)	Human BMMSC, Aggregate pellet 10 % Fetal bovine serum	5.03	1	4	1	4	= proteoglycan = collagen	
				4	7	28	+ proteoglycan + collagen	
Finger 2007 (Finger et al. 2007)	Human BMMSC, Agarose gel Type VII Growth medium Cambrex	7.5	1	4	14	56		= Sox9

Bader 2007; Spiller et al. 2011). Four different constructs were used to culture chondrocytes: a) explants, which consist of a complete section of cartilage that is excised from a cadaver and embedded in a culture medium (Parkkinen et al. 1993) (Table 1), b) tissue engineered meshes that have a structural 3D shape (Table 2), c) monolayers that consist of isolated chondrocytes from full thickness pieces of cartilage seeded onto a plate (Jortikka et al. 2000; Smith et al. 2000) (Tables 3–4), d) hydrogels that have a softer structure compared to meshes (Carver and Heath 1999b; Hu and Athanasiou 2006) (Tables 3–4). One study used serum free medium (Li et al. 2013), one study added human serum (Nebelung et al. 2012), three added calf serum, and twenty one studies added bovine serum, with thirteen studies also adding L-ascorbic acid and two also adding growth factors in conjunction (Tables 1, 2, 3, 4).

Second, BMMSCs were harvested from bone marrow, and centrifuged to become a pellet culture (Miyanishi et al. 2006a; Kawanishi et al. 2007) (Table 5). Two cultivated constructs were used onto which BMMSCs were seeded : a) a gel or pellet composition and b) tissue engineered meshes (Luo and Seedhom 2007; Wagner et al. 2008) (Table 5). Bovine serum was added in five out of 6 studies, with four studies also adding 50 μg/mL L-ascorbic acid and dexamethasone.

Loading regime

Two types of cyclic compression were applied: hydrostatic or direct compression (Fig. 2). Hydrostatic pressure is applied by compressing the fluid surrounding the tested culture with a piston (Elder and Athanasiou 2009) (Tables 1, 2, 3 and 5). Direct compression implies that a piston directly presses on the tissue, which is commonly expressed in percentage of strain (Demarteau et al. 2003) (Tables 1,2 and 4). Except the studies by Torzelli et al. (Torzilli et al. 1996; Torzilli et al. 2011) and De Croos et al. (De Croos et al. 2006), all other eleven studies required conversion from strain to pressure (Tables 1, 2 and 4).

The loading magnitude, frequency and regime varied highly. For example Carver and Heath stimulated their samples with 6.9 MPa at 0.25Hz for 2 h per day over a period of 35 days (Carver and Heath 1999b), while Démarteau et al. applied a loading of 5 % of strain with 0.1Hz for 4 h per day over a period of 3 days (Démarteau et al. 2003). In contrast to this, five out of six studies with human derived BMMSC used 1 Hz as loading frequency for 4 h per day (Table 5) (Angele et al. 2003; Miyanishi et al. 2006a, 2006b; Finger et al. 2007; Wagner et al. 2008).

Cartilage cellular, signaling and mechanical response parameters

Three types of methods were found to document cartilage quality response: cellular, signaling, and mechanical responses (Tables 1, 2, 3, 4, 5). Cellular response is routinely determined with histology, which allows identification of specific (macro) molecules that typically represent healthy cartilage (proteoglycans, glucosaminoglycans (GAGs) and sulfated glucosaminoglycans (sGAGs), collagen type II). An increase of proteoglycans is typically determined using staining with Safranin O (Darling and Athanasiou 2003; Schulz and Bader 2007). Similarly, the increase of GAGs and sGAGs is determined with dimethylmethylene blue assay staining (Farndale et al. 1986; Carver and Heath 1999b; Shelton et al. 2003; Heyland et al. 2006; Hilz et al. 2014). The increase in collagens is determined by staining with Picrosirius red, Masson's trichrome stain, or antibody-staining such as anti-collagen antibodies or monoclonal antibodies, and/or the use of polarized light (Angele et al. 2003; Darling and Athanasiou 2003; Heyland et al. 2006; Elder and Athanasiou 2008; Nicodemus and Bryant 2010). After staining, the histologic samples

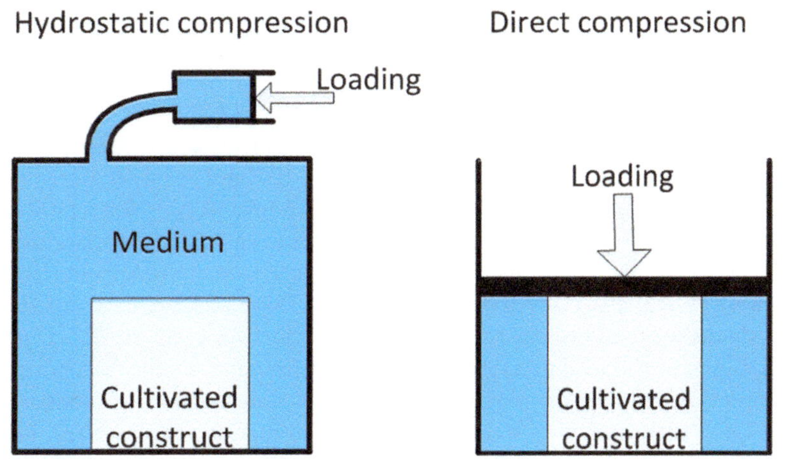

Fig. 2 Difference between hydrostatic compression (left) and direct compression (right). The arrows indicate the loading direction

are further interpreted with histologic scores and compared to control samples to indicate relative cellular responses. The type of collagen is assessed with immunohistochemistry (Elder and Athanasiou 2008). Finally, cellular response in the form of proteoglycan synthesis is routinely determined by assessing the radioactive labeled ^{35}Sulfate-uptake by the proteoglycans (Parkkinen et al. 1993; Torzilli et al. 2011; Li et al. 2013).

Signaling response indirectly indicates the potential of the cells to (de)differentiate into cartilage, because it assesses changes in the level of mRNA expression as produced by the chondrocyte cells with a reverse transcription polymerase chain reaction (RT-PCR) (Darling and Athanasiou 2003; Schulz and Bader 2007). A change in proteoglycan production is commonly documented as an increase in aggrecan mRNA that is the core protein backbone to which GAGs chains are attached (Tables 1, 2, 3, 4) (Démarteau et al. 2003; Ikenoue et al. 2003; Schulz and Bader 2007). With the same method other relevant expressions are assessed: collagen type II, the gene sex determining region box 9 (Sox9) and Matrix metalloproteinases (MMP). Sox9 is indicative for the regulation of chondrogenic differentiation and plays a role in expression of collagen type II and aggrecan (Démarteau et al. 2003; Miyanishi et al. 2006a; Finger et al. 2007; Wagner et al. 2008; Hilz et al. 2014). MMP plays a major role in ECM turnover and degradation (Hilz et al. 2014). MMP-3 has shown to be a key player in degrading matrix and inactivating other degrading enzymes (Cawston and Wilson 2006; Echtermeyer et al. 2009), and MMP-13 seems to influence the progress of osteoarthritis (Hilz et al. 2014).

Mechanical responses were documented by compression tests of the samples and determining the Young's (or E-) modulus from the linear range of the stress–strain curve (Carver and Heath 1999b; Hung et al. 2004; Heyland et al. 2006; Hu and Athanasiou 2006; Elder and Athanasiou 2008; Omata et al. 2012). Cartilage quality response was given as change of cellular response (including synthesis) by 27 of 33 studies, as change of signaling response by 21 of 33 studies, and as change of mechanical response by 9 of 33 studies.

Responses to mechanical stimuli

Due to the difference in cell sources, cultivated constructs, compression and outcome measures only qualitative comparison could be performed. Bovine explant testing mimics the *in vivo* case most closely especially the study by Li et al. (Li et al. 2013), since they used bruised explants (Table 1). The studied variations in the loading regime of the explants suggest a certain threshold for the magnitude of loading (>10 % or > 1.2 MPa) and the frequency (>0.5 Hz) to stimulate increased proteoglycan synthesis (Table 1). Only Okuda et al. (Okuda et al. 2013) confirmed that this was correlated to increased mechanical response. Studies that tested equine chondrocyte-seeded meshes by hydrostatic compression support the need for a loading threshold (Table 2), since increased cell density was observed by higher loading magnitudes and correlated to increased mechanical response (Carver and Heath 1999b). The three studies of chondrocyte-seeded meshes by direct compression presented too much variation to point in a specific loading regime (Table 2).

The studies that use monolayer and gel cultivated constructs and test variations in loading magnitude, frequency or loading regime (Tables 3–4) also suggest the need for thresholds in magnitude and frequency with a trend towards higher values (up to 5–10 MPa and up to 1 Hz) compared to the explant studies to achieve increased responses (Parkkinen et al. 1993; Smith et al. 2000; Ikenoue et al. 2003; Shelton et al. 2003; Waldman et al. 2004; Elder and Athanasiou 2008). Tables 3–4 also highlight the effect of different loading regimes, which seems to suggest that prolonged duration and loading at intervals (no continuous intermittent loading) increase cell density and synthesis, signaling response as well as mechanical response (e.g. (Shelton et al. 2003; Hung et al. 2004)). Exceptions are the studies by De Croos (De Croos et al. 2006) who find increased response at a low magnitude of 0.001 MPa applied for less than 1 h, and by Hu and Athanasiou (Hu and Athanasiou 2006) who did not find a change in the E-modulus after prolonged loading for 160 h.

The studies using BMMSCs as cell source support the suggestion that the largest increase in cellular and signaling response is achieved for larger loading magnitudes (>5 MPa) at a frequency of 1 Hz for a prolonged period (>7 days) at intermittent intervals (Table 5). However, no mechanical responses were measured for these constructs.

Discussion

Five studies mimicked the *in vivo* case most closely by testing bovine explants. Only two of these varied the loading magnitude or frequency, which suggest the need of a certain threshold (>20 % strain and > 0.5 Hz) for increased proteoglycan synthesis (Table 1). A careful qualitative interpretation of the results suggests that for chondrocyte-seeded cultivated constructs a loading pressure between 5–10 MPa and a loading frequency of 1 Hz exerted at intermittent intervals for a period of a week or longer are recommended as appropriate mechanical stimulus. These values are in the physiologic range of normal gait (Waters et al. 1988; Giddings et al. 2000; Brand 2005; Doke et al. 2005; van Dijk et al. 2010a). Due to the variety of testing conditions and methods to express cartilage quality response, only qualitative comparison was possible, which poses limitations to the study. First, differences in sample tissue, sample preparation, donor type and donor age all accounted for differences in the outcome of these studies

(Parkkinen et al. 1993; Carver and Heath 1999a; Darling and Athanasiou 2003; Chung and Burdick 2008). Still, fourteen of the 33 studies did measure the cartilage quality response to varying loading parameters within the same set up. Even though, signaling response does not always reflect actual cellular and mechanical changes, the studies that report them also report cellular and/or mechanical response in conjunction (Tables 2, 3, 4, 5), with in the majority of the cases showing corresponding in- or decreases. With this, the decision was made to include studies that only present signaling response (four in total), since two have varied the loading regime (intermittent vs continuous loading (Smith et al. 2000); and loading magnitude and duration (Ikenoue et al. 2003)) as needed to answer our main research question (Table 3). Second, two different types of compression were applied: hydrostatic (Tables 1, 2, 3 and 5) and direct compression (Tables 1,2 and 4). There is an on-going debate which type of loading is more physiological. Some are in favor of direct compression (Buschmann et al. 1995; Mauck et al. 2000; Waldman et al. 2004). Also, direct compression allows continuous measurement of mechanical responses, but needs some tricks to be applied to soft constructs by placing the samples in bags (De Croos et al. 2006). Bachrach et al. (Bachrach et al. 1998) suggest that hydrostatic pressure seems to be more representative for the *in vivo* loading case, because it mimics the viscoelastic multiphasic cartilage behavior closest. A drawback is that it also stimulates the sides of the samples. An advantage of applying hydrostatic compression is that it allows for harmonization of the applied load, and it allows mechanical stimulation of different types of cultivated constructs including the softer ones. The proposed transformation procedure from strain to pressure seems to make sense, because the calculated pressure values are in line with the values found in other studies: 3.6 MPa leads to a 29 % strain (Herberhold et al. 1999) vs 20 % strain (Hilz et al. 2014) (Tables 2 and 4). However, it still remains an approximation, which needs to be interpreted with care. Third, biologic demonstration of the increase in cartilage quality response is highly important, since it indicates parameters (signals, cells types, cell synthesis) that should be triggered to stimulate the cell activity and behave like cartilage. However, documentation of actual mechanical response would be expected as well, since this determines performance. In one quarter of the studies (9 out of 33) the mechanical response was measured, which is a rather low percentage. Some of the cultivated constructs (monolayer, pellet) do not resemble the actual ECM structure, which makes mechanical testing difficult or impossible (Tables 1, 2, 3, 4, 5). Full characterization is difficult, because of its highly complex viscoelastic behavior (Mow et al. 1999; Schulz and Bader 2007; Khan and Scott 2009; Madry et al. 2010). Furthermore, constructs can also change due to the loading or do not necessarily mimic mechanical cartilage behavior (Nebelung et al. 2011). This latter is supported by conflicting results that were found for two studies in which agarose gel was used: Hu and Athanasiou (Hu and Athanasiou 2006) show that a 20 % increase in collagen type II does not seem to influence the mechanical properties (Table 3), and others (Hung et al. 2004; Elder and Athanasiou 2008; Omata et al. 2012) did not find a relation between histologic and mechanical parameters.

In vivo tissue engineering cartilage repair techniques (e.g. Matrix-Induced Autologous Chondrocyte Implantation or cell-seeded hydrogel plugs (Brittberg 2010; Fortier et al. 2011; Hildner et al. 2011; Spiller et al. 2011)) make use of similar scaffolds. This review gives a summary of current evidence, which can be used for future development of on *in vivo* application rehabilitation protocol. Several factors are fundamentally different for the *in vivo* case, including the fact that the ECM is not intact as result of the cartilage lesion, and that the access to essential biologicals (e.g. cytokines, growth factors) is different in the physiologic situation compared to the *in vitro* situation. Especially, the boundary between the healthy cartilage and tissue engineered scaffold is a vulnerable spot (Khan et al. 2008), which most likely cannot withstand the suggested loading magnitude (Guettler et al. 2004; Khan et al. 2008; van Dijk et al. 2010a, 2010b; Spiller et al. 2011; Hunt et al. 2012). However, the results could be used to optimize preconditioning of tissue engineered scaffolds before implantation into patients (Shelton et al. 2003; Nebelung et al. 2012; Omata et al. 2012). Therefore, the timing of loading could be a critical factor that needs to be further explored. For example the testing period might be even further extended (Waldman et al. 2004), since *in vivo* studies with animal models evaluated the cartilage quality response after long testing periods (56 days or longer), much longer than those found in this review (Saris et al. 2003; Kok et al. 2013; Miller et al. 2014; Ortved et al. 2015). Finally, studying the dynamic compression of damaged explants (e.g. (Li et al. 2013)), should be elaborated to identify the best magnitude, frequency and loading regime, since these constructs mimic the *in vivo* cartilage lesion closest. This will facilitate the translation of the found combination of mechanical parameters to patients.

Conclusions

Overall, the results seem to suggest that a certain threshold exits for enhanced cartilage *in vitro* cultivation of explants, and that chondrocyte-seeded cultivated constructs show best results when loaded with physiological mechanical stimuli. This seems a reasonable conclusion, because nature is highly optimized for daily activities such as normal walking. Critical aspects remain to be answered for translation of the results into *in vivo* therapies.

Competing interests

The authors declare that they have no competing interests.

Authors' contributions

JN, GT: have made substantial contributions to conception and design, or acquisition of data, or analysis and interpretation of data; JN, AK, JD, GT: have been involved in drafting the manuscript or revising it critically for important intellectual content; AK, JD, GT: have given final approval of the version to be published.

References

Angele P, Yoo JU, Smith C, Mansour J, Jepsen KJ, Nerlich M, Johnstone B (2003) Cyclic hydrostatic pressure enhances the chondrogenic phenotype of human mesenchymal progenitor cells differentiated *in vitro*. J Orthop Res 21(3):451–457

Arokoski JP, Jurvelin JS, Vaatainen U, Helminen HJ (2000) Normal and pathological adaptations of articular cartilage to joint loading. Scand J Med Sci Sports 10(4):186–198

Bachrach NM, Mow VC, Guilak F (1998) Incompressibility of the solid matrix of articular cartilage under high hydrostatic pressures. J Biomech 31(5):445–451

Bahuleyan B, Cheung HS, Huang CYC (2009) Role of biomechanical force in stem cell-based therapy for cartilage repair. Curr Rheumatol Rev 5(1):34–39

Bonassar LJ, Grodzinsky AJ, Frank EH, Davila SG, Bhaktav NR, Trippel SB (2001) The effect of dynamic compression on the response of articular cartilage to insulin-like growth factor-I. J Orthop Res 19(1):11–17

Brand RA (2005) Joint contact stress: a reasonable surrogate for biological processes? Iowa Orthop J 25:82–94

Brittberg M (2010) Cell carriers as the next generation of cell therapy for cartilage repair: a review of the matrix-induced autologous chondrocyte implantation procedure. Am J Sports Med 38(6):1259–1271

Buckwalter JA, Mankin HJ (1998) Articular cartilage: tissue design and chondrocyte-matrix interactions. Instr Course Lect 47:477–486

Buschmann MD, Gluzband YA, Grodzinsky AJ, Hunziker EB (1995) Mechanical compression modulates matrix biosynthesis in chondrocyte/agarose culture. J Cell Sci 108(Pt 4):1497–1508

Carver SE, Heath CA (1999a) Increasing extracellular matrix production in regenerating cartilage with intermittent physiological pressure. Biotechnol Bioeng 62(2):166–174

Carver SE, Heath CA (1999b) Influence of intermittent pressure, fluid flow, and mixing on the regenerative properties of articular chondrocytes. Biotechnol Bioeng 65(3):274–281

Cawston TE, Wilson AJ (2006) Understanding the role of tissue degrading enzymes and their inhibitors in development and disease. Best Pract Res Clin Rheumatol 20(5):983–1002

Chu CR, Szczodry M, Bruno S (2010) Animal models for cartilage regeneration and repair. Tissue Eng Part B Rev 16(1):105–115

Chung C, Burdick JA (2008) Engineering cartilage tissue. Adv Drug Deliv Rev 60(2):243–262

Cohen NP, Foster RJ, Mow VC (1998) Composition and dynamics of articular cartilage: structure, function, and maintaining healthy state. J Orthop Sports Phys Ther 28(4):203–215

Darling EM, Athanasiou KA (2003) Biomechanical strategies for articular cartilage regeneration. Ann Biomed Eng 31(9):1114–1124

De Croos JN, Dhaliwal SS, Grynpas MD, Pilliar RM, Kandel RA (2006) Cyclic compressive mechanical stimulation induces sequential catabolic and anabolic gene changes in chondrocytes resulting in increased extracellular matrix accumulation. Matrix biology : journal of the International Society for Matrix Biology 25(6):323–331

Demarteau O, Jakob M, Schafer D, Heberer M, Martin I (2003) Development and validation of a bioreactor for physical stimulation of engineered cartilage. Biorheology 40(1–3):331–336

Démarteau O, Wendt D, Braccini A, Jakob M, Schäfer D, Heberer M, Martin I (2003) Dynamic compression of cartilage constructs engineered from expanded human articular chondrocytes. Biochem Biophys Res Commun 310(2):580–588

Doke J, Donelan JM, Kuo AD (2005) Mechanics and energetics of swinging the human leg. J Exp Biol 208(Pt 3):439–445

Echtermeyer F, Bertrand J, Dreier R, Meinecke I, Neugebauer K, Fuerst M, Lee YJ, Song YW, Herzog C, Theilmeier G, Pap T (2009) Syndecan-4 regulates ADAMTS-5 activation and cartilage breakdown in osteoarthritis. Nat Med 15(9):1072–1076

El-Ayoubi R, DeGrandpre C, DiRaddo R, Yousefi AM, Lavigne P (2011) Design and dynamic culture of 3D-scaffolds for cartilage tissue engineering. J Biomater Appl 25(5):429–444

Elder BD, Athanasiou KA (2008) Synergistic and additive effects of hydrostatic pressure and growth factors on tissue formation. PLoS One 3(6), e2341

Elder BD, Athanasiou KA (2009) Hydrostatic pressure in articular cartilage tissue engineering: from chondrocytes to tissue regeneration. Tissue Eng Part B Rev 15(1):43–53

Fan JC, Waldman SD (2010) The effect of intermittent static biaxial tensile strains on tissue engineered cartilage. Ann Biomed Eng 38(4):1672–1682

Farndale RW, Buttle DJ, Barrett AJ (1986) Improved quantitation and discrimination of sulphated glycosaminoglycans by use of dimethylmethylene blue. Biochim Biophys Acta 883(2):173–177

Finger AR, Sargent CY, Dulaney KO, Bernacki SH, Loboa EG (2007) Differential effects on messenger ribonucleic acid expression by bone marrow-derived human mesenchymal stem cells seeded in agarose constructs due to ramped and steady applications of cyclic hydrostatic pressure. Tissue Eng 13(6):1151–1158

Fortier LA, Barker JU, Strauss EJ, McCarrel TM, Cole BJ (2011) The role of growth factors in cartilage repair. Clin Orthop Relat Res 469(10):2706–2715

Giddings VL, Beaupre GS, Whalen RT, Carter DR (2000) Calcaneal loading during walking and running. Med Sci Sports Exerc 32(3):627–634

Grodzinsky AJ, Levenston ME, Jin M, Frank EH (2000) Cartilage tissue remodeling in response to mechanical forces. Annu Rev Biomed Eng 2:691–713

Guettler JH, Demetropoulos CK, Yang KH, Jurist KA (2004) Osteochondral defects in the human knee: influence of defect size on cartilage rim stress and load redistribution to surrounding cartilage. Am J Sports Med 32(6):1451–1458

Hannon CP, Smyth NA, Murawski CD, Savage-Elliott I, Deyer TW, Calder JD, Kennedy JG (2014) Osteochondral lesions of the talus: aspects of current management. The bone & joint journal 96-B(2):164–171

Heath CA, Magari SR (1996) Mini-review: Mechanical factors affecting cartilage regeneration *in vitro*. Biotechnol Bioeng 50(4):430–437

Herberhold C, Faber S, Stammberger T, Steinlechner M, Putz R, Englmeier KH, Reiser M, Eckstein F (1999) In situ measurement of articular cartilage deformation in intact femoropatellar joints under static loading. J Biomech 32(12):1287–1295

Hess R, Douglas T, Myers KA, Rentsch B, Rentsch C, Worch H, Shrive NG, Hart DA, Scharnweber D (2010) Hydrostatic pressure stimulation of human mesenchymal stem cells seeded on collagen-based artificial extracellular matrices. J Biomech Eng 132(2):021001

Heyland J, Wiegandt K, Goepfert C, Nagel-Heyer S, Ilinich E, Schumacher U, Portner R (2006) Redifferentiation of chondrocytes and cartilage formation under intermittent hydrostatic pressure. Biotechnol Lett 28(20):1641–1648

Hildner F, Albrecht C, Gabriel C, Redl H, van Griensven M (2011) State of the art and future perspectives of articular cartilage regeneration: a focus on adipose-derived stem cells and platelet-derived products. J Tissue Eng Regen Med 5(4):e36–51

Hilz FM, Ahrens P, Grad S, Stoddart MJ, Dahmani C, Wilken FL, Sauerschnig M, Niemeyer P, Zwingmann J, Burgkart R, von Eisenhart-Rothe R, Südkamp NP, Weyh T, Imhoff AB, Alini M, Salzmann GM (2014) Influence of extremely low frequency, low energy electromagnetic fields and combined mechanical stimulation on chondrocytes in 3-D constructs for cartilage tissue engineering. Bioelectromagnetics 35(2):116–128

Hu JC, Athanasiou KA (2006) The effects of intermittent hydrostatic pressure on self-assembled articular cartilage constructs. Tissue Eng 12(5):1337–1344

Hung CT, Mauck RL, Wang CC, Lima EG, Ateshian GA (2004) A paradigm for functional tissue engineering of articular cartilage via applied physiologic deformational loading. Ann Biomed Eng 32(1):35–49

Hunt KJ, Lee AT, Lindsey DP, Slikker W 3rd, Chou LB (2012) Osteochondral lesions of the talus: effect of defect size and plantarflexion angle on ankle joint stresses. Am J Sports Med 40(4):895–901

Ikenoue T, Trindade MCD, Lee MS, Lin EY, Schurman DJ, Goodman SB, Smith RL (2003) Mechanoregulation of human articular chondrocyte aggrecan and type II collagen expression by intermittent hydrostatic pressure *in vitro*. J Orthop Res 21(1):110–116

Jortikka MO, Parkkinen JJ, Inkinen RI, Karner J, Jarvelainen HT, Nelimarkka LO, Tammi MI, Lammi MJ (2000) The role of microtubules in the regulation of proteoglycan synthesis in chondrocytes under hydrostatic pressure. Arch Biochem Biophys 374(2):172–180

Kawanishi M, Oura A, Furukawa K, Fukubayashi T, Nakamura K, Tateishi T, Ushida T (2007) Redifferentiation of dedifferentiated bovine articular chondrocytes enhanced by cyclic hydrostatic pressure under a gas-controlled system. Tissue Eng 13(5):957–964

Khan IM, Gilbert SJ, Singhrao SK, Duance VC, Archer CW (2008) Cartilage integration: evaluation of the reasons for failure of integration during cartilage repair. A review. Eur Cell Mater 16:26–39

Khan KM, Scott A (2009) Mechanotherapy: how physical therapists' prescription of exercise promotes tissue repair. Br J Sports Med 43(4):247–252

Kok AC, Tuijthof GJ, den Dunnen S, van Tiel J, Siebelt M, Everts V, van Dijk CN, Kerkhoffs GM (2013) No effect of hole geometry in microfracture for talar osteochondral defects. Clin Orthop Relat Res 471(11):3653–3662

Li Y, Frank EH, Wang Y, Chubinskaya S, Huang HH, Grodzinsky AJ (2013) Moderate dynamic compression inhibits pro-catabolic response of cartilage to mechanical injury, tumor necrosis factor-α and interleukin-6, but accentuates degradation above a strain threshold. Osteoarthritis Cartilage 21(12):1933–1941

Luo ZJ, Seedhom BB (2007) Light and low-frequency pulsatile hydrostatic pressure enhances extracellular matrix formation by bone marrow mesenchymal cells: an in-vitro study with special reference to cartilage repair. Proc Inst Mech Eng H J Eng Med 221(5):499–507

Madry H, Grün UW, Knutsen G (2011) Cartilage repair and joint preservation: Medical and surgical treatment options. Deutsches Arzteblatt 108(40):669–677

Madry H, van Dijk CN, Mueller-Gerbl M (2010) The basic science of the subchondral bone. Knee surgery, sports traumatology, arthroscopy: official journal of the ESSKA 18(4):419–433

Magnussen RA, Dunn WR, Carey JL, Spindler KP (2008) Treatment of focal articular cartilage defects in the knee: a systematic review. Clin Orthop Relat Res 466(4):952–962

Mauck RL, Nicoll SB, Seyhan SL, Ateshian GA, Hung CT (2003) Synergistic action of growth factors and dynamic loading for articular cartilage tissue engineering. Tissue Eng 9(4):597–611

Mauck RL, Soltz MA, Wang CC, Wong DD, Chao PH, Valhmu WB, Hung CT, Ateshian GA (2000) Functional tissue engineering of articular cartilage through dynamic loading of chondrocyte-seeded agarose gels. J Biomech Eng 122(3):252–260

Meachim G, Stockwell RA (1973) The Matrix. Freeman MA (ed) Adult articular cartilage. Pitman medical, London, pp 1–5.

Miller RE, Grodzinsky AJ, Barrett MF, Hung HH, Frank EH, Werpy NM, McIlwraith CW, Frisbie DD (2014) Effects of the combination of microfracture and self-assembling Peptide filling on the repair of a clinically relevant trochlear defect in an equine model. J Bone Joint Surg Am 96(19):1601–1609

Miyanishi K, Trindade MC, Lindsey DP, Beaupre GS, Carter DR, Goodman SB, Schurman DJ, Smith RL (2006a) Dose- and time-dependent effects of cyclic hydrostatic pressure on transforming growth factor-beta3-induced chondrogenesis by adult human mesenchymal stem cells *in vitro*. Tissue Eng 12(8):2253–2262

Miyanishi K, Trindade MC, Lindsey DP, Beaupre GS, Carter DR, Goodman SB, Schurman DJ, Smith RL (2006b) Effects of hydrostatic pressure and transforming growth factor-beta 3 on adult human mesenchymal stem cell chondrogenesis *in vitro*. Tissue Eng 12(6):1419–1428

Mizuno S, Ogawa R (2011) Using changes in hydrostatic and osmotic pressure to manipulate metabolic function in chondrocytes. Am J Physiol Cell Physiol 300(6):C1234–1245

Mow VC, Wang CC, Hung CT (1999) The extracellular matrix, interstitial fluid and ions as a mechanical signal transducer in articular cartilage. Osteoarthritis and cartilage / OARS, Osteoarthritis Research Society 7(1):41–58

Nebelung S, Gavenis K, Luring C, Zhou B, Mueller-Rath R, Stoffel M, Tingart M, Rath B (2012) Simultaneous anabolic and catabolic responses of human chondrocytes seeded in collagen hydrogels to long-term continuous dynamic compression. Annals of anatomy = Anatomischer Anzeiger: official organ of the Anatomische Gesellschaft 194(4):351–358

Nebelung S, Gavenis K, Rath B, Tingart M, Ladenburger A, Stoffel M, Zhou B, Mueller-Rath R (2011) Continuous cyclic compressive loading modulates biological and mechanical properties of collagen hydrogels seeded with human chondrocytes. Biorheology 48(5):247–261

Nicodemus GD, Bryant SJ (2010) Mechanical loading regimes affect the anabolic and catabolic activities by chondrocytes encapsulated in PEG hydrogels. Osteoarthritis Cartilage 18(1):126–137

Okuda Y, Konishi R, Miyata S (2013) Effect of cyclic compressive stimuli on mechanical anisotropy of chondrocyte-seeded agarose gel culture. Nihon Kikai Gakkai Ronbunshu, C Hen/Transactions of the Japan Society of Mechanical Engineers, Part C 79(801):1736–1743

Omata S, Sonokawa S, Sawae Y, Murakami T (2012) Effects of both vitamin C and mechanical stimulation on improving the mechanical characteristics of regenerated cartilage. Biochem Biophys Res Commun 424(4):724–729

Ortved KF, Begum L, Mohammed HO, Nixon AJ (2015) Implantation of rAAV5-IGF-I Transduced Autologous Chondrocytes Improves Cartilage Repair in Full-thickness Defects in the Equine Model. Molecular therapy: the journal of the American Society of Gene Therapy 23(2):363–373

Parkkinen JJ, Ikonen J, Lammi MJ, Laakkonen J, Tammi M, Helminen HJ (1993) Effects of cyclic hydrostatic pressure on proteoglycan synthesis in cultured chondrocytes and articular cartilage explants. Arch Biochem Biophys 300(1):458–465

Potier E, Noailly J, Ito K (2010) Directing bone marrow-derived stromal cell function with mechanics. J Biomech 43(5):807–817

Saris DB, Dhert WJ, Verbout AJ (2003) Joint homeostasis. The discrepancy between old and fresh defects in cartilage repair. J Bone Joint Surg 85(7):1067–1076

Schulz RM, Bader A (2007) Cartilage tissue engineering and bioreactor systems for the cultivation and stimulation of chondrocytes. European biophysics journal : EBJ 36(4–5):539–568

Shelton JC, Bader DL, Lee DA (2003) Mechanical conditioning influences the metabolic response of cell-seeded constructs. Cells Tissues Organs 175(3):140–150

Shepherd DE, Seedhom BB (1999) The 'instantaneous' compressive modulus of human articular cartilage in joints of the lower limb. Rheumatology (Oxford) 38(2):124–132

Smith RL, Lin J, Trindade MC, Shida J, Kajiyama G, Vu T, Hoffman AR, van der Meulen MC, Goodman SB, Schurman DJ, Carter DR (2000) Time-dependent effects of intermittent hydrostatic pressure on articular chondrocyte type II collagen and aggrecan mRNA expression. J Rehabil Res Dev 37(2):153–161

Smith RL, Rusk SF, Ellison BE, Wessells P, Tsuchiya K, Carter DR, Caler WE, Sandell LJ, Schurman DJ (1996) *In vitro* stimulation of articular chondrocyte mRNA and extracellular matrix synthesis by hydrostatic pressure. J Orthop Res 14(1):53–60

Spiller KL, Maher SA, Lowman AM (2011) Hydrogels for the repair of articular cartilage defects. Tissue Eng Part B Rev 17(4):281–299

Suh JK, Baek GH, Aroen A, Malin CM, Niyibizi C, Evans CH, Westerhausen-Larson A (1999) Intermittent sub-ambient interstitial hydrostatic pressure as a potential mechanical stimulator for chondrocyte metabolism. Osteoarthritis and cartilage / OARS, Osteoarthritis Research Society 7(1):71–80

Torzilli PA, Bhargava M, Chen CT (2011) Mechanical Loading of Articular Cartilage Reduces IL-1-Induced Enzyme Expression. Cartilage 2(4):364–373

Torzilli PA, Tehrany AM, Grigiene R, Young E (1996) Effects of misoprostol and prostaglandin E2 on proteoglycan biosynthesis and loss in unloaded and loaded articular cartilage explants. Prostaglandins 52(3):157–173

van Dijk CN, Reilingh ML, Zengerink M, van Bergen CJ (2010a) The natural history of osteochondral lesions in the ankle. Instr Course Lect 59:375–386

van Dijk CN, Reilingh ML, Zengerink M, van Bergen CJ (2010b) Osteochondral defects in the ankle: why painful? Knee surgery, sports traumatology, arthroscopy : official journal of the ESSKA 18(5):570–580

Wagner DR, Lindsey DP, Li KW, Tummala P, Chandran SE, Smith RL, Longaker MT, Carter DR, Beaupre GS (2008) Hydrostatic pressure enhances chondrogenic differentiation of human bone marrow stromal cells in osteochondrogenic medium. Ann Biomed Eng 36(5):813–820

Waldman SD, Spiteri CG, Grynpas MD, Pilliar RM, Kandel RA (2004) Long-term intermittent compressive stimulation improves the composition and mechanical properties of tissue-engineered cartilage. Tissue Eng 10(9–10):1323–1331

Waters RL, Lunsford BR, Perry J, Byrd R (1988) Energy-speed relationship of walking: standard tables. J Orthop Res 6(2):215–222

Zengerink M, Szerb I, Hangody L, Dopirak RM, Ferkel RD, van Dijk CN (2006) Current concepts: treatment of osteochondral ankle defects. Foot Ankle Clin 11(2):331–359, vi

Experimental articular cartilage repair in the Göttingen minipig: the influence of multiple defects per knee

Bjørn Borsøe Christensen[1*], Casper Bindzus Foldager[1], Morten Lykke Olesen[1], Louise Vingtoft[1], Jan Hendrik Duedal Rölfing[1], Steffen Ringgaard[2] and Martin Lind[3]

Abstract

Background: A gold standard treatment for articular cartilage injuries is yet to be found, and a cost-effective and predictable large animal model is needed to bridge the gap between *in vitro* studies and clinical studies. Ideally, the animal model should allow for testing of clinically relevant treatments and the biological response should be reproducible and comparable to humans. This allows for a reliable translation of results to clinical studies.This study aimed at verifying the Göttingen minipig as a pre-clinical model for articular cartilage repair by testing existing clinical cartilage repair techniques and evaluating the use of two defects per knee.

Methods: Sixteen fully mature Göttingen minipigs were used. The minipigs received bilateral trochlear osteochondral drill-hole defects or chondral defects (Ø 6 mm), either one defect per knee or two defects per knee. The defects were treated with one of the following: Matrix-induced autologous chondrocyte implantation (MACI), microfracture (MFx), autologous-dual-tissue transplantation (ADTT), autologous bone graft, autologous cartilage chips. Empty chondral and osteochondral defects were used as controls. MRI and CT were performed 3 and 6 month, histology was performed 6 month postoperative.

Results: The repair tissue varied in morphology from non-cartilaginous fibrous tissue to fibrocartilaginous tissue as seen on MRI, CT and histology at 6 month. The worst results were seen in the empty controls, while the best results were achieved with the MACI and ADTT treatment. The use of two defects per knee did not have any significant effect on the repair response.

Conclusion: The outcomes of the applied treatments were consistent with the outcomes in clinical studies and it was possible to apply two defects per knee. The Göttingen minipig model was easy to handle, cost-effective and provided predictable outcome. Based on this study the use of two defects per knee, one in the medial and one in the lateral trochlear facet, in male Göttingen minipigs is recommended.

Keywords: Animal model; Articular cartilage; Göttingen minipig; Bone graft; Cartilage chips

Background

Articular cartilage does not heal spontaneously, and so far no treatment method has been able to regenerate hyaline cartilage in a consistent and predictable manner (Bae et al. 2006; Knutsen et al. 2007; Bentley et al. 2012; Gobbi et al. 2013; Bekkers et al. 2013; Christensen et al. 2015a). Several well established cartilage repair methods are available including microfracture (MFx) and matrix-induced autologous chondrocyte implantation (MACI). MFx results in short-term clinical improvements, but due to the fibrocartilaginous and fibrous nature of the repair tissue, the improvements tend to deteriorate after 2–5 years (Kreuz et al. 2006; Gobbi et al. 2013). MACI results in similar clinical improvements, and the results are longer lasting than with MFx (Behrens et al. 2006; Ventura et al. 2012), but the MACI treatment is limited by the need for two separate surgeries and the high cost of cell culturing. Recently, the use of cartilage chips is

* Correspondence: bjornbc@gmail.com
[1]Orthopedic Research Laboratory, Aarhus University Hospital, Nørrebrogade 44, building 1A, 1. Floor, Aarhus, Denmark
Full list of author information is available at the end of the article

emerging as a potential treatment method. Studies have been published on particulated juvenile cartilage, and autologous cartilage chips in combination with scaffolds or embedded in fibrin glue (Cole et al. 2011; Farr et al. 2011; Marmotti et al. 2013; Farr et al. 2014; Christensen et al. 2015b), but long-term results are pending. To develop new surgical treatment methods and to test existing methods, cost-effective, reliable, and predictable large animal models are needed.

The Göttingen mini-pig has previously been used for cartilage repair research. Skeletal maturity is reached at the age of 18 months, defined by closing of the distal femoral growth plates and the characteristics of mature cartilage (Hurtig et al. 2011). Defects with a diameter of 5 mm has been shown to be critically sized (Gotterbarm et al. 2008). Skeletal maturity is important in order to prevent overestimation of repair response due to endogenous healing. The size of the animal, the joint size and the docile nature of the animal make the Göttingen minipig an appealing animal model in cartilage research. Nevertheless, possibility of application of clinical treatments and their repair responses has not been characterized sufficiently. Healing responses in the animal model as evaluated by histology and imaging should be comparable to those found in humans to allow for reliable translation of results from large animal studies to the clinical setting. Furthermore, the use of multiple cartilage defects per animal is important, both economically and ethically, since the utilization of multiple defects will allow the researcher to reduce the number of animals needed. However, the influence of multiple cartilage defects in one joint on cartilage repair response has not been investigated.

The present study aimed to 1) Validate the Göttingen minipig as a pre-clinical model for chondral and osteochondral repair using existing clinical cartilage repair techniques, and 2) Investigate whether or not two defects per knee (double-defect knees) will affect the repair outcome compared to single-defect knees.

We hypothesized that clinically available cartilage repair techniques could be applied in the Göttingen minipig and that the repair response would be similar to that found in clinical trials. Furthermore, we hypothesized that the repair outcome would not be affected by doubling the number of defects per knee, thereby reducing the number of Göttingen minipigs needed.

Methods

Study design

The study design is outlined in Fig. 1. The hypotheses were tested in two separate studies. All animals involved underwent bilateral knee surgery. One study focused on one defect per knee. Ten Göttingen minipigs were used (5 male, 5 female). The applicability and repair response of five different treatment methods and two different empty controls were tested in one defect per knee. The second study focused on the use of two defects per knee. Six Göttingen minipigs (6 male) received two defects in each knee. The outcome was compared between the neighboring defects, and between single-defect knees and double-defect knees.

The average age of the Göttingen minipigs was 21.0 months (18.5–23.7 months). The average weight was 41.9 kg (32.4–47 kg). The study complied with the Danish Law on Animal Experimentation and was approved by the Danish Ministry of Justice Ethical Committee, J.nr. 2012-15-2934-00301.

Anesthesia

The animals were pre-medicated with Azaperone (Stresnil, 0.1 mL/kg, Janssen Pharmaceutica, Belgium) and Midazolam (Dormicum, 0.1 mL/kg, Hoffmann-La Roche AG, Switzerland) administrated subdermally. By an intravenous access was gained through the auricular vein general anesthesia was established with etomidate (Hypnomidate, 0.25 mL/kg, Janssen Pharmaceutica, Belgium), and a standard tracheal tube, size 6.5, was inserted. General anesthesia was maintained with Sevoflurane® (3 %, AbbVie, Denmark) and fentanyl (0.175 mL/kg/h, Hameln pharmaceuticals, Germany). Prior to the surgery, the animal was treated with prophylactic antibiotics (Penicillinprokain, Ceva Sante Animale, France) 0.03 mL/kg).

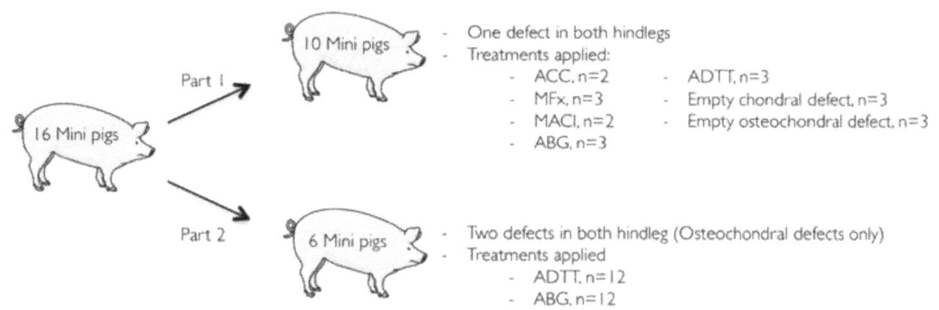

Fig. 1 The study design. *ACC*, Autologous cartilage chips. *MFx*, Microfracture. *MACI*, Matrix induced autologous chondrocyte implantation. *ABG*, Autologous boe graft. *ADTT*, Autologous Dual-Tissue Transplantation. Pig sketch from www.servier.com

Surgery

Local analgesics were administrated to the skin and periarticular tissue (Xylocain, 10 mL, 20 mg/mL, Astra Zeneca, Denmark). The location of the distal patella pole and the tibial tuberosity was marked on the skin, and a 5 cm midline skin incision directly over the patella ligament was made. The patella ligament was exposed, and access to the knee joint was gained by a trans-patella-ligamental incision from the distal patella pole to the tibial tuberosity. Through this access the intercondylar notch and trochlea was exposed.

In the single-defect knees, the Göttingen minipigs received chondral or osteochondral defects in the medial facet of the trochlear groove approximately two cm proximal to the intercondylar notch. In the double-defects knees, one osteochondral defect was made in the medial facet of the trochlear grove, approximately two cm proximal to the intercondylar notch, while the other osteochondral defect was made in the lateral facet of the trochlear grove, approximately 1 cm proximal to the medial defect. The chondral defects were outlined using a 6-mm skin biopsy punch and the cartilage was carefully stripped off using a curette until all cartilage including the calcified cartilage layer was removed, without any subchondral bleeding observed. Osteochondral defects 6 mm in diameter and 8 mm in depth were created using a cannulated 6 mm drill bit, which was preceded by drilling with a 2 mm guide wire. Low speed manual drilling was performed carefully to avoid heat damage to the tissue. After treatment was applied (Table 1) the patella ligament, subcutaneous tissue and skin were sutured. The animals were treated postoperatively with Finadyne 5 % (Flunixin meglumin, 1.1 mg/kg, oral paste, Intervet, Denmark) for five days, and were allowed free cage activity immediately after the operation.

The defects of the single-defect knees were randomized into one of seven groups presented in Table 1. The double-defect knees were randomized to either autologous bone graft (ABG) or Autologous Dual-Tissue Transplantation (ADTT).

Magnetic resonance imaging (MRI)

To evaluate the repair tissue surface, the subchondral tissue and the repair tissue signal intensity, each Göttingen minipig was MRI scanned prior to surgery, and three and six month postoperative using a 3 T whole-body MRI scanner (Magnetom Skyra; Siemens, Erlangen, Germany). The following sequences were used: Double Echo Steady State (DESS, 3D imaging with field-of-view (FOV) 151 × 180 × 90 mm; acquisition matrix 216 × 256 × 128; TR 13.5; TE 5.0; flip angle 28°; acquisition time 5 min 25 s), SPACE (3D imaging with FOV 98 × 180 × 78 mm; acquisition matrix 140 × 256 × 112; TR 1000; TE 40.0; ETL 52; acquisition time 3 min 57 s) and MPRAGE (3D imaging with FOV 120 × 183 × 99.8 mm; acquisition matrix 168 × 256 × 128; TR 2200; TE 2.65; TI 900; acquisition time 3 min 49 s).

For all the 3D imaging sequences an isotropic voxel of $0.7 \times 0.7 \times 0.7$ mm^3 was used.

OsiriX v. 5.8.5 64-bit (Pixmeo SARL, Bernex, Switzerland) was used for the analyses. An experienced, independent radiologist evaluated the images.

Table 1 Description of the five different treatment groups and the empty chondral- and osteochondral control groups

Treatment	Type	*n*	Details
Empty full-thickness chondral defect	Full thickness chondral	3	Ø 6 mm full thickness chondral defect left untreated.
Autologous cartilage chips (ACC)	Full thickness chondral	2	This treatment was applied to a full-thickness chondral defect. A 6 mm chondral defect was created using a skin biopsy punch, and the harvested cartilage was cut into chips approximately 0.5 mm^2, using a scalpel. The cartilage chips were embedded in fibrin glue and added to the defect, secured using fibrin glue.
Microfracture (MFx)	Full thickness chondral	3	The 6 mm defect was debrided so only the subchondral bony plate was left. Small perforations of the subchondral bone plate were made (Ø 1 mm), and the mesenchymal stem cells from the bone marrow cells were allowed to enter the full-thickness chondral defect.
Matrix-induced articular cartilage implantation (MACI)	Full thickness chondral	2	A collagen I/III membrane seeded with autologous chondrocytes was placed in a full-thickness chondral defect and secured using suture. Cartilage biopsies were performed one month prior to the surgery. The cartilage biopsies were cultured as previously described (Christensen *et al.* [2012]; Hansen *et al.* [2013]), and seeded onto the collagen I/III membranes one week prior to the surgery.
Empty osteochondral defect	Osteochondral	3	Ø 6 mm, 8 mm deep defect left untreated.
Autologous bone graft (ABG)	Osteochondral	15	A drill hole was made using a hand drill to avoid heat damage. The bone was collected and morselized into a paste and press-fitted into the osteochondral defect. Finally, the defect was sealed using fibrin glue (Tissel Duo Quick, Baxter Denmark).
Autologous Dual-Tissue Transplantation (ADTT)	Osteochondral	15	As above ABG is press-fitted into the osteochondral defect. A cartilage biopsy, taken before drilling, was cut into cartilage chips approximately 0.5 mm^2 in size. The autologous cartilage chips (ACC) were then embedded in fibrin glue, and added onto the ABG

Computed tomography (CT)

To evaluate the bone repair of the osteochondral lesion, repair tissue structure and presence of subchondral bone cysts, each animal was CT scanned three and six months postoperative using a SOMATOM Definition CT scanner (Siemens AG Medical Solutions, Erlangen, Germany). A clinical CT scanner was chosen over a Micro-CT due to its clinical relevance. In order to achieve the best-technically possible isotropic resolution of $0.6 \times 0.6 \times 0.6$ mm^3 the following scanning parameters were applied: 120 kV, 200 mAs, slice thickness 0.6 mm, spiral pitch factor 0.5 mm and reconstructed with a field of view of 307 mm^2, an increment of 0.3 mm and filters of either B40f or B80f. The images were analyzed using OsiriX v. 5.8.5 64-bit (Pixmeo SARL, Bernex, Switzerland). To determine the bone defect volume in cm^3, a region of interest (ROI) corresponding to the bone defect was drawn onto each 2D slide, and using the Osirix ROI volume tool the bone defect volume was computed. The bone defect repair percentage was calculated by comparing the remaining defect volume with the original drill hole defect. An experienced, independent radiologist evaluated the images.

Histology

The animals were euthanized 6 months postoperative and the gross appearances of the defects were photographed. The samples were dehydrated in increasing concentrations of ethanol (70–96 %) at 4 °C. Clearing in 2-isopropanol and xylene preceded infiltration with methyl methacrylate (MMA) at 4 °C. The final polymerization of MMA was accelerated with N,N-dimethyl-p-toluidine at −20 °C. The samples were cut into 10 μm serial sections from the center of the defect using a microtome (Reichert Jung polycot).

Before staining the sections were deplasticized in dimetoxyethylacetate and rehydrated. The samples were stained with hematoxylin and eosin (HE), safranin-O, and toluidine blue.

In the first study the sample size of each treatment group allowed for evaluation according to cell morphology, glycosaminoglycan (GAG) staining and repair tissue surface. In the second study, blinded evaluation of the repair response was performed by two experienced staff members using the ICRS II scoring system (Mainil-Varlet et al. 2010).

Animal welfare

Trained animal keepers, supervised by a veterinarian, closely observed each animal thrice daily. If the animal keepers assessed the Göttingen minipig to be limping or to be unwell, the animal was further evaluated according to general appearance, appetite, clinical findings (temperature, stool evaluation) and behavior, both when alone and when interacting with the animal keeper, each category was assigned a score of 1–4. Slight limping and decreased appetite and activity level was accepted for the first four days post-operative.

Statistics

Residuals were checked for normal distribution using QQ-plots. Bone defect fill from CT scans was evaluated using two-way ANOVA (time*treatment) with repeated measures (Prism 6, GraphPad Software, Inc., La Jolla, CA, USA). No interaction between the independent variables was observed and their effects were measured independently. Part 1: Due to high risk of a type 1 error, statistical tests were not used to investigate a difference between treatment methods. Part 2: All defects treated with ADTT and autologous bone graft were ICRS II scored. The treatments were grouped according to whether the defect was from a single-defect knee (Fig. 2, circle 1), if the defect was the proximal defect of double-defect knees (Fig. 2, circle 2) or if the defect was the distal defect of double-defect knees (Fig. 2, circle 3).

As the groups differed in size, and non-normal data distribution was confirmed using QQ-plots, Kruskal-Wallis one-way analysis of variance was used to test for a difference in repair response between the neighboring defects in the double-defect knees, and between the defects in single-defect knees and the defects in double-defect knees. For post-hoc evaluation, Dunn's test was used. P-values less than 0.05 were considered significant.

Results

No animals were limping, had reduced appetite nor reduced activity level after the initial five days of analgesic treatment. The trans-patella-ligament surgical approach provided adequate access to both the medial and lateral trochlear facet. Both the medial and the lateral trochlear facet were well suited for 6 mm defects.

Part 1: The histological results are presented in Table 2 and Fig. 3 and the radiological results are presented in Table 3, Figs. 4–5. Complete regeneration of hyaline cartilage was not observed in any treatment group.

The *chondral* treatment groups all had a smooth, but depressed repair tissue surface, and very little GAG-positive staining. The worst results were found in the empty defects (Fig. 3a) where the tissue was predominantly fibrous, whereas the best results were found in the MACI group with a mixture of hyaline tissue and fibrocartilage (Fig. 3d). The defects were clearly distinguishable on MRI three and six months postoperative with a persistent large defect in the empty defects and smooth and slightly depressed surface of non-hyaline tissue in the MACI group (Fig. 4).

In the *osteochondral* treatment groups the worst results were also found in the empty defects, where fibrous

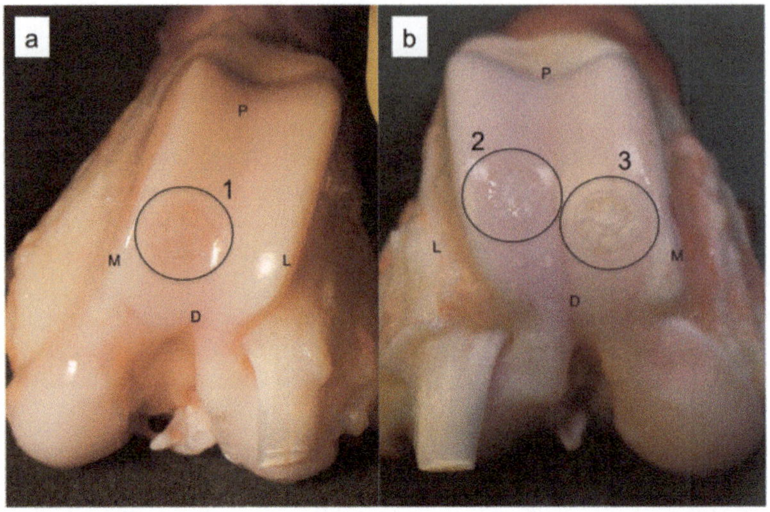

Fig. 2 Macroscopic images of (**a**) a single defect knee, and (**b**) a double defect knee. The defects have been marked with circles 1–3. The defects in these images have all been treated with ADTT. Remains of cartilage chips can be seen in all three defects as white areas in the defect. *P*, Proximal, *D*, Distal, *M*, Medial and *L*, Lateral

tissue was predominant (Fig. 3b). The best osteochondral repair results were found in the ADTT group where a combination of hyaline tissue and fibrocartilage was predominant (Fig. 3g). MRI showed a marked surface depression in the empty defects while defect filling in the ADTT group was almost complete with repair tissue resembling healthy cartilage. CT imaging showed a significant increase in bone volume from 3 to 6 month ($p = 0.033$) indicating continuous subchondral bone regeneration after 3 months follow-up. The average increase in subchondral bone volume from 3 to 6 month was 36 % and the average bone deficit after 6 month was only 0.06 cm^3 (SD $\pm$ 0.04) compared with the native subchondral bone level.

Part 2: In the ADTT and ABG treated knees there were no significant difference in ICRS II score between the neighboring defects nor were there any significant difference between the neighboring defects and the single-defect knees in any subcategory. The results of each ICRS II subcategory can be seen in Table 4.

Discussion

The primary findings of the present study was that the histological and radiological outcomes of clinically applied chondral and osteochondral repair techniques exhibited similar healing characteristics as seen in previous studies on the Göttingen minipig and in clinical situations. Furthermore, we found no change in outcome having

Table 2 The histological results of all treatment groups, assessed according to cellular morphology, GAG staining and repair tissue surface

Treatment	Cellular Morphology	GAG-Staining	Repair tissue surface
Empty chondral defect (Fig. 3a)	Mixture of *fibrous* tissue and *fibrocartilage*	Negative	Smooth, but depressed
Autologous cartilage chips (Fig. 3e)	Predominantly *fibrocartilage*. Areas with *hyaline-like* tissue dispersed throughout the defect area	Negative	Smooth
MFx (Fig. 3c)	*Fibrocartilage*	<50 %	Smooth, but depressed
MACI (Fig. 3d)	*Hyaline* cartilage in the periphery, *fibrocartilage* in the center	Negative	Smooth, but depressed
Empty osteochondral defect (Fig. 3b)	Predominantly *fibrous* tissue. Fibrocartilage present profoundly. Rich vascularity	<10 %	Smooth, but depressed
Autologous bone graft (Fig. 3f)	Mixture of *fibrous* tissue and *fibrocartilage*. Rich vascularity	<50 %	Smooth, but depressed. Slight fissuring observed
ADTT (Fig. 3g)	*Hyaline cartilage and fibrocartilaginous* tissue profoundly. *Fibrocartilage* and *fibrous* tissue superficially	<50 %	Smooth, but slightly depressed

GAG, Glycosaminoglycan. GAG staining percentage was assessed semi-quantitatively. *MFx*, Microfracture, *MACI*, Matrix-induced autologous chondrocyte implantation, *ADTT*, Autologous dual-tissue transplantation

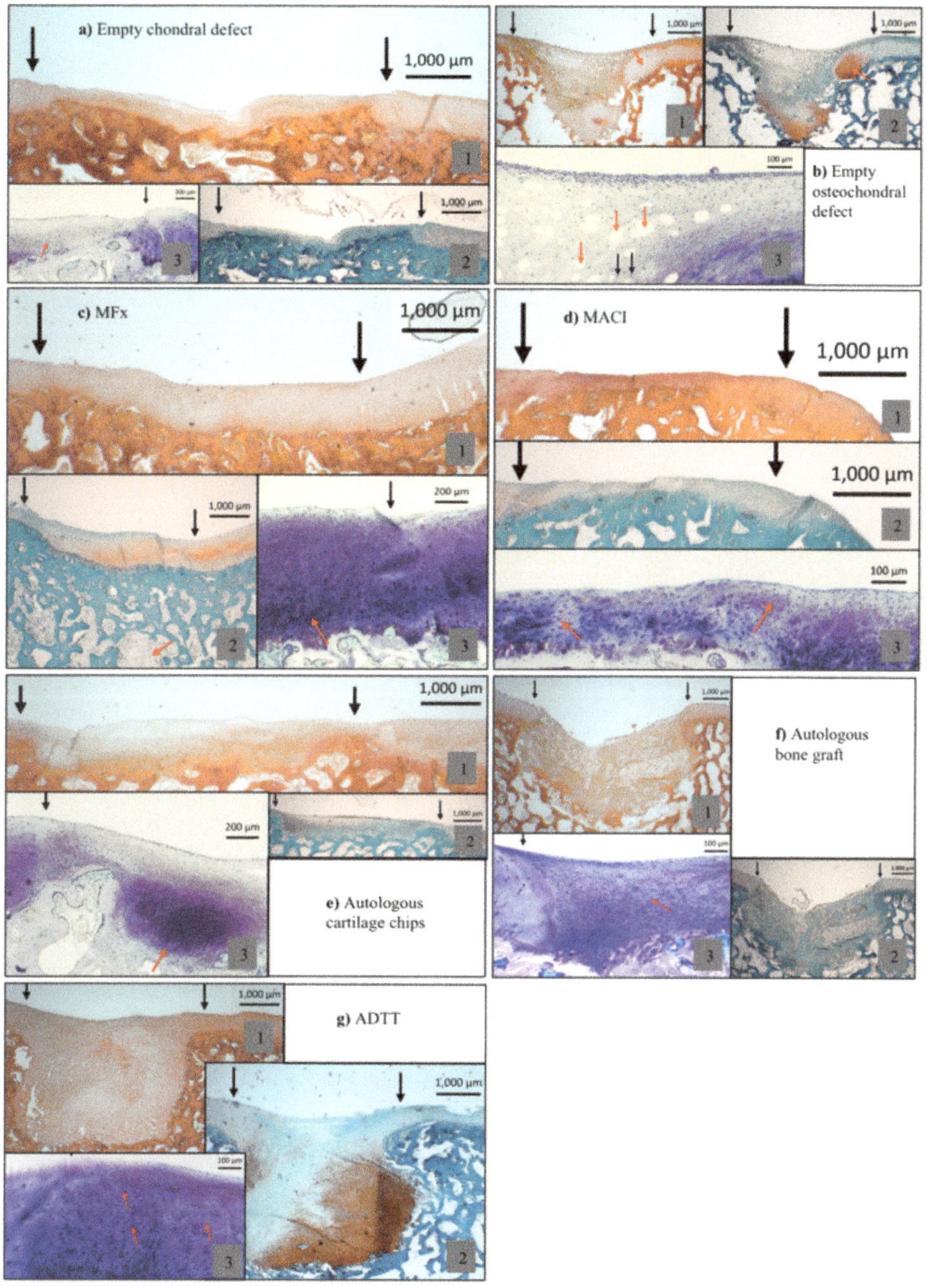

Fig. 3 Histological images of the seven groups. In each group (**1**) is HE stained, (**2**) is Safranin-O stained and (**3**) is a higher magnification stained with Toluidine blue. **a1-3** Black arrows: Defect area. Red arrow: fibrous tissue. **b1** Black arrows: Defect area. Red arrow: An example of cartilage flow phenomenon. **b2** Black arrows: Defect area. **b3** Red arrows: vascular tissue, Black arrows: fibrocytes. **c1** Black arrows: Defect area, **c2** Black arrows: Defect area, red arrow: MFx drill tunnel. **c3** Black arrow: Transition area from healthy tissue to repair tissue. Red arrow: Fibrocartilage. **d1-3** Black arrows: Defect area. Red arrows: Chondrocytes in lacunaes embedded in fibrous tissue. **d1-3** Black arrows: Defect area. Red arrow: Cartilage chip. **f1-3** Black arrows: Defect area. red arrow: fibrocytes. **g1-3** Black arrows: Defect area, red arrows: Chondrocytes in lacunae embedded in fibrous tissue

two defects in per knee joint as compared to one, thus advocating the use of two defects in future studies.

The aim of surgical treatment of cartilage injuries in humans is the relief of symptoms and the return to normal daily activities and sports. Inherently these parameters cannot directly be measured in animal models, and a successful outcome is ultimately based on the biological healing response evaluated by histology and radiology. In a recent study on Yukatan minipigs, Fisher *et al.* found that untreated full-thickness chondral defects were incompletely filled with fibrous and fibrocartilaginous tissue 6 weeks post-operative (Fisher et al. 2015). Similar results

Table 3 The radiological results of all treatment groups

Treatment method	Time-point	Bone defect repair (CT)	Repair tissue surface (MRI)	Subchondral tissue – MRI and CT
Empty chondral defect, (Fig. 4a)	3 months	NA	Persistent full-diameter chondral defect	Slight subchondral signal changes
	6 months	NA	Small persistent chondral defect, with surface fissuring	Slight subchondral signal changes
Autologous cartilage chips, (Fig. 4c)	3 months	NA	Intact surface, slightly irregular, with slight signal changes.	No subchondral signal changes
	6 months	NA	Intact surface, with slight signal changes.	No subchondral signal changes
MFx, (Fig. 4b)	3 months	NA	Slight surface depression, and surface fissuring. Repair tissue non-cartilaginous, non-bony	Signal changes around the MFx holes, and signs of subchondral cyst formation
	6 months	NA	Slight surface depression. No surface fissuring. Repair tissue non-cartilaginous, non-bony	Marked subchondral signal changes. No subchondral cyst formation
MACI, (Fig. 4d)	3 months	NA	Slight surface depression, but smooth surface covered with non-cartilaginous, non-bony tissue	Subchondral signal changes
	6 months	NA	Slight surface depression, but smooth surface covered with non-cartilaginous, non-bony tissue	No subchondral signal changes
Empty Osteochondral defect, (Fig. 5a, d)	3 months	50 %	Persistent defect	Persistent bone defect. The surrounding bone were less dense than native subcortical bone
	6 months	67 %	Marked surface depression with non-cartilaginous, non-bony tissue	Persistent bone defect. Sclerotic edge, and subchondral bone cyst formation
Autologous bone graft, (Fig. 5b, e)	3 months	63 %	Slight surface depression. Repair tissue non-cartilaginous, non-bony	Persistent bone defect, with fibrous repair tissue. No cyst formation or edema
	6 months	76 %	Slight surface depression. Repair tissue non-cartilaginous, non-bony	Persistent bone defect with fibrous repair tissue. No cyst formation or edema
ADTT, (Fig. 5c, f)	3 months	83 %	Slight surface depression. Defect partially covered by cartilage-like tissue	Superficial fibrous tissue, with profound bone repair. Small persistent bone defect
	6 months	92 %	Slight surface depression. Defect almost completely covered with cartilage-like tissue	Almost complete bone repair

The repair tissue surface was assessed using MRI, while the subchondral tissue was assessed using MRI and CT. The bone defect repair percentage is a measure of the degree of repair compared to the original defect volume. *MFx*, Microfracture, *MACI*, Matrix-induced autologous chondrocyte implantation, *ADTT*, Autologous dual002Dtissue transplantation

have been reported by Gotterbarm *et al.* who investigated the histological outcome of untreated chondral- and osteochondral defects in the Göttingen minipig. The authors evaluated empty chondral and osteochondral defects from 62 Göttingen minipigs. They found that empty chondral defects were filled mainly with fibrous and partially fibrocartilaginous tissue. The empty osteochondral defects were concavely depressed and filled with fibrous tissue and fibrocartilage with blood vessels present in the defect and signs of the cartilage flow phenomenon (Gotterbarm et al. 2008). These results were mirrored in the untreated chondral- and osteochondral defects of the present study as seen in Table 2 and Fig. 3a and b. However, chondral and osteochondral repair techniques were not tested in the study by Gotterbaum *et al.*.

In a clinical situation MFx will often result in a significant short-term clinical improvement with deterioration of long-term outcome. The repair tissue morphology, as seen in the present study as well, is fibrous or at best fibrocartilaginous (Gobbi et al. 2005; Saris et al. 2008; Vanlauwe et al. 2011; Gobbi et al. 2013). Both Zuo *et al.* and Fisher *et al.* studied MFx in adolescent minipigs and found that defects treated with MFx were filled with fibrocartilage with rounded cells in lacunae situated in disarranged fibrous matrix, as seen in the present study (Fig. 3c) (Zuo et al. 2007; Fisher et al. 2015). These findings are comparable to clinical histological outcome as seen by Gudas *et al.*, who found that 57 % of MFx repair tissue was fibrocartilaginous, while 43 % was fibrous (Gudas et al. 2005a). Karthikyan *et al.*, found the MFx repair tissue to be fibrocartilaginous

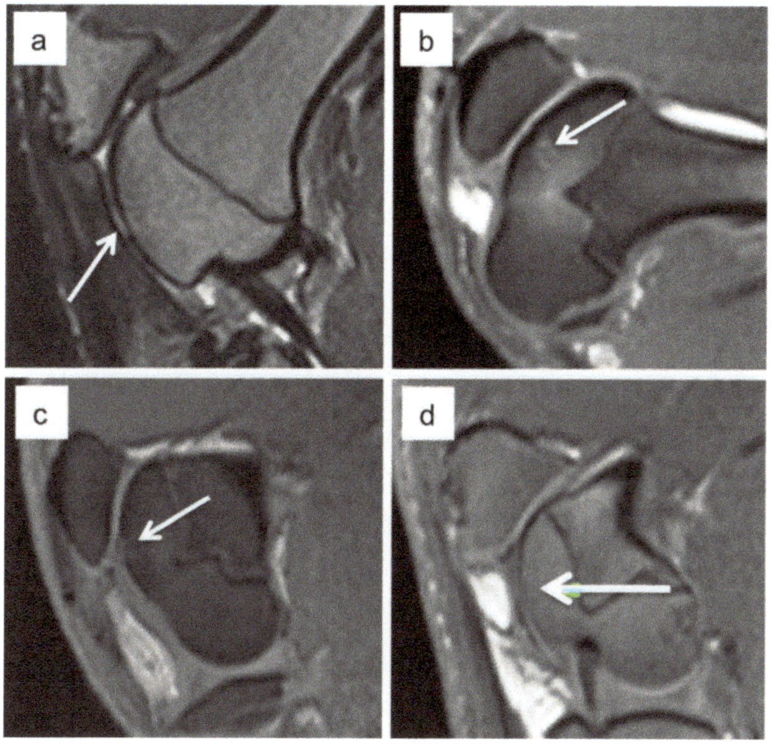

Fig. 4 MRI of the four chondral treatment groups. **a** Empty chondral defect, **b** Microfracture. The MFx drill holes can be seen in the subchondral area. **c** Autologous cartilage chips and **d** MACI. The white arrows mark the defects

(Karthikeyan et al. 2012) while Bae *et al.*, found a mixture of fibrocartilage and hyaline-like tissue (Bae et al. 2006).

In the present study MACI produced predominantly hyaline tissue and fibrocartilaginous repair tissue (Fig. 3d). This is also well established in clinical studies. Zheng *et al.*, reported 75 % hyaline-like cartilage 6 months after surgery, and Bartlett *et al.* reported 36 % of the repair tissue to be hyaline-like, the remainder being fibrous (Bartlett et al. 2005; Zheng et al. 2007). Anders *et al.* found 33 % to be a mixture of hyaline-like tissue and fibrous tissue, with 41 % being fibrocartilaginous (Anders et al. 2008).

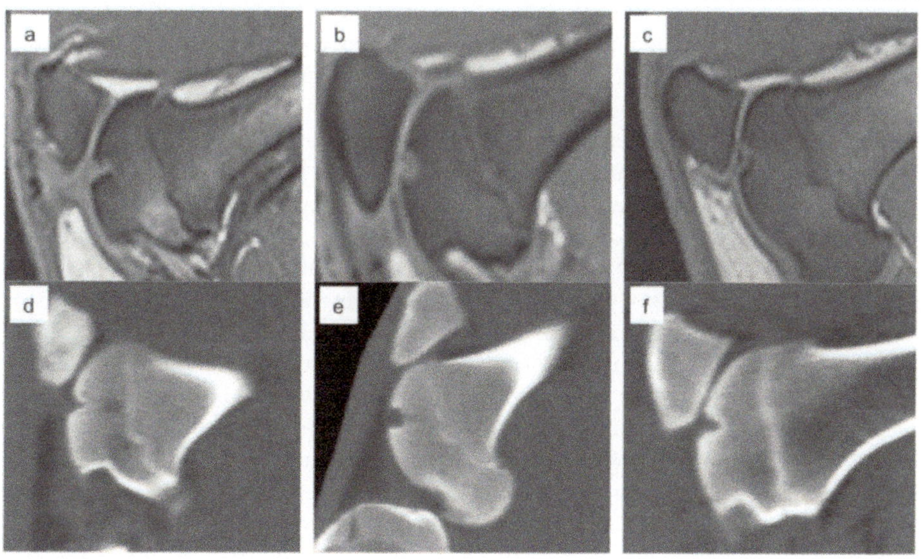

Fig. 5 MRI and corresponding CT for the empty osteochondral defects (**a** and **d**), autologous bone graft (**b** and **e**) and the ADTT treated defects (**c** and **f**). Incomplete subchondral bone repair with a cyst-like appearance is seen in d)

Table 4 The ICRS II subcategories for the single defect knees and the double defect knees of study 2

ICRS II category	ADTT proximal	ADTT distal	ADTT single	ABG proximal	ABG distal	ABG single
Tissue morphology	38.3 ± 8.2	41.7 ± 7.3	36.7 ± 1.7	15.8 ± 6.4	20.0 ± 7.7	11.7 ± 3.3
Material staining	67.3 ± 11.2	70.0 ± 11.3	86.6 ± 8.8	40.0 ± 10	51.7 ± 15.5	35.0 ± 27.8
Cell morphology	40.0 ± 7.2	40.0 ± 8.2	36.7 ± 1.7	16.7 ± 6.3	20.8 ± 7.7	11.7 ± 3.3
Clusters	55.8 ± 14.5	67.6 ± 17.5	90.0 ± 5.7	69.2 ± 12.7	57.5 ± 19	58.3 ± 26.8
Surface architecture	35.0 ± 6.7	38.3 ± 11.1	36.7 ± 18.6	64.2 ± 10.4	40.1 ± 5.5	23.3 ± 13.7
Basal integration	60.0 ± 5.2	52.5 ± 8.7	40.0 ± 0	64.2 ± 5.2	54.2 ± 10.7	25.0 ± 7.6
Tidemark formation	24.2 ± 10.8	20.8 ± 9.3	21.7 ± 8.3	8.3 ± 3.3	19.2 ± 11.6	8.3 ± 4.4
Subchondral bone	23.3 ± 9.4	25.8 ± 9.6	35.0 ± 7.6	45.8 ± 6.9	49.2 ± 10.5	18.3 ± 7.3
Vascularization	58.3 ± 18.5	65.0 ± 14.3	40.0 ± 23.1	35.8 ± 15.1	49.2 ± 21.3	33.3 ± 33
Surface assessment	30.8 ± 7.9	26.7 ± 9.1	31.7 ± 15.9	35.0 ± 11.4	34.2 ± 9.2	21.7 ± 14.8
Deep assessment	47.5 ± 7.3	43.3 ± 7.6	43.3 ± 12	46.7 ± 8.3	58.3 ± 6	18.3 ± 4.4
Overall assessment	48.8 ± 3	50.0 ± 3.3	52.0 ± 3	48.1 ± 3.4	49.4 ± 4.4	31.0 ± 3.7

"Single", "proximal" and "distal" corresponds to Fig. 2, circle 1, 2 and 3 respectively. No significant difference was found between any defect location in neither the ADTT group nor the ABG group

One of the main responsibilities of researchers performing animal experiments is to minimize the suffering of the animal by considering: 1) *Reducing* the number of animals used. 2) *Refining* the surgical technique and the care and housing facilities and 3) *Replacing* the animal studies with *in vitro* studies when possible. This was introduced by Russell *et al.* in 1959 and is known as "the three R's" (Russell and Burch 1959). In the present study we established that doubling the number of defects per knee did not affect the repair outcome or cause postoperative mortality. This enables researchers to achieve the same number of defects while halving the number of animals used. This reduces the cost of the studies and addresses ethical concerns, however one must remember that the biological variation is reduced in the process.

Several animal models are available for articular cartilage research. As described in the above, the biological repair response must resemble what is seen in a clinical situation, but the size of the animal, the cartilage thickness, and ethical concerns must also be considered before choosing a suitable model. Small animal models as the rabbit are frequently used in articular cartilage research, but the model suffers from a high level of endogenous repair making the model best suited for proof-of-concept studies rather than clinical translation (Chu et al. 2010). The dog, sheep and goat models are roughly the same size as the minipig, and all have been used in cartilage repair studies. The articular cartilage of the dog and minipig shares the same collagen arrangement as in humans (Kaab et al. 1998). Furthermore, dogs, unlike rabbits, goats, sheep and minipigs, can be trained to accept braces to limit weight bearing, to further mimic the clinical situation. While the dogs' status as a family pet complicates its use from an ethical standpoint, the fact that goats and sheep are ruminant animals limits the available housing and surgical facilities due to the risk of prion disease transmission. The horse model has an articular cartilage thickness of 1.5–2 mm which is significantly closer to humans (2–2.5 mm) than rabbits (<0.3 mm), sheep (0.4–0.5 mm), dogs and minipigs (0.5–0.8 mm) or goats (0.9–1.5 mm) (Shortkroff et al. 1996; Hunziker 2002; Frisbie et al. 2006; Gotterbarm et al. 2008). This makes the horse model an obvious choice if human-like cartilage thickness is required, however, the acquisition cost and handling difficulties significantly limits a more widespread use.

The Göttingen minipig is close, but not equal, to humans regarding weight, joint size and articular cartilage collagen arrangement. The docile nature of the minipig, and the fact that a stable weight of 30–50 kg is maintained in adulthood makes handling the animal very easy. Furthermore, the blood count, blood clotting parameters, electrolytes and liver enzymes have similar values to those found in humans (Marshall et al. 1972; Rispat et al. 1993). However, the Göttingen minipig is limited by the relatively thin articular cartilage, which complicates the use of radiological follow-up due to resolution limitations of MRI. Furthermore, the Göttingen minipig does not accept braces to limit postoperative weight bearing.

The present study is limited by the small sample size per treatment method. This prevents comparison of results between groups but allows for a larger number of treatments methods to be tested. The number of Göttingen minipig knees assigned to each treatment group did not allow for statistical analysis between treatment outcomes, however, the high consistency in outcome within each treatment group was an important finding since the outcomes reported are consistent with the results of current clinical studies. The use of both male and female pigs is an important study limitation. However, Rispat *et al.*

showed that no biochemical or haematological differences between male and female Yucatan minipigs existed and to further minimize the risk of gender bias, the treatments were randomization. Still, the existence of a gender bias must be considered.

Additional surgical experience using the Göttingen minipig was achieved in a pilot study where a medial parapatellar approach was tested. This approach was more time demanding, caused greater surgical trauma and resulted in more postoperative pain as observed by limping on the operated leg in the animals. The parapatellar approach was therefore abandoned for the transpatella-ligament approach. Furthermore, the surgeons found that the male Göttingen minipig had a more slender hind leg, which improved surgical access to the trochlea compared with the female.

Conclusion

Based on the results of this study, the authors recommend the Göttingen minipig as a suitable model for cartilage repair. At six months follow-up of clinically relevant treatment methods, histology was comparable to that found in humans. CT imaging proved crucial to the monitoring of subchondral bone repair, and is recommended in the evaluation of all osteochondral treatments. The use of two defects in each knee on male Göttingen minipigs proved to be the most cost-effective approach.

Abbreviations

ACC: Autologous cartilage chips; MACI: Matrix-induced autologous chondrocyte implantation; MFx: Microfracture; ADTT: Autologous Dual-Tissue Transplantation; MRI: Magnetic resonance imaging; CT: Computed tomography; DESS: Double echo steady state; FOV: Field of view; ETL: Echo train length; SPACE: 3D turbo spin echo with variable flip angle; TE: Echo time; TR: Repetition time; MMA: Methyl methacrylate; HE: Hematoxylin and eosin; BSA: Albumin bovine serum; PBS: Phosphate buffered saline; GAG: Glycosamino glycane.

Competing interests

The authors declare that they have no competing interests.

Authors' contributions

BBC conceived the study, participated in the study design, performed the surgery, performed the MRI, performed interpretation of data, assisted in histological preparation and drafted the manuscript. CBF conceived the study, participated in the study design, performed the surgery, performed interpretation of data and performed the statistical analysis and revised the manuscript. MLO assisted in surgery and euthanization and revised the manuscript. CEB participated in the study design, interpretation of data and revised the manuscript. LV assisted in surgery, performed histological preparation and contributed to drafting the manuscript. JHDR assisted in euthanization, performed the CT scans, performed interpretation of data and contributed to drafting the manuscript. SR supervised on MRI and contributed to drafting the manuscript. ML conceived the study, participated in the study design, performed interpretation of data and revised the manuscript. All authors have given final approval of this manuscript.

Acknowledgements

The authors would like to thank The Novo Nordisk Foundation and The Danish Rheumatish Association for financial support. We thank Kasper Sandager Mikkelsen for surgical assistance, Anette Baatrup, Jane Pauli and Vibeke Skovhus Nielsen for technical assistance and Jonas Jensen for radiological assistance.

Author details

[1]Orthopedic Research Laboratory, Aarhus University Hospital, Nørrebrogade 44, building 1A, 1. Floor, Aarhus, Denmark. [2]MR Research Center, Aarhus University Hospital, Skejby, Denmark. [3]Department of Sports Traumatology, Department of orthopedic surgery, Aarhus University Hospital, Aarhus, Denmark.

References

Anders S, Schaumburger J, Schubert T, Grifka J, Behrens P (2008) Matrix-associated autologous chondrocyte transplantation (MACT). Minimally invasive technique in the knee. Oper Orthop Traumatol. doi:10.1007/s00064-008-1303-1

Bae DK, Yoon KH, Song SJ (2006) Cartilage Healing After Microfracture in Osteoarthritic Knees. Arthroscopy 22:367–374. doi:10.1016/j.arthro.2006.01.015

Bartlett W, Skinner J, Gooding C, Carrington R, Flanagan A, Briggs T, Bentley G (2005) Autologous chondrocyte implantation *versus* matrix-induced autologous chondrocyte implantation for osteochondral defects of the knee: a prospective, randomised study. J bone Jt Surg Br Vol 87:640–645

Behrens P, Bitter T, Kurz B, Russlies M (2006) Matrix-associated autologous chondrocyte transplantation/implantation (MACT/MACI)–5-year follow-up. Knee 13:194–202. doi:10.1016/j.knee.2006.02.012

Bekkers JEJ, Bartels LW, Vincken KL, Dhert WJA, Creemers LB, Saris DBF (2013) Articular Cartilage Evaluation After TruFit Plug Implantation Analyzed by Delayed Gadolinium-Enhanced MRI of Cartilage (dGEMRIC). Am J Sports Med 41:1290–5. doi:10.1177/0363546513483536

Bentley G, Biant LC, Vijayan S, Macmull S, Skinner JA, Carrington RW (2012) Minimum ten-year results of a prospective randomised study of autologous chondrocyte implantation *versus* mosaicplasty for symptomatic articular cartilage lesions of the knee. J Bone Jt Surg Br 94:504–509. doi:10.1302/0301-620X.94B4.27495

Christensen BB, Foldager CB, Hansen OM, Kristiansen AA, Le DQS, Nielsen AD, Nygaard JV, Bünger CE, Lind M (2012) A novel nano-structured porous polycaprolactone scaffold improves hyaline cartilage repair in a rabbit model compared to a collagen type I/III scaffold: In vitro and in vivo studies. Knee Surgery, Sport Traumatol Arthrosc 20:1192–1204. doi:10.1007/s00167-011-1692-9

Christensen BB, Foldager CB, Jensen J, Jensen NC, Lind M (2015a) Poor osteochondral repair by a biomimetic collagen scaffold: 1- to 3-year clinical and radiological follow-up. Knee Surg Sports Traumatol Arthrosc. doi:10.1007/s00167-015-3538-3

Christensen BB, Foldager CB, Jensen J, Lind M (2015b) Autologous Dual-Tissue Transplantation for Osteochondral Repair: Early Clinical and Radiological Results. Cartilage. doi:10.1177/1947603515580983

Chu CR, Szczodry M, Bruno S (2010) Animal models for cartilage regeneration and repair. Tissue Eng Part B Rev 16:105–115. doi:10.1089/ten.TEB.2009.0452

Cole BJ, Farr J, Winalski CS, Hosea T, Richmond J, Mandelbaum B, De Deyne PG (2011) Outcomes after a single-stage procedure for cell-based cartilage repair: a prospective clinical safety trial with 2-year follow-up. Am J Sports Med 39:1170–1179. doi:10.1177/0363546511399382

Farr J, Yao JQ, Jack Farr JQY (2011) Chondral Defect Repair with Particulated Juvenile Cartilage Allograft. Cartilage 2:346–353. doi:10.1177/1947603511405838

Farr J, Tabet SK, Margerrison E, Cole BJ (2014) Clinical, Radiographic, and Histological Outcomes After Cartilage Repair With Particulated Juvenile Articular Cartilage: A 2-Year Prospective Study. Am J Sports Med 42:1417–1425. doi:10.1177/0363546514528671

Fisher MB, Belkin NS, Milby AH, Henning EA, Bostrom M, Kim M, Pfeifer C, Meloni G, Dodge GR, Burdick JA, Schaer TP, Steinberg DR, Mauck RL (2015) Cartilage Repair and Subchondral Bone Remodeling in Response to Focal Lesions in a Mini-Pig Model: Implications for Tissue Engineering. Tissue Eng Part A 21:850–860. doi:10.1089/ten.tea.2014.0384

Frisbie DD, Cross MW, McIlwraith CW (2006) A comparative study of articular cartilage thickness in the stifle of animal species used in human pre-clinical studies compared to articular cartilage thickness in the human knee. Vet Comp Orthop Traumatol 19:142–146

Gobbi A, Nunag P, Malinowski K (2005) Treatment of full thickness chondral lesions of the knee with microfracture in a group of athletes. Knee Surg Sports Traumatol Arthrosc 13:213–221. doi:10.1007/s00167-004-0499-3

Gobbi A, Karnatzikos G, Kumar A (2013) Long-term results after microfracture treatment for full-thickness knee chondral lesions in athletes. Knee Surg Sports Traumatol Arthrosc. doi:10.1007/s00167-013-2676-8

Gotterbarm T, Breusch SJ, Schneider U, Jung M (2008) The minipig model for experimental chondral and osteochondral defect repair in tissue engineering : retrospective analysis of 180 defects. 71–82. doi: 10.1258/la.2007.06029e

Gudas R, Kalesinskas RJ, Kimtys V, Stankevicius E, Toliusis V, Bernotavicius G, Smailys A (2005a) A prospective randomized clinical study of mosaic osteochondral autologous transplantation *versus* microfracture for the treatment of osteochondral defects in the knee joint in young athletes. Arthroscopy 21:1066–75. doi:10.1016/j.arthro.2005.06.018

Hansen OM, Foldager CB, Christensen BB, Everland H, Lind M (2013) Increased chondrocyte seeding density has no positive effect on cartilage repair in an MPEG-PLGA scaffold. Knee Surgery, Sport Traumatol Arthrosc 21:485–493. doi:10.1007/s00167-012-1996-4

Hunziker EB (2002) Articular cartilage repair: basic science and clinical progress. A review of the current status and prospects. Osteoarthr Cartil 10:432–463. doi:10.1053/joca.2002.0801

Hurtig MB, Buschmann MD, Fortier LA, Hoemann CD, Hunziker EB, Jurvelin JS, Mainil-Varlet P, McIlwraith CW, Sah RL, Whiteside RA (2011) Preclinical Studies for Cartilage Repair: Recommendations from the International Cartilage Repair Society. Cartilage 2:137–152. doi:10.1177/1947603511401905

Kaab MJ, Gwynn IA, Notzli HP (1998) Collagen fibre arrangement in the tibial plateau articular cartilage of man and other mammalian species. J Anat 193(Pt 1):23–34

Karthikeyan S, Roberts S, Griffin D (2012) Microfracture for acetabular chondral defects in patients with femoroacetabular impingement: results at second-look arthroscopic surgery. Am J Sports Med 40:2725–30. doi:10.1177/0363546512465400

Knutsen G, Drogset JO, Engebretsen L, Grøntvedt T, Isaksen V, Ludvigsen TC, Roberts S, Solheim E, Strand T, Johansen O (2007) A randomized trial comparing autologous chondrocyte implantation with microfracture. Findings at five years. J Bone Joint Surg Am 89:2105–12. doi:10.2106/JBJS.G.00003

Kreuz PC, Steinwachs MR, Erggelet C, Krause SJ, Konrad G, Uhl M, Sudkamp N (2006) Results after microfracture of full-thickness chondral defects in different compartments in the knee. Osteoarthr Cartil 14:1119–1125. doi:10.1016/j.joca.2006.05.003

Mainil-Varlet P, Van Damme B, Nesic D, Knutsen G, Kandel R, Roberts S (2010) A new histology scoring system for the assessment of the quality of human cartilage repair: ICRS II. Am J Sports Med 38:880–890. doi:10.1177/0363546509359068

Marmotti A, Bonasia DE, Bruzzone M, Rossi R, Castoldi F, Collo G, Realmuto C, Tarella C, Peretti GM (2013) Human cartilage fragments in a composite scaffold for single-stage cartilage repair: An *in vitro* study of the chondrocyte migration and the influence of TGF-??1 and G-CSF. Knee Surgery, Sport Traumatol Arthrosc 21:1819–1833. doi:10.1007/s00167-012-2244-7

Marshall M, Lydtin H, Krawietz W, Hagen R, Schuckert G, Hess H, Zåollner N (1972) Das Miniaturschwein als Versuchstier in der experimentellen Medizin. Res Exp Med 316:300–316

Rispat G, Slaoui M, Weber D, Salemink P, Berthoux C, Shrivastava R (1993) Haematological and plasma biochemical values for healthy Yucatan micropigs. Lab Anim 27:368–373. doi:10.1258/002367793780745561

Russell W, Burch R (1959) The Principles of Humane Experimental Technique. Methuen, London

Saris DBF, Vanlauwe J, Victor J, Haspl M, Bohnsack M, Fortems Y, Vandekerckhove B, Almqvist KF, Claes T, Handelberg F, Lagae K, van der Bauwhede J, Vandenneucker H, Yang KGA, Jelic M, Verdonk R, Veulemans N, Bellemans J, Luyten FP (2008) Characterized chondrocyte implantation results in better structural repair when treating symptomatic cartilage defects of the knee in a randomized controlled trial *versus* microfracture. Am J Sports Med 36:235–246. doi:10.1177/0363546507311095

Shortkroff S, Barone L, Hsu HP, Wrenn C, Gagne T, Chi T, Breinan H, Minas T, Sledge CB, Tubo R, Spector M (1996) Healing of chondral and osteochondral defects in a canine model: The role of cultured chondrocytes in regeneration of articular cartilage. Biomaterials 17:147–154. doi:10.1016/0142-9612(96)85759-0

Vanlauwe J, Saris DBF, Victor J, Almqvist KF, Bellemans J, Luyten FP, Bohnsack M, Claes T, Fortems Y, Handelberg F, Haspl M, Jelic M, Lagae K, Vandekerckhove B, Vandenneucker H, van der Bauwhede J, Verdonk R (2011) Five-Year Outcome of Characterized Chondrocyte Implantation *Versus* Microfracture for Symptomatic Cartilage Defects of the Knee: Early Treatment Matters. Am J Sports Med 39:2566–2574. doi:10.1177/0363546511422220

Ventura A, Memeo A, Borgo E, Terzaghi C, Legnani C, Albisetti W (2012) Repair of osteochondral lesions in the knee by chondrocyte implantation using the MACI(R) technique. Knee Surg Sport Traumatol Arthrosc 20:121–126. doi:10.1007/s00167-011-1575-0

Zheng M-H, Willers C, Kirilak L, Yates P, Xu J, Wood D, Shimmin A (2007) Matrix-induced autologous chondrocyte implantation (MACI): biological and histological assessment. Tissue Eng. doi:10.1089/ten.2006.0246

Zuo ZH, Yang L, Duan XJ, Guo L (2007) Repair of articular cartilage defects in minipigs by microfracture surgery and BMSCs transplantation. J Med Coll PLA 22:288–292. doi:10.1016/S1000-1948(07)60059-8

22

Comparative study of subtalar arthrodesis after calcaneal frature malunion with autologous bone graft or freeze-dried xenograft

Carlo Henning, Gabriel Poglia*, Murilo Anderson Leie and Carlos Roberto Galia

Abstract

Background: Calcaneal fracture malunion may evolve into arthrosis and severe foot deformities. The aim of this study was to identify differences in bony union following corrective subtalar arthrodesis with interposition of autologous tricortical bone graft or freeze-dried bovine xenograft.

Methods: We prospectively evaluated 12 patients who underwent subtalar arthrodesis, six patients received autografts and 6 received freeze-dried bovine xenografts. After a mean followup of 58 weeks, the patients were clinical assessed using AOFAS scale and the visual analog scale (VAS) for pain and for final radiographic parameters measurement. Two blind raters evaluated the length of time required for solid union of the arthrodesis and graft integration by retrospective radiographic examination.

Results: In the autograft group, AOFAS score improved from a preoperative average of 37 to 64 points postoperatively ($p = 0.02$) and mean VAS score improved from 4.7 to 1.9 ($p = 0.028$). In the xenograft group, AOFAS score improved from 38 to 74 points ($p = 0.02$) and VAS from 5.5 to 2.7 ($p = 0.046$). Solid union was achieved in all cases in the autograft group at an average of 5.3 weeks and in five cases in the xenograft group at 8.8 weeks ($p = 0.077$). Graft integration occurred after an average of 10.7 weeks in the autograft group and 28.8 weeks in the xenograft group ($p = 0.016$).

Conclusion: With the numbers available, no significant difference could be detected in the length of time required for solid union of subtalar arthrodesis between groups, although time to integration of freeze-dried bovine xenografts was statistically higher. Clinical and functional improvement was observed in both groups.

Keywords: Calcaneus; Malunion; Arthrodesis; Bone graft; Xenograft; Freeze-dried

Background

Late complications of calcaneal fracture malunion are related to: arthrosis of the talocalcaneal joint, and possibly of the calcaneocuboid joint, due to joint incongruity or chondral lesion; widening of the calcaneus, which may lead to changes in the peroneal tendons, calcaneofibular impingement, and shoe wear difficulties; and often varus deformity of the calcaneus, loss of hindfoot height, and foot flattening (Chandler et al. 1999; Nickisch and Anderson 2006). In addition, neurovascular and heel pad injuries may be responsible for chronic pain and functional limitation in these patients (Lim and Leung 2001).

Several authors have described subtalar arthrodesis with bone graft block interposition in the treatment of post-traumatic arthrosis of this joint along with lateral calcaneal wall prominence resection in order to correct deformities and hindfoot malalignment with good clinical and radiographic outcomes (Amendola and Lammens 1996; Bednarz et al. 1997; Burton et al. 1998; Chan and Alexander 1997; Chen et al. 1998; Clare et al. 2005; Easley et al. 2000; Garras et al. 2008; Marti et al. 1999; Myerson and Quill 1993; Rammelt et al. 2004; Thermann et al. 1999; Trnka et al. 2001).

Solid union of this type of subtalar arthrodesis using autologous tricortical iliac crest graft has been achieved in

* Correspondence: gabrielpoglia@gmail.com
Department of Orthopaedics, Hospital de Clínicas de Porto Alegre, Medicine School, Universidade Federal do Rio Grande do Sul, Rua Ramiro Barcelos, 2350, Zip Code 90035-003 Porto Alegre Rio Grande do Sul, Brazil

86 to 100% of cases (Amendola and Lammens 1996; Bednarz et al. 1997; Burton et al. 1998; Chan and Alexander 1997; Chen et al. 1998; Marti et al. 1999; Myerson and Quill 1993; Rammelt et al. 2004; Thermann et al. 1999). However, complications associated with bone graft harvest from the iliac crest have been estimated to occur in up to 49% of cases (Finkemeier 2002; Seiler and Johnson 2000). The most common donor site complications include chronic pain, nerve injury, hematoma and infection (Scranton 2002). Furthermore, it is an additional procedure that may increase operative time, length of hospital stay and costs (Salama 1983; Seiler and Johnson 2000). With the use of allografts in this type of arthrodesis, union rates may vary considerably, from 20 to 90.5% (Easley et al. 2000; Garras et al. 2008; Seiler and Johnson 2000). No studies using xenografts in this particular type of surgery were identified by the authors in the literature.

The need to use large quantities of bone graft in hip surgeries at our department encouraged research and use of bone substitutes, specifically freeze-dried bovine xenografts (Galia et al. 2009a; Macedo et al. 1999). The bovine bone is considered a natural hydroxyapatite with chemical composition, porosity, size and shape similar to the human bone, providing structural and osteoconductive support for new bone formation (Galia et al. 2008). Defatting, cell removal and dehydration by freeze-drying decrease graft antigenicity, maintaining its structural characteristics and protein-mineral matrix. At the end of the process, grafts can be sterilized and easily stored (Kakiuchi et al. 1996). The advantages of xenografts include good availability, easy handling and potentially favorable clinical performance. The xenografts currently used in orthopedic surgery have proven to be safe and reliable (Laurencin and El-Amin 2008).

The main objective of this study was to identify whether there are differences in bony union following subtalar arthrodesis, after calcaneal fracture malunion, with interposition of autologous tricortical iliac crest bone graft or freeze-dried bovine xenograft. Secondary objectives included clinical and radiographic parameters.

Methods

Between September 2006 and October 2007, twelve consecutive non randomized patients underwent subtalar arthrodesis with interposition of a bone graft block for the treatment of calcaneal fracture malunion. Autologous tricortical iliac crest graft (autograft group) was used in six patients (six cases) and freeze-dried cancellous bovine xenograft bone block (xenograft group) in six patients (six cases) (Figure 1). A total of twelve nonrandomized patients were prospectively analyzed with a mean followup of 58.17 weeks (range, 42 to 82 weeks). A bone graft of each type was used in the first two operated cases. Tricortical autograft was then used in the next five cases, and freeze-dried bovine xenograft was subsequently used in the other five cases. The study was approved by the institutional review board (Group for Research and Graduate Studies of Hospital de Clínicas de Porto Alegre) and all patients gave their informed consent.

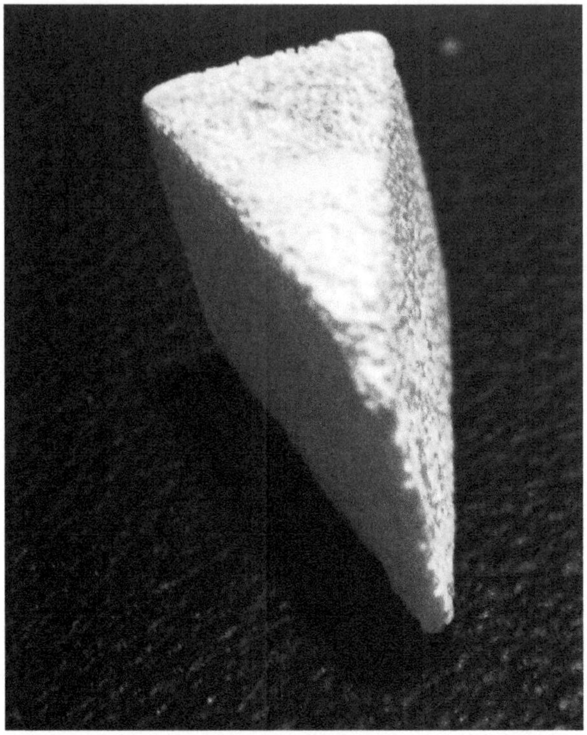

Figure 1 Freeze-dried bovine xenograft.

The sample was composed of patients aged between 20 and 60 years of age with talocalcaneal joint arthrosis after calcaneal fracture who showed significant loss of calcaneal height, limitation of hindfoot range of motion, hindfoot pain, and limitation to perform daily activities. Patients with open calcaneal fracture or osteomyelitis, or those with rheumatic disease, peripheral neuropathy or other diseases or deformities that hinder walking were excluded.

Table 1 summarizes the patients' data. There was one case of bilateral fracture of the calcaneus in each group, but only one side was operated on in this study. All patients were conservatively treated for the index calcaneal fracture. One case in the autograft group and two cases in the xenograft group had previously undergone lateral calcaneal wall decompression.

Clinical assessment was performed using the American Orthopedic Foot and Ankle Society (AOFAS) Ankle-Hindfoot Scale and the visual analog scale (VAS) for pain pre and postoperatively. Postoperative iliac donor site pain was independently assessed by the visual analog scale.

The following parameters were measured on the lateral weight bearing radiograph of the foot without

Table 1 Description of sample data

	Autograft	Xenograft
Sex*	4 F, 2 M	6 M
Age†	44.2 years (29–57)	47.2 years (31–56)
Side	4 right	4 right
Smoking	1 patient	3 patients
Time from fracture to surgery†	138 weeks (19–330)	134.3 weeks (36–362)
Follow-up†**	68 weeks (62–82)	48.3 weeks (38–58)

F: female, M: male. *p = 0.014. **p = 0.001. †Mean (minimum-maximum).

plaster at final followup: talocalcaneal angle, calcaneal-to-floor angle, talus-first metatarsal angle, talar tilt angle (in degrees), and talar height (in millimeters). Calcaneal width was measured (in millimeters) on the axial heel view of the calcaneus. The opposite side was considered normal for radiographic comparison purposes in all patients but the two with bilateral calcaneal fracture. Clinical and radiographic parameters assessments were done by third year orthopaedic residents with close supervision of the orthopedic surgeon instructor. Two independent blind raters retrospectively examined all lateral radiographs for evidence of solid union of the arthrodesis and graft integration, in addition to signs of loosening of the osteosynthesis material and type of bone graft used (autologous or xenograft). Solid union of the arthrodesis was defined as radiographic union of the talus, bone graft and the calcaneus, and graft integration was defined as the presence of host bone trabeculae replacing graft trabeculae, thus hiding individualization of the graft on radiographs (Easley et al. 2000). Length of time (in weeks) required for solid union of the arthrodesis or graft integration was defined as the first record agreed on by the two raters as long as both raters confirmed radiographic evidence of solid union or graft integration at the final follow-up evaluation. If there was no agreement between raters at the final radiographic evaluation, the case was considered as nonunion or not integrated, regardless of previous assessments. Radiographs were done monthly after surgery until arthrodesis union was considered and at final followup.

The following data were abstracted from the patients' medical records: duration of surgery, duration of cast immobilization, and postoperative complications.

Operative technique

Surgery was done by one single foot and ankle surgeon (HC). The patient was positioned supine with a pad under the ipsilateral hip. The lower limb was exsanguinated using an elastic bandage, and a pneumatic tourniquet was placed in the proximal third of the thigh. Calcaneal tendon lengthening was indicated in cases of ankle dorsiflexion less than 10°. An extended lateral L-shaped incision was made to approach the talocalcaneal joint with a single dissection toward the bone plane in all cases. The prominence in the lateral calcaneal wall was then resected. After opening and releasing the talocalcaneal joint capsule, cartilage of the posterior facet of the calcaneus and the talus was removed to expose the subchondral bone. The talocalcaneal space was opened with a distractor until correction of hindfoot bone relationships was achieved, as assessed by intraoperative radiographic control, and a graft block was interposed to fill the space obtained. A single 7.0 mm partially threaded cannulated screw was inserted from the calcaneus to the talus for fixation through the graft block. At the end of the procedure, the tourniquet was released for hemostasis and rinsing with saline, followed by subcutaneous closure with bioabsorbable suture and skin closure with nonabsorbable suture and placement of a plaster splint.

Bone graft was harvested from the anterolateral aspect of the iliac crest. The periosteum was elevated of the internal and external iliac wall, 3 cm posterior to the anterior superior iliac spine. A tricortical bone graft block of the desired size was harvested using an osteotome. Routine closure was performed after rinsing and hemostasis.

The plaster splint was applied for two postoperative weeks until sutures were removed, when the splint was replaced with a non-weight-bearing cast boot. After six weeks, partial weight-bearing was allowed with the cast boot until there was clinical and radiographic evidence of solid union of the arthrodesis, when weight-bearing was allowed as tolerated without immobilization and the motor rehabilitation program started.

Statistical analysis was performed using the following tests: the chi-square test to verify association between variables; the Student *t* test to compare means; Wilcoxon, Mann–Whitney and Levene's nonparametric tests to compare scores; and the kappa coefficient to assess interrater agreement. The significance level was set at 5%.

Results

According to the AOFAS Ankle-Hindfoot Scale, there was a significant improvement between preoperative and final followup scores in the autograft and xenograft groups ($p = 0.02$). There was no statistically significant difference between groups. A statistically significant difference was observed between preoperative and final followup VAS scores in the autograft group ($p = 0.028$) and in the xenograft group ($p = 0.046$), with no difference between groups (Table 2).

None of the patients who underwent the procedure to harvest autologous bone graft from the iliac crest had preoperative pain at the donor site. At the final followup, two patients were free of pain and four patients had pain with VAS scores ranging from 0.1 to 0.6. All patients

Table 2 Scores on the American Orthopedic Foot and Ankle Society (AOFAS) Ankle-Hindfoot Scale and visual analog scale (VAS) for pain

Group	n	AOFAS scale†		p*	VAS for pain†		p*
		Preop.	Postop.		Preop.	Postop.	
Autograft	6	37 (11.08)	63.83 (9.58)	0.02	4.73 (2.17)	1.87 (1.33)	0.028
Xenograft	6	38 (14.92)	73.83 (9.54)	0.02	5.53 (1.91)	2.72 (2.4)	0.046
Both	12	37.83 (12.56)	68.33 (10.77)	0.002	5.13 (1.99)	2.29 (2.01)	0.006

*Wilcoxon nonparametric test. †Mean (standard deviation).

showed a small area of hypoesthesia around the wound, without hindering the performance of daily activities. No major complications were observed in these patients.

Talocalcaneal height showed a statistically significant difference between pre and postoperative values in the autograft group ($p = 0.04$) and in the xenograft group ($p = 0.03$). There was a statistically significant difference between pre and postoperative talocalcaneal angle ($p = 0.04$) and talus-first metatarsal angle ($p = 0.04$) in the autograft group. In the xenograft group, calcaneal width ($p = 0.04$) showed a statistically significant difference pre and postoperatively. When each group was evaluated separately, no statistically significant difference was observed between postoperative radiographic parameters in relation to the contralateral side (Table 3).

The retrospective evaluation performed by the two blind raters revealed no statistically significant difference in time to union of the arthrodesis, which was achieved at an average of 5.33 weeks in the autograft group and 8.8 weeks in the xenograft group ($p = 0.077$). A statistically significant difference was observed for graft integration, which occurred after an average of 10.67 weeks in the autograft group and 28.8 weeks in the xenograft group ($p = 0.016$) (Table 4). Solid union of the arthrodesis and graft integration were achieved in all six cases in the autograft group and in five out of six cases in the xenograft group (Figure 2). One case in the xenograft group was considered as nonunion (Figure 3). The raters did not identify signs of loosening of the osteosynthesis material in any case. Interrater agreement for identification of the type of graft used was poor (kappa coefficient 0.17) for rater #1 and substantial (kappa coefficient 0.67) for rater #2.

Mean duration of cast immobilization was 10.33 weeks (range, 8 to 12) in the autograft group and 13.33 weeks (range, 10 to 18) in the xenograft group ($p = 0.054$). Mean duration of surgery was 114.67 (SD 8.14) minutes in the autograft group and 96.67 (SD 6.83) minutes in the xenograft group ($p = 0.002$).

At the index procedure the posterior calcaneal tuberosity was removed in one patient of each group because it was still proeminent over the Achilles tendon after realignment of the hindfoot. Calcaneal tendon lengthening was performed in two cases in the autograft group and in three cases in the xenograft group. There was one case of wound dehiscence in the autograft group and two cases in the xenograft group, which were not related with previous surgery. In all patients, wounds were allowed to heal by secondary intention after serial dressing changes, with no need for further surgical intervention. In two patients in the autograft group the screw used for internal fixation was removed after 60 weeks, because its head was prominent in the calcaneus and caused discomfort wearing regular shoes. One patient in the autograft group persisted with a varus hindfoot and underwent a calcaneus valgus osteotomy with cannulated screw fixation to restore hindfoot alignment. One patient in the autograft group developed complex regional pain syndrome (CRPS) in the immediate postoperative period and had the cannulated screw removed in the 18th week, since it appeared to be prominent dorsally into the body of the talus. The patient continued with pain and daily activities restriction afterwards, despite use of pain medication, shoe modification and physical therapy. In one patient in the xenograft group a bony prominence in the medial wall of the calcaneus was resected in the 54th week, as it was causing friction against the flexor hallucis longus tendon, which alleviated symptoms promptly. There was involvement of the sural nerve with complaints of paresthesia and hypoesthesia on the lateral aspect of the hindfoot in four patients in the autograft group and in three in the xenograft group. Five out of six patients in the autograft group and four out of six patients in the xenograft group complained of diffuse pain in the hindfoot on physical examination at the final followup. None of the patients that entered the study were excluded from data analisys.

Based on the data obtained in our study, a power calculation indicated that eleven cases in each group would be required to assess time to union of the arthrodesis and five cases in each group to assess time to graft integration with a study power of 80% at a significance level of 5%.

Discussion

In the surgical treatment of sequelae of calcaneal fractures, all possible causes of pain should be considered and the anatomy of the hindfoot restored (Nickisch and Anderson 2006; Paley and Hall 1993; Savva and Saxby 2007). Carr *et al.* (Carr et al. 1988) described the subtalar

Table 3 Radiographic parameters

Group	X-ray	TC height*†	Calcaneal width†	CF angle*††	TC angle*††	TFM angle*††	Talar tilt angle††
Autograft	Contralateral	67 (63.5/69.75) [p = 0.18]¶	31.5 (22.5/34.75)	17 (12.25/22.5) [p = 0.11]	41 (32.5/49.5) [p = 0.11]	3 (−6.25/10) [p = 0.18]	21.5 (15.75/28.75) [p = 1.0]
	Preoperative	64 (60/71) [p = 0.04]¶	42 (35/49)¶[p = 0.47]	14 (10.5/21) [p = 0.85]	29 (22/33) [p = 0.04]	12.5 (7.5/17) [p = 0.04]	13.5 (9/18) [p = 0.07]
	Postoperative	69 (63.5/80)	40.5 (36/45.75)	20 (7/23)	36 (30/42)	10 (0/11.5)	18 (16/25)
Xenograft	Contralateral	78 (77.25/79.5) [p = 0.11]	35 (29/35)¶[p = 0.1]	21 (18.5/23.5) [p = 0.14]	46.5 (42.75/51) [p = 0.07]	1.5 (0/3.75) [p = 0.1]	24 (24/28.5) [p = 0.11]
	Preoperative	71.5 (69.5/75) [p = 0.03]	48 (39.75/50.5) [p = 0.04]	13 (11.5/19.75) [p = 0.6]	32 (22/42.5) [p = 0.1]	5.5 (0/13.25) [p = 0.89]	17.5 (9.75/24.75) [p = 0.79]
	Postoperative	76.5 (72.75/80.75)	42 (39/45.25)	15 (10/22)	38 (30.5/44.5)	8.5 (3/10)	18 (16.25/21)
Both	Contralateral	73.5 (66/78) [p = 0.04]	33 (29.5/35) [p = 0.07]	20.5 (14.25/22.75) [p = 0.04]	43.5 (40.5/51) [p = 0.02]	1.5 (−3/8.5) [p = 0.04]	24 (19.5/28.75) [p = 0.11]
	Preoperative	69 (63/72.75) [p = 0.003]	45 (37/50) [p = 0.07]	13 (11.25/19.5) [p = 0.54]	29 (22.5/36) [p = 0.01]	10.5 (0.5/15.25) [p = 0.12]	16 (10/18) [p = 0.06]
	Postoperative	76 (69/79)	42 (37/50)	18 (10/22)	36 (30/44)	10 (4/10)	18 (17/22)

*TC height: talocalcaneal height; CF angle: calcaneal-to-floor angle; TC angle: talocalcaneal angle; TFM angle: talus-first metatarsal angle. †Height and width in millimeters. ††Angle in degrees. ¶ Median (25th percentile/75th percentile) [p value in relation to the postoperative period]: Wilcoxon nonparametric test.

Table 4 Length of time for solid union of the arthrodesis and bone graft integration

Group	Union*	Integration*
Autograft	5.33 (2/8)	10.67 (6/28)
Xenograft	8.8 (6/14)	28.8 (10/38)
p†	0.077	0.016

*Mean in weeks (range). †P value: Levene's test.

arthrodesis with interposition of bone graft to restore normal alignment of the hindfoot and thus achieve functional improvement, since they believed that loss of talocalcaneal height leads to painful anterior tibiotalar impingement. Myerson and Quill (Myerson and Quill 1993) indicate this type of arthrodesis when there is more than 8 mm loss of talocalcaneal height in relation to the contralateral side or when there is evidence of anterior ankle impingement demonstrated by a talar tilt angle less than 20°. Chandler *et al.* (Chandler et al. 1999) suggest that this type of arthrodesis should be performed in cases of anterior ankle pain and ankle dorsiflexion less than 10°.

Radiographic evaluation of union of the arthrodesis and graft integration is subjective. The length of time required for union of the arthrodesis was higher in the xenograft group (average 8.8 weeks) then in the autograft group (average 5.33), although not statistically significant (p = 0.077), as evaluated by two independent blind raters. Our patients were placed in a non-weight-bearing cast for 6 weeks followed by partial weight-bearing until there was clinical and radiographic evidence of union. Mean immobilization time was 10.33 weeks in the autograft group and 13.33 weeks in the xenograft group, which difference was not statistically significant. The mean immobilization time employed by the authors was longer than the mean time required for union of the arthrodesis according to the radiographic criteria used by both blind raters. Time to arthrodesis union considered as the time of immobilization favors the results described in the literature that range from 12 to 20 weeks (mean, 14 weeks) with fresh-frozen allografts and from 10 to 30 weeks with autografts for a solid union to be obtained (Bednarz et al. 1997; Easley et al. 2000; Trnka et al. 2001).

Other factors that may be related to the occurrence of nonunion include smoking and presence of avascular necrosis of bone (Clare et al. 2005; Easley et al. 2000; Trnka et al. 2001). In the present study, the only case of nonunion occurred in one of the three smokers in the xenograft group that also showed signs of calcaneal bone sclerosis, suggestive of bone necrosis, at final x-ray evaluation (Figure 3).

Time to graft integration, 28.8 weeks in the xenograft group and 10.67 weeks in the autograft group, had a statistically significant difference (p = 0.016). Freeze-dried bone grafts, due to the process which they undergo, are considered to have osteoconductive properties, with no osteoinductive or osteogenic characteristics, which might delay graft integration (Hartl et al. 2004). Even fresh-frozen allograft need 24 to 48 weeks to revascularizate and integrate (Garras et al. 2008; Myerson et al. 2005). The association of osteoinductive properties to freeze-dried xenograft bones, to maybe increase union rate and accelerate graft integration, is open to further research.

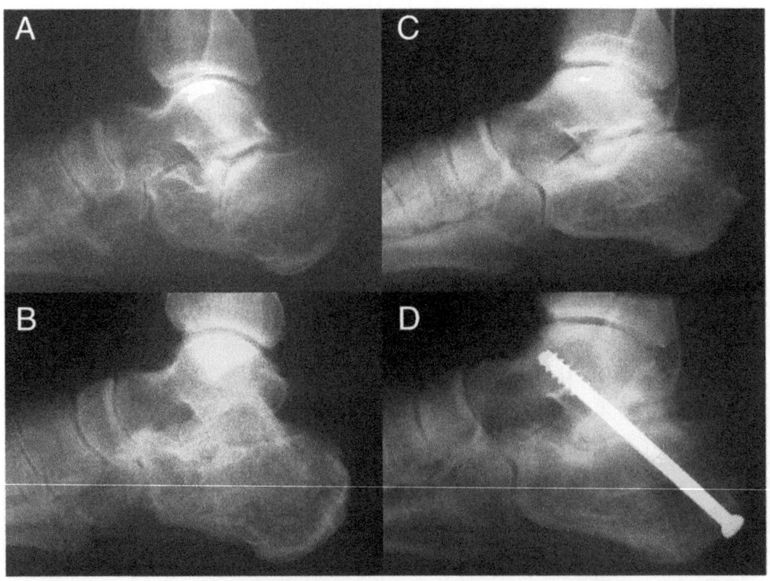

Figure 2 Lateral radiograph focused on rearfoot showing evidence of solid union of subtalar arthrodesis with use of autologous iliac crest graft (preoperative (A), last followup (B)) and freeze-dried bovine xenograft (preoperative (C), last followup (D)).

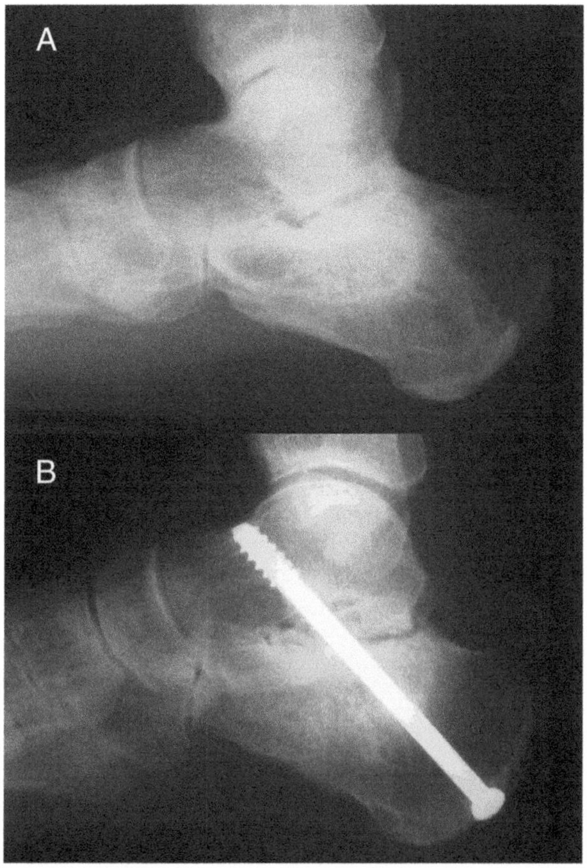

Figure 3 Preoperative (A) and final postoperative (B) lateral radiograph of subtalar arthrodesis with interposition of freeze-dried bovine xenograft in the case considered as nonunion.

The AOFAS scale is a validated, widely accepted rating scale (Schepers et al. 2008). In our series, patients showed a statistically significant improvement as assessed by the AOFAS scale or VAS for pain. AOFAS scores improved 30.5 points, from a preoperative average of 37.8 to 68.3 points postoperatively ($p = 0.002$), and VAS scores improved 2.84, from a preoperative average of 5.13 to 2.29 postoperatively ($p = 0.006$). These values are close to those described in the literature, with the improvement in AOFAS scores ranging from 32 to 50 points, from a preoperative average between 20 and 40 points to an average between 69 and 75 points postoperatively (Amendola and Lammens 1996; Bednarz et al. 1997; Garras et al. 2008; Rammelt et al. 2004; Trnka et al. 2001). VAS scores range from a preoperative average between 6.07 and 8.1 to an average between 2.0 and 2.56 postoperatively (Amendola and Lammens 1996; Trnka et al. 2001). Nevertheless, all six patients in the autograft group and four patients in the xenograft group complained of pain in the operated foot at the final followup. Persistent residual pain after arthrodesis with interpositional graft was described by Clare *et al.* (Clare et al. 2005) in 64% of 45 patients after a mean followup of 5.3 years and by Marti *et al.* (Marti et al. 1999) in 82% of 19 patients after a mean followup of nine years. We agree with Chan and Alexander (Chan and Alexander 1997) who stated that, although pain relief is neither complete nor universal, patient satisfaction is high.

The analysis of radiographic parameters revealed a statistically significant improvement in talocalcaneal height from pre to postoperative values in both groups. This improvement, however, was not sufficient to equal the talocalcaneal height obtained postoperatively with the contralateral side, regarded as the normal parameter for the patient, with a persisting statistically significant difference ($p = 0.04$) when data from both groups were analyzed together. However, when groups were evaluated separately, no significant difference was found between postoperative and contralateral side values. This may be due to a small number of cases in each group. The talar tilt angle did not show significant differences at any time point. The calcaneus was found to be significantly narrower, as measured by its width, only between the pre and postoperative periods in the xenograft group (Table 3). The amount of correction of these radiographic variables is not uniform in the literature (Burton et al. 1998; Pollard and Schuberth 2008; Rammelt et al. 2004) and has not shown, in some studies, correlation with clinical findings (Chandler et al. 1999; Flemister et al. 2000). Chen *et al.* (Chen et al. 1998) observed that correction of the talocalcaneal height was achieved in 80.1% of cases with good functional results and in only 47.6% of cases with fair results. Marti *et al.* (Marti et al. 1999) did not find correlation between radiological measurements and clinical findings, except for the height of the calcaneal fat pad. The time from fracture to arthrodesis is also indicated by some authors as a factor that may influence the amount of correction possible due to retraction of periarticular tissues of the hindfoot (Amendola and Lammens 1996; Burton et al. 1998; Rammelt et al. 2004). In our series, the mean time from fracture to arthrodesis was 136.17 weeks, which may have influenced the non-correction of some radiographic parameters.

Solid union of subtalar arthrodesis with interposition of autologous iliac crest bone graft in the treatment of malunited fractures of the calcaneus is described in the literature as occurring in 86 to 100% of cases (Amendola and Lammens 1996; Bednarz et al. 1997; Burton et al. 1998; Chan and Alexander 1997; Chen et al. 1998; Myerson and Quill 1993; Rammelt et al. 2004; Thermann et al. 1999). The procedure to harvest bone graft from the iliac crest can cause complications in up to 49% of cases (Finkemeier 2002; Seiler and Johnson 2000). This complication rate is lower for foot arthrodesis cases, affecting only up to 6% (Burton et al. 1998; Trnka et al. 2001). Because it is a surgical procedure that adds the possibility of comorbidities, iliac crest bone graft harvesting is not always easily accepted by patients (Pollard and Schuberth 2008), and is also likely to result in longer operative time and higher costs (Scranton 2002). The duration of surgery was 18% higher in the group undergoing iliac crest bone graft harvesting which was statistically significant (p = 0.002).

Other sources of bone graft have been described in the literature (Kalamchi and Evans 1977). Clare *et al.* (Clare et al. 2005) described good results in 40 patients (45 feet) who underwent subtalar arthrodesis with interposition of autologous bone graft harvested from the lateral wall of the calcaneus, achieving a 93.5% union rate. The use of allografts in this situation showed, in some studies, solid union in only 20 to 40% of cases (Easley et al. 2000; Trnka et al. 2001). Other authors, however, have reported better results using allografts, with union rates similar to those achieved using autografts (Myerson et al. 2005; Pollard and Schuberth 2008; Scranton 2002). Nickisch and Anderson (Nickisch and Anderson 2006) indicate the use of allografts when bone grafts over 1 cm in height are needed for interposition in the subtalar arthrodesis. Garras *et al.* (Garras et al. 2008) described a series of 21 cases using fresh-frozen allografts for interposition in the subtalar arthrodesis with 90.5% union rate, although, in seven cases, grafts were used in association with platelet-rich plasma.

Due to limited availability of fresh-frozen allografts in our department, we have started research and development of a bone bank with freeze-dried bovine bone grafts (Galia et al. 2009a; Galia et al. 2009b; Macedo et al. 1999). In the medical literature, there are only a few studies describing the use of xenografts (Laurencin and El-Amin 2008; Zabeu and Mercadante 2008). Their use in different situations has yielded good results concerning incorporation of the graft and union of the arthrodesis (Malca et al. 1996; Salama 1983; Säveland et al. 1994). In the only study found in the literature on the use of bone xenograft in arthrodeses of the foot and ankle, Thompson *et al.* (Thompson et al. 2002) described five cases that developed nonunion and required further surgical intervention using autografts to achieve solid union of the arthrodesis. Those authors contraindicated the use of xenografts. In our experience, solid union of subtalar arthrodesis with interposition of freeze-dried xenograft bone block was achieved in five out of six cases (83% union rate) and in all six cases (100% union rate) with autologous tricortical iliac crest bone graft after a mean followup of 58.17 weeks.

The use of an extended lateral L-shaped approach allows adequate visualization of the peroneal tendons and calcaneocuboid and subtalar joints, also allowing the lateral calcaneal wall prominence to be easily resected (Clare et al. 2005). However, this approach poses a potential risk for incision closure, mainly when grafts of great height are used, therefore more vertical incisions are preferred in these cases (Pollard and Schuberth 2008). In our study, three cases (25%) developed wound dehiscence. Clare *et al.* (Clare et al. 2005), using this approach, reported the occurrence of wound healing problems in 24% of 45 operated feet. Another common complication is sural nerve injury, which may occur in up to 17% of cases (Rammelt et al. 2004), and may result from direct injury or stretch injury due to increased talocalcaneal height. (Garras et al. 2008) Complaints related to sural nerve injury in our series accounted for seven cases (58%), a complaint rate higher than expected, which might be related to the surgical learning curve for this technique.

Conclusion

Solid union of subtalar arthrodesis after calcaneal fracture was achieved in all six cases that we used autologous iliac crest graft and in five out of six cases that we used freeze-dried bovine xenograft. There was no statistically significant difference in the length of time required for solid union to occur with the numbers available. Time to integration of freeze-dried bovine xenografts was statistically higher than that of autologous iliac crest grafts. The limited number of patients is a weakness of this study and the results are preliminary, but promising, which stimulates further research using freeze-dried bovine xenografts as a bone substitute.

Competing interests
None of the authors have competing interests. The authors declare that they have no competing interests.

Authors' contributions
CH carried out surgeries and drafted the article. GP grouped and analysed data and drafted the article. MAL grouped and analysed data. CRG supervised the study and drafted the article. All authors read and approved the final manuscript.

References

Amendola A, Lammens P (1996) Subtalar arthrodesis using interposition iliac crest bone graft after calcaneal fracture. Foot Ankle Int 17(10):608–614
Bednarz PA, Beals TC, Manoli A II (1997) Subtalar distraction bone block fusion: an assessment of outcome. Foot Ankle Int 18(12):785–791
Burton DC, Olney BW, Horton GA (1998) Late results of subtalar distraction fusion. Foot Ankle Int 19(4):197–202
Carr J, Hansen S, Benirschke SK (1988) Subtalar distraction bone block fusion for late complications of os calcis. Foot Ankle 9(2):81–86
Chan SCF, Alexander IJ (1997) Subtalar arthrodesis with interpositional tricortical iliac crest graft for late pain and deformity after calcaneus fracture. Foot Ankle Int 18(10):613–615
Chandler JT, Bonar SK, Anderson RB, Davis H (1999) Results of in situ subtalar arthrodesis for late sequelae of calcaneus fractures. Foot Ankle Int 20(1):18–24
Chen YJ, Huang TJ, Hsu KTY, Hsu RW, Chen CW (1998) Subtalar distractional realignment arthrodesis with wedge bone grafting and lateral decompression of calcaneal malunion. J Trauma 45(4):729–737
Clare MP, Lee WE, Sanders RW (2005) Intermediate to long-term results of a treatment protocol for calcaneal fracture malunions. J Bone Join Surg Am 87-A(5):963–973
Easley ME, Trnka H-J, Schon LC, Myerson MS (2000) Isolated subtalar arthrodesis. J Bone Joint Surg Am 82-A(5):613–624

Finkemeier CG (2002) Bone-grafting and bone-graft substitutes. J Bone Join Surg Am 84-A(3):454–464
Flemister ASJR, Infante AF, Sanders RW, Walling AK (2000) Subtalar arthrodesis for complications of intra-articular calcaneal fractures. Foot Ankle Int 21(5):392–399
Galia CR, Macedo CA, Rosito R, Mello TM, Camargo LMAQ, Moreira LF (2008) *In vitro* and *in vivo* evaluation of lyophilized bovine bone biocompatibility. Clinics 63:801–806
Galia CR, Macedo CAS, Rosito R, Moreira LF (2009a) Osteointegração de enxertos liofilizados impactados. Acta Ortop Bras 17(2):24–28
Galia CR, Macedo CA, Rosito R, Camargo LM, Marinho DR, Moreira LF (2009b) Femoral and acetabular revision using impacted nondemineralized freeze-dried bone allografts. J Orthop Sci 14(3):259–265
Garras DN, Santangelo JR, Wang DW, Easley ME (2008) Subtalar distraction arthrodesis using interpositional frozen structural allograft. Foot Ankle Int 29(6):561–567
Hartl A, Bitzan P, Wanivenhaus A, Kotz R (2004) Faster integration of human allograft bone than of the bovine substitute Lubboc. Acta Orthop Scand 75(2):217–220
Kakiuchi M, Ono K, Nishimura A, Shiokawa H (1996) Preparation of bank bone using defatting, freeze-drying and sterilization with ethylene oxide gas. Part 1. Experimental evaluation of its efficacy and safety. Int Orthop 20(3):142–146
Kalamchi A, Evans JG (1977) Posterior subtalar fusion. J Bone Joint Surg Br 59-B(3):287–289
Laurencin CT, El-Amin SF (2008) Xenotransplantation in orthopaedic surgery. J Am Acad Orthop Surg 16(1):4–8
Lim EVA, Leung JPF (2001) Complications of intraarticular calcaneal fractures. Clin Orthop Relat Res 391:7–16
Macedo CAS, Galia CR, Silva ALB, César PC, Sanches PRS, Duarte LS, Müller LM (1999) Comparação de resistência à compressão do osso bovino congelado e liofilizado. Rev Bras Ortop 34(9/10):529–533
Malca SA, Roche PH, Rosset E, Pellet W (1996) Cervical interbody xenograft with plate fixation: evaluation of fusion after 7 years of use in post-traumatic discoligamentous instability. Spine 21(6):685–690
Marti RK, Heus JAC, Roolker W, Poolman RW, Besslaar PP (1999) Subtalar arthrodesis with correction of deformity after fractures of the os calcis. J Bone Joint Surg Br 81-B(4):611–616
Myerson MS, Quill GE (1993) Late complications of fractures of the calcaneus. J Bone Joint Surg Am 75-A(3):331–341
Myerson MS, Neufeld SK, Uribe J (2005) Fresh-frozen structural allografts in the foot and ankle. J Bone Joint Surg Am 87-A(1):113–120
Nickisch F, Anderson RB (2006) Post-calcaneus fracture reconstruction. Foot Ankle Clin N Am 11:85–103
Paley D, Hall H (1993) Intra-articular fractures of the calcaneus. A critical analysis of results and prognostic factors. J Bone Joint Surg Am 75-A(3):342–354
Pollard JD, Schuberth JM (2008) Posterior bone block distraction arthrodesis of the subtalar joint: a review of 22 cases. J Foot Ankle Surg 47(3):191–198
Rammelt S, Grass R, Zawadski T (2004) Biewener. A; Zwipp, H: Foot function after subtalar distraction bone-block arthrodesis. J Bone Joint Surg Br 86-B(5):659–668
Salama R (1983) Xenogeneic bone grafting in humans. Clin Orthop Relat Res 174(4):113–121
Säveland H, Aspenberg P, Zygmunt S, Herrlin K, Cristensson D, Rydholm U (1994) Bovine bone grafting in occipito-cervical fusion for atlanto-axial instability in rheumatoid arthritis. Acta Neurochir 127:186–190
Savva N, Saxby TS (2007) In Situ arthrodesis with lateral-wall ostectomy for the sequelae of fracture of the os calcis. J Bone Joint Surg Br 89-B(7):919–925
Schepers T, Heetveld MJ, Mulder PGH, Patka P (2008) Clinical outcome scoring of intra-articular calcaneal fractures. J Foot Ankle Surg 47(3):213–218
Scranton PE Jr (2002) Use of bone graft substitutes in lower extremity reconstructive surgery. Foot Ankle Int 23(8):689–692
Seiler JG III, Johnson J (2000) Iliac crest autogenous bone grafting: donor site complications. J South Orthop Assoc 9(2):91–97
Thermann H, Hüfner T, Schratt H-E, Held C, Tscherne H (1999) Die subtalare Fusion nach konservativ oder operativ behandelter intraartikulärer Kalkaneusfraktur. Unfallchirurg 102:13–22
Thompson NS, Swain WD, Thompson RD, Dilworth GR (2002) Non-union in ankle and hindfoot arthrodeses using xenograft. Foot Ankle Surg 8:239–244
Trnka H-J, Easley ME, Lam PW-C, Anderson CD, Shon LC, Myerson MS (2001) Subtalar distraction bone block arthrodesis. J Bone Joint Surg Br 83-B(6):849–854
Zabeu JLA, Mercadante MT (2008) Substitutos ósseos comparados ao enxerto ósseo autólogo em cirurgia ortopédica - Revisão sistemática da literatura. Rev Bras Ortop 43(3):59–68

A new graphical method to display data sets representing biomechanical knee behaviour

Silvia Pianigiani[1*], Jos Vander Sloten[2], Walter Pascale[1], Luc Labey[3] and Bernardo Innocenti[4]

Abstract

Background: When researchers describe data from their studies, there is no rule defining the best way to represent results. Therefore, collecting and explaining results from personal research or understanding data from publications is not always straightforward. These issues are even worse in fields such as biomedical engineering, where researchers from different backgrounds, usually engineers and surgeons, need to interact and exchange information. For these reasons, the purpose of this study is to introduce and illustrate an innovative method to represent, concisely and intuitively, biomechanical knee behavior, called KneePrints.

Methods: To test the KneePrints method, a huge amount of data from previously published sensitivity analyses were used and represented both with conventional techniques and with this new graphical method. Then, a survey has been distributed among different international specialists in the orthopedic field, such as surgeons and researchers. In the survey, interviewees were asked to select the favorite method that addressed to be the most effective to show the same results.

Results: Collecting the outcomes from the survey, the KneePrints method resulted to be more effective than standard graphs, such as tables and histograms. KneePrints method has been selected to be clearer in representing outputs and more immediate in results understanding independently from the occupation of the interviewees by the survey. The general preference for the KneePrints is 63 %, up to 74 % being surgeons' choice.

Conclusions: The innovative KneePrints method has been endorsed to be effective in representing and making more understandable knee joint outputs. This method can be extended also to other topics.

Keywords: Graphical method; Biomechanical analysis; Knee

Background

When researchers describe data from their study, there is no accepted rule that defines the best way to represent results. Therefore, collecting and explaining results from personal study, or understanding data from the literature, is not always straightforward. These issues are even worse in the biomedical engineering field in which people with different backgrounds, usually engineers and clinicians, need to interact and exchange information.

By definition, graphical displays complement verbal discourse in written documents and in oral presentations as a more powerful form of effective redundancy. Through spatial relationships and potential richness of detail, they provide insights in ways that text cannot hope to match (Doumont 2009).

Graphs are mainly used to show comparisons between data sets, overlapping of data, compositions of data, correlations among variables, or evolutions of a variable (Best 2005).

The graph is a visually reproduced concept that is aimed to bridge the gap between meaning across languages and different research fields.

Designing good charts presents more challenges than tabular display as it draws also on the artistic talent of the scientist; in fact, the complete knowledge and understanding of own data is necessary together with a good sense of how the audience will visualize and understand the chart's graphical elements independently from the structure of the dataset as, often, the structure of the data set largely suggests the type

* Correspondence: silvia.pianigiani84@gmail.com
[1]IRCCS Istituto Ortopedico Galeazzi, via via R. Galeazzi 4, 20161 Milan, Italy
Full list of author information is available at the end of the article

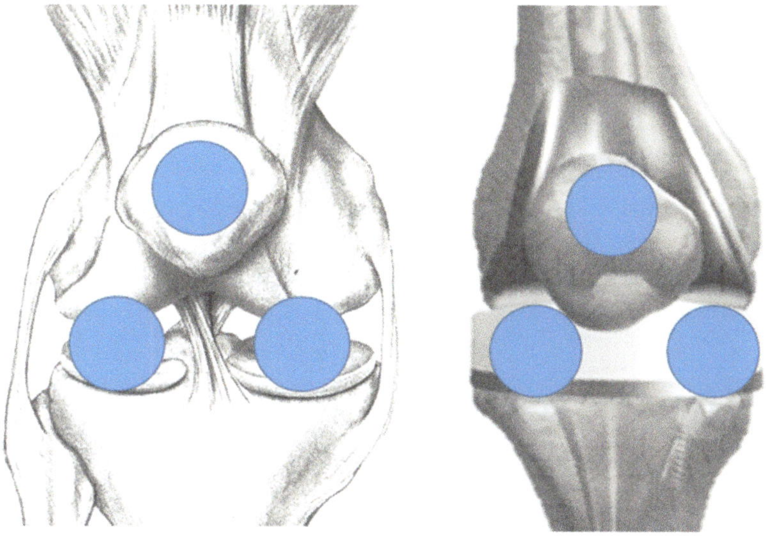

Fig. 1 On the selected background, the position of the circle graphs indicates directly which response is described, for example, the medial tibio-femoral contact force graphic is placed on the medial interface between the femur and the tibia bones for the native joints and femoral and tibial component for a knee with a total knee arthroplasty

of graph to be selected (Coles 1997, Few 2004). Poor structure ruins otherwise effective graphs by accidentally distorting the data, making them hard to read, or distracting the readers if purposefully misleading (Doumont 2009).

Unfortunately, it could happen that researchers have a straightforward overview of their represented results while the reader can not immediately understand the meaning of the results section of these papers, especially when there are mainly graphs and images to show the outputs.

As there is no standard method to be used to show data, authors can decide which is the best method for presenting their work, but the chosen method may not be fully understandable for the readers.

Sometimes, a compromise between details and accuracy is made in showing results, especially when a big amount of data has been collected.

In literature, papers usually present data through tables, pie charts, and histograms to show all the results, but often confuse the reader or overflow him with information (Innocenti et al. 2011, Pianigiani et al. 2012).

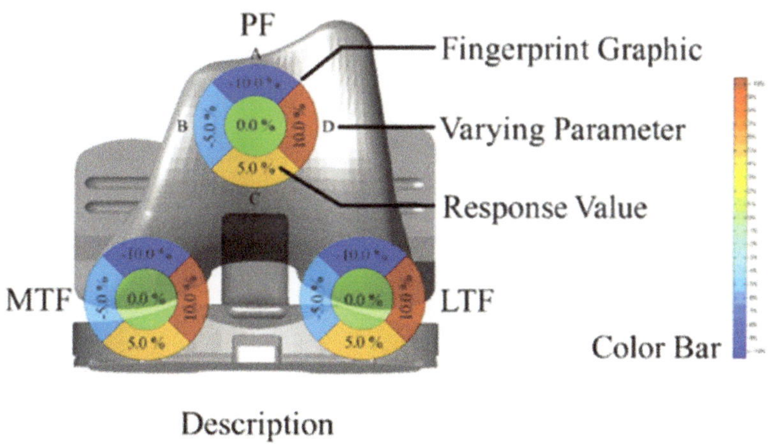

Fig. 2 The standard graphic proposed in this study consists of circular graphics overlaid to a specific background. For example, for the KneePrints after a sensitivity analysis, circular graphs are sited on a specific total knee arthroplasty design at the patellofemoral (PF), medial tibiofemoral (MTF) and lateral tibiofemoral (LTF) locations. The description may indicate a fixed parameter for combined configurations studies or the varying parameter for single configurations. A, B, C, and D indicate the varying parameter configuration and the response value is displayed in text and in colour (according to the colour bar)

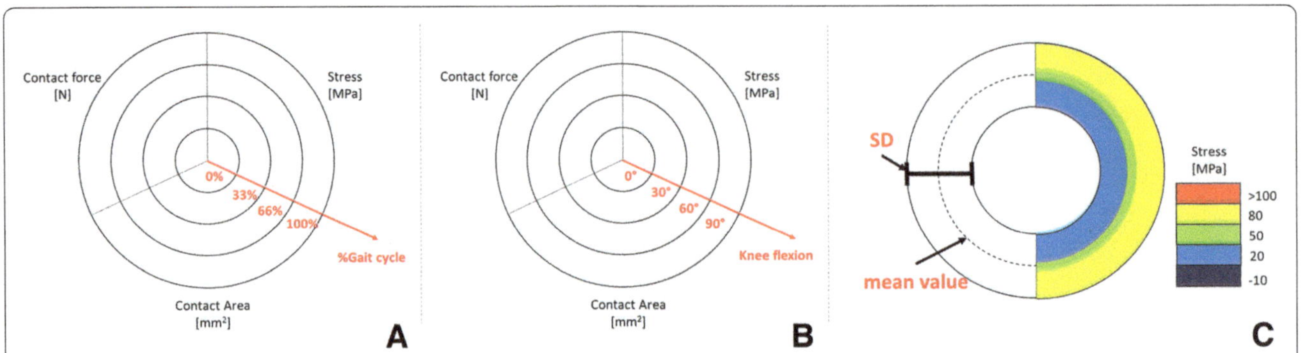

Fig. 3 Possible solutions to express different outcomes in function of the percentage of a simulated task, i.e. gait cycle (**a**), or a certain knee flexion (**b**). Data can be expressed as absolute values (**a**,**b**) or expressed as mean values and their standard deviations (**c**). **c** shows an example of application for stress outputs for which, i.e., mean value is 50 and SD =30

Looking at literature about biomechanics of knee joint, a large number of studies has been published. These studies are based on different techniques such as experimental tests and in vitro tests (Arnout et al. 2014, Delport et al. 2013, Heesterbeek et al. 2014), in vivo measurements (Battaglia et al. 2014, Fregly et al. 2012, Kutzner et al. 2011), numerical analyses (Fitzpatrick and Rullkoetter 2014, Innocenti et al. 2014, Zelle et al. 2011), imaging or biologic tests (Victor et al. 2009, Worsley et al. 2011, Zdero et al. 2001). In these works, knee movements and forces are expressed in function of several motor tasks that can be performed both during daily activities and in some extreme situations, such as sport activities, and comparing healthy or pre-operative knee conditions with post-operative configurations. The method of representation is often typical for that specific area in which the analysis has been performed, but less common in other fields and sometimes also dependent on the technique in use.

Aiming to find an innovative graphical method to show datasets representing knee biomechanics, a new technique called "KneePrints" has been proposed. Thanks to its customizable nature, the KneePrints graph can be adopted for several situations and also to represent data from sensitivity analyses.

Introducing the KneePrints, the first aim is to define a new methodology to bridge the gap between making presentable and explainable data, about knee biomechanics, for the writer and so, making the readers able to manage the full flow of represented biomechanics data and to improve its comprehension.

To demonstrate the efficacy of this new method, it has been tested on an already published set of data (Innocenti et al. 2011). To evaluate the perception of different audiences in the biomedical field, a survey was proposed to surgeons and researches. In the survey, this new technique has been compared with more conventional presentation methods for the same data set. In the survey, distributed by hand and on line to international operators in the

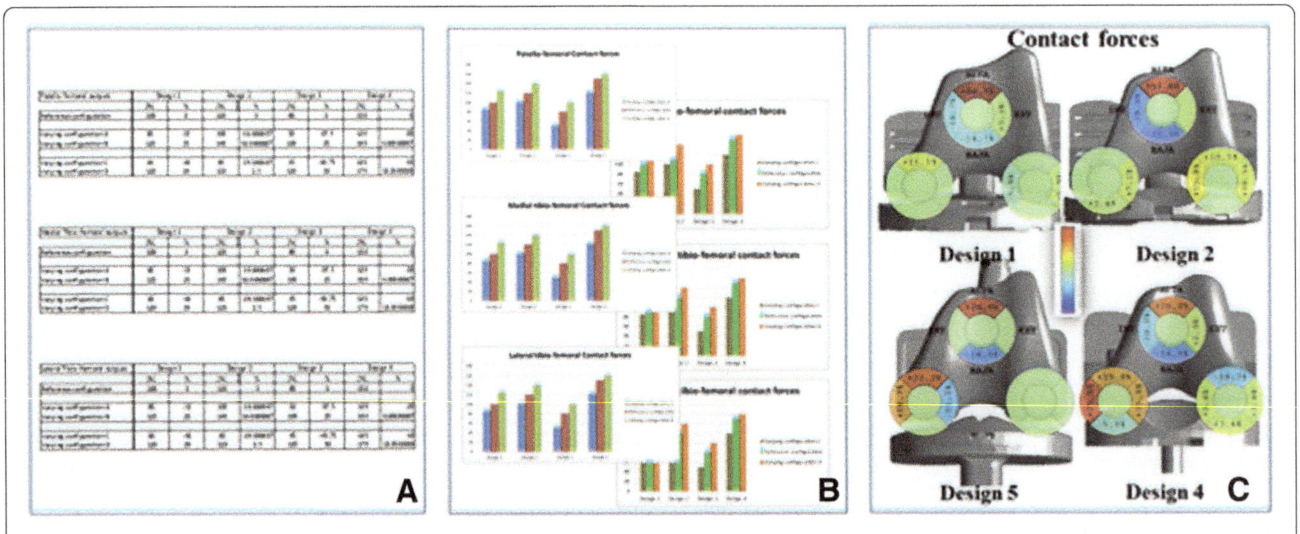

Fig. 4 Possible graphical methods to represent the outputs after the same sensitivity analysis: **a** table, **b** histogram, **c** KneePrints

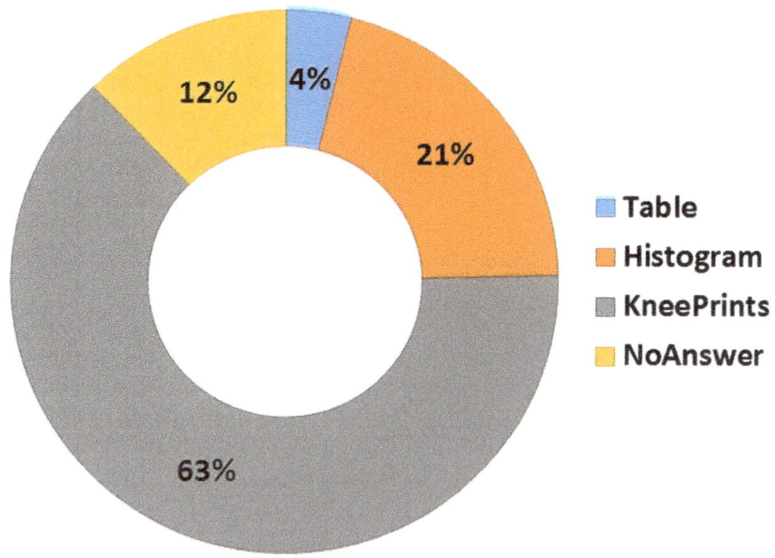

Fig. 5 Results from the survey about the preferred method, among table, histogram or Kneeprints, for representing data outputs after the same sensitivity analysis

biomechanical field, a detailed description of the proposed method was also provided.

Methods

The KneePrints graph aims to represent how the joint's biomechanics changes according to daily motor tasks inputs or any other variations, such as, but not limited to, changes in anatomical factors or knee implant component types and positions.

As shown in the template in Fig. 1, the outputs are directly represented in a circle positioned over the analyzed structures located in the background both for a native knee and for a knee with a total knee arthroplasty.

The KneePrints can be made after a conventional table is filled with all the outputs recorded from standard or sensitivity analyses. Once all the calculations are terminated, in case of standard analysis, a relative coloured bar can be defined to take into account the range and the values of the outputs. The coloured bar can indicate,

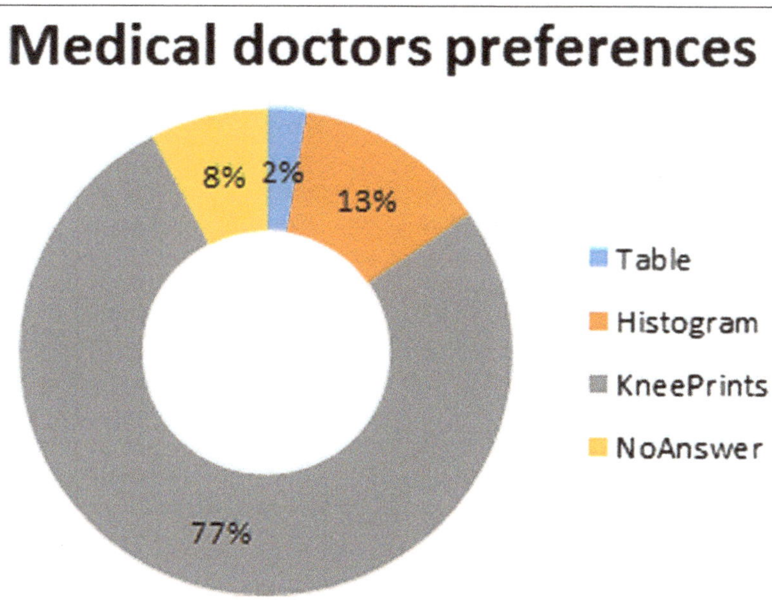

Fig. 6 Results from the survey about the preferred method of representation by medical doctors

for example, with a green colour the reference configuration, and with a red and a blue colour respectively an increase or a decrease of the output value with respect to the reference value.

In the case of sensitivity analyses, a comparison among each deviated configuration and the reference can be performed and the result can eventually be represented in percentage of variation. While filling the KneePrints graph is quite straightforward for standard analysis, for a multi-parametric analysis more details should be added to improve the findings understanding. For example, the circle graphs could consist of two (or more) concentric circles indicating, for example, the inner circle the reference configuration, while the outer rings can be subdivided to account for multiple simulated configurations considered. An example is shown in Fig. 2. For the sake of clarity, in each section of the circular graph, the value of the outputs or its change expressed in percentage should be optionally indicated. Then, according to the previously defined coloured bar, that indicates different thresholds of changes, the inner part of the graph is green filled, while each section of the outer ring is coloured to indicate the relative change of the output. Moreover, a label describing which altered configuration is considered in each part of the ring could be added (Fig. 2).

The previous description is mainly dedicated to sensitivity analysis, however the KneePrints can also be adopted to express data from other analysis such as in-vivo or in-vitro tests. In these situations it is often important to provide an overview of one or several outputs with respect to the knee flexion achieved during a specific task. For these cases, Fig. 3a and 3b show how the ring to be imposed on the back ground could be subdivided. In detail, both figures are subdivided in three main regions that are dedicate to different outputs. Each region is then subdivided in portions of rings that are referred to different percentage of the analyzed motion, i.e. Fig. 3a shows a possible subdivision for the gait cycle, or different knee flexions (Fig. 3b) achieved during the simulated task. On the other hand, often it is important to express mean values outputs and their standard deviations. Figure 3c show a possible template for such data representation.

To generate a KneePrints graph, the user can decide to use the favorite graphical software. The method is not strictly linked to a particular software.

Once the KneePrints is obtained, there is a large amount of information to could be extracted. First of all, looking at the picture, the reader will see if the analysis is about a native knee or a knee with a prosthesis. In the case of a knee with a prosthesis, the reader can visualize its design and its features. Second, in the case of a standard analysis, data concerning knee contact forces or knee kinematics are described in the areas relative to tibio-femoral and patello-femoral responses, or also ligaments outputs, if it is needed. Third, if outputs from a sensitivity analysis are shown, the reader can obtain additional multiple information: reading only the green circle he can understand the standard behavior of the joint, while by observing the outer ring he can understand how and how much a varying parameter can affect the analyzed output. The use of such coloured bar will help the reader in understanding more intuitively which is the most affecting parameter and in which area of the joint.

To prove the efficacy of the KneePrints method, the characteristic responses of the maximum patello-femoral and medial and lateral tibio-femoral contact forces after a sensitivity analysis, as reported in Innocenti et al. (2011), have been considered. In this published paper, conventional representation methods, such as tables and histograms, have been used to represent a huge amount of data after 96 analyzed configurations.

In order to detect if the proposed method is valid and more understandable for the readers than standard graphical methods, a survey among people in the bio-medical field was conducted. Face to face interviews took place during international conferences and trough an on-line survey (accessible by www.surveymonkey.-com/s/PM6SYNL). The interviewed people were not conditioned during the survey and their results are anonymous.

People were asked to answer three questions after being provided with an explanation about KneePrints.

The questions were:

- The gender (male, female, prefer to not reply);
- The occupation (Medical doctor, Engineer/Researcher, Other);
- The preference among Tables, Histograms or KneePrints to represent the same outputs from a sensitivity analysis (Innocenti et al. 2011).

Figure 4 shows how the final question of the survey that has been proposed to compare three different graphical methods in expressing the same outputs.

Replies from the survey were collected and subdivided by gender and occupation of the interviewees. In order to calculate the probability distribution of the outcomes, a multinomial distribution statistical analysis has been performed determining, for all the groups, singularly and overall an interval of confidence at 95 %.

Results and discussion

A total of 130 people replied to the survey. 80 % were male and 17 % were female (3 % preferred to not indicate his/her gender), 30 % were medical doctors, 63 % were engineers or scientists, 6 % were other kind of

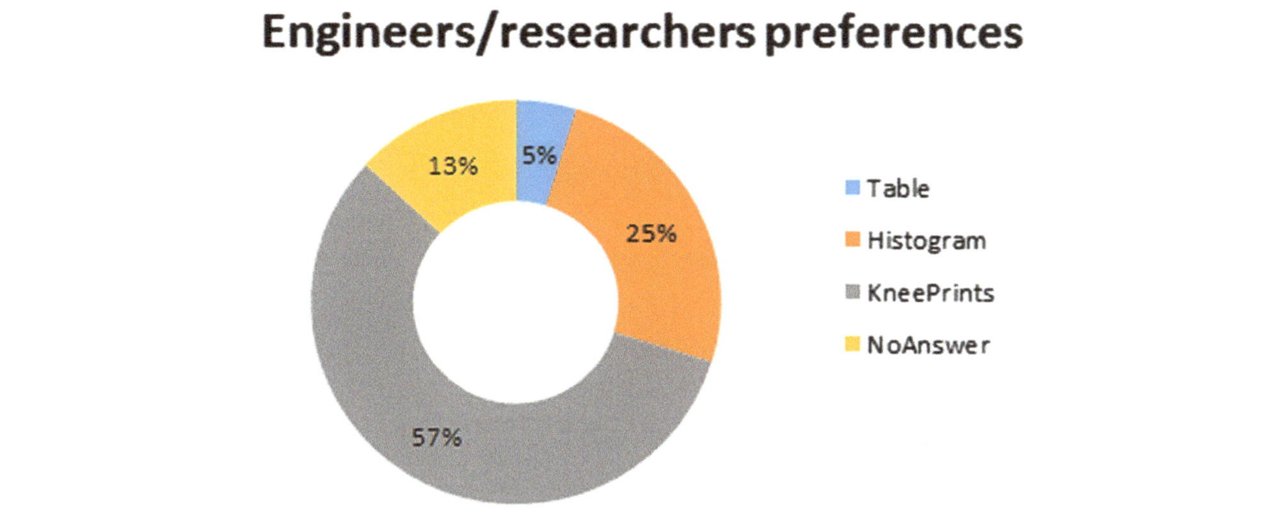

Fig. 7 Results from the survey about the preferred method of representation by engineers/researchers

workers in the biomedical field and 1 % preferred not to answer.

Figures 5 shows that the KneePrints method is the favourite among the proposed data presentation formats in the survey with a preference of 63 %. The Kneeprints is the favourite independently from the type of interviewed operator: 77 % of the medical doctors (Fig. 6), 57 % of the engineers/researchers (Fig. 7) and 57 % of the other group (Fig. 8) preferred the KneePrints to the other two graphical methods.

After performing a multinomial distribution, based on the 95 % confidence interval, KneePrints is expected to be selected with a probability of 62–77 % for the overall group; in particular surgeons are expected to choose it with a probability of 75–97 %.

As parameter variation studies for knee biomechanics understanding become more common, standardized graphical representations of the results will become necessary for the comparison and the validation of different analyses.

In this paper, the concept of KneePrints has been introduced as a tool to characterize and graphically convey outputs, also from a sensitivity analysis, describing possible knee biomechanics alterations related to patient anatomical

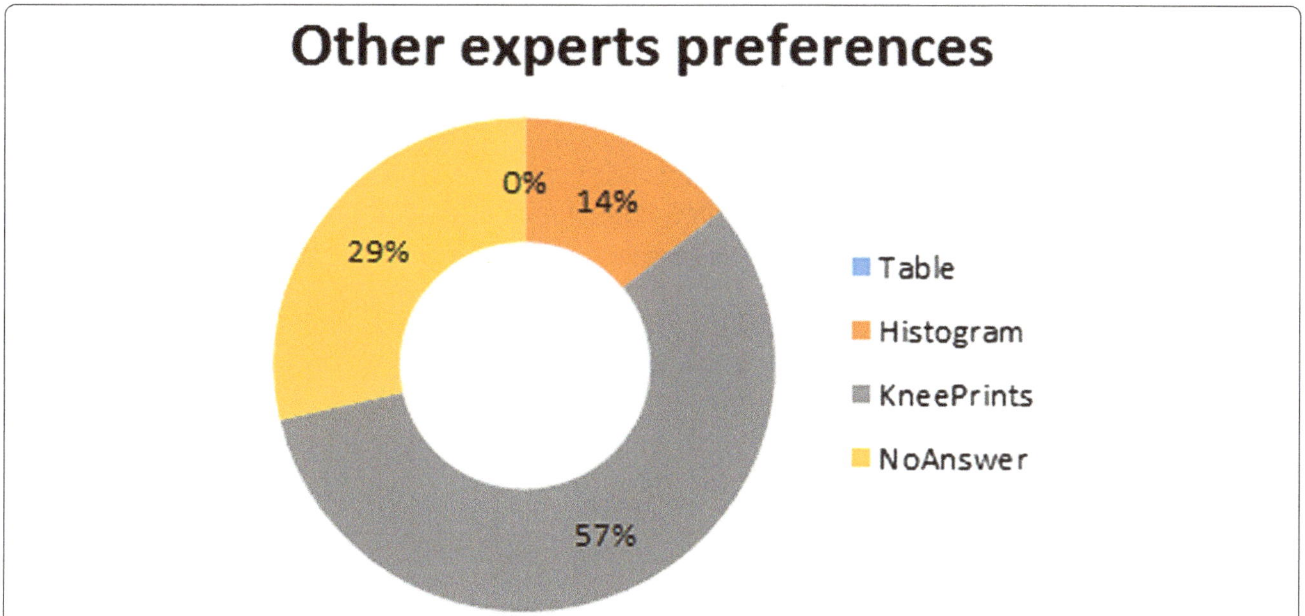

Fig. 8 Results from the survey about the preferred method of representation by other expert in the biomedical field

factors and/or surgical variability in implant component position and orientation of a possible implanted total knee arthroplasty design.

The challenge of a method to represent results intuitively is dual because it must suit the writers' needs and the readers' perception. In particular, readers' perception can be affected by different backgrounds, such as in the biomedical field where both medical doctors and engineers are mutually involved. A graphical approach which all at once prints the responses of a specific case to same factors variability is strongly suggested.

To show how the standard KneePrints developed graphic should be used to report future numerical sensitivity studies, the maximum patello-femoral and tibiofemoral contact force, after commonly reported surgical variations in total knee arthroplasty components alignment obtained in a recent study (Innocenti et al. 2011), were presented as application example.

According to the results, related to the proposed survey, the KneePrints method is generally the preferred, with respect to the standard used graph methods, from 7 on 10 interviewed people. Hence, KneePrints covers the aim to be concise and intuitive for different kinds of operators in the biomedical field.

The new proposed graphical method has been tested in the survey reporting only one case of already published data for a sensitivity analysis. However, testing it with different data sets could help in understanding its efficacy also for other typologies of outcomes, i.e. experimental outcomes describing mean values and standard deviations.

On the other hand, from the audience comments, the KneePrints resulted more effective, especially for the way results are directly reported in the region of interest, without many labels or captions, and for the use of intuitive colors that immediately highlight the worst scenarios, so can be hypnotized that similar preference can be achieved also representing other datasets. In particular, the feedbacks from the interviewed clinicians were the most favorable expressing that finally also data from studies leaded by engineers were immediately and clearly understandable and could be used as a guideline to improve the clinical research.

In this paper an application based on a numerical analysis was introduced, but the method can be also used for other kinds of analysis, such as experimental tests and gait analysis for the knee. For the sake of clarity, the authors would like to suggest the use of this new method also in representing already published data from different papers in order to employ a unique graphic method to compare them.

Moreover, the KneePrints is a particular application of a more general graphical method. The suggestion of its application for other joints biomechanics understanding or other research fields is thus foreseen. When the same approach is needed for other fields, the same indications provided to obtain the KneePrints should be followed changing some features accordingly to the content, such as, for example, the background of the graph or the labels of the different rings.

Depending on the demand of using the new proposed method, future developments of this study, that mainly provides guidelines on how obtaining this representation of data, should include the generation of an ad-hoc software that could be helpful to quickly generate this sort of graphs and let them even more standardized.

Conclusions

The purpose of this study was to introduce and illustrate an innovative method to represent, concisely and intuitively, biomechanical knee behavior, called KneePrints. KneePrints has been endorsed to be more efficient than standard graphical methods. For these reasons, the KneePrints method can be proposed to bridge the gap between research outputs and applications in the orthopedic field.

Competing interests

The authors declare that they have no competing interests.

Authors' contributions

SP conceived of the study planning and development, managed the survey, analyzed the results, and wrote the manuscript; JVS participated in the study planning and in writing the draft of the manuscript; WP participated in the underling the clinical need of such study and in writing the manuscript; LB participated in the design of the study and in drafting the manuscript; BI supported the conceiving of the study, and participated in its design and coordination and helped in writing the manuscript. All authors read and approved the final manuscript.

Acknowledgements

This work was supported by FNRS (Fonds National de la Recherche Scientifique, CDR 19545501). The funders had no role in study design, data collection and analysis, decision to publish, or preparation of the manuscript.

Author details

[1]IRCCS Istituto Ortopedico Galeazzi, via via R. Galeazzi 4, 20161 Milan, Italy. [2]KU Leuven, Biomechanics Section, Celestijnenlaan 300 - bus 2419, Leuven, Belgium. [3]KU Leuven, Mechanical Engineering Technology TC, Kleinhoefstraat 4, Geel, Belgium. [4]BEAMS Department, Université Libre de Bruxelles, Av. F. Roosevelt, 50 CP165/56, Bruxelles, Belgium.

References

Arnout N, Vanlommel L, Luyckx JP, Labey L, Innocenti B, Victor J, Bellemans J (2014) Post-cam mechanics and tibiofemoral kinematics: a dynamic in vitro analysis of eight posterior stabilized total knee designs. Knee Surg Sport Tr A 22:135–137

Battaglia S, Belvedere C, Abdel Jabera S, Affatato S, D'Angeli V, Leardini A (2014) A new protocol from real joint motion data for wear simulation in total knee arthroplasty: Stair climbing. Med Eng Phy 36:1605–1610

Best J (2005) Lies, Calculations and Constructions: Beyond How to Lie with Statistics. Statist Sci 20:210–204

Coles S (1997) Creating effective graphs and charts. Industrial management & data systems. Nat Biotechnol 97:114–118

Delport H, Labey L, Innocenti B, De Corte R, Vander Sloten J, Bellemans J (2013) Collateral ligament strains during knee joint laxity evaluation before and after TKA. Clin Biomech 28:777–782
Doumont JL (2009) Tree, maps, and theorems. Effective communication for rational minds. Principiae Structuring thoughts
Few S (2004) Show me the numbers: Designing tables and graphs to enlighten. Analytics Press 1, Oakland, CA
Fitzpatrick CK, Rullkoetter PJ (2014) Estimating total knee replacement joint load ratios from kinematics. J Biomech 47:3003–3011
Fregly BJ, Besier TF, Lloyd DG, Delp SL, Banks SA, Pandy MG, D'Lima D (2012) Grand challenge competition to predict in vivo knee loads. J Orthopaed Res 30:503–513
Heesterbeek PJC, Labey L, Wong P, Innocenti B, Wymenga AB (2014) A new spacer-guided, PCL balancing technique for cruciate-retaining total knee replacement. Knee Surg Sport Tr A 22:650–659
Innocenti B, Pianigiani S, Labey L, Victor J, Bellemans J (2011) Contact forces in several TKA designs during squatting: A numerical sensitivity analysis. J Biomech 44:1573–1581
Innocenti B, Bilgen ÖF, Labey L, van Lenthe HG, Vander Sloten J, Catani F (2014) Load sharing and ligament strains in balanced, overstuffed and understuffed UKA. A validated finite element analysis. J Arthroplasty 29:1481–1489
Kutzner I, Heinlein B, Graichen F, Rohlmann A, Halder A, Beier A, Bergmann G (2011) Loading of the knee joint during activities of daily living measured in vivo in five subjects. J Biomech 43:2167–2173
Pianigiani S, Chevalier Y, Labey L, Pascale V, Innocenti B (2012) Tibio-femoral kinematics in different total knee arthroplasty designs during a loaded squat: A numerical sensitivity study. J Biomech 45:2315–2323
Victor J, Van Doninck D, Labey L, Innocenti B, Parizel PM, Bellemans J (2009) How precise can bony landmarks be determined on a CT scan of the knee? Knee 16:358–365
Worsley P, Stokes M, Taylor M (2011) Predicted knee kinematics and kinetics during functional activities using motion capture and musculoskeletal modelling in healthy older people. Gait Posture 33:268–273
Zdero R, Fenton PV, Rudan J, Bryant JT (2001) Fuji film and ultrasound measurement of total knee arthroplasty contact areas. J Arthroplasty 16:367–375
Zelle J, Janssen D, Van Eijden J, De Waal Malefijt M, Verdonschot N (2011) Does high-flexion total knee arthroplasty promote early loosening of the femoral component? J Biomech 29:976–83

24

Biomechanical properties of five different currently used implants for open-wedge high tibial osteotomy

Arnaud Diffo Kaze[1*], Stefan Maas[1], Danièle Waldmann[1], Andreas Zilian[1], Klaus Dueck and Dietrich Pape

Abstract

Background: As several new tibial osteotomy plates recently appeared on the market, the aim of the present study was to compare mechanical static and fatigue strength of three newly designed plates with gold standard plates for the treatment of medial knee joint osteoarthritis.

Methods: Sixteen fourth-generation tibial bone composites underwent a medial open-wedge high tibial osteotomy (HTO) according to standard techniques, using five TomoFix standard plates, five PEEKPower plates and six iBalance implants. Static compression load to failure and load-controlled cyclic fatigue failure tests were performed. Forces, horizontal and vertical displacements were measured; rotational permanent plastic deformations, maximal displacement ranges in the hysteresis loops of the cyclic loading responses and dynamic stiffness were determined.

Results: Static compression load to failure tests revealed that all plates showed sufficient stability up to 2400 N without any signs of opposite cortex fracture, which occurred above this load in all constructs at different load levels. During the fatigue failure tests, screw breakage in the iBalance group and opposite cortex fractures in all constructs occurred only under physiological loading conditions (<2400 N). The highest fatigue strength in terms of maximal load and number of cycles performed prior to failure was observed for the ContourLock group followed by the iBalance implants, the TomoFix standard (std) and small stature (sm) plates. The PEEKPower group showed the lowest fatigue strength.

Conclusions: All plates showed sufficient stability under static loading. Compared to the TomoFix and the PEEKPower plates, the ContourLock plate and iBalance implant showed a higher mechanical fatigue strength during cyclic fatigue testing. These data suggest that both mechanical static and fatigue strength increase with a wider proximal T-shaped plate design together with diverging proximal screws as used in the ContourLock plate or a closed-wedge construction as in the iBalance design. Mechanical strength of the bone-implant constructs decreases with a narrow T-shaped proximal end design and converging proximal screws (TomoFix) or a short vertical plate design (PEEKPower Plate). Whenever high mechanical strength is required, a ContourLock or iBalance plate should be selected.

Keywords: High tibial osteotomy (HTO); Osteoarthritis; Biomechanics; Mechanical test; Cyclic and static loading; TomoFix; ContourLock; PEEKPower; iBalance; Stiffness; Valgus malrotation

* Correspondence: arnaud.diffokaze@uni.lu
[1]Faculty of Science, Technology and Communication, University of Luxembourg, 6, rue R. Coudenhove-Kalergi, L-1359 Luxembourg, Luxembourg
Full list of author information is available at the end of the article

Background

High tibial osteotomy (HTO) is a well-established method for the treatment of unicompartmental varus gonarthrosis. Both lateral closing and medial opening techniques exist to produce a valgus alignment (Staubli 2008; Staubli and Jacob 2010). The latter is becoming increasingly popular when performed in a biplanar fashion. Since the introduction of long and rigid-angle stable plates, the frequency of non-unions after an open-wedge HTO has declined significantly (Staubli and Jacob 2010). Apart from a good vascularization of the bone, solid plate fixation is mandatory for rapid bone healing (Staubli 2008; Staubli and Jacob 2010). Although clinical results after HTO often are encouraging some factors associated with a poor long-term outcome such as imprecise osteotomy or loss of the primary correction angle due to poor primary fixation stability of the implant (Spahn et al. 2006; Pornrattanamaneewong et al. 2012).

There are many different implants from different manufacturers available. Biomechanical (Luo et al. 2013; Spahn and Wittig 2002; Stoffel et al. 2004; Zhim et al. 2005; Agneskirchner et al. 2006; Maas et al. 2013; Watanabe et al. 2014) and clinical (Pape et al. 2011; Saeed and Rae 2009; Valkering et al. 2009; Cotic et al. 2014; Woon-Hwa et al. 2013) comparative studies are often performed to help surgeons choose the most appropriate fixation device for the osteotomy.

TomoFix, the long and rigid T-shaped titanium internal fixator with uniaxial locking system (Synthes GmbH, Oberdorf, Switzerland), is currently the gold standard. It combines biomechanical properties that are held accountable for fast bone healing: (1) high primary fixation stability; (2) a compliant bone-implant construct which allows residual micromotion within the osteotomy gap to promote a "callus massage". TomoFix plates exist in two versions, such as the small stature (sm) version designed for lighter patients and the standard (std) version without weight restriction. Both plates have a narrow proximal design which allows for a biplanar osteotomy, thus enlarging the surface for rapid contact healing (Pape et al. 2010, 2011).

PEEKPower (carbon-fiber reinforced polyetheretherketone (PEEK)) and iBalance (non-absorbable polyetheretherketone)–two implants also indicated for a biplanar osteotomy–were recently designed by Arthrex, a company based in Munich (Germany). The PEEKPower plate is T-shaped, shorter than the TomoFix but coming with a multidirectional locking system. The iBalance implant, a PEEK spacer, is inserted into the osteotomy gap in a uniplanar and closed-wedge-like technique with immediate close contact between the PEEK material and the proximal and distal cortical and spongious bone surface (Pape et al. 2012).

In our previously performed comparative biomechanical study (Maas et al. 2013) comparing the TomoFix sm plate and the Contour Lock plate (Arthrex, Munich, Germany) (Fig. 1) Static and fatigue strength for both plates were investigated. The same materials and methods were used in this study to perform static and cyclic tests on bone-implant constructs with the TomoFix std, the PEEK Power and the iBalance fixators (Fig. 2). The results obtained were then compared to those of our previous study, thus allowing a comparison between (1) the TomoFix sm plate, (2) the Contour Lock plate, (3) the iBalance implant, (4) the PEEK Power plate and (5) the TomoFix std plate. The hypothesis of the present study was that implants well attached with a wide proximal end to the tibial head provide better stability to the bone-implant construct.

Except for the iBalance system thermoplastic (PEEK), screws were used whereas all other fixation plates used metal screws (titanium alloy or stainless steel).

Methods

Sixteen large-size fourth-generation composite analogue tibia bone models (Sawbones, Pacific Research Laboratories, Inc., Vashon Island, Washington, USA) were used in this study since these composite bones have mechanical properties similar to human bones (Chong et al. 2007; Gardner et al. 2010; Heiner 2008). Using artificial composite bones has the advantage of minimizing biomechanical variability between the specimens, which can arise when using cadaveric bones.

Specimen preparation

Each specimen tested was prepared in the same standardized manner as described in the following four steps (Maas et al. 2013). (a) Open-wedge high tibial osteotomies were performed on each of the sixteen composite bones in the same way by an experienced surgeon, according to standard techniques of each implant (Fowler et al. 2000; Lobenhoffer and Agneskirchner 2003). (b) The composite tibias were then cut. Only the proximal part of 300 mm length was fixed in a cylindrical mold. All specimens were identically positioned with the help of a template and a centrical pinion at the bottom of the mold form. The inclination angle in the frontal and sagittal direction was such chosen that the tibial plateau was horizontal in both directions. The repeatability of the described positioning system was checked with different specimens and found to be less than 1 mm in all three dimensions. (c) The cylindrical pot was filled with a two-component polyurethane casting resin (FC 52) formed by reacting an isocyanate with a polyol in a 1:1 ratio (Huntsman Advanced Materials GmbH, Basel, Switzerland). (d) After the hardening of the resin, the specimens were turned 180° and the tibial heads with the osteotomy plates were positioned in shallow cylindrical molds. Two small thin-metal plates were added in the molds in order to attach the displacement sensors later on (Fig. 3).

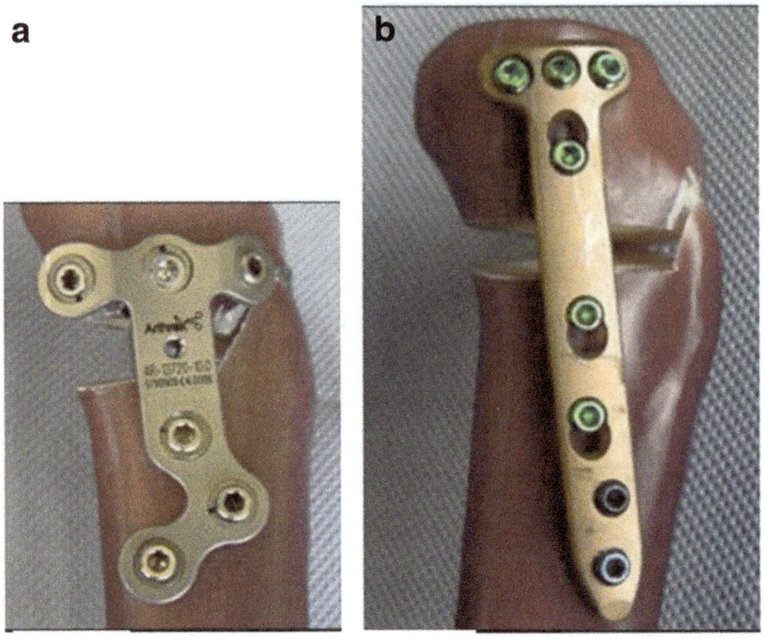

Fig. 1 Fixation devices compared by Maas et al. (Maas et al. 2013). (**a**) The ContourLock HTO plate is applicable to patients without weight limitation. (**b**) The TomoFix sm plate is indicated only for small stature patients

Mechanical testing system

Purely vertical loading was applied to the tibia head through a freely movable support (Fig. 4-a), allowing only horizontal motion in the transversal plane, using three freely rolling metal balls. Hence a rotational movement or tilting of the tibia head was not possible. The tibial plateau always remained horizontal in both directions though no mechanical guiding rail was used. The deformations of the specimens were captured using six displacement sensors. A medial sensor MS measured the vertical displacement in the frontal plane on the medial side of the tibial head and the second sensor LS at the lateral side. The distal ends of the tibias were fixed to the vertical moving piston of the hydraulic testing machine with constrained motions in the transversal plane. Three displacement sensors DX, DY1 and DY2 were attached to the easily sliding support in order to measure the horizontal displacements of the tibial head in two horizontal perpendicular directions X (medial-lateral) and Y (proximal-distal) in the transverse plane.

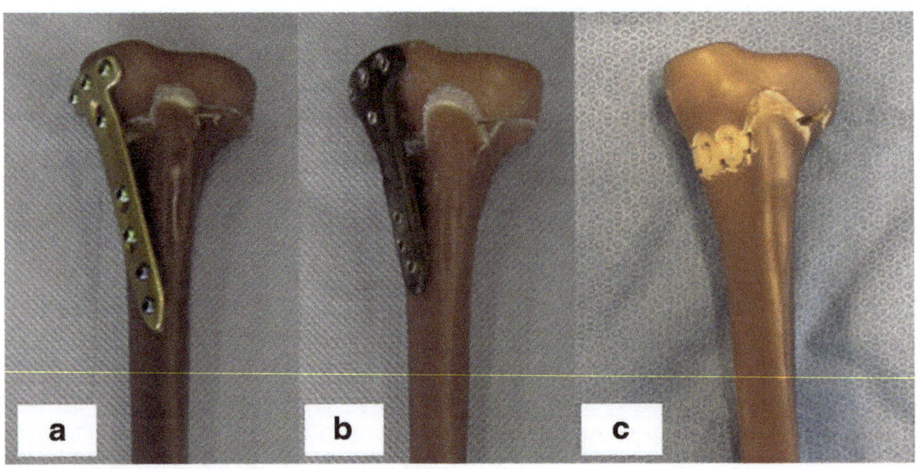

Fig. 2 Fixation devices compared during the last tests performed. (**a**) TomoFix std plate, (**b**) PEEKPower HTO plate and (**c**) iBalance HTO implant. All this implants are indicated with no weight restriction

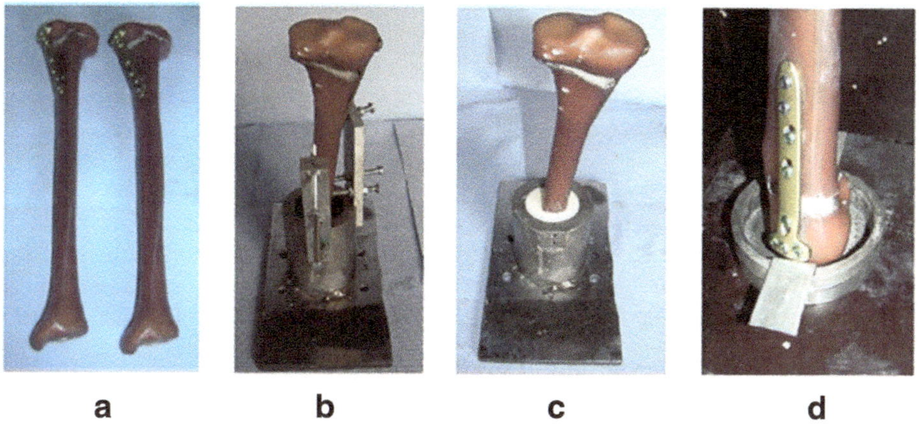

Fig. 3 Different steps of a specimen preparation (Maas et al. 2013). (**a**) The composite bones after the osteotomy; (**b**) Fixation in the cylindrical mold; (**c**) Specimen after casting with polyurethane resin FC 52; (d) Preparation of tibial head with pre-insertion of sensor attachments

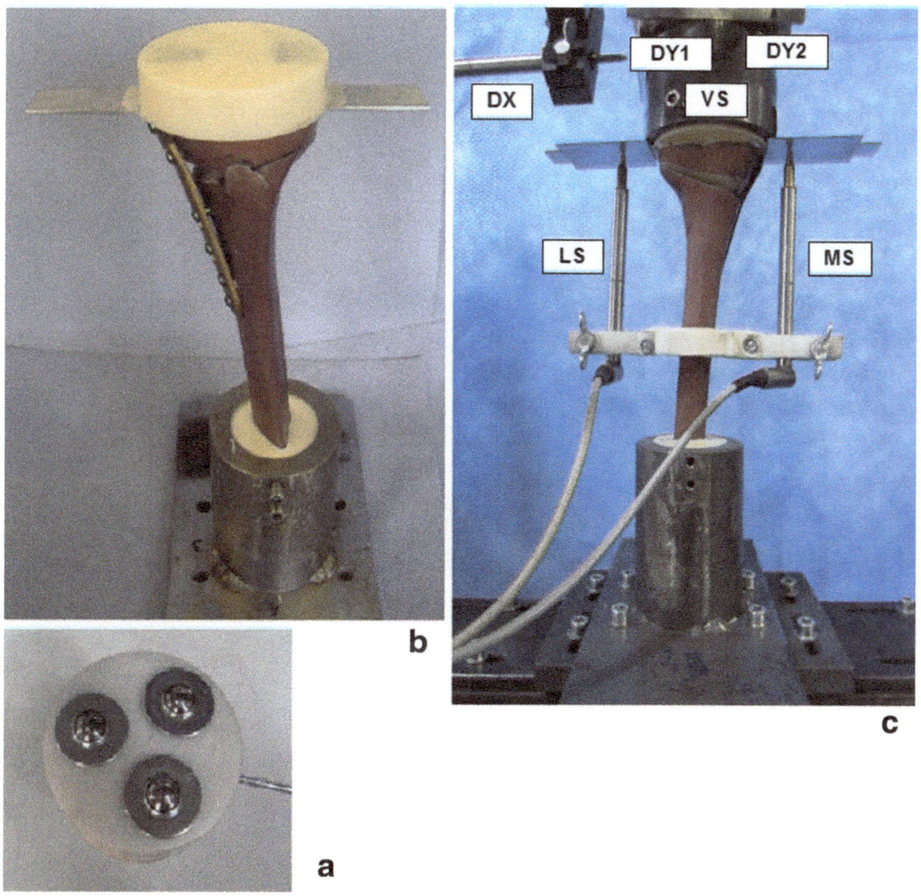

Fig. 4 Materials and test setting-up. (**a**) Low friction sliding support to apply purely vertical forces. (**b**) Specimen before mounting to hydraulic press. (**c**) Specimen under test: the lateral and the medial sensor (LS and MS) registered the relative lateral and medial vertical displacements from the tibial head, while VS measured its vertical displacement. The DX, DY1 and DY2 sensors registered the horizontal displacements of the tibial head; along the transverse axis for the first and the sagittal axis for the latters

The sensors DY1 and DY2 were positioned in a way to detect rotation of the tibial head in the transversal plane. A sixth displacement sensor VS embedded in the testing hydraulic machine (INSTRON, Darmstadt, Germany) measured the vertical displacement of its piston (Fig. 4-c).

Testing procedure

The bone-implant-constructs were subjected to static and cyclic tests. The static tests consisted of applying quasi-static compression displacement-controlled single loading to failure at a speed of 0.1 mm/s. The dynamic tests consisted of load-controlled cyclic fatigue testing, with stepwise compression sinusoidal (frequency = 5Hz) loading where the force amplitude of each step was kept constant with feed-back control of the force signal within the hydraulic machine. The lower compressive force limit of each load step was kept constant at 160 N. Starting with 800 N for the first step, the upper compressive force limit was increased stepwise by 160 N after N = 20000 cycles if no failure occurred (Fig. 5). The failure criteria considered in this study are summarized in Table 1. The present testing procedure is similar to the standardized testing protocol for hip joints (ISO 7206-4, 1989; ISO 7206-6, 1992; ISO 7206-8, 1995) and was also used in a study by Agneskirchner et al. (Agneskirchner et al., 2006).

The sixteen specimens were regrouped as follows: group 1 (n = 5, TomoFix standard plates (TomoFix std)), group 2 (n = 5, PEEKPower plates) and group 3 (n = 6, iBalance implants). The groups were further subdivided depending on the performed test (Table 2). Group 4 (n = 5, TomoFix small stature plates (TomoFix sm)) and group 5 (n = 5, ContourLock plates) were composed from the specimens used in our previous study (Maas et al. 2013). It is important to recall here that the specimens used in the previous study were prepared in the same standardized manner as indicated in the previous paragraph.

Type and definition of failure

Defining the failure criteria is decisive since the specimens were never completely damaged. The failure criteria that were used in this biomechanical study are summarized in Table 1 and were already used by Pape et al. (Pape et al., 2010). With type 3 failure the wobble degree or the stability of the sample during the cyclic testing was quantified. This was checked by plotting the force versus the displacement; for nonlinear cases this plot is ideally an elliptical curve with a slope proportional to the stiffness and an enclosed area proportional to the damping of the structure tested. If the specimen becomes unstable and starts to wobble, e. g. after a failure, the width of this curve representing the maximal displacement range increases.

Mechanical stiffness

Changes in stiffness are frequently used as an additional damage indicator in fatigue tests of complex structures. Therefore the evolution of the dynamic stiffness of the specimens subjected to the cyclic testing was determined as the ratio of peak-to-peak force $\Delta F = F_{max}\text{-}F_{min}$ to the peak-to-peak displacement ΔX measured in the same period T (Fig. 6):

$$k = \frac{F_{max} - F_{min}}{\Delta X}.$$

Lateral and vertical stiffness were defined by considering the lateral and the vertical displacements registered by the lateral (LS) and the vertical (VS) sensors respectively. Medial stiffness depends on the implants' stiffness and is thus not considered.

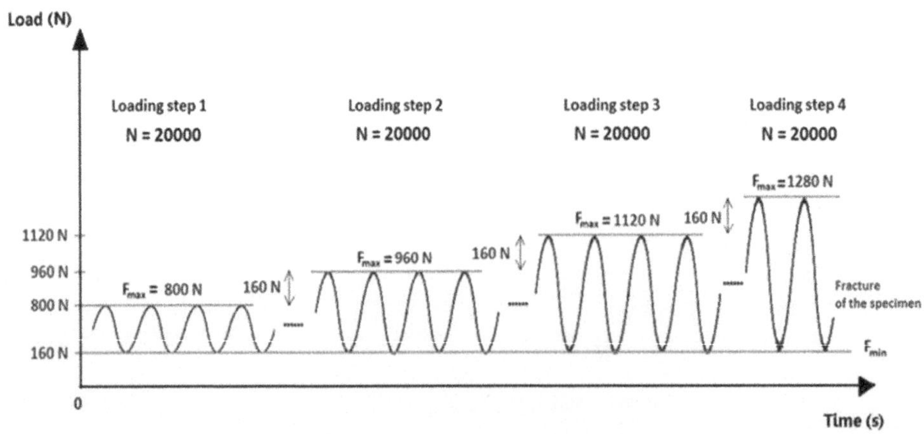

Fig. 5 Scheme of the applied vertical sinusoidal force loading (load-controlled) (Maas et al. 2013). After N = 20000 cycles the upper force was increased stepwise by 160 N until failure. The loading frequency was constant and set to 5 Hz

Table 1 The failure types used and their defining criteria

Failure type	Criteria
1	Medial or lateral displacements of the tibial head in relation to the tibial shaft greater than 2 mm. This criterion can only be checked in the unloaded condition.
2	Visible collapse of the lateral cortex. Small hairline cracks are not considered as failure.
3	Maximal displacement range greater than 0.5 mm within one hysteresis loop in the case of cyclic testing only.
4	Cracks of the screws greater than 1 mm

For the static loading to failure test static stiffness was defined as the ratio of the measured force to the measured displacement at a given time.

Permanent plastic deformation of the specimen

Any permanent plastic deflection and the correlated permanent plastic deflection angle would lead to an alteration of correction and had to be checked to quantify type 1 failure as the criterion can only be checked in the unloaded condition. Permanent plastic deformation (Fig. 7) was estimated here as the irrecoverable displacement with a minimal force of 160 N, considered as nearly zero force, at the start of the tests. Permanent plastic deformations could therefore be measured online during the cyclic tests at any time, for example before failure (U_{PB}) and additionally after the gross failure, i.e. the collapse of the lateral cortex (U_{PA}) in general.

The permanent plastic valgus malrotation of the tibial head, which corresponds to the permanent plastic deflection angle of the tibial plateau at a given time, was defined as the resulting permanent plastic displacements on the medial and the lateral sides in the specimens' frontal plane.

As already indicated, the two sensors LS and MS registered the lateral displacement d_L and the medial displacement d_M of the tibial head respectively. Though the test force was strictly vertical, it was observed that the specimens deformed not purely vertically, which resulted in unequal displacement values for d_L and d_M (Fig. 8). The valgus malrotation of the tibia was then defined as the deflection angle (in radians) in the frontal plane and could be calculated at any time as

$$\alpha = \frac{|d_L - d_M|}{D}.$$

According to the definitions of permanent plastic deformations type 1 failure occurs when

$$\frac{d}{D}\left|d_{Lp} - d_{Mp}\right| > 2\ \text{mm};$$

that is if $\alpha_p > 0.024$ rad or 1.4°, with the index "*p*" meaning permanent plastic.

The displacements in the direction of the loading (e.g. the vertical descending direction) were considered as to be positive and negative in the opposite direction.

Results and discussion

Results

Static loading to failure tests

All specimens failed due to a fracture of the contralateral cortical bone, which represents type 2 failure (Fig. 9). Before the final collapse there were crack formations observed in the cases of the TomoFix std 1 (Fig. 10) and PEEKPower 2 (Fig. 11). For the others specimens the abrupt fractures of the contralateral cortex were not preceded by observable crack formations.

While considering the vertical descending displacements as positive, the medial displacement (MS) was negative in the cases of the TomoFix std 1 (Fig. 10), TomoFix std 2, PeekPower 1 and iBalance 2. The lateral displacement (LS) was always positive and its absolute value remained greater than the medial displacement. The same applies when the latter was positive for PEEKPower 2 (Fig. 11) and iBalance 1, meaning that the tibial plateau of all specimens rotated during the static loading.

The crack and ultimate loads of the specimens were determined as indicated in Fig. 10 and are summarized with the corresponding medial and lateral displacement, valgus malrotation of the tibial head and static lateral stiffness in Table 3. The values of the specimens of groups 4 and 5

Table 2 Specimen grouping and assignment, depending on the implants used and the tests performed

Test	Group 1; n = 5 Specimens	Group 2; n = 5 Specimens	Group 3; n = 6 Specimens	Group 4; n = 5 Specimens	Group 5; n = 5 Specimens
Static: Single loading to failure test	TomoFix 1	PEEKPower 1	iBalance 1	TomoFix sm 1	ContourLock 1
	TomoFix 2	PEEKPower 2	iBalance 2	TomoFix sm 2	ContourLock 2
Dynamic: cyclic fatigue failure test	TomoFix 3	PEEKPower 3	iBalance 3	TomoFix sm 3	ContourLock 3
	TomoFix 4	PEEKPower 4	iBalance 4	TomoFix sm 4	ContourLock 4
	TomoFix 5	PEEKPower 5	iBalance 5	TomoFix sm 5	ContourLock 5
			iBalance 6		

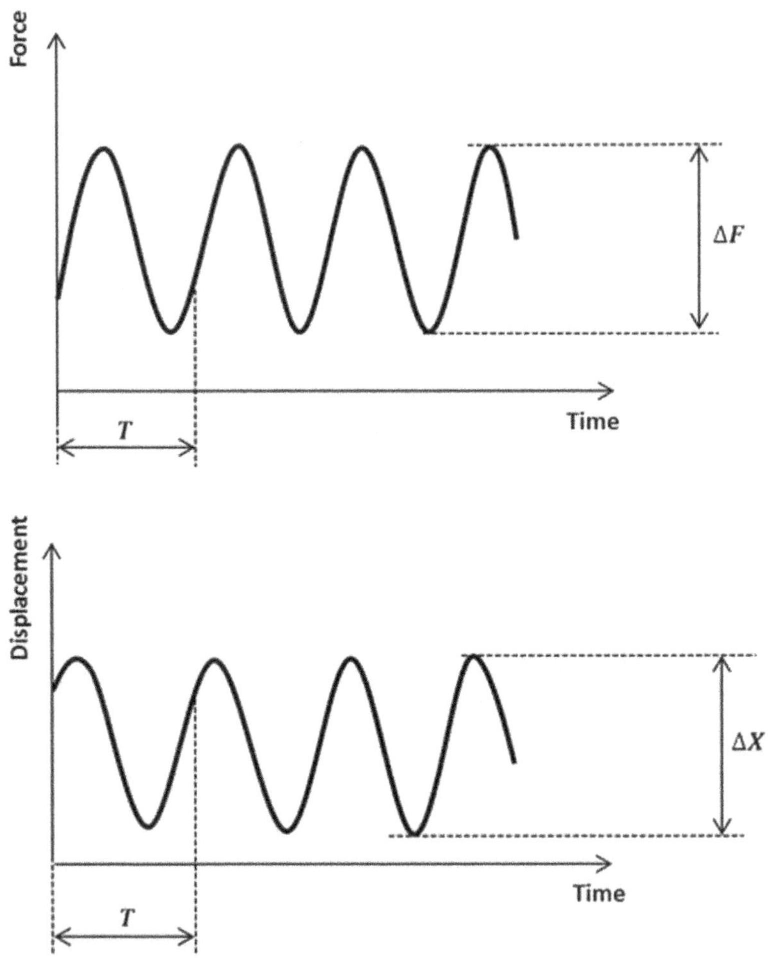

Fig. 6 Definition of ΔF and ΔX to calculate dynamic stiffness in the cyclic fatigue to failure tests (Maas et al. 2013). ΔF and ΔX are the peak-to-peak force and the corresponding peak-to-peak displacement in the same period T. This allows to determine the time history of the specimen stiffness during loading

(TomoFix sm and ContourLock) are from our previous study and presented here for sake of comparison.

The PEEKPower 2, ContourLock 1, TomoFix std 1 & 2 and ContourLock 2 specimens showed the largest lateral displacements at collapse time. The average displacement on the medial compared to the lateral side was always smaller for all implant types. The determined valgus malrotation of the tibial head was greater or equal to the fixed limit of 1.4° of the permanent deflection angle for all implants, except for the iBalance specimen which showed a mean value of 0.9° (Table 3). The iBalance specimens were the stiffest bone-implant constructs for the performed static loading to failure tests with an average lateral stiffness of 3.1 kN/mm at ultimate load.

Fatigue loading to failure tests

As for the static tests all the specimen failed in the fatigue tests due to the fracturing of the contralateral cortical bone. Damage of the implant occurred only in the case of the iBalance 3, for which a rupture of the screw and fracture of the medial cortex as indicated in Fig. 12 was observed.

The breakage of the screw occurred at the transition zone of elasticity modulus difference between the stiffer cortical bone and the PEEK screw. The applied loads versus the resulting lateral displacements were plotted in order to check type 3 failures (Table 1). The maximal displacement ranges within the hysteresis loops were determined as showed by the examples in Figs. 13, 14 and 15 in cases of the iBalance 5, PEEKPower 5 and TomoFix std 5 respectively. The values obtained were always below the predefined limit of 0.5 mm. Hence there was no type 3 failure observed for the specimens of group 1, 2 and 3. The lateral displacement (LS) was always used since it was higher than the medial displacement (MS) and the rupture occurred always on that side.

Permanent plastic valgus malrotations just before and after the collapse of the lateral cortex had been determined

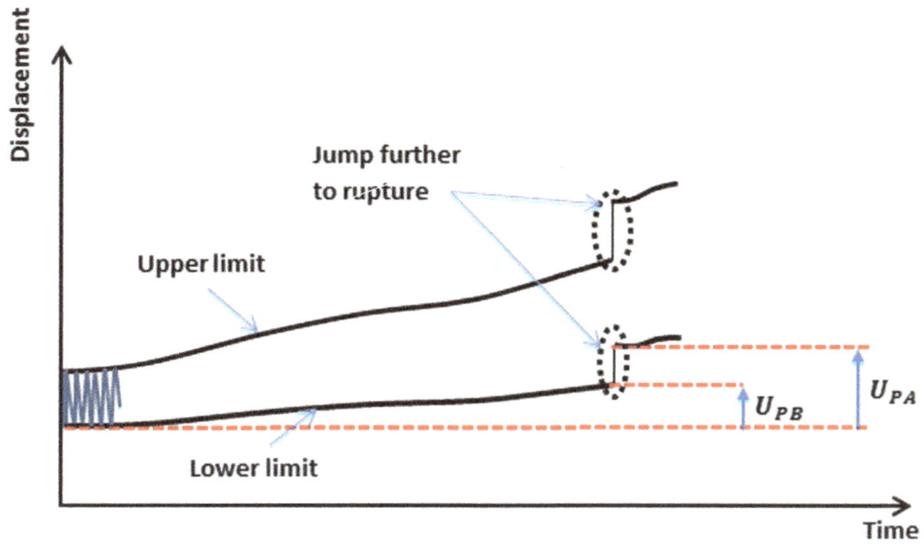

Fig. 7 Definition of permanent plastic deformation before and after failure (Maas et al. 2013): creep deformations of the specimens were observed. This allowed defining permanent plastic deformations before (UPB) and after failure (UPA) as the irrecoverable displacement with respect to the initial instantaneous displacements

for the specimens of the first three groups (TomoFix std, PEEKPower and iBalance) and are represented in Fig. 16. The load history according to Fig. 5 is indicated with the Load Step number (LSn) at which the failure occurred. As stated above, a type 1 failure occurred when the permanent plastic valgus malrotation was greater than 1.4°. Only the iBalance 6 exceeded this limit, but only after the failure of the specimen. The graph in Fig. 17 retrieved from our previous study and presented for sake of comparison shows the permanent plastic valgus malrotations for the TomoFix sm and ContourLock specimens.

Tables 4 and 5 summarize the results of the cyclic fatigue to failure tests by listing the maximal compressive force, lateral and the vertical stiffness of the specimens at the beginning of the first load step, the number of cycles performed prior to failure and the types of failure. The data displayed in Table 5 are from our previous study. Table 6 shows mean values, including the standard deviations, per group of the characteristic values given in Tables 4 and 5 of the individual specimens.

Based on Table 6 and taking the TomoFix std group as reference, average relative values per groups of the cyclic tests are shown in Fig. 18. Regarding the parameters investigated for cyclic tests, the iBalance group showed the highest values compared to groups 1 and 2. The PEEK-Power group showed higher stiffness compared to the

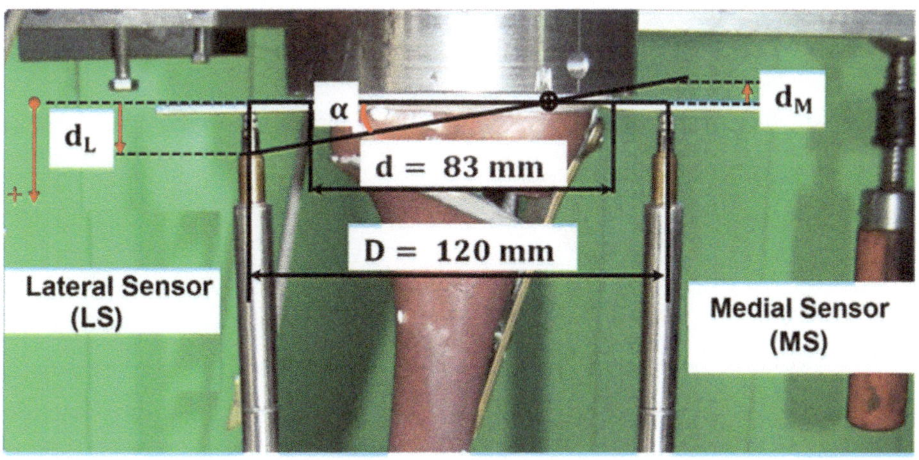

Fig. 8 Definition of the deflection angle (Maas et al. 2013). In general the lateral displacement d_L was found to be positive with greater magnitude than the medial displacement d_M that was counted as negative. Hence the deflection angle *a* was defined by means of the difference (d_L-d_M)

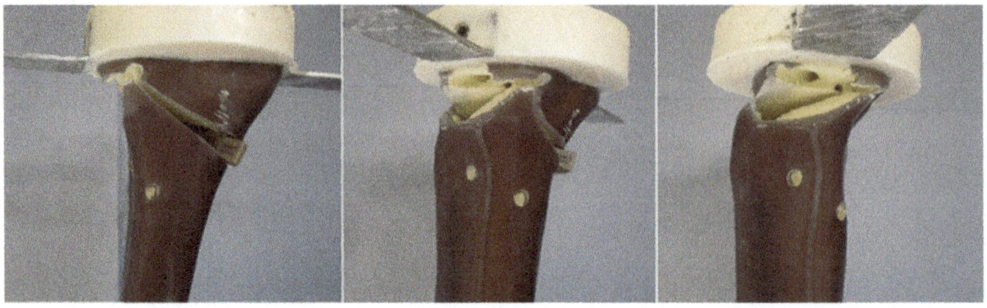

Fig. 9 Fracture of the contralateral cortex (specimen with the iBalance implant). The opposite cortex appeared to be the weak point of the bone-implant constructs

TomoFix plates. The vertical stiffness of the iBalance group was on average around 1.7 higher than the one of the TomoFix std group.

Discussion

In this study three implants were investigated and compared to our previous study using the same experimental setup and protocol, thus comparing the static and fatigue fixation stability provided by the following five different medial open-wedge HTO plates: the TomoFix std plate, the PEEK Power plate, the iBalance implant, the Contour Lock HTO plate and the TomoFix sm plate. The key findings of the present study were the following: (1) the stiffest bone-implant construct was found to be the iBalance implant followed by the Contour Lock plate. (2) The Contour Lock plate provided highest fatigue strength under cyclic loading conditions. (3) Static loading until failure tests revealed superior strength for the iBalance implant followed by the TomoFix std, the PEEK Power plate, the Contour Lock and the TomoFix sm plates. (4) All implants withstood the maximal physiological vertical tibiofemoral contact force while slow walking. This force corresponds to

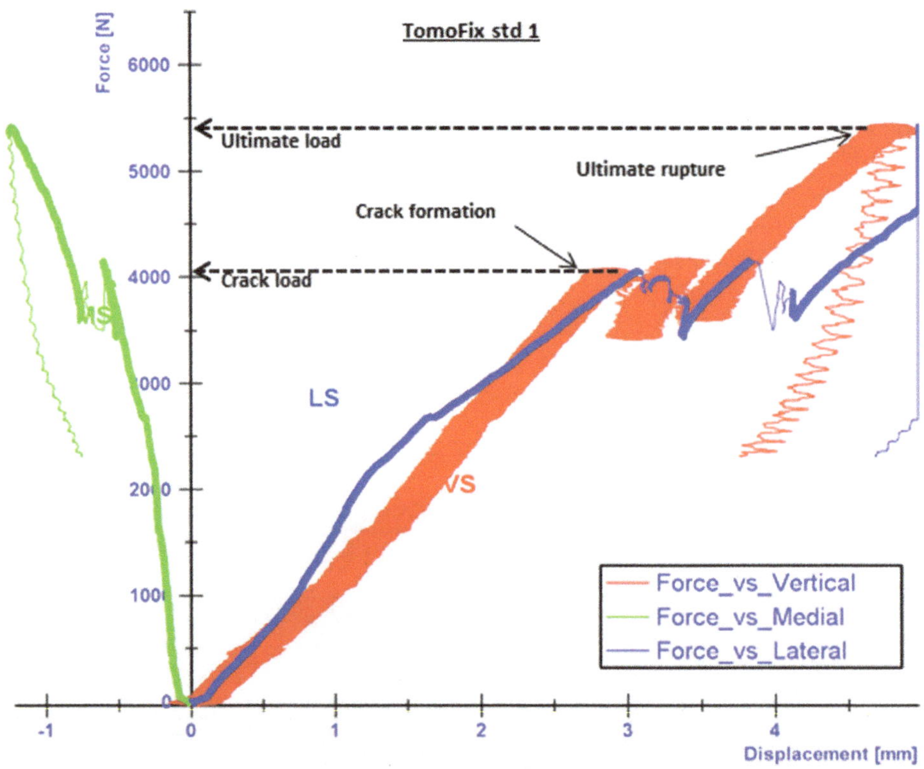

Fig. 10 Curves of the force versus the displacements in cases of TomoFix std1. The final rupture of the specimen occurred quite promptly after the crack formations, which were characterized by a drop in the registered applied force. The crack and the ultimate loads were considered as the approximate loads at the moment the crack formations and collapse of the contralateral cortex occurred respectively

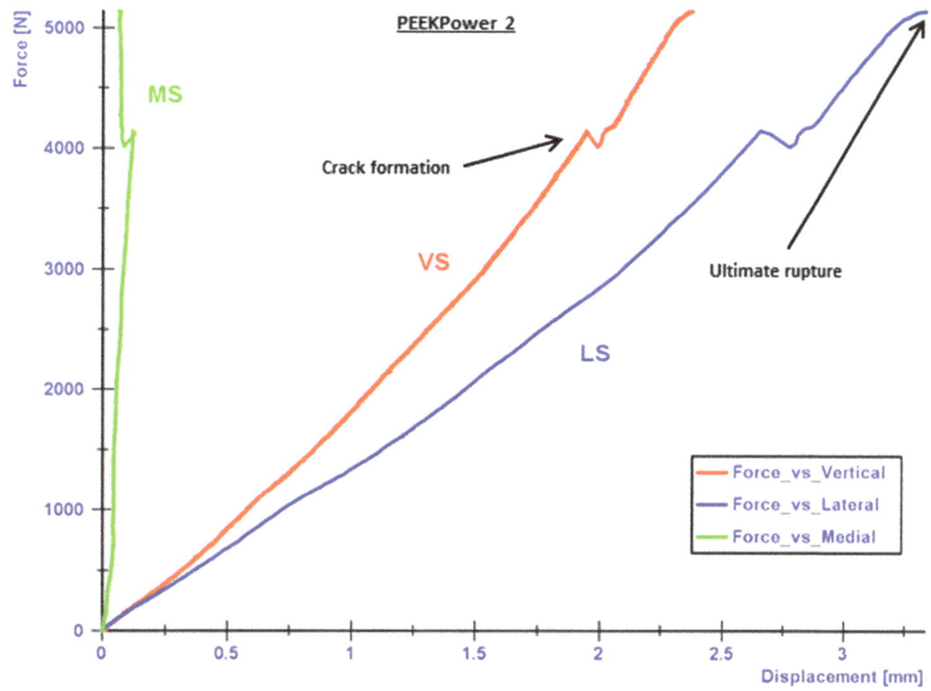

Fig. 11 Curves of the force versus the displacements in cases of PEEKPower 2. The final rupture of the specimen occurred quite promptly after the crack formations. The medial displacement (MS) was positive contrary to e.g. the TomoFix std 1

about three times the body weight (Heinlein et al. 2009; Taylor et al. 2004), e.g. 2400 N for a patient weighing 80 kg.

The principal failure mode of all bone-implant-constructs tested was the collapse of the opposite cortex, which generally occurred quickly after the initial opposite cortex crack. This behavior was observed regardless whether a static or cyclic failure test was applied. This finding correlates with previous studies with the lateral cortex being a medial HTO's weakest point (Spahn and Wittig 2002; Stoffel et al. 2004; Zhim et al. 2005; Agneskirchner et al. 2006; Maas et al. 2013; Watanabe et al. 2014). The displacements of the lateral side of the osteotomy were more pronounced than the medial displacement, which explains the valgus rotation in the frontal plane of the tibial head during the static and the cyclic loading tests.

The mean ultimate forces were 5.5 kN, 5.3 kN, 4.4 kN, 3.6 kN and 3.4 kN for the iBalance, the TomoFix std, the PEEK Power, the Contour Lock and the TomoFix sm group respectively. Hence, the iBalance and the TomoFix std are superior regarding static performance. The iBalance implant showed however the smallest mean lateral displacement (1.9 mm) at the time of opposite cortex fracture indicating a certain superiority compared to the TomoFix std plates, which failed at the largest mean lateral displacement of 4.7 mm and the largest valgus malrotation of the tibial head of 2.8° thus exceeding the limit of 1.4°, which corresponds to the occurrence of type 1 failure.

Static loading simulates only the standing of a patient. After medial HTO however, patients are also supposed to perform calm activities. The repetitive loadings of the knee are better simulated by fatigue tests. The maximal loads at failure observed during the fatigue tests were all smaller than the threshold value of 2.4 kN (Table 6). Full loading of the knee directly after an osteotomy should therefore be avoided. When considering these maximum loads at failure and the number of cycles carried out, the ContourLock plate performed best with 2.2 kN and 173000 cycles and the PEEKPower plate worst with 1.4 kN and 73000 cycles. Based on these two parameters a ranking for the dynamic analysis would place the iBalance in the second position after the ContourLock, followed by the TomoFix std and the TomoFix sm.

The maintenance of the primary correction is decisive for a positive outcome of the osteotomy. When considering the deformation mode of the specimens during the cyclic loading, a permanent plastic valgus malrotation of the tibial head occurred which caused a valgus deformation of the knee, consequently altering the localization of the mechanical axis and the primary performed correction. The valgus malrotation of the tibial head can be considered as an overcorrection. There was no permanent plastic valgus malrotation of the tibial head observed

Table 3 Static tests summary: displacements, valgus malrotation of the tibial head and their corresponding cracks and ultimate loads, including mean values and standard deviations (SD)

Specimen	Crack / ultimate load [kN]	Medial displ. at crack / ultimate load [mm]	Lateral displ. at crack / ultimate load [mm]	Valgus malrotation of the tibial head at crack / ultimate load (°)	Lateral stiffness at crack / ultimate load [kN/mm]	Failure types
TomoFix std 1	4.1 / 5.4	0.6 / 1.2	3.1 / 5.0	1.8 / 2.9	1.3 / 1.1	1 and 2
TomoFix std 2	5.1 / 5.2	1.0 / 1.1	4.2 / 4.4	2.5 / 2.6	1.2 / 1.2	1 and 2
Mean:	4.6 / 5.3	0.8 / 1.2	3.7 / 4.7	2.1 / 2.8	1.3 / 1.1	
SD ±:	0.7 / 0.1	0.3 / 0.1	0.8 / 0.4	0.5 / 0.2	0.1 / 0.1	
PEEKPower 1	-/ 3.7	-/ 0.5	-/ 2.9	-/ 1.6	-/ 1.3	1 and 2
PEEKPower 2	4.2 / 5.1	0.1 / 0.1	2.7 / 3.3	1.3 / 1.5	1.6 / 1.5	1 and 2
Mean:	-/ 4.4	-/ 0.3	-/ 3.1	-/ 1.6	-/ 1.4	
SD ±:	-/ 0.1	-/ 0.3	-/ 0.3	-/ 0.1	-/ 0.1	
iBalance 1	-/ 5.7	-/ 0.3	-/ 1.6	-/ 0.6	-/ 3.6	2
iBalance 2	-/ 5.4	-/ 0.3	-/ 2.1	-/ 1.1	-/ 2.6	2
Mean:	-/ 5.5	-/ 0.3	-/ 1.9	-/ 0.9	-/ 3.1	
SD ±:	-/ 0.2	-/ 0	-/ 0.4	-/ 0.4	-/ 0.7	
TomoFix sm 1	3.1 / 3.2	0.6 / 0.9	1.3 / 1.8	0.9 / 1.3	2.4 / 1.8	2
TomoFix sm 2	3.2 / 3.6	0.4 / 0.6	1.6 / 2.3	0.9 / 1.4	2.0 / 1.6	2
Mean:	3.2 / 3.4	0.5 / 0.8	1.5 / 2.1	0.9 / 1.4	2.2 / 1.7	
SD ±:	0.1 / 0.3	0.1 / 0.2	0.2 / 0.4	0 / 0.1	0.3 / 0.1	
ContourLock 1	2.4 / 3.2	0.6 / 0.5	2.5 / 3.9	1.5 / 2.1	1.0 / 0.8	1 and 2
ContourLock 2	-/ 3.9	-/ 0.5	-/ 4.2	-/ 2.2	-/ 0.9	1 and 2
Mean:	-/ 3.6	-/ 0.5	-/ 4.1	-/ 2.2	-/ 0.9	
SD ±:	-/ 0.5	-/ 0	-/ 0.2	-/ 0.1	-/ 0.1	

There were no cracks observed prior to the ultimate failure in the case of PEEKPower 1, iBalance 1 & 2 (all values rounded to the 1st decimal)

before the collapse of the specimens, just for the iBalance 6 specimen after failure (Fig. 16). As shown in Fig. 17 retrieved from (Maas et al. 2013), permanent plastic valgus malrotation after failure was observed in the TomoFix sm (group 4) and ContourLock (group 5) groups. As a result we can assume that the TomoFix std and the PEEKPower plates conserve correction better. Therefore the number of load steps performed before failure needs also be taken into account. However this observation is only valid if there was no bone healing prior to the fatigue failure, which is not a realistic scenario.

As indicated in Figs. 13, 14 and 15 the hysteresis loops are growing with damage but do not reach the critical threshold of 0.5 mm (Table 1) for the specimens of the TomoFix std, PEEKPower and iBalance groups. Maas et al. (Maas et al. 2013) reported the occurrence of type 3 failure for the ContourLock group (group 5) and twice within the TomoFix sm (group 4). Thus they concluded that the ContourLock plate was superior to the TomoFix sm plate as far as this parameter is concerned. This result was correlated to the fact that the ContourLock plate is wider and that the fixation screws are more

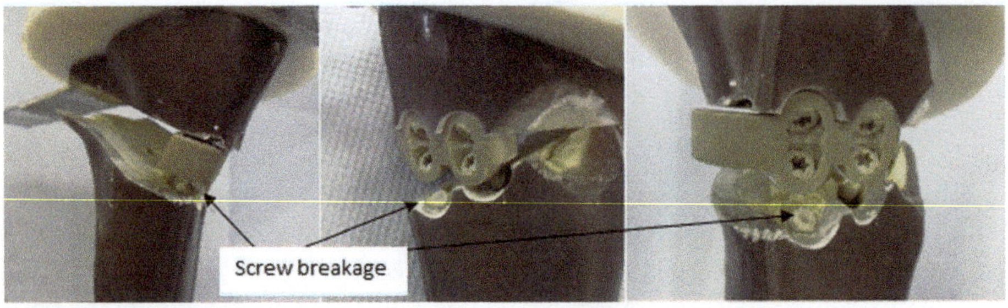

Fig. 12 Damage of the iBalance 3 specimen. The iBalance implant damaged once during the cyclic test. Ruptures of the screws were observed. There was only one type 4 failure observed

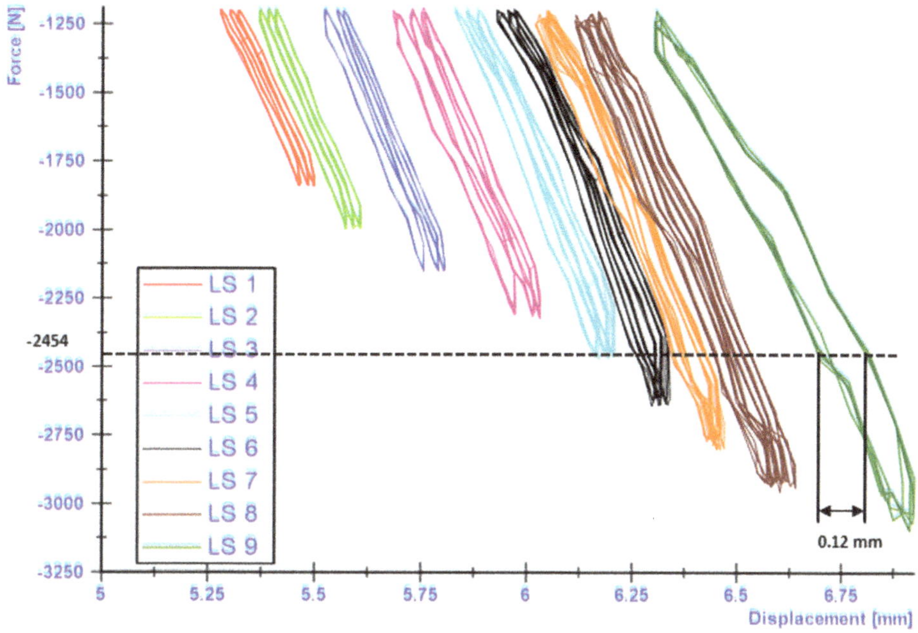

Fig. 13 Hysteresis loops: lateral displacement (iBalance 5 specimen). The higher the loads, the more the maximal displacement range within the loops grew but was never bigger than 0.5 mm

widely spaced than those of the TomoFix sm. In other words, the ContourLock plate is better anchored to the tibial head.

The high mechanical strength of the iBalance construct is most likely due to its higher stiffness compared to other specimens since it is screwed within the osteotomy gap. It thus fills a part of the gap and provides a closed-wedge design with a higher stiffness compared to all other bone-implant constructs (Table 6 and Fig. 18). However there was damage of the iBalance system's

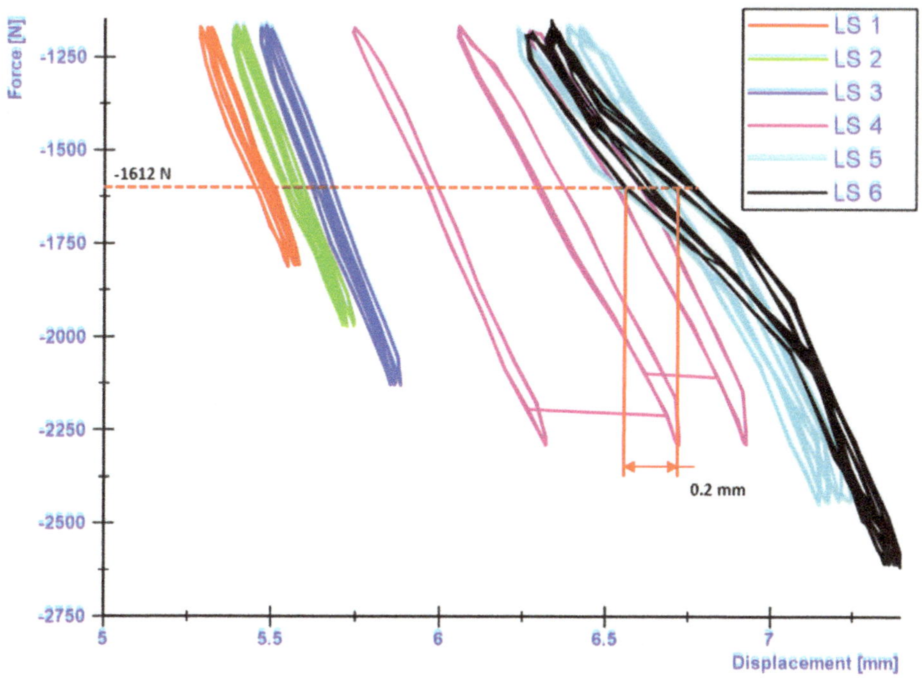

Fig. 14 Hysteresis loops: lateral displacement (PEEKPower 5 specimen). The higher the loads, the more the maximal displacement range within the loops grew but was never bigger than 0.5 mm

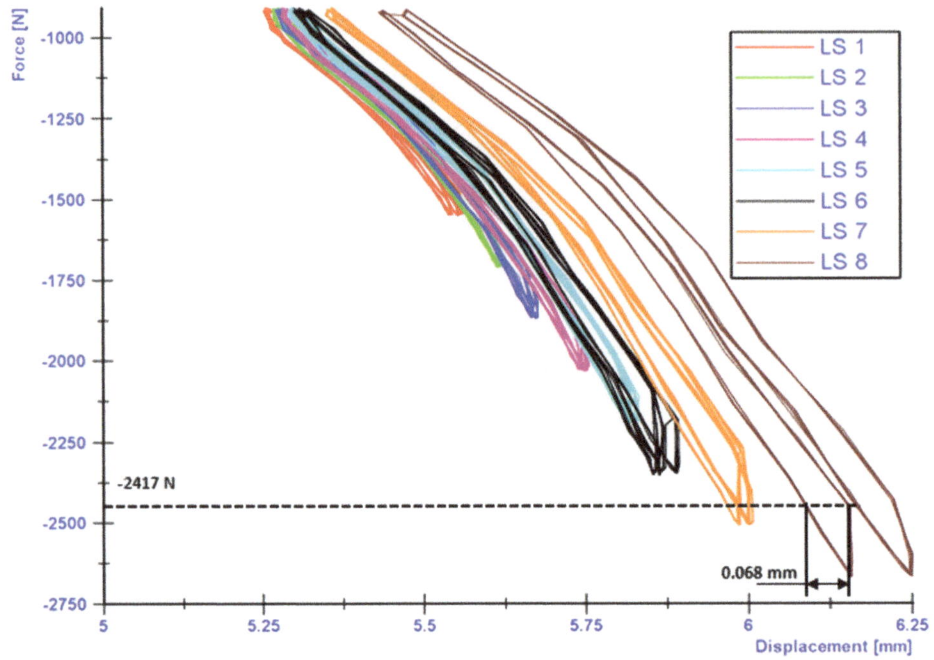

Fig. 15 Hysteresis loops: lateral displacement (TomoFix 5 specimen). The higher the loads, the more the maximal displacement range within the loops grew but was never bigger than 0.5 mm

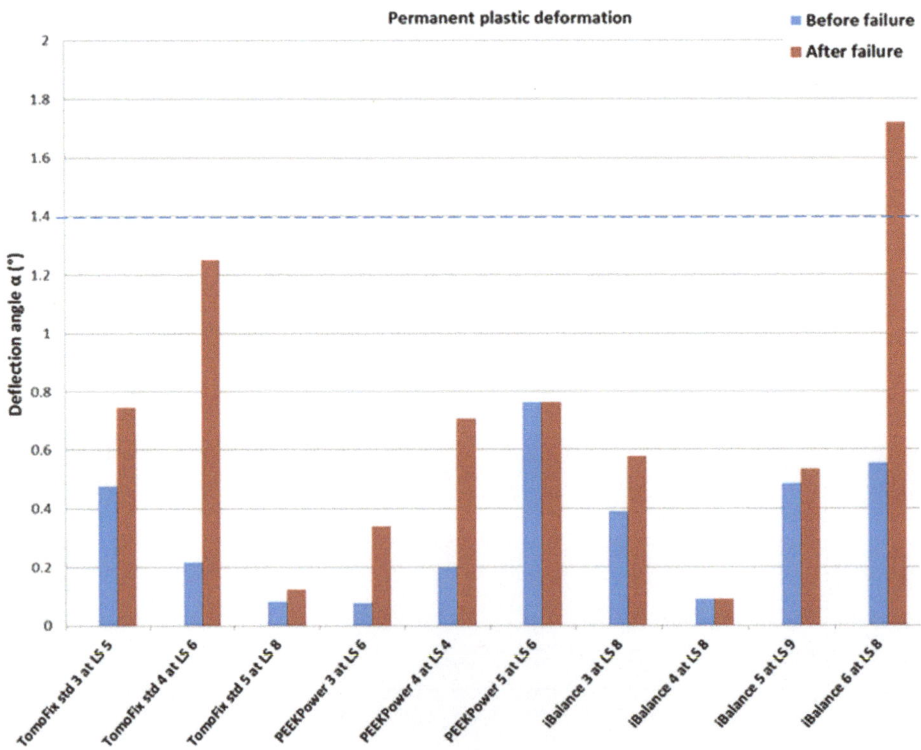

Fig. 16 Deflection angle or valgus malrotation of the tibial head before and after failure for groups 1, 2 and 3. A type 1 failure was only observed in the case of the iBalance 6 specimen after the collapse of the opposite cortex

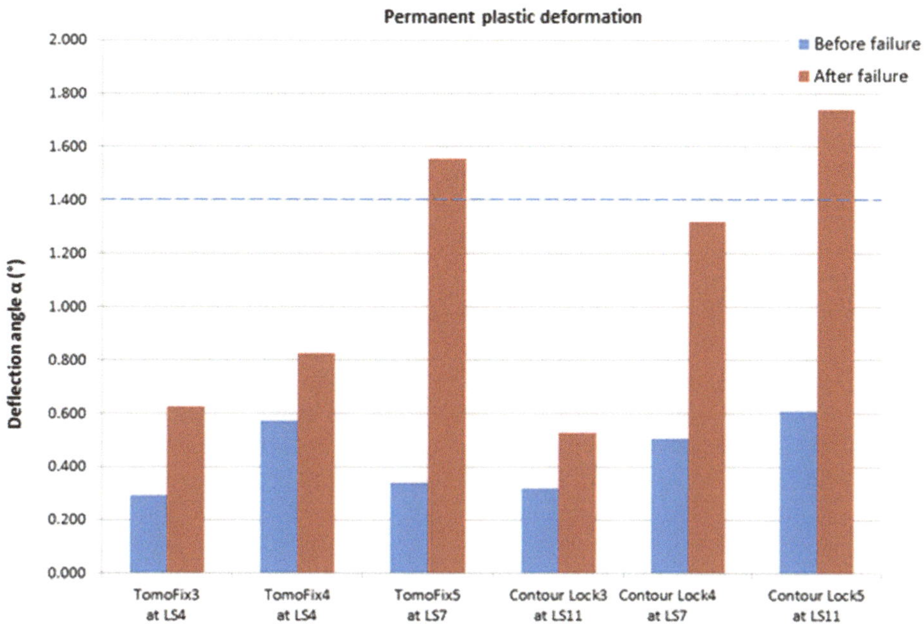

Fig. 17 Deflection angle or valgus malrotation of the tibial head before and after failure for groups 4 and 5 (the graph is retrieved from our previous study and showed here for sake of comparison). The TomoFix specimens here are the TomoFix small stature of group 4 in the present study

screws observed at very high number of cycles and loading. This underlines the importance of a good positioning of the screws and their anchorage in the tibial head. Though the loading was only vertical the screws and fixation had undergone complex tridimensional loading which is surely even more pronounced in reality than it was in this simplified test. It should be repeated that the screws of the iBalance are thermoplastics (PEEK) and not metallic materials like for the other fixation systems tested.

Agneskirchner et al. (Agneskirchner et al. 2006) also performed static compression load to failure and cyclical load to failure tests using composite bones and compared the stability of four different implants: three spacer plates and a TomoFix plate. The spacer plates were shorter than the TomoFix plate. The loads were also applied vertically to the bone-implant-constructs as it was done in the present study. They reported longer resistance to failure of the specimens for the TomoFix during the static tests. Stoffel et al. (Stoffel et al. 2004) also performed axial compression load to failure tests to compare the TomoFix plate to the Puddu plate (rectangular short spacer plate) by using composite bones and also reported a better axial stability for the TomoFix. Watanabe et al. (Watanabe et al. 2014) also performed a comparative study of the TomoFix and the Puddu plates by using cadaveric bones and reported the highest failure load for the TomoFix. None of the previously cited studies included the iBalance and the

Table 4 Summary of fatigue failure tests (groups 1, 2 & 3): max. load, vertical & lateral stiffness, number of cycles (all values prior to failure) and failure types

Specimen	Maximal load [N]	Vertical stiffness K_V [N/mm]	Lateral stiffness K_L [N/mm]	Number of cycles	Failure types
TomoFix std 3	1280	1350	2000	>60 000	2
TomoFix std 4	1440	2000	2500	>80 000	2
TomoFix std 5	1760	2500	2200	>120 000	2
PEEKPower 3	1440	2000	2500	>80 000	2
PEEKPower 4	1280	1950	2140	>60 000	2
PEEKPower 5	1440	2785	2250	>80 000	2
iBalance 3	1760	4000	3600	>120 000	2,4
iBalance 4	1760	3000	3400	>120 000	2
iBalance 5	1920	3000	2952	>140 000	2
iBalance 6	1760	3500	2500	>120 000	1,2

Table 5 Summary of fatigue to failure tests (groups 4 & 5): max. load, vertical & lateral stiffness, number of cycles (all values prior to failure) and failure types

Specimen	Maximal load [N]	Vertical stiffness K_V [N/mm]	Lateral stiffness K_L [N/mm]	Number of cycles	Failure types
TomoFix sm 3	1280	2200	2000	>60 000	2,3
TomoFix sm 4	1280	1750	1500	>60 000	2,3
TomoFix sm 5	1760	2000	2300	>120 000	1,2
ContourLock 3	2400	2100	4400	>200 000	2
ContourLock 4	1760	2300	2400	>120 000	2
ContourLock 5	2400	2700	2600	>200 000	1,2,3

From our previous study and reported here for purposes of comparison

Table 6 Average mean values, including the standard deviations (SD) per group of the cyclic fatigue to failure tests (all decimal values rounded to the 1st decimal)

Groups	Maximal load [kN]		Vertical stiffness K_V [N/mm]		Lateral stiffness K_L [N/mm]		Number of cycles prior to failure	
	Mean	SD ±	Mean	SD ±	Mean	SD ±	Mean	SD ±
TomoFix std	1.5	0.2	1950	577	2233	252	>86 000	30 550
PEEKPower	1.4	0.1	2245	468	2297	184	>73 000	11 500
iBalance	1.8	0.1	3375	479	3113	490	>125 000	10 000
TomoFix sm	1.4	0.3	1983	184	1933	330	>80 000	28 300
ContourLock	2.2	0.4	2367	250	3133	900	>173 000	37 700

PEEKPower implants, whereas we did not include the Puddu plate. The TomoFix plate fixator yielded the best fatigue strength during the cyclic load to failure tests performed by Agneskirchner et al. (Agneskirchner et al. 2006), who reported that a rigid long plate fixator with stable locking bolts provides the best results in open-wedge HTO. Maas et al. (Maas et al. 2013) reported higher fatigue strength for the ContourLock plates when compared to the TomoFix sm plates. This observation diverges somewhat with the findings of Agneskirchner et al. (Agneskirchner et al. 2006). With regard to the results of our study, it can be concluded that the ContourLock was also superior to the TomoFix std regarding the cyclic load to failure tests (Table 6 and Fig. 18). Furthermore the iBalance group showed superior stability than the TomoFix groups in the cyclic loading hence one may conclude that stability provided by a plate is not correlated only to its length, but also to the kind of fixation, which seems to be the governing feature since the plates already have sufficient stiffness and strength.

Clinical studies reported better clinical results in terms of implant-related complications, non-unions and stability (Saeed and Rae 2009; Valkering et al. 2009; Woon-Hwa et al. 2013; Cotic et al. 2014; Staubli et al. 2003) for the TomoFix plates. This high healing rate is supposedly due to the callus-massage effect of the implant, meaning no compression between plate and bone (Staubli et al. 2003), which promotes osteogenesis thanks to the elastic bone-implant construct (Staubli 2008; Staubli and Jacob 2010). This fact is in accord with the present results since the TomoFix plates did not show the highest stiffness in this study. Nevertheless the question of the correlation between the best osteotomy outcomes and the stiffness provided by the implants could be discussed.

The limited number of specimens per group should also be taken into account. The testing procedure differs from reality where muscle forces, bending moments and ligament act together in the knee biomechanics and

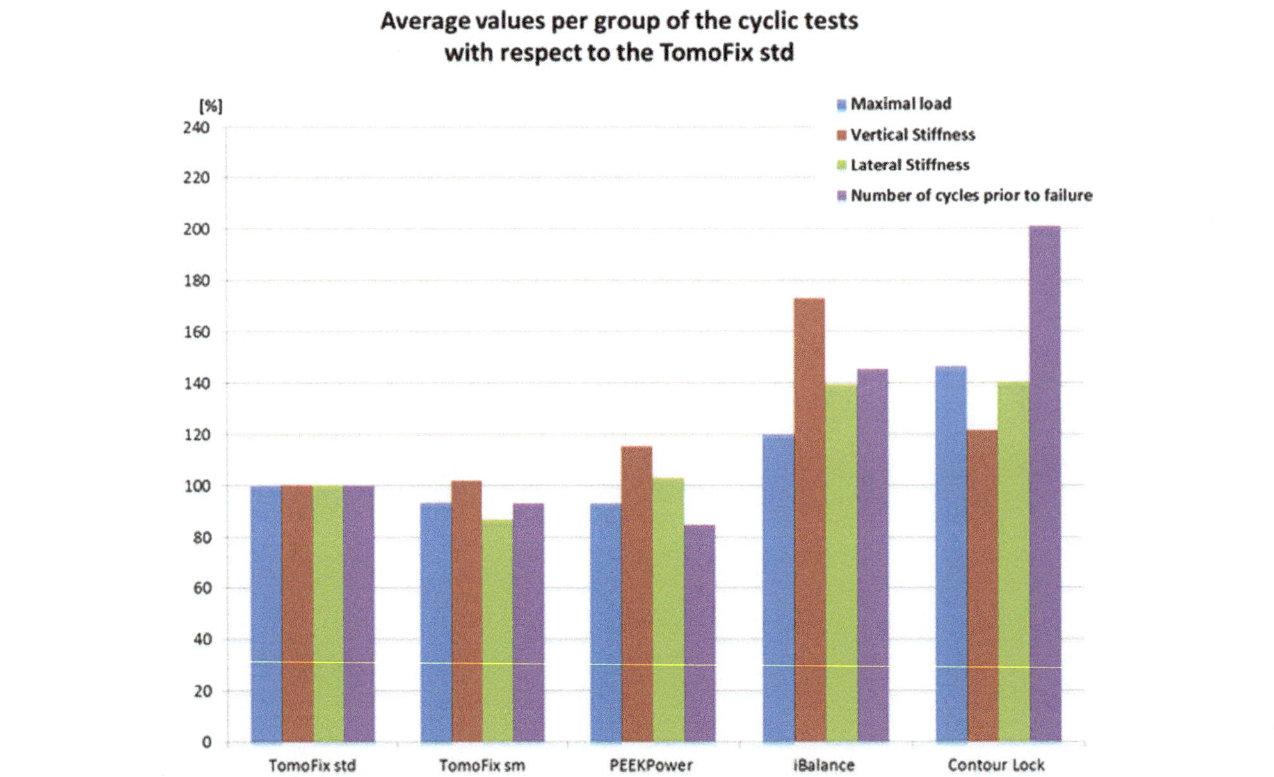

Fig. 18 Average relative strength values of Table 6. The TomoFix std group was taken as reference

hence alter the real charging of the plates. As already stated by (Brinkman et al. 2014), it is important to consider life-like test conditions while performing biomechanical testing of implants. The loads applied during the cyclic fatigue testing resemble the physiological loads like when slow walking. However if bone healing takes place before high cycle numbers as those in this study can be reached. Hence one should proceed with caution when applying the results of the present study to clinical settings.

Conclusions

In summary all the tested plates showed sufficient strength during static loading. All specimens failed due to a fracture of the opposite cortical bone. The TomoFix std showed a higher degree of stability than the small stature version. The results of the cyclic load to failure tests show that the stability of the bone-implant constructs is correlated with the fixation design. The ContourLock plate with its wider T-shaped proximal end showed a higher lifespan prior to failure, followed by the iBalance implants due their closed-wedge design which provides higher stiffness to the bone-implants constructs. The TomoFix and the PEEKPower plates with their narrow T-shaped proximal ends showed less rigidity compared to the ContourLock and the iBalance implants. Since healing rates are reported to be high after TomoFix fixation, which is supposedly due to the callus-massage effect of the implant and the elastic bone-implant construct, it remains to be seen whether constructs with a higher mechanical strength have higher bone healing rates with an equal amount of intraoperative safeness than the TomoFix plate, the current golden standard.

Competing interests

There is no financial relation to the commercial parties mentioned directly or indirectly in this paper. All the authors report no conflict of interest.

Authors' contributions

All authors have contributed to writing and correcting this manuscript. ADK: principal author, study planning, performing tests, analyzing test results, writing manuscript; SM: study planning, analyzing test results, writing manuscript; DW: study planning, writing manuscript; AZ: study planning, writing manuscript; KD: study planning, performing tests, writing manuscript; DP: study planning, analyzing test results, writing manuscript. All authors have read and approved the final manuscript.

Acknowledgements

Supported by the INTERREG IV Programme of the European Union, Stefan Maas and Dietrich Pape are partners in the project "Experimentelle und klinische Orthopädie der Großregion / Orthopédie Expérimentale et Clinique de la Grande Région" at the Universität der Großregion / Université de la Grande Région (UGR).

Author details

[1]Faculty of Science, Technology and Communication, University of Luxembourg, 6, rue R. Coudenhove-Kalergi, L-1359 Luxembourg, Luxembourg. [2]Department of Orthopedic Surgery, Centre Hospitalier de Luxembourg, L-1460 Luxembourg, Luxembourg. [3]Sports Medicine Research Laboratory, Public Research Centre for Health, Luxembourg, Centre Médical de la Fondation Norbert Metz, 76, rue d'Eich, L-1460 Luxembourg, Luxembourg.

References

Agneskirchner J, Freiling D, Hurschler C, Lobenhoffer P (2006) Primary stability of four different implants for opening wedge high tibial osteotomy. Knee Surg Sports Traumatol Arthrosc 14:291–300

Brinkman J-M, Hurschler C, Agneskirchner J, Lobenhoffer P, Castelein RM, Van Heerwaarden RJ (2014) Biomechanical testing of distal femur osteotomy plate fixation techniques: The role of simulated physiological loading. J Exp Orthop 1:1

Chong AC, Miller F, Buxton M, Friis EA (2007) Fracture Toughness and fatigue crack propagation rate of short fiber reinforced epoxy composites for analogue cortical bone. J Biomech Eng 129(4):487–493

Cotic M, Vogt S, Hinterwimmer S, Feucht MJ, Slotta-Huspenina J, Schuster T, Imhoff AB (2014) A matched-pair comparison of two different locking plates for valgus-producing medial open-wedge high tibial osteotomy: peek-carbon composite plate versus titanium plate. Knee Surgery, Sport Traumatology, Arthroscopy, doi: 10.1007/s00167-014-2914-8

Fowler PJ, Tan JL, Brown GA (2000) Medial opening wedge high tibial osteotomy: how I do it. Oper Tech Sports Med 8:32–38

Gardner MP, Chong ACM, Pollock AG, Wooley PH (2010) Mechanical Evaluation of Large-Size Fourth-Generation Composite Femur and Tibia Models. Ann Biomed Eng 38(3):613–620

Heiner AD (2008) Structural properties of fourth-generation composite femurs and tibias. J Biomech 41:3282–3284

Heinlein B, Kutzner I, Graichen F, Bender A, Rohlmann A, Halder AM, Beier A, Bergmann G (2009) ESB clinical biomechanics award 2008: Complete data of total knee replacement loading for level walking and stair climbing measured in vivo with a follow-up of 6-101 months. Clin Biomech 24:315–326

ISO 7206-4 (1989) Implants for surgery: Determination of endurance properties of stemmed femoral components with application of torsion

ISO 7206-6 (1992) Implants for surgery: Determination of endurance properties of head and neck region of stemmed femoral components

ISO 7206-8 (1995) Implants for surgery: Endurance performance of stemmed femoral components with application of torsion

Lobenhoffer P, Agneskirchner JD (2003) Improvements in surgical technique of valgus high tibial osteotomy. Knee Surg Sports Traumatol Arthrosc 3(11):132–138

Luo C-A, Hua S-Y, Lin S-C, Chen C-M, Tseng C-S (2013) Stress and stability comparison between different systems for high tibial osteotomies. Muscoskel Disord 14:110. doi:10.1186/1471-2474-14-110

Maas S, Diffo Kaze A, Dueck K, Pape D (2013) Static and Dynamic Differences in Fixation Stability between a Spacer Plate and a Small Stature Plate Fixator Used for High Tibial Osteotomies: A Biomechanical Bone Composite Study. ISRN Orthopedics, Volume 2013. doi: 10.1155/2013/387620

Pape D, Lorbach O, Schmitz C, Busch LC, Van Giffen N, Seil R, Kohn DM (2010) Effect of a biplanar osteotomy on primary stability following high tibial osteotomy: a biomechanical cadaver study. Knee Surg Sports Traumatol Arthrosc 18:204–211

Pape D, Kohn D, Van Giffen N, Hoffman A, Seil R, Lorbach O (2011) Differences in fixation stability between spacer plate and plate fixator following high tibial osteotomy. Knee Surg Sports Traumatol Arthrosc, PubMed. doi: 10.1007/s00167-011-1693-8

Pape D, Dueck K, Haag M, Lorbach O, Seil R, Madry H (2012) Wedge Volume and osteotomy surface depend on surgical technique for high tibial osteotomy. Knee Surg Sports Traumatol Arthrosc 21(1):127–133

Pornrattanamaneewong C, Harnroongroj T, Chareancholvanich K (2012) Loss of correction after medial opening wedge high tibial osteotomy: a comparison of locking plate without bone grafts and non-locking compression plates with bone grafts. J Med Assoc Thai 95(9):21–28

Saeed HZ, Rae PJ (2009) High tibial valgus osteotomy using the Tomofix plate–medium-term results in young patients. Acta Orthop Belg 75(3):360–367

Spahn G, Wittig R (2002) Primary stability of various implants in tibial opening wedge osteotomy: a biomechanical study. J Orthop Sci 7:683–687

Spahn G, Kirschbaum S, Kahl E (2006) Factors that influence high tibial osteotomy results in patients with medial gonarthritis: a score to predict the results. OsteoArthritis and Cartilage 14:190–195

Staubli AE (2008) Radiological examination of bone healing after open-wedge tibial osteotomy. In: Osteotomies around the knee. Thieme, AO Foundation Publishing, Stuttgart, New York, pp 131–146

Staubli AE, Jacob H (2010) Evolution of open-wedge high tibial osteotomy: experience with a special angular stable device for internal fixation without interposition material. Int Orthop 34:167–172

Staubli AE, De Simoni C, Babst R, Lobenhoffer P (2003) TomoFix: a new LCP-concept for open wedge osteotomy of the medial proximal tibia - early results in 92 cases. Injury 34:55–62

Stoffel K, Stachowiak G, Markus K (2004) Open wedge high tibial osteotomy: biomechanical investigation of the modified Arthrex Osteotomy Plate (Puddu Plate) and the TomoFix Plate. Clin Biomech 19:944–950

Taylor WR, Heller MO, Bergmann G, Duda GN (2004) Tibio-femoral loading during human gait and stair climbing. J Orthop Res 22:625–632

Valkering KP, Van den Bekerom MPJ, Kappelhoff FM, Albers GHR (2009) Complications after tomofix medial opening wedge high tibial osteotomy. J Knee Surg 22(3):218–225

Watanabe K, Kamiya T, Suzuki D, Otsubo H, Teramoto A, Suzuki T, Yamashita T (2014) Biomechanical stability of open-wedge high tibial osteotomy: comparison of two locking plates. Open J Orthoped 4:257–262

Woon-Hwa J, Chung-Woo C, Ji-Hoon L, Ha J-H, Ji-Hyae K, Jae-Heon J (2013) Comparative Study of Medial Opening-Wedge High Tibial Osteotomy Using 2 Different Implants. Arthroscopy: J Arthroscopic Related Surgery 29(6):1063–1071

Zhim F, Laflamme GY, Viens H, Saidane K, Yahia L (2005) Biomechanical stability of high tibial opening wedge osteotomy: Internal fixation versus external fixation. Clinical Biomechanics 20:871–876

An intra-bone axial load transducer: development and validation in an in-vitro radius model

Nikolas K. Knowles[1,3], Michael Gladwell[1,2] and Louis M. Ferreira[1,2*]

Abstract

Background: Accurate measurement of forces through the proximal radius can assess the effects of some surgical procedures on radioulnar load sharing, but is difficult to achieve given the redundant loading nature of the musculoskeletal system. Previously reported devices have relied on indirect measurements that may alter articular joint location and function. An axial load transducer interposed in the diaphysis of the radius may accurately quantify unknown axial loads of the proximal radius, and maintain articular location.

Methods: An *in-vitro* radius model was developed by interposing an axial load transducer in the diaphysis of the proximal radius. Static loads of 20, 40, 60, 80, and 100 N were applied with a servo-hydraulic actuator to the native radial head at angles of 10°, 20°, 30°, and 40° in the anterior, posterior, medial and lateral directions.

Findings: Linear regression of five repeatability trials showed excellent agreement between the transducer and applied loads ($R^2 = 1$ for all trials). For off-axis net joint loads, the majority of measured loading errors were within the inter-quartile range for mean loads up to 80 N. Loads below 80 N and outside the inter-quartile range had errors of less than 1 N.

Conclusions: The repeatability and off-axis net joint load results of this study validate the effectiveness of the interposed axial load transducer to accurately quantify proximal radius loads. The surgical technique preserves the native articular location and soft-tissue constructs, like the annular ligament. The modular design allows for testing the effects of length-changing osteotomies in subsequent biomechanical studies.

Keywords: Axial load transducer, Radiocapitellar joint, Bone-bridge, Radial head, Forearm loading, Radioulnar load sharing, Joint loading

Introduction

Load-sharing between the radius and ulna can be altered by some orthopaedic procedures as a result of implant placement during total elbow arthroplasty, replacement of the radial head with a prosthesis, or radial head and capitellum surgery (Markolf et al. 1998). In many clinical cases, length changes of the radius occur (Markolf et al. 1998), altering loads through the articulation and soft tissues. Length changes of the radius alter the natural kinematics of the elbow, intuitively increasing or decreasing radioulnar load sharing as a function of increasing or decreasing radial length. Although it has been suggested that failure to restore the joint to its native condition has unknown consequences (Shaaban et al. 2006), altered loads may increase the risk of cartilage wear and degenerative changes at the radiocapitellar and ulnohumeral articulations. As such, post-traumatic arthritis has been well-described and is a common complication of complex elbow injuries, even following appropriate bone and ligament repair (Ring et al. 2002). To ensure native load-sharing is maintained following surgical procedures to minimize the risk of the aforementioned suboptimal outcomes, it is essential to isolate intra-articular loads. Isolating loads through the proximal radius is impossible without interposing a measurement device within

* Correspondence: louis.ferreira@sjhc.london.on.ca
[1]Roth|Mcfarlane Hand and Upper Limb Centre, Surgical Mechatronics Laboratory, St. Josephs Health Care, 268 Grosvenor St., London N6A 4V2, ON, Canada
[2]Schulich School of Medicine and Dentistry, The University of Western University, 1151 Richmond St., N6A3K7 London, ON, Canada
Full list of author information is available at the end of the article

the bone due to the redundant loading scenario imposed by soft-tissues and osseous contacts.

Multiple studies have assessed elbow load sharing, and describe devices capable of measuring in-vitro radial and ulnar loads (Ekenstam et al. 1984; Markolf et al. 1998; Palmer et al. 1984; Palmer and Werner 1981; Pfaeffle and Fischer 1999; Rabinowitz and Light 1994; Trumble and Glisson 1987); however these devices disrupt soft tissues, especially the annular ligament, which are significant contributors to the net load vector through the radial head. Such a device which does not disrupt soft tissues, or alter the native location of the radial head, has yet to be described. This study describes the validation of a custom axial load transducer implanted in the proximal radius. The device was tested in an in-vitro radius model with a servo-hydraulic testing frame to assess the devices accuracy in measuring a wide range of proximal radius loading vector magnitudes and directions. Following validation of the device, its use in biomechanical studies assessing radiocapitellar and ulnar load sharing as a function of length changes of the radius will be performed.

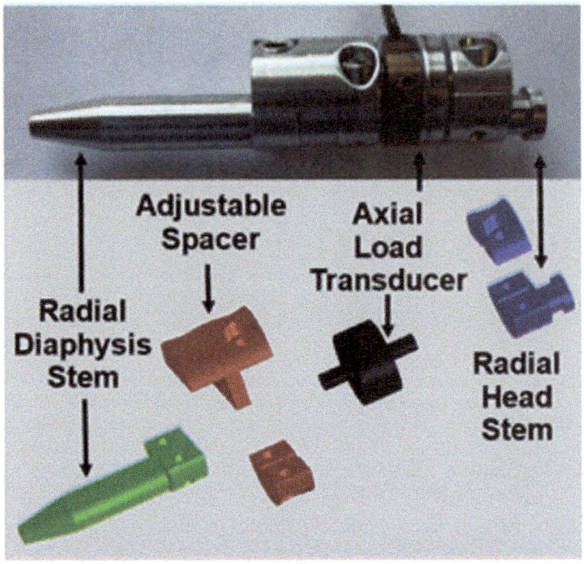

Fig. 1 Modular axial load transducer components. The radial and diaphysis stems are cemented in-situ. The adjustable spacer was changed to assess the effect of lengthening and shortening in subsequent cadaveric biomechanical studies

Methods

The *in-vitro* model consisted of one fresh-frozen cadaveric radius (age: 62, male) and an interposed modular axial load transducer device (Fig. 1). The device was custom manufactured to allow for stem fixation in the diaphysis and head of the radius. An adjustable spacer was included as part of the design to allow for the effect of radial length changes on radial loads to be measured in subsequent cadaveric biomechanical studies. The device uses a commercially available axial load transducer (Subminiature Model 11, Honeywell, Morristown, NJ, USA) and the modular design allows for installation while maintaining a bone bridge to preserve the native radial head articular location.

The surgical procedure (Fig. 2) consisted of first opening a cortical window in the radial neck to expose the intermedullary canal. Bone cement was then inserted in the diaphysis and radial head, the respective stems were placed, and the load transducer was assembled in-situ, prior to cement hardening. At this time a section of the radial neck remained, termed the 'bone-bridge,' in order to preserve the native radial head articular location. The proximal radius osteotomy was completed after the cement hardening by removing the bone-bridge. The radius was then excised from the forearm and denuded of all soft-tissue for validation testing of the implanted device.

The radius was rigidly mounted in a clamp for digitization of the load transducer and bony landmarks using a rigid body stylus with an optical tracking system (Optotrak Certus, NDI, Waterloo, CAN). These landmarks were used to derive an anatomical coordinate system about the long-axis of the radius. The anatomical coordinate system was derived using the mid-point of the dorsal and volar aspects of the distal radial ulnar joint (DRUJ), and radial styloid point, as well as the center of the radial head. The proximal and distal coordinates of the load transducer within the bone were also digitized to determine its relative offset with the anatomical long-axis. This coordinate system allowed for alignment of the anatomical long-axis relative to the actuator of a servo-hydraulic testing frame (Instron® 8501, Norwood, MA, USA). Transducer offset was 3.61° in the anterior-posterior and 3.50° in the medial-lateral planes relative to the anatomical long-axis.

The radius was aligned and fixed in an ABS tube using the same previously digitized anatomical landmarks. Bone cement was placed in the ABS tube to secure the radius and maintain alignment of the anatomical long-axis. The ABS tube with the proximal radius protruding was mounted on a custom base within an angle jig mounted to an X-Y stage (Fig. 3). This jig allowed for a range of simulated net load vector angles of the model, and the X-Y stage ensured proper alignment of the servo-hydraulic actuator with the anatomical long-axis. The native capitellum diameter was simulated using a metal hemisphere mounted to the servo-hydraulic actuator. The base of the ABS tube pivoted on a smooth spherical bearing, aligned with the digitized anatomical long-axis of the radius, to nullify reaction moments.

Repeatability was assessed using five independent trials with the anatomical long-axis aligned with the servo-hydraulic actuator (0° position) (Fig. 4a). Loads were applied at 10 Hz from 0 to 450 N and corresponding

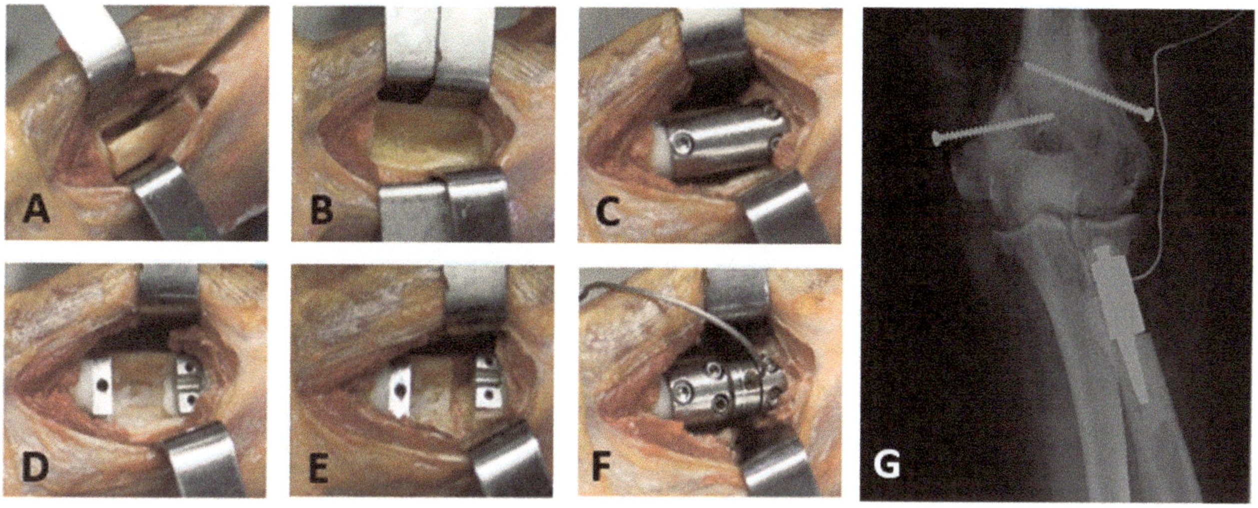

Fig. 2 The bone-bridge surgical technique. Removal of cortical window (**a**). Exposed intermedullary canal (**b**). Head and diaphysis stem placement using spacer to ensure alignment (**c**). Spacer removed and stems cemented in-situ (**d**). Removal of bone-bridge (**e**). Implantation of load transducer and re-alignment of native anatomical position (**f**). Radiograph of implanted load transducer device in a cadaveric radius (**g**)

transducer loads were collected at 10 Hz. Linear regression was used to assess linearity of the applied load and measured transducer loads for each trial. This repeatability test represented a 4.5 fold increase in desired maximum validation testing load, and was also used to assess the durability of the device under extreme loading conditions.

For validation testing of a variety of simulated net joint load directions and magnitudes, static loads were applied from 20 to 100 N at 20 N increments at angles of 10°, 20°, 30° and 40° to the anatomical long-axis. The radius model was rotated in quarter turn increments to assess loads in the anterior-posterior and medial-lateral planes, resulting in 16 separate loading conditions. Axial load transducer values were collected using custom software (Labview, National Instruments, Austin TX, USA).

External loads of 20, 40, 60, 80, and 100 N were applied using the Instron servo-hydraulic actuator. The Instron load cell provided the 'gold standard' load measurement, which was corrected for the angle between the actuator applied load and the anatomical long-axis, to calculate the radial axis load (Fig. 4b). The transducer axis offset of 3.61° was added to the off-axis net joint load angle in the anterior direction and subtracted in the posterior

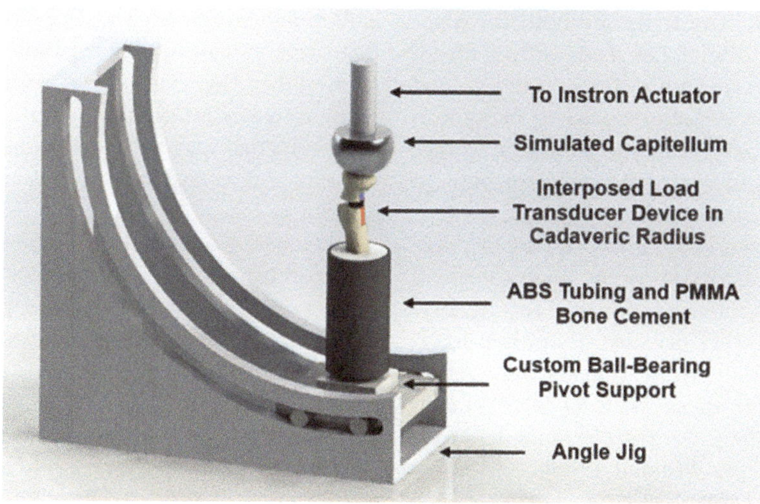

Fig. 3 Experimental set-up of the in-vitro radius model with interposed axial load transducer. The angle jig was mounted to an X-Y stage on a servo-hydraulic testing frame (not shown) for alignment of the actuator and simulated capitellum with the radial head. Note the support base could be fixed at the desired angle along the angle jig

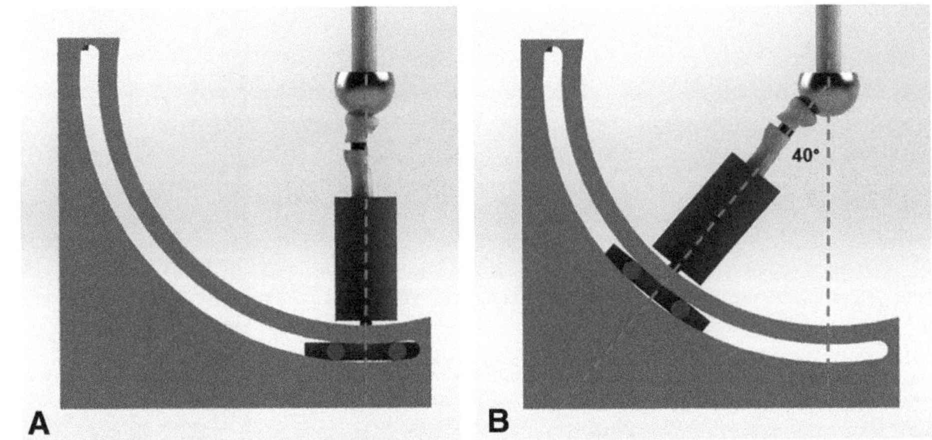

Fig. 4 Alignment of the servo-hydraulic actuator with the anatomical long-axis of the radius. Zero degree applied load direction (**a**). The anatomical long-axis alignment of 40° to the servo-hydraulic actuator (**b**). Note that the radius was tested at angles of 10°, 20°, 30° and 40° and four rotations of the radius for net loads in the anterior, posterior, medial, and lateral directions

direction, and transducer axis offset of 3.50° was added in the medial direction and subtracted in the lateral direction (i.e. for 10° off-axis load in the anterior direction, radial axis load $= \frac{\text{applied load (20,40,60,80,100N)}}{\cos(10^\circ + 3.61^\circ)}$). The measured transducer loads and known radial axis loads were plotted as Bland-Altman plots to assess variations in transducer and Instron loads, and to visualize systematic bias. Correlations between load transducer and radial axis loads at each net load position were calculated using Pearson Product Moment Correlations. Significance was set at $p < 0.05$.

Findings

Linear regression of the five repeatability trials with the actuator and anatomical long-axis aligned (0° position), showed linear trends for all five trails and both the measured load transducer and radial axis loads ($R^2 = 1$ for all trials). There was no variation in the measured load transducer values with the 4.5 fold increase in maximum load, indicating the device's ability to withstand forces greater than experienced in-vivo, without disruption to device fixation or the load transducer.

Differences in transducer and radial axis loads were less than 6 N for off-axis angles up to 30° in all four load directions. Differences increased linearly for linearly applied static loads, and were greatest at applied loads greater than 80 N. Most differences in loads were within the inter-quartile range for mean loads of 80 N. Loads below 80 N and outside the inter-quartile range had load differences of less than 1 N. Pearson Product Moment Correlations showed significant relationships between transducer and radial axis loads for all 16 net joint load directions ($r = 1.00$ and $p < 0.001$ for each net joint load). Largest differences between transducer and radial axis loads occurred at 40° in the medial and anterior directions (Fig. 5).

Conclusions

The majority of differences between transducer and known radial axis loads below load magnitudes of 80 N fell within the inter-quartile range for each net load direction. Loads below 80 N outside of this range had load magnitudes of less than 1 N. This result, as well as the results of the repeatability trials, validate the effectiveness of the interposed transducer device to accurately quantify intra-articular loading of the proximal radius.

It is important to keep in mind that the range of angles tested does not represent the joint range, but rather a range of loading vectors due to articular contact and soft tissue supports. This does not suggest that possible load vectors can be this extreme. As such, this validation shows that this device can accurately represent a wide cone range of internally generated net loads.

The medial and anterior loading directions are perpendicular, and as such the increased error in these positions cannot be explained by reduced implant fixation or stiffness of the overall construct. In accounting for misalignment of the load transducer measurement axis with the anatomical long-axis, it was noted that the transducer was positively misaligned in these directions. Although this misalignment was accounted for, and was constant throughout testing, it may interact with the load transducers off-axis measurement error to produce a non-linear response, contributing to the larger differences observed at these two positions.

Strengths of this study include the modular design of the axial load transducer, which allows for in-vitro real-time dynamic testing of radial length changes. The bone-bridge surgical technique ensures proper alignment of the device

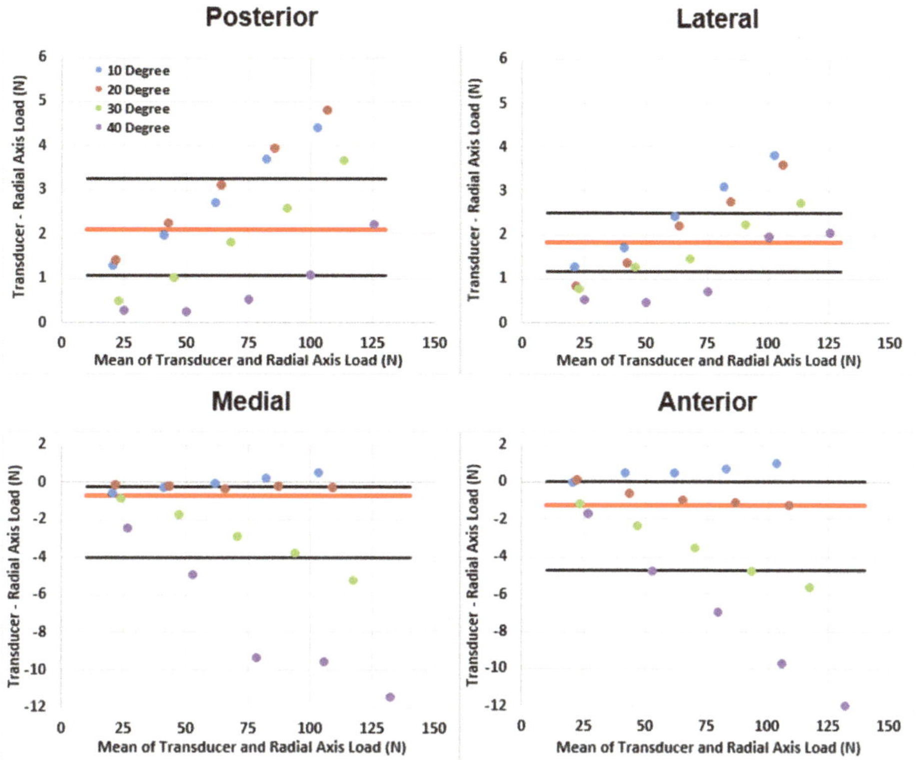

Fig. 5 Bland-Altman plots of four load angles and four rotations of the in-vitro radius model. The red line indicates the median and the black lines indicate the 25th and 75th quartiles for the non-parametric data

with the anatomical long-axis of the radius while maintaining the articular locations and soft-tissue constructs, such as the annular ligament. Furthermore, validation with the Instron servo-hydraulic testing frame and an external 'gold standard' load cell, provided a highly repeatable and controlled testing platform to measure loading of the interposed device. The ball-bearing pivot support nullified reaction moments and ensured only desired loads were measured.

Limitations of this study include the requirement to calculate the radial axis load partly based on the off-axis loading angle. Of course, it was not possible to directly measure the applied radial axis load because that was the novel function of the transducer. However, although the misalignment of the load transducer was determined with a highly accurate digitizer, any error in these angle measurements may have contributed a systematic bias.

This study provides a validated in-vitro interposed axial load transducer to be used in cadaveric biomechanical studies. Its modular design allows assessment of length-changing osteotomies, and its compactness provides for minimal soft-tissue disruption, including the annular ligament. Additionally, it allows preservation of the native articular alignment. Maintaining the native articulations using the bone bridge technique ensures physiologic loads are measured.

Competing interests
The authors declare that they have no competing interests.

Authors' contributions
NK developed the testing protocol, collected data, performed data analysis, and wrote manuscript. MG developed the testing protocol, performed surgical procedures and edited manuscript. LF developed the testing protocol, performed data analysis and edited manuscript. All authors read and approved the final manuscript.

Author details
[1]Roth|Mcfarlane Hand and Upper Limb Centre, Surgical Mechatronics Laboratory, St. Josephs Health Care, 268 Grosvenor St., London N6A 4V2, ON, Canada. [2]Schulich School of Medicine and Dentistry, The University of Western University, 1151 Richmond St., N6A3K7 London, ON, Canada. [3]Department of Biomedical Engineering, The University of Western Ontario, 1151 Richmond St., N6A3K7 London, ON, Canada.

References
af Ekenstam F, Palmer AK, Glisson RR (1984) The load on the radius and ulna in different positions of the wrist and forearm: a cadaver study. Acta Orthop Scand 55(3):363–365
Markolf KL, Lamey D, Yang S, Meals ROY, Hotchkiss R (1998) Radioulnar load-sharing in the forearm. J Bone Joint Surg Am 80(6):879–888

Palmer A, Werner F (1981) The triangular fibrocartilage complex of the wrist—anatomy and function. J Hand Surg Am 6(2):153–162
Palmer AK, Werner FW, Eng MM (1984) Biomechanics of the distal radioulnar joint. Clin Orthop Relat Res 187:26–35
Pfaeffle HJ, Fischer K (1999) A new methodology to measure load transfer through the forearm using multiple universal force sensors. J Biomech 32(12):1331–1335
Rabinowitz R, Light T (1994) The role of the interosseous membrane and triangular fibrocartilage complex in forearm stability. J Hand Surg Am 19(3):385–393
Ring D, Jupiter J, Zilberfarb J (2002) Posterior dislocation of the elbow with fractures of the radial head and coronoid. J Bone Joint Surg Am 84(4):547–551
Shaaban H, Giakas G, Bolton M, Williams R, Wicks P, Scheker LR, Lees VC (2006) The load-bearing characteristics of the forearm: pattern of axial and bending force transmitted through ulna and radius. J Hand Surg Br 31(3):274–279
Trumble T, Glisson R (1987) Forearm force transmission after surgical treatment of distal radioulnar joint disorders. J Hand Surg Am 12(2):196–202

26

Surgical-experimental principles of anterior cruciate ligament (ACL) reconstruction with open growth plates

Romain Seil[1,2*], Frederick K Weitz[3] and Dietrich Pape[1,2]

Abstract

Objective: To review surgical and animal experimental studies performed with open growth plates in relation with pediatric anterior cruciate ligament (ACL) reconstruction.

Backround: When it comes to the treatment of ACL injured children, there is a lack of current international guidelines, leaving the treating physicians with a therapeutic dilemma. A variety of surgical and animal experimental studies have been undertaken over the last decades in relation with open growth plates and ACL-reconstruction.

Method: Based on our own previous animal experimental data, we highlighted 15 specific points concerning pediatric ACL-reconstruction and reviewed additional literature concerning these individual items.

Results: Pediatric ACL-reconstruction could be proven to be safe in animal models. Growth abnormalities, risk factors and factors, which were specifically related to biological healing processes in children, were identified. From them surgical principles for safe pediatric ACL replacements can be deducted. Applying these principles through a correct technical execution of surgery may prevent clinically significant growth changes.

Conclusion: Over the last 2 decades it has been shown that a technically correct pediatric ACL reconstruction has little risk in creating clinically significant growth abnormalities. Animal experiments support this hypothesis despite the fact that the gained knowledge cannot be fully generalized to humans. More long time follow-up is needed to fully understand the complete risk factors related to ACL surgery with open growth plates.

Introduction

Anterior cruciate ligament (ACL) injuries are among the most frequent severe knee injuries affecting physically active children and adolescents. They have both short and long-term consequences, affecting future knee structure and function with subsequent meniscus and cartilage injuries, early development of osteoarthritis and a serious economic burden to civil society due to potentially shortened professional careers and later surgeries. McConkey et al. (2011) reported that 0.5-3% of all ACL injuries occur in children and adolescents and the incidence is increasing due to increased sports participation. Shea et al. (2004) reviewed the insurance claims in football over a 5 years period in athletes aged from 5 to 18. Of 8215 total claims, knee injuries accounted for 22% and from the knee claims ACL injuries accounted for 31%. At the end of the growth period, the incidence of ACL injuries increases dramatically, reaching a peak in the group of 15–20 years old female athletes who participate in sports that require sudden deceleration, landing and pivoting movements (Engelman et al. 2014; Arendt and Dick 1995; Yu and Garrett 2007). Altogether, ACL injuries in children, adolescents and young adults are increasing (Aichroth 2002; Mohtadi and Grant 2006). The main reasons for this are participation in organized youth sports, increased female participation in high risk sports, potentially decreased motoric skills in this population and the physicians' improved diagnostic skills.

When it comes to the treatment of ACL injured children, there is a lack of current international guidelines, leaving the treating physicians with a therapeutic dilemma.

* Correspondence: rseil@yahoo.com
[1]Department of Orthopaedic Surgery, Centre Hospitalier Luxembourg, Clinique d'Eich. 78, rue d'Eich, L-1460 Luxembourg, Luxembourg
[2]Sports Medicine Research Laboratory, Luxembourg Institute of Health, 78 rue d'Eich, L-1460 Luxembourg, Luxembourg
Full list of author information is available at the end of the article

On the one hand, nonoperative treatment has shown to be successful in some patients (Woods and O'Connor 2004; Moksnes et al. 2013), but the reasons for this are poorly understood (Funahashi et al. 2014). Furthermore, a strong association between the delay of surgery and the occurrence of meniscus and cartilage lesions strongly suggests that a nonoperative treatment may be detrimental to the intra-articular soft tissues. On the other hand, surgery is difficult and highly specialized due to the specific anatomy of children's knees and its serious complication potential. Therefore, anterior cruciate ligament replacement surgery in children is controversial and many operative techniques have been described (Figure 1). All of them bear a specific risk for growth disturbances, either through indirect growth changes in extraepiphyseal surgical procedures or through growth plate injuries in epiphyseal or transphyseal techniques (Mohtadi and Grant 2006; McConkey et al. 2011; Kocher et al. 2007; Frosch et al. 2010; Lo et al. 1997).

Every surgical procedure or injury near to growth plate may lead to growth abnormalities. Experimental studies on the growth plate cartilage helps understanding the risk of such growth changes (Ollier 1867; Bidder 1873; Haas 1945a,b; Ford and Key 1956). The purpose of the present review article is (1) to illustrate the surgical and experimental knowledge on growth plate injuries related to pediatric ACL reconstruction and (2) show the relation between routinely used tibial and femoral tunnels of an intra-articular, transphyseal ACL replacement technique, the tibial and femoral growth plate and relevant soft-tissue structures around the knee.

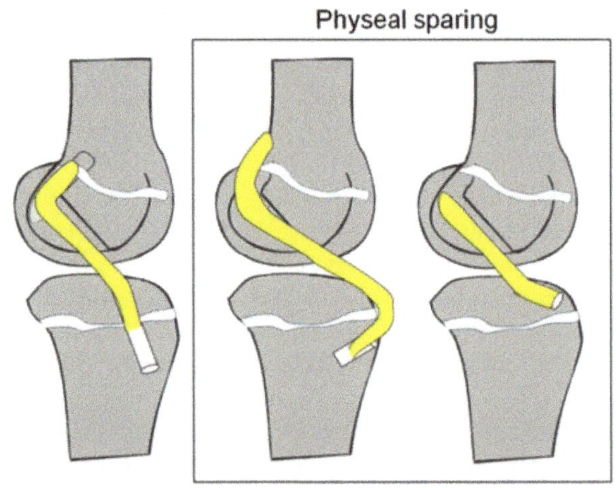

Figure 1 Representation of different pediatric ACL reconstruction techniques in lateral knee views. Surgeons differentiate between transphyseal and physeal sparing techniques. The former implicate drilling of a bone tunnel through the femoral and tibial growth plate whereas the latter do not cause any direct iatrogenic physeal injuries, but bear the risk of indirect damage to the growth plate. The ACL grafts are placed either within the epiphysis or turn around the physis. Many surgeons use different techniques on the femoral and the tibial side.

Anatomy and function of the growth plate

The growth plate is located between the epiphysis and the metaphysis of long bones. It regulates endochondral growth and has in its center a complex anatomy with the following cellular layers (from the epiphyses to the metaphysis): the reserve zone, the proliferative zone, the layer with prehypertrophic chondrocytes and the hypertrophic zone which is subdivided in cellular layers of maturation, degeneration and calcification (Jouve et al. 1998; Mackie et al. 2011) (Figure 2). The review does not intend to give a detailed overview of the cellular and molecular levels of the growth plate cartilage, recently described in details by Mackie et al. (2011) and Michigami (2013). Vascularisation is separated between the epi- and the metaphysis and as a consequence the growth plate represents a frontier between these 2 structures playing an important role in the physeal pathology of certain tumors and infections. At its periphery we find the presence of the perichondral structures. They are composed by the perichondral ring of Lacroix (Lacroix 1951) providing mechanical support and the ossification groove of Ranvier (Ranvier 1889) which provides cells for growth in width. In a newer study, Karlsson et al. (2009) exposed 3 month old New Zealand white rabbits to bromodeoxyuridine (BrdU). They could find BrdU positive cells i.e. proliferative cells in the perichondral zone of Ranvier and in all zones of cartilage. After wash out, a small amount of progenitor cells were present in the cartilage and in the perichondral groove

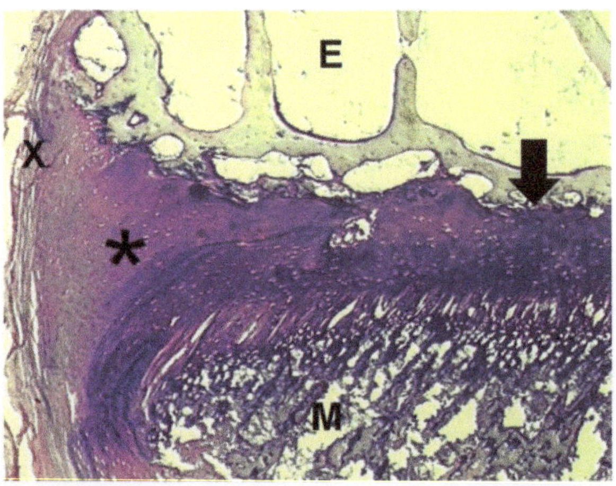

Figure 2 Distal femoral growth plate of a 10 months old sheep (x = perichondral fibrous ring of LaCroix; * = ossification groove of Ranvier; E = epiphysis; M = metaphysis; arrow = center of the growth plate with columnal chondrocyte structure) (Giemsa staining; magnification x 25).

of Ranvier, showing that the latter is also a stem cell niche. They have an important physiologic role thus constituting the crossroads between longitudinal growth and growth in width of the bone. Furthermore, their presence plays an important role in the stabilization of this transitional zone between the epi- and the metaphysis. The perichondral structures do also play an important role from a pathologic point of view through the specific pediatric fractures classified as #6 in the Ogden classification system (Ogden 1981).

Experimental principles on surgery with open growth plates

The question of remaining endochondral growth after growth plate injuries has been of great interest for orthopaedic surgeons for more than 150 years. Already in 1867 Ollier performed surgical experiments on cats in which he sectioned the growth plate longitudinally. He noticed that the superficial sections did not influence longitudinal growth whereas deep cuts did induce growth abnormalities. Haas noted in 1945 that a cerclage wire which was slung around the growth plate resulted in a decrease of longitudinal growth. In case of a breakage of the wire, growth continued normally. Based on the first clinical experiences with epiphysiodesis (Phemister 1933; Blount and Clarke 1949) in the first half of the 20th century, many experimental studies were published with the goal to develop treatments regulating longitudinal growth like temporary epiphysiodesis, epiphysiolysis capitis femoris and their respective fixation principles (Haas 1945a,b, 1950; Campbell et al. 1959; Friedenberg 1957; Ford and Key 1956; Key and Ford 1958; Siffert 1956; Barash and Siffert 1966; Nordentoft 1969). With the development of ACL reconstruction techniques and the identification of the problem of ACL injuries in children, several specific surgical-experimental studies analysing paediatric ACL replacements were published during the last 3 decades. They were conducted in rabbits, pigs, sheep and dogs with open growth plates (Stadelmaier et al. 1995; Guzzanti et al. 1994; Janarv et al. 1998; Ono et al. 1998; Edwards et al. 2001; Seil et al. 2008; Meller et al. 2008a,b, 2009a,b, Chudik et al. 2007; Murray et al. 2010). They allowed recognizing the risks related to specific surgical techniques and especially the fact, that a technically correct anterior cruciate ligament surgery in a pediatric patient bears little risk of a clinically relevant secondary growth change. From these experimental studies on the growth plate as well as clinical experiences from the past, a certain number of surgical principles can be applied either directly or indirectly to ACL reconstruction with open growth plates. The surgical principles, which will be discussed in this review paper, are represented in Table 1.

The cartilage of the growth plate does generally not regenerate after a drill injury

Based on their animal experiments in rabbits and pigs, Langenskiöld and colleagues have shown between the 1950's and the 1980's that central lesions of the growth plate had the capacity to regenerate in very young animals if a transphyseal bone bridge formation was prevented (Langenskiöld (1993); Langenskiöld 1987; Langenskiöld 1986; Langenskiöld 1981; Langenskiöld 1975; Langenskiöld 1979). In their experiments, regeneration took place by interstitial proliferation of cells from the germinal layer of the adjacent uninjured parts of the growth plate. The extent of this process was inversely proportional to the size of the used animal species. However, if a bone bridge developed after a transphyseal drill injury, the lesion of the growth plate cartilage was irreversible. This could be shown in the 1950's by Siffert (1956) et al. in 6 weeks old rabbits. Despite this bone bridge, longitudinal growth often did not get altered. Similar findings were repeatedly noted in many other animal experiments (Figure 3).

Leaving a transphyseal drill hole empty results in the formation of a bone bridge (Figure 4)

Siffert (1956) analyzed the effect of a transphyseally placed 2.0 mm K-wire on the medial epiphysis of the proximal tibia in rabbits. In none of the animals growth changes could be noted. The wire grew distally from the physis and the cartilage resulting from the drill injury of the growth plate was replaced by bone. In 1960, Johnson and Southwick (1960) drilled bone tunnels (Ø 2,8 mm, corresponding to approximately 11% of the surface of the physis) through the distal femoral growth plate of 6 weeks old rabbits. In all of their 32 cases, they noticed the formation of a transphyseal bone bridge which induced a complete or a partial closure of the growth plate in 3 animals. In 21 cases the bone bridge was partially resorbed whereas resumption was complete in 8 rabbits.

These localized bone bridge formations must be differentiated from the bony transformation of the growth plate occurring at the end of the growth period. At this stage, the entire growth plate cartilage is progressively replaced by cancellous bone (Synder et al. 1994).

Small bone bridges may resolve spontaneously

The impact of the transphyseal bone bridge on longitudinal growth is depending on several variables. Small bone bridges may be resorbed without influencing the remaining growth process. The absence of a macroscopic growth abnormality does not mean that there are no microscopic changes of the growth plate after surgically or traumatic induced injuries. Guzzanti et al. (1994) found that microscopic changes occurred within the growth plate after injury. They found a hyperplasia of the growth plate and a loss of the classical cellular

Table 1 Surgical-experimental principles of pediatric ACL-reconstruction

1.	Growth plate cartilage does generally not regenerate after a drill injury.
2.	Leaving a transphyseal drill hole empty results in the formation of a bone bridge.
3.	Small bone bridges may resolve spontaneously.
4.	The formation of a bone bridge may be prevented by the transphyseal placement of a tendon graft.
5.	Permanent transphyseal hardware placement can result in a growth abnormality.
6.	A central growth plate lesion may result in a symmetric shortening whereas a peripheral growth plate lesion may result in an axial deformity.
7.	The critical size for a growth abnormality due to a central growth plate lesion is 7-9% of the size of the growth plate.
8.	The critical size for a growth abnormality due to a peripheral growth plate lesion is 3-5% of the circumference of the growth plate.
9.	The size of the growth plate injury increases with drilling obliquity.
10.	The risk of a growth deformity is inversely proportional to the remaining growth potential.
11.	The force of the growth plate is associated with body weight.
12.	An excessive graft tension may lead to a tenoepiphysiodesis.
13.	During femoral tunnel drilling, iatrogenic injury to perichondral structures should be avoided.
14.	Epiphyseal and transphyseal ACL reconstructions may induce rotational deformities at the distal femur.
15.	Graft incorporation is faster in immature specimen as compared to adults.

architecture of this specific cartilage. This could be confirmed by other studies (Seil 2002). Filling a bony tunnel completely by a tendon graft could not prevent the formation of a bone bridge on a systematic basis. On the contrary, an incomplete filling of the tunnel by a tendon graft of a lesser diameter did not systematically result in the formation of a bone bridge (Seil 2002).

The formation of a bone bridge may be prevented by the transphyseal placement of a soft-tissue graft

Stadelmaier et al. (1995) analyzed the effects of filling transphyseal bone tunnels with tendon grafts in 10 weeks old dogs. Leaving the tunnel (Ø 4 mm) empty resulted in the formation of a transphyseal bone bridge as early as two weeks postoperatively. When the tunnel was filled with a soft tissue graft bridging could be avoided. In the study the tunnels were located in the center of the proximal tibia and in the distal femur. Growth abnormalities could not be found over a four-month observation period. Janarv et al. (1998) implanted a free tendon autograft (patellar tendon or Extensor digitorum longus tendon) into distal femoral tunnels (Ø 1,7; 2,5 and 3,4 mm) in rabbits. Bone bridge developments could be diminished through the implantation of the tendon grafts and growth abnormalities could be avoided. Österman (1994) created large surgical defects in the central part of distal femoral epiphysis on 37 rabbits. If the injured physis was left without grafting, it lead to significant growth disturbance. After filling the large growth plate defect with a fatty tissue augmentation at least a partial regeneration of longitudinal growth was restored and no significant deformities of the joint contours were seen.

Permanent transphyseal hardware placement can result in a growth abnormality

Based on early clinical experiences with permanent or temporary epiphysiodesis (Phemister 1933; Blount and Clarke 1949) many experimental articles were published in the mid-20th century with the goal to improve growth regulation of long bones, but also to evaluate the risk of epiphyseal fractures or epiphysiolysis on the remaining longitudinal growth (Haas 1948, Haas 1945a,b, 1950; Campbell et al. 1959; Ford and Key 1956; Friedenberg 1957; Siffert 1956; Barash and Siffert 1966; Nordentoft 1969). At the end of the 20th century, first experiments were conducted with biodegradable materials. Mäkelä et al. (1987) studied the reaction of growth plates to a polyglactin 91 rod that was placed in the central portion of distal femoral growth plate in rabbits. Six weeks after implantation, the distal femoral physis showed similar growth disturbance as a drill hole which was left empty. In a later study, the same author (Mäkelä et al. 1989) showed that the size of the implant played a significant role in the development of growth disturbances. In rabbits with transphyseally placed 2.0 mm polydioxanone (PDS) implants no permanent growth disturbances could be found, whereas 3.2 mm PDS implants caused a growth disturbance similar to a drill hole. In a large animal study on sheep, placing a biodegradable interference screw over the growth plate resulted in a deformity of the proximal tibial growth plate. The fact that no major growth changes were observed may have been related to the fact that the inteference screw was placed centrally in the growth plate of the proximal tibia, similar to Stadelmaier's study (Stadelmaier et al. 1995). This revealed that microscopic growth plate deformities may also occur with the

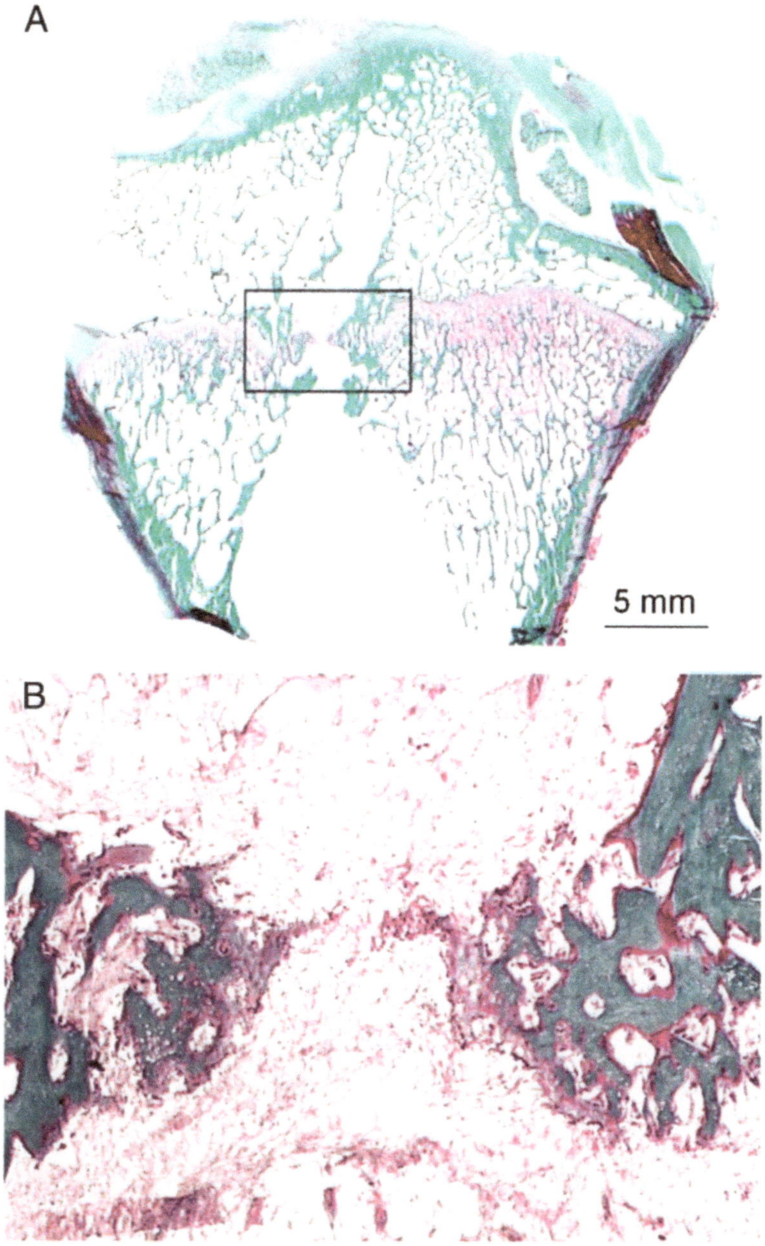

Figure 3 Sagittal section through a proximal tibia after drilling of a 5 mm tunnel in 4 months-old sheep. Six months later the growth plate cartilage did not recover and a bone bridge occurred. Below: Magnification X 25 (Masson-Goldner staining).

implantation of biodegradable materials and the authors did not recommend the use of such transphyseally placed implants in pediatric ACL reconstruction (Seil 2002).

A central growth plate lesion may result in a symmetric shortening whereas a peripheral lesion may result in an axial deformity

In 1956, Ford and Key showed that a central lesion of the distal femoral growth plate in rabbits of a significant size could be responsible for a symmetric shortening. In one group of animals they made a simple drill hole whereas a complete destruction of the growth plate was performed in a second group of animals. The disturbance of longitudinal growth was maximal in group 2. In a third group of animals they destroyed the perichondral structures completely and found that these lesions induced severe axial deviations. In the same year Siffert (1956) drilled a 2.8 mm K-wire through the medial physis of the proximal tibia in rabbits or created an injury with a curette. He noted that that the central lesions caused decreased longitudinal growth whereas axial deformities could be seen in the group with the peripheral

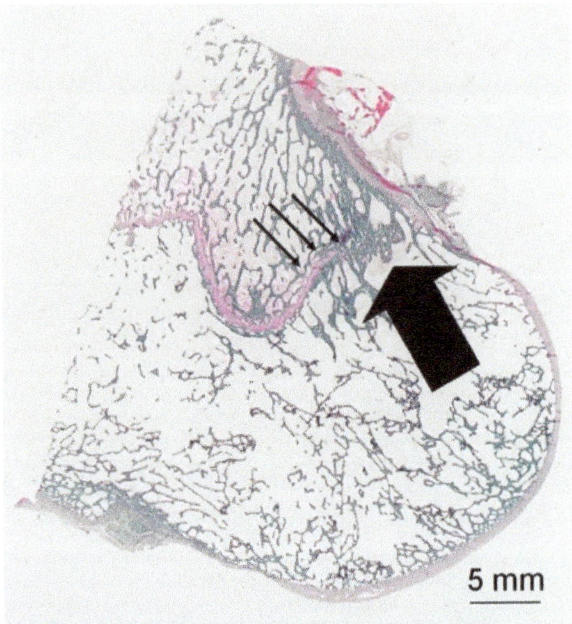

Figure 4 Sagittal section through the distal lateral femur of a 10 month old sheep. At 4 months a 5 mm tunnel had been drilled through the growth plate and the drill hole was not filled with a soft tissue graft. The growth plate cartilage did not recover (small arrows). A strong bone bridge occurred (large arrow) resulting in a femoral valgus deformity of 12°. Masson-Goldner staining.

injuries. While these early studies documented a difference between peripheral and central physeal lesions in terms of axial malalignment, little is known about the regional differences of an injury within the physis. Since most of these experimental data resulted from small animal studies, it remains questionable whether their conclusions may be extrapolated to larger animals or even to the human knee. Nevertheless, animal experiments (Seil et al. 2008; Edwards et al. 2001) and clinical reports on complications (Koman and Sanders 1999; Robert and Casin 2010; Kocher et al. 2002) showed that the anatomical location of a peripheral growth plate lesion (medial, lateral, anterior or posterior) might have an impact on specific growth abnormalities.

The critical size for a growth abnormality caused by a central growth plate lesion is 7-9% of the size of the growth plate

The cut-off point from which a bone bridge cannot be spontaneously resorbed and from which the amount of injury or the cellular destruction may create growth abnormalities has not been completely evaluated yet (Pous et al. 1979; Bonnel et al. 1984; Seil 2002). A first attempt to quantify the critical size of the growth plate injury susceptible to create a growth abnormailty was undertaken by Johnson and Southwick (1960) in a rabbit model. They estimated it at 11% of the physeal surface. Nordentoft (1969) estimated the diameter of a bone tunnel to 20% of the width of the physis in the frontal plane which corresponded to approximately 10% of the physeal surface. Mäkelä et al. (1988) evaluated the size of a growth plate lesion of 2 respectively 3,2 mm bone tunnels at 13% (20%) of the width of the distal femoral physis in the frontal plane and 3% (7%) of the physeal surface. The larger diameter tunnels created growth abnormalities with significant shortening in 19 of 20 animals, whereas only minor shortening (<0,5 mm) occurred in 3 of 20 animals in the group with tunnel diameters of 2 mm. Janarv et al. (1998) confirmed these findings in another rabbit model and postulated that the relative size of a physeal drill injury necessary to cause growth disturbance starts at an injury of 7-9% of the physeal surface. Similarly, Garces et al. (1994) found no growth disturbances with surface lesions of 3,2% in the rat model.

In the human knee, Janarv et al. (1998) measured the surface of the tibial growth plate and estimated that a drill injury with a diameter of 8 mm corresponds to a lesion of 3-4% of the physeal surface. Using an MRI module for adolescent ACL reconstructive surgery (MAARS), Kercher et al. (2009) confirmed this finding in 10–15 years old children. Their module allowed for creating a 3-dimensional representation of the distal femoral and proximal tibial physis. They found that a variation of graft diameter from 6 mm to 11 mm increased the volume percent removed from 2.3% to 7.8%, corresponding to which approximately 1.1% for every 1 mm increase in tunnel diameter.

The critical size for a growth abnormality caused by a peripheral growth plate lesion is 3-5% of the circumference of the growth plate

Little has been published so far on this specific subject. In contrast to the amount of injured central growth plate, the minimum size of a lesion of the perichondral structures causing a localized growth disturbance or even a complete growth arrest has not been completely investigated yet. In a previous animal study on 4 months old sheep, we obtained a severe malalignment of the distal femoral physis by drilling a 5 mm tunnel through the perichondral structures and by avoiding to fill the tunnel with a tendon graft. An MRI analysis of the injured bones at 10 months revealed that the injured size of the perichondral structures was 3-5% of the size of the entire perichondral circumference (Seil 2002). Further studies need to confirm these data and to evaluate more precisely at which time point of the growth period and from which amount a localized peripheral growth plate injury may become deleterious for further longitudinal growth.

The size of the growth plate injury increases with drilling obliquity

If the growth plate is perforated perpendicularly during tunnel drilling, the drill injury is round and its size can be deducted from the following formula (Figure 5a and b):

$$A = \pi x\ r^2,$$
$$\text{where } r = a/2.$$

However, the drilled tunnel is almost never perpendicular to the growth plate, leading to bigger drill injury to the growth plate than the actual diameter of the drill. Seil (2002) showed an elliptical deformation of the round drill canal with the increase of the inclination angle (Figure 5 a and b). The area of the ellipse could be calculated with following formula:

$$z = a/\cos\alpha$$
$$A = \pi\ x\ (a/2)\ x\ (z/2)$$
$$= {}^1/_4\ x\ \pi\ x\ a\ x\ z$$
$$= {}^1/_4\ x\ \pi\ x\ a\ x\ (a/\cos\ \alpha)$$
$$= (\pi\ x\ a2)/4\ \cos\ \alpha$$

In the following this theoretical example will be transposed to the femoral growth plate for either transphyseal or anteromedial portal drilling: The angle between the inclination of the drill and the femoral tunnel with transtibial drilling is approximately 25°, whereas it increases to 75° with drilling through the anteromedial portal. Considering a tunnel diameter of 7 mm, the former will result in a growth plate injury of 42 mm^2, whereas it will result in a 3-fold increase of 148 mm^2 with the latter. Increasing the tunnel diameter to 9 mm will result in a growth plate injury of 70 or 245 mm^2 respectively. In terms of volume of the growth plate Kercher et al. showed in a specific MRI module that increasing the tunnel drill angle from 45 degrees to 70 degrees decreased the volume percent removed from 4.1% to 3.1%, which averages 0.2% removed for each 5 degrees increase in drill angle. These examples show that both inclination and tunnel diameter are critical.

The risk of a growth deformity is inversely proportional to the remaining growth potential

The probability of a bone bridge development is supposed to be higher in older children in whom the activity of the growth plate has already decreased. It is well known that severe growth arrests may be transitional in younger children in whom the large remaining growth potential may counteract a strong localized bone bridge. In these cases, the growth plate is able to develop a sufficient force to break a bone bridge early on (Ford and Key 1956; Friedenberg 1957; Campbell et al. 1959; Nordentoft 1969; Pous et al. 1979). A similar process can be deducted from animal experiments performed by Barash and Siffert (1966)). They splitted the distal radial epiphysis cats and dogs and interposed a synthetic membrane. At the time of operation the animals were aged from several days to 8 ½ weeks. The trend to develop a bone bridge was highest in those animals with the largest epiphyseal bone core and hence the smallest distance between this epiphyseal bone core and the metaphyseal bone (Figure 6). In these animals a dip deformity of the growth plate could be documented. 5.

As a consequence of these findings one could assume that due to the low remaining growth potential in older patients with little growth remaining, the risk of a significant growth deformity is also reduced in these patients. In fact, adolescents are at a higher risk of epiphysiodesis but with little clinical consequences in terms of growth disturbances, whereas young children are at a lower risk of

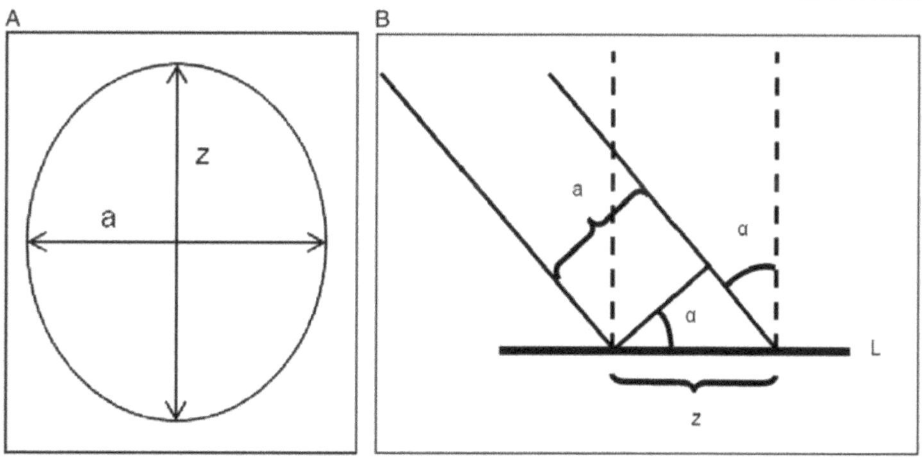

Figure 5 a: The inclination of a round drill leads to an elliptic drill injury (a = drill diameter; z = longitudinal diameter of drill injury proportional to the drill inclination). b: Representation of the calculation of the longest diameter of an ellipse (a = drill diameter; α = angle between tunnel and growth plate [L]; z = length of the elliptic drill injury).

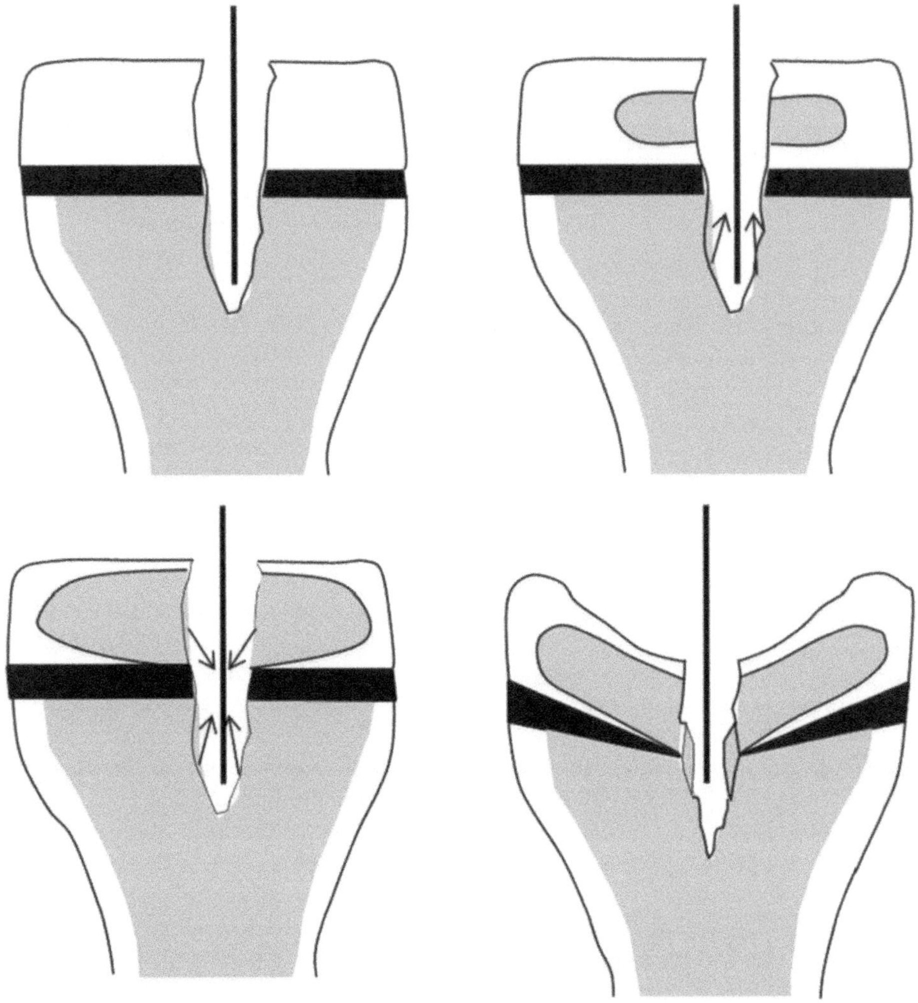

Figure 6 In the absence of an epiphyseal bone core or at the beginning of its formation (above), and the risk to develop a transphyseal bone bridge is lower in comparison to a situation where the bone core has developed further. In these cases a transphyseal bone formation with the development of a dip deformity could be observed (below) (modified from Barash and Siffert 1966).

epiphysiodesis but sometimes with dramatic clinical consequences if the physeal bridge persists and continues to develop until the end of growth. Pediatric ACL reconstructions, and especially the transphyseal technique, in adolescents close to knee skeletal maturity may not be a benign procedure and should be performed with great care in this period.

The force of the growth plate is associated with the body weight

Friedenberg (1957) resected the periphery of the growth plate and its neighboring bone. He noted not only the formation of bone bridges over the resected area but also a frequent resumption of longitudinal growth. This indicated that the bone bridge may be resorbed by the distraction forces induced by the cartilage of the growth plate. An attempt to quantify this distraction force was made by Strobino et al. (1952). They found that the force which was necessary to cause a growth arrest of the bovine proximal tibial growth plate approximated 11,5 to 19,2 mg/mm^2. In rabbits this amount seems to be much higher (15 g/mm^2) (Bonnel et al. 1984). By analyzing the resistance of bone cement which was used for tumor prosthesis in 7–13 years old children, Safran et al. (1992) estimated the force induced by the growth plate to 58 kg per square centimeter.

An excessive graft tension may lead to a tenoepiphysiodesis

Ono et al. (1998) performed ACL reconstructions with iliotibial tract tendons in 25 rabbits and with patellar tendons in 31 rabbits. Despite the fact that most of the grafts were ruptured, significant growth abnormalities with limb shortening and axial deformities could be found in 10 animals in which the grafts remained intact. It was concluded that these abnormalities were secondary to the high tensioning of the grafts. The authors created the term tenoepiphysiodesis which describes the fact that an excessively tensioned graft which is thoroughly fixed both proximally and distally may be able to create compression forces on the growth plate and slow down the growth process according to the HUETER-VOLKMANN-principle (Hueter (1862); Volkmann (1862); Volkmann (1869)). This principle showed that an increasing pressure on the physis might inhibit longitudinal growth and vice versa. A similar effect could be found by Edwards et al. (2001) who performed ACL reconstructions with autologous fascia lata grafts on twelve 8 weeks old dogs. The authors tensioned their fascia lata autografts to 80 N and found a significant femoral valgus deformity. In these animals limp shortening could be found on the lateral femoral and the medial tibial side. Even if the ideal tension of ACL grafts is unknown to date, it is reasonable to believe that a tension of 80 N is excessive in skeletally immature patients. In our own findings we could show that an intraoperative tensioning of Achilles tendon autografts to 40 N did not result in major growth disturbances (Seil et al. 2008). Similar clinical complications in pediatric patients could be described by Kocher et al. (2002) and Robert and Casin (2010)). Both found a valgus deformity after ACL reconstruction in children. Similarly, placing a transphyseal synthetic graft material may lead to the same type of complication (Kurosaka 2013).

Following the description of the HUETER-VOLKMANN principle, numerous clinical examples which were reinforced by further experimental work among else by Bonnel et al. (1984), showed a rebound effect of longitudinal bone growth. This means that a transitional stimulation of longitudinal growth may occur after the removal of a supra physiological constraint. Chudik et al. (2007) found a significant increase in longitudinal growth compared to the control side in the tibia in transphyseal ACL reconstructions in dogs. This longitudinal overgrowth process can also be observed on a regular basis in children, be it in association with tibial fractures or with pediatric ACL reconstructions and may be transient (Chotel et al. 2010). So far it is not clear to which extent rebound and overgrowth effects are related to each other.

Iatrogenic injury to perichondral structures should be avoided

We analyzed the risk of growth abnormalities after injuries of the perichondral structures of the distal femur in sheep (Seil et al. 2008). In those cases in which the perichondral structures were injured and the bone tunnel was left empty, a strong valgus deformity could be observed. On the contrary, if the ACL reconstruction procedure was technically correct with extracortical graft fixations and bone tunnels which were filled with autologous tendon grafts, no growth changes could be found even if the perichondral structures were injured. A similar development could not be observed on the tibial side, indicating that the femoral tunnel has the potential to cause more severe growth abnormalities than the tibial tunnel. (Seil et al. 2008). Figure 7 illustrates the critical location of the femoral tunnel in transphyseal pediatric ACL reconstructions in a specimen of a 10-year-old girl. The transphyseal tunnel was drilled with an adult drill guide with an offset of 5 mm. This creates an eccentrically located bone tunnel, which is very close to the peripheral perichondral structures. Not filling this peripheral tunnel with a tendon graft may create a large bone bridge gapping the perichondral structures with a resulting significant valgus deformity (Seil et al. 2008).

Epiphyseal and transphyseal ACL reconstructions may induce rotational deformities

Chudik et al. (2007) studied the reaction of growth in rapidly growing 10-week-old dogs with three different variations of femoral drill holes. They used a central tibial tunnel and three variations of femoral graft placement: epiphyseal, over the top, or transphyseal. All techniques had a high rate of graft failure and none of them was shown to be superior. There were no significant differences in femoral longitudinal growth. The epiphyseal technique reproduced the anatomic position of the ACL graft most closely but resulted in the development of rotational deformities, a growth abnormality that had not been reported before. MRI revealed more

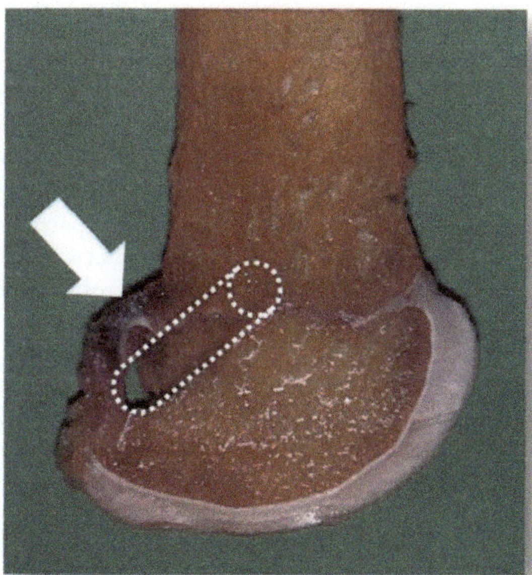

Figure 7 Specimen of a 10-years old girl: The arrow marks the perichondral ring of Ranvier. The dotted cylinder represents the posterolaterally located transphyseal femoral bone tunnel with a 5-mm diameter.

chondral and subchondral damage on the lateral femoral condyle with the epiphyseal technique. Further investigation is needed to understand this observation and its clinical implications. So far, this deformity has not been described in the human knee.

Graft incorporation is faster in immature specimen

There are several experimental studies analyzing the graft incorporation in animals with open growth plates. Meller et al. (2008a,b, 2009a,b) found that in immature sheep Sharpey-like fibers develop after 3 weeks post operatively at the passing site of the graft. The maximum load to failure was decreased to 37.8 +/– 17.8 N after 3 weeks, but restored to 522.9+/– 113 N after 24 weeks. At 24 weeks, the knee had regained 69% of its biomechanical strength. The authors could demonstrate that the remodeling of the soft tissue graft is faster and more complete in immature sheep than in mature sheep. Further biological investigations were performed by Magarian et al. (2011) who studied the age related function of ACL-fibroblasts. They could prove that cellular migration and proliferation of human ACL-fibroblasts is age determined in a similar way as described in large animal models. The findings indicate that immature patients are more likely to benefit from tissue engineering than adolescent or adults. This presumption needs to be still verified in future studies. Murray et al. (2010) did their research on minipigs that concluded the better and faster healing of soft tissue in immature individuals. The research group from Murray (Murray 2009, Fleming et al. 2009) has done its work over better understanding the ACL healing in biological-cellular level. They could show promising results in minipigs after using Collagen-platelet composites around the standard ACL graft. After a dissected ACL was sutured and grafted with CPC, the control group was treated with suture alone. Load at yield, maximum load and ACL tangent modulus were all significantly higher in the suture repairs augmented with collagen-platelet composite than in repairs performed with suture alone. This work confirms the bigger biological potential of pediatric soft-tissues as compared to adults. However, its clinical relevance in the field of pediatric ACL reconstruction is still under investigation (Proffen et al. 2013).

Summary

The risks related to different techniques of pediatric ACL reconstruction are increasingly recognized and scientific research in the field is growing. In the last decade it has been shown that a technically correct pediatric ACL reconstruction has little risk in creating growth abnormalities. Animal experiments support this hypothesis. They have helped to identify specific risk factors related to pediatric ACL reconstruction. Nevertheless, the understanding of the pathophysiologic changes of an iatrogenic injury to the growing cartilaginous structures in the knee is still incomplete and the gained knowledge in animals cannot be fully generalized in humans. Further knowledge could be gained from animal experiments by assessing complete follow-ups until the end of the growth period.

Competing interests

The authors declare that they have no competing interests.

Authors' contributions

All authors participated in drafting the manuscript. All of the authors read and approved the final manuscript.

Author details

[1]Department of Orthopaedic Surgery, Centre Hospitalier Luxembourg, Clinique d'Eich. 78, rue d'Eich, L-1460 Luxembourg, Luxembourg. [2]Sports Medicine Research Laboratory, Luxembourg Institute of Health, 78 rue d'Eich, L-1460 Luxembourg, Luxembourg. [3]Department of Pediatric Surgery, University of Tampere, Teiskontie 35, 33521 Tampere, Finland.

References

Aichroth P (2002) The natural history and treatment of ACL rupture in children and adolescents. J Bone Joint Surg (Br) 84:38–41

Arendt E, Dick R (1995) Knee injury patterns among men and women in collegiate basketball and soccer. NCAA data and review of literature. Am J Sports Med 23:694–701

Barash ES, Siffert RS (1966) The potential for growth of experimentally produced hemiepiphyses. J Bone Joint Surg-A 48:1548

Bidder A (1873) Experimente über die künstliche Hemmung des Längenwachstums von Röhrenknochen durch Reizung und Zerstörung des Epiphysenknorpels. Naunyn-Schmiedebergs Arch Exp Path Pharmak 1:248–263

Blount WP, Clarke GR (1949) Control of bone growth by epiphyseal stapling. A preliminary report. J Bone Joint Surg 31-A:464–478

Bonnel F, Dimeglio A, Baldet P, Rabischong P (1984) Biomechanical activity of the growth plate. Clinical incidences. Anat Clin 6:53–61

Campbell CJ, Grisolia A, Zanconato G (1959) The effects produced in the cartilaginous epiphyseal plate of immature dogs by experimental surgical traumata. J Bone Joint Surg 41-A:1212–1242

Chotel F, Henry J, Seil R, Chouteau J, Moyen B, Bérard J (2010) Growth disturbances without growth arrest after ACL reconstruction in children. Knee Surg Sports Traumatol Arthrosc 18:1496–1500

Chudik S, Beasley L, Potter H, Wickiewicz T, Warren R, Rodeo S (2007) The influence of femoral technique for graft placement on anterior cruciate ligament reconstruction using a skeletally immature canine model with a rapidly growing physis. Arthroscopy 23:1309–1319

Edwards TB, Green CC, Baratta RV (2001) The effect of placing a tension graft across open growth plates. J Bone Joint Surg Am 83:725–734

Engelman GH, Carry PM, Hitt KG, Polousky JD, Vidal AF (2014) Comparison of allograft versus autograft anterior cruciate ligament reconstruction graft survival in an active adolescent cohort. Am J Sports Med 42:2311–2318

Fleming BC, Spindler KP, Palmer MP, Magarian EM, Murray MM (2009) Collagen-platelet composites improve the biomechanical properties of healing anterior cruciate ligament grafts in a porcine model. Am J Sports Med 37:1554–1563

Ford LT, Key JA (1956) A study of experimental trauma to the distal femoral epiphysis in rabbits. J Bone Joint Surg 38-A:84–92

Friedenberg ZB (1957) Reaction of the epiphysis to partial surgical resection. J Bone Joint Surg-A 39:332–340

Frosch KH, Stengel D, Brodhun T, Stietencron I, Holsten D, Jung C, Reister D, Voigt C, Niemeyer P, Maier M, Hertel P, Jagodzinski M, Lill H (2010) Outcomes and risks of operative treatment of rupture of the anterior cruciate ligament in children and adolescents. Arthroscopy 26:1539–1550

Funahashi KM, Moksnes H, Maletis GB, Csintalan RP, Inacio MC, Funahashi TT (2014) Anterior cruciate ligament injuries in adolescents with open physis:

effect of recurrent injury and surgical delay on meniscal and cartilage injuries. Am J Sports Med 42:1068–1073
Garces GL, Mugica-Garay I, Lopez-Goncalves Coviella N, Guerardo E (1994) Growth-plate modifications after drilling. J Pediatr Orthop 14:225–228
Guzzanti V, Falciglia F, Gigante A, Fabbriciani C (1994) The effect of intra-articular ACL reconstruction on the growth plates of rabbits. J Bone Joint Surg Br 76:960–963
Haas SL (1945a) The changes produced in the growing bone after injury to the epiphyseal cartilage plate. J Orthop Surg 1:67–99
Haas SL (1945b) Retardation of bone growth by a wire loop. J Bone Joint Surg-Am 27:25–36
Haas SL (1948) Mechanical retardation of bone growth. J Bone Jointt Surg-Am 30:506–512
Haas SL (1950) Restriction of bone growth by pins through the epiphyseal cartilaginous plate. J Bone Joint Surg-Am 32:338
Hueter C (1862) Anatomische Studien an den Extremitätengelenken Neugeborener und Erwachsener. Virchow's Arch 25:575–599
Janarv PM, Wikström B, Hirsch G (1998) The influence of transphyseal drilling and tendon grafting on bone growth: an experimental study in the rabbit. J Pediatr Orthop 18:149–154
Johnson JTH, Southwick WO (1960) Growth Following Transepiphyseal Bone Grafts An Experimental Study to Explain Continued Growth Following Certain Fusion Operations. J Bone Joint Surg Am 42:1381–1395
Jouve JL, Mottet V, Cottalorda J, Frayssinet P, Bollini G (1998) Reimplantation of growth plate chondrocyte cultures in central growth plate defects: Part I. Characterization of cultures. J Pediatr Orthop B 7:167–173
Karlsson C, Thornemo M, Barreto Henriksson H, Lindahl A (2009) Identification of a stem cell niche in the zone of Ranvier within the knee joint. J Anat 215:355–363
Kercher J, Xerogeanes J, Tannenbaum A, Al-Hakim R, Black JC, Zhao J (2009) Anterior Cruciate Ligament Reconstruction in the Skeletally Immature: An Anatomical Study Utilizing 3-Dimensional Magnetic Resonance Imaging Reconstructions J Pediatr Orthop 29(2):124–129
Key JA, Ford LT (1958) A study of experimental trauma to the distal femoral epiphysis in rabbits. II. J Bone Joint Surg Am 40-A:887–896
Kocher MS, Saxon HS, Hovis WD, Hawkins RJ (2002) Management and complications of ACL injuries in skeletally immature patients: survey of the Herodicus Society and the ACL study group. J Pediatr Orthop 22:452–457
Kocher MS, Smith JT, Zoric BJ, Lee B, Micheli LJ (2007) Transphyseal anterior cruciate ligament reconstruction in skeletally immature pubescent adolescents. J Bone Joint Surg Am 89:2632–2639
Koman JD, Sanders JO (1999) Valgus deformity after reconstruction of the anterior cruciate ligament in a skeletally immature patient. A case report. J Bone Joint Surg-A 81:711–715
Kurosaka M (2013)Dramatic growth abnormality after paediatric ACL reconstruction with transphyseal synthetic graft placement. Instructional course, ISAKOS meeting, Toronto
Lacroix P (1951) The organization of bone. Churchill, London, pp 131–133
Langenskiöld A (1993) Partial closure of the epiphyseal plate. Principles of treatment. 1978. Clin Orthop Relat Res 297:4–6
Langenskiöld A, Osterman K, Valle M (1987) Growth of fat grafts after operation for partial bone growth arrest: demonstration by computed tomography scanning. J Pediatr Orthop 7:389–394
Langenskiöld A, Videman T, Nevalainen T (1986) The fate of fat transplants in operations for partial closure of the growth plate. Clinical examples and an experimental study. J Bone Joint Surg-B 68:234–238
Langenskiöld A (1981) Surgical treatment of partial closure of the growth plate. J Pediatr Orthop 1:3–11
Langenskiöld A (1975) An operation for partial closure of an epiphysial plate in children, and its experimental basis. J Bone Joint Surg-B 57:325–330
Langenskiöld A, Osterman K (1979) Surgical treatment of partial closure of the epiphysial plate. Reconstr Surg Traumatol 17:48–64
Lo IK, Kirkley A, Fowler P, Miniaci A (1997) The outcome of operatively treated ACL disruption in the skeletally immature child. Arthroscopy 13:627–634
Mackie EJ, Tatarczuch L, Mirams M (2011) The skeleton: a multi-functional complex organ. The growth plate chondrocyte and endochondral ossification. J Endocrinol; 211:109–121
Magarian EM, Vavken P, Murray MM (2011) Human anterior cruciate ligament fibroblasts from immature patients have a stronger in vitro response to platelet concentrates than those from mature individuals. Knee 18:247–251
Mäkelä EA, Vainionpää S, Vihtonen K, Mero M, Laiho J, Tormala P, Rokkanen P (1987) The effect of a penetrating biodegradable implant on the epiphyseal plate: an experimental study on growing rabbits with special regard to polyglactin 910. J Pediatr Orthop 7:415–420
Mäkelä EA, Vainionpaa S, Vihtonen K, Mero M, Rokkanen P (1988) The effect of trauma to the lower femoral epiphyseal plate. An experimental study in rabbits. J Bone Joint Surg Br 70(2):187–191
Mäkelä EA, Vainionpää S, Vihtonen K, Mero M, Helevirta P, Törmälä P, Rokkanen P (1989) The effect of a penetrating biodegradable implant on the growth plate. An experimental study on growing rabbits with special reference to polydioxanone. Clin Orthop Relat Res 241:300–308
McConkey MO, Bonasia DE, Amendola A (2011) Pediatric anterior cruciate ligament reconstruction. Curr Rev Musculoskelet Med 4:37–44
Meller R, Brandes G, Drögemüller C, Fritz F, Schiborra F, Fehr M, Hankemeier S, Krettek C, Hurschler C (2009a) Graft remodeling during growth following anterior cruciate ligament reconstruction in skeletally immature sheep. Arch Orthop Trauma Surg 129:1037–1046
Meller R, Haasper C, Westhoff J, Brand J, Knobloch K, Hankemeier S, Hesse E, Krettek C, Jagodzinski M (2009b) An animal model to study ACL reconstruction during growth. Technol Health Care 17:403–410
Meller R, Willbold E, Hesse E, Dreymann B, Fehr M, Haasper C, Hurschler C, Krettek C, Witte F (2008a) Histologic and biomechanical analysis of anterior cruciate ligament graft to bone healing in skeletally immature sheep. Arthroscopy 24:1221–1231
Meller R, Kendoff D, Hankemeier S, Jagodzinski M, Grotz M, Knobloch K, Krettek C (2008b) Hindlimb growth after a transphyseal reconstruction of the anterior cruciate ligament: a study in skeletally immature sheep with wide-open physes. Am J Sports Med 36:2437–2443
Michigami T (2013) Regulatory mechanisms for the development of growth plate cartilage. Cell Mol Life Sci 70:4213–4221
Mohtadi N, Grant J (2006) Managing anterior cruciate ligament deficiency in the skeletally immature individual: a systematic review of the literature. Clin J Sport Med 16:457–464
Moksnes H, Engebretsen L, Risberg MA (2013) Prevalence and incidence of new meniscus and cartilage injuries after a nonoperative treatment algorithm for ACL tears in skeletally immature children: a prospective MRI study. Am J Sports Med 41:1771–1779
Murray MM, Magarian EM, Harrison SL, Mastrangelo AN, Zurakowski D, Fleming BC (2010) The effect of skeletal maturity on functional healing of the anterior cruciate ligament. J Bone Joint Surg-Am 1(92):2039–2049
Murray MM (2009) Current status and potential of primary ACL repair. Clin Sports Med 28:51–61
Nordentoft EL (1969) Experimental epiphyseal injuries: grading of traumas and attempts at treating traumatic epiphyseal arrest in animals. Acta Orthop Scand 40:176–192
Ogden JA (1981) Injury to the growth mechanisms of the immature skeleton. Skeletal Radiol 6:237–253
Ollier L (1867) Traité expérimental et clinique de la régénération des os et de la production artificielle du tissu osseux, vol 1 und 2. Masson, Paris
Ono T, Wada Y, Takahashi K, Tsuchida T, Minamide M, Moriya H (1998) Tibial deformities and failures of anterior cruciate ligament reconstruction in immature rabbits. J Orthop Sci 3:150–155
Österman K (1994) Healing of large surgical defects of the epiphyseal plate. An experimental study. Clin Orthop 300:264–268
Phemister DB (1933) Operative arrestment of longitudinal growth in the treatment of deformities. J Bone Joint Surg 15:1–15
Pous JG, Baldet P, Dimeglio A, Bonnel F (1979) Les traumatismes du cartilage de conjugaison. Notions fondamentales. Rev Chir Orthop Reparatrice Appar Mot 65:259–265
Proffen BL, Fleming BC, Murray MM (2013) Histologic Predictors of Maximum Failure Loads Differ between the Healing ACL and ACL Grafts after 6 and 12 Months In Vivo. Orthop J Sports Med. 2013 Nov;1(6). doi:10.1177/2325967113512457
Ranvier L (1889) Traité technique d'histologie. 2. Ausg. Savy, Paris, pp 356–357
Robert HE, Casin C (2010) Valgus and flexion deformity after reconstruction of the anterior cruciate ligament in a skeletally immature patient. Knee Surg Sports Traumatol Arthrosc 18:1369–1373
Safran MR, Eckardt JJ, Kabo JM, Oppenheim WL (1992) Continued growth of the proximal part of the tibia after prosthetic reconstruction of the skeletally immature knee. J Bone Joint Surg-Am 74:1172–1179
Seil R, Pape D, Kohn D (2008) The risk of growthchanges during transphysealdrilling in sheep with open physes. Arthroscopy 24:824–833
Seil R (2002) Die Ersatzplastik des vorderen Kreuzbandes bei offenen Wachstumsfugen: Eine experimentelle Untersuchung. Habilitationsschrift.

Vorgelegt zur Erlangung der Venia legendi für das Fach Orthopädie an der medizinischen Fakultät der Universität des Saarlandes, Homburg / Saar, Germany
Shea KG, Pfeiffer R, Wang JH, Curtin M, Apel PJ (2004) Anterior cruciate ligament injury in pediatric and adolescent soccer players: an analysis of insurance data. J Pediatr Orthop 24:623–628
Siffert RS (1956) The effect of staples and longitudinal wires on epiphyseal growth. An experimental study. J Bone Joint Surg-A 38:1077
Stadelmaier DM, Arnoczky SP, Dodds J, Ross H (1995) The effect of drilling and soft tissue grafting across open growth plates. Am J Sports Med 23:431–435
Strobino LJ, French GO, Colonna PC (1952) The effect of increasing tension on the growth of epiphyseal bone. Surg Gynecol Obstet 95:694–700
Synder M, Harcke T, Bowen R, Caro PA (1994) Evaluation of physeal behavior in response to epiphyseodesis with the use of serial magnetic resonance imaging. J Bone Joint Surg-Am 76:224–229
Volkmann R (1862) Chirurgische Erfahrungen über Knochenverbiegungen und Knochenwachstum. Arch f Pathol Anat 24:512–540
Volkmann R (1869) Die Krankheiten der Bewegungsorgane. In: Pitas F, Billroth CAT (Hrsg.): Handbuch der allgemeinen und speziellen Chirurgie, Bd II, Abt. 1. Ferdinand Enke Verlag, Erlangen, 350–351
Woods GW, O'Connor DP (2004) Delayed anterior cruciate ligament reconstruction in adolescents with open physes. Am J Sports Med 32:201–210
Yu B, Garrett WE (2007) Mechanisms of non-contact ACL injuries. Br J Sports Med 41(Suppl 1):i47–i51

Mechanical tensile properties of the anterolateral ligament

Martin Zens[1,2*†], Matthias J Feucht[2†], Johannes Ruhhammer[1], Anke Bernstein[2], Hermann O Mayr[2], Norbert P Südkamp[2], Peter Woias[1] and Philipp Niemeyer[2]

Abstract

Background: In a noticeable percentage of patients anterolateral rotational instabilities (ALRI) remain after an isolated ACL reconstruction. Those instabilities may occur due to an insufficiently directed damage of anterolateral structures that is often associated with ACL ruptures. Recent publications describe an anatomical structure, termed the anterolateral ligament (ALL), and suggest that this ligament plays a significant role in the pathogenesis of ALRI of the knee joint. However, only limited knowledge about the biomechanical characteristics and tensile properties of the anterolateral ligament exists.

Methods: The anterolateral ligament was dissected in four fresh-frozen human cadaveric specimens and all surrounding tissue removed. The initial length of the anterolateral ligament was measured using a digital caliper. Tensile tests with load to failure were performed using a materials testing machine. The explanted anterolateral ligaments were histologically examined to measure the cross-sectional area.

Results: The mean ultimate load to failure of the anterolateral ligament was 49.90 N (± 14.62 N) and the mean ultimate strain was 35.96% (± 4.47%). The mean length of the ligament was 33.08 mm (± 2.24) and the mean cross-sectional area was 1.54 mm^2 (± 0.48 mm^2). Including the areal measurements the maximum tension was calculated to be 32.78 $\frac{N}{mm^2}$ (± 4.04 $\frac{N}{mm^2}$).

Conclusions: The anterolateral ligament is an anatomical structure with tensile properties that are considerably weaker compared to other peripheral structures of the knee. Knowledge of the anterolateral ligament's tensile strengths may help to better understand its function and with graft choices for reconstruction procedures.

Keywords: Anterolateral ligament; ALL; Biomechanics; Load to failure; Tensile testing; Mechanical properties; Histology

Background

Traumatic injuries to the anterior cruciate ligament (ACL) are one of the most common reasons for clinical presentation in sports medicine. Its surgical repair follows standard procedures which evolved over several decades. However, in a noteworthy percentage of patients anterolateral rotational instabilities (ALRI) remain following state-of-the-art surgery. Reasons for this observation are discussed in current literature and several research groups suggest that injury to anterolateral structures of the knee joint may result in ALRI. Baker et al. (1983); Hughston et al. (1976); Tanaka et al. (2012); Terry et al. (1993), Wroble et al. (1993) in an anatomical study, Claes et al. (2013) recently investigated a ligamentous structure that had primarily been described by Segond (1879) in 1879. This structure, termed anterolateral ligament (ALL), connects the lateral epicondylus of the femur with the anterolateral proximal tibia and was found in 40 of 41 examined specimen. Those findings were confirmed by other research groups. Caterine et al. (2014); Dodds et al. (2014); Helito et al. (2013); Parsons et al. (2015); Zens et al. (2014) independently, various authors suggested that

*Correspondence: martin.zens@imtek.uni-freiburg.de
†Equal contributors
[1]Albert-Ludwigs-University Freiburg, Department of Microsystems Engineering (IMTEK), Design of Microsystems, Georges-Koehler-Allee 102, 79110 Freiburg i. Brsg., Germany
[2]University Medical Center Freiburg, Department of Orthopaedics and Trauma Surgery, Hugstetter Str. 55, 79106 Freiburg i. Brsg., Germany

the ALL may be a significant stabilizer in the knee. Reconstruction was proposed to be necessary to avoid or diminish ALRI, especially for revision cases and primary cases with gross positive pivot-shifts (Claes et al. 2013; Helito et al. 2014, 2013; Rezansoff et al. 2014, Sonnery-Cottet et al. 2014). However, before implying such a necessity a thorough biomechanical analysis ought to be conducted. Knowledge about the ligaments tensile properties may serve a better understanding of the ligaments behavior, allows a fact-based assessment of its possible contribution to ALRI and is essential for the selection of a suitable transplant and reconstruction technique. Up until now only very few studies have been published regarding the mechanical properties of the ALL. All of those studies have investigated the length changes of the ALL during passive knee motion. The purpose of this study was to determine typical mechanical properties of the ALL through tension testing. No previous study has measured the maximum load to failure of the ALL. By comparing this data with values previously determined for other ligaments and considering the absolute values, such as ultimate tensile stress, ultimate strain and Young's modulus, a better evaluation of the ligaments significance can be given. Furthermore, possible reconstruction grafts with similar mechanical features can be identified.

Methods

Dissection technique

Four fresh-frozen human cadaveric knees were included in this study (3 male, 1 female). The cadaveric knees were obtained from the Institut of Anatomy, Friedrich-Alexander-University of Erlangen-Nuremberg, with written consent from all donors and in accordance with ethical approval of the University of Freiburg (Ref. 45/15). The mean age of the specimen was 86.5 $\pm$ 1.7. None of the studied knees had undergone significant surgery or showed signs of bone deformity. Before testing, the specimens were thawed for 48 hours. All tests were performed at room temperature and the specimens were constantly kept moist with saline solution. Initially the ALL was carefully dissected using a standardized procedure described by Claes et al. (2013). This was done by a single investigator with the knee in 90° of flexion. Bony landmarks of the ALL, being the lateral epicondyle, the fibular head and Gerdy's tubercle, were identified through palpation. A hand sized, rectangular cuteness flap was removed above this area. After removal of subcutaneous fat the iliotibial tract, extensor apparatus and the short head of the biceps femoris were displayed. Subsequently, the iliotibial tract was cut through approximately 60 mm proximal of the lateral epicondyle and delicately released to its tibial attachment by cutting the Kaplan fibers attached to the lateral intermusculare septum and the lateral retinaculum. Following this step the lateral collateral ligament (LCL) was identified and the distal tibia rotated in interior direction, thus allowing an identification of the ALL. In all four specimen a ligamentous structure, as described in previous publications, was identified connecting the lateral femoral epicondyle and the anterolateral proximal tibia (Figure 1). The initial length L_0 of the ALL was measured in 0° flexion using a digital caliper and documented. Afterwards the ALL was carefully isolated and undermined with a surgical vessel loop. Tibia and femur were thoroughly fixated in two hollow aluminum cylinders that were used to mount the knee joints in the materials testing machine. This step was succeeded by a radical removal of all connecting structures between thigh and lower leg, except the ALL, leaving the anterolateral ligament as the only connecting tissue bridge.

Testing procedure

Uniaxial tensile failure tests were conducted on a servo-hydraulic materials testing machine (Zwick/Roell Amsler HC 10, Zwick/Roell AG, Ulm, Germany) at an extension rate of 0.5 mm/s. The fiber course of the ALL was in line with the direction of force thereby simulating a worst-case scenario. All four specimen were tested without preconditioning cycles. The stop criterion was a relative drop in force of 90%. A force-distance curve, ultimate load to failure (in N) and ultimate extension distance (in mm) were recorded for each specimen. The sampling rate was set to 100 Hz. Stress-strain curves, ultimate tensile stress (in N/mm^2), ultimate strain (in %) and Young's modulus at 20% strain were calculated by taking the initial length L_0 and the cross-sectional area A_0 into account.

Cross-sectional area measurement

Accurate cross-sectional measurements of the ALL were performed by obtaining and dimensioning histological cross-sectional cuts. For this purpose the torn ALL of each cadaveric knee was explanted after tensile testing and quick-frozen in liquid isopentane ($T < -80$°C). Tissue

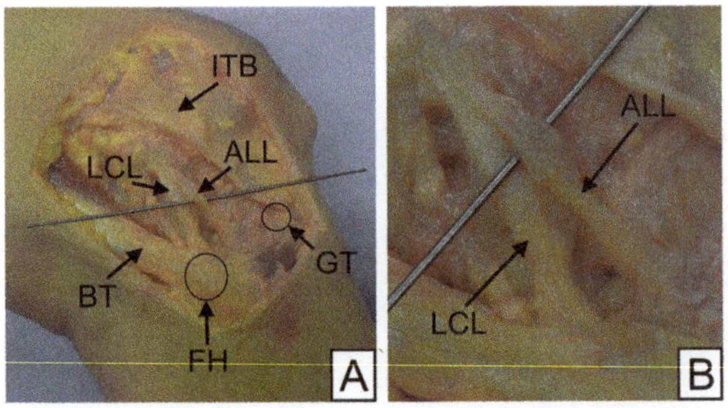

Figure 1 Dissected ALL. A: Dissected anterolateral ligament (ALL) with surrounding structures in a right knee; ITB: iliotibial band, LCL: lateral collateral ligament, GT: Gerdy's tubercle, BT: biceps tendon, FH: fibular head. **B**: Detailed view of the dissected ALL.

Freezing Medium® (Leica Biosystems Nussloch GmbH, Nussloch, Germany) was used to embed the quick-frozen ALL. Cuts along approximately five equidistant sections of each ALL were fixated on a specimen holder. A Leica CM3050 S cryostat (Leica Biosystems Nussloch GmbH, Nussloch, Germany) was utilized for this task. Following fixation, representative cuts of each section were stained with HE and Giemsa. AxioVision (Carl Zeiss AG, Oberkochen, Germany) software was used to acquire images and measure the cross-sectional area. The mean was determined from cuts of the five equidistant sections.

Statistical analysis

Measurements were plotted and analyzed using OriginPro® 9.0 (OriginLab Corp., Northampton, MA, USA). Correlations between initial length, cross-sectional area, ultimate load to failure, ultimate stress and ultimate distance were revealed by calculating correlation coefficients. Subsequently, Student's t-tests were performed to test significance. Significance was set at $P < 0.05$.

Results

All four specimen showed an interligamentous failure at approximately one third of the ALL's length distal from the femorial insertion site. A force-distance curve with an average of 2,399 (± 318) data points was recorded for each specimen. The resulting curves are shown in Figure 2A. The mean ultimate load to failure was 49.90 N ± 14.62 N and the mean ultimate extension distance was 11.89 mm ± 1.56 mm. Hence, resulting in a mean extensional stiffness of 2.60 N ± 0.93 N.

In order to calculate stress-strain curves the initial length L_0 and the average cross-sectional area A_0 per ligament were included. Whereas the initial length was measured prior to the tensile tests, the cross-sectional area was determined by measuring five cuts of each ALL and calculating their average. The mean initial length was 33.1 mm ± 2.2 mm and the mean cross-sectional area 1.54 mm^2 ± 0.48 mm^2. Dividing force by the cross-sectional area and distance by the initial length results in the stress-strain curves displayed in Figure 2B. The mean ultimate stress was 32.78 $\frac{N}{mm^2}$ ± 4.04 $\frac{N}{mm^2}$ and the mean ultimate strain 35.96% ± 4.47%. A Young's modulus was calculated at 20% strain with a mean value of 1.20 $\frac{N}{mm^2}$ ± 0.44 $\frac{N}{mm^2}$. Specimen 3 and 4 show a partial failure between 25 and 30% strain prior to ultimate failure of the ligament. Statistical analysis revealed a significant correlation between ultimate load to failure and cross-sectional area ($r = 0.897$; $P < 0.05$) as well as ultimate stress and ultimate distance ($r = -0.990$; $P < 0.01$). The initial length of the ALL has no significant effect on the ultimate strain ($r = -0.126$; $P > 0.1$). All measurement results are summarized in Table 1.

Besides cross-sectional area measurements the histological cuts were further investigated regarding the composition of the anterolateral ligament. Using polarization microscopy a unique crimping pattern was found for the ALL. This proves the existence of a ligamentous structure. Figure 3A shows the crimping of the ALL along with detailed images of HE stained (Figure 3B) and Giemsa stained (Figure 3C) histological samples.

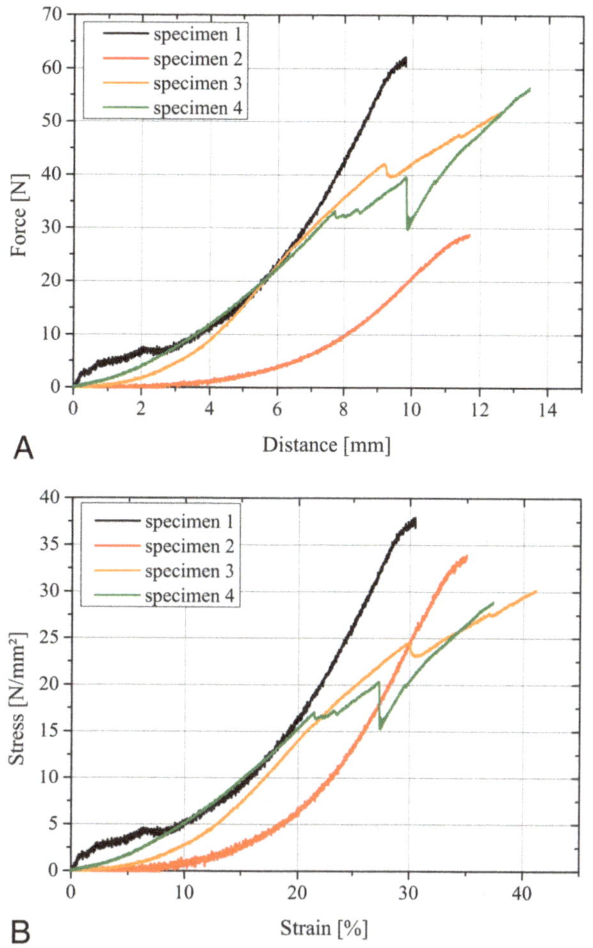

Figure 2 Measurement results. A: Force-distance-curve directly recorded using the materials testing machine; **B**: Stress-strain-curve calculated by taking relative length changes and cross-sectional areas into account.

Discussion

The purpose of this study was to determine the tensile mechanical properties of the anterolateral ligament. Terry et al. (1993) do not consider the ALL to be a distinct ligamentous structure and use this term for a synergistically acting combination of superficial, deep and capsulo-osseous layers of the ilitibial tract. The results of this study are consistent with previous studies (Claes et al. 2013; Helito et al. 2013) and show a clearly distinguishable fibre course with evidently defined insertion sites for the four knees investigated. Hence, the ALL can be considered as a self-contained anatomical structure.

Table 1 Measurement results of tensile tests of the anterolateral ligament

Parameter	Specimen 1	Specimen 2	Specimen 3	Specimen 4	Mean	SD
Data points [*n*]	1,961	2,379	2,569	2,686	2,399	± 318
Length L_0 [*mm*]	32.2	33.4	30.7	36.0	33.1	± 2.2
Cross-sectional area A_0 [mm^2]	1.64	0.85	1.72	1.95	1.54	± 0.48
Max. force [*N*]	62.21	28.88	52.01	56.48	49.90	± 14.62
Max. distance [*mm*]	9.80	11.69	12.62	13.43	11.89	± 1.56
Max. stress [$\frac{N}{mm^2}$]	37.93	33.98	30.24	28.96	32.78	± 4.04
Max. strain [%]	30.43	34.99	41.12	37.31	35.96	± 4.47
Extensional stiffness [*N*]	3.99	2.04	2.24	2.15	2.60	± 0.93
Young's modulus (20%) [$\frac{N}{mm^2}$]	1.80	1.14	1.13	0.74	1.20	± 0.44

However, findings and supposed interaction of iliotibial band layers suggest that not a single stabilizer, but rather a complex system of anterolateral structures is responsible for rotational stability with the ALL being one element of this system. Further actors of this system are the iliotibial band and the anterolateral capsule. Kittl et al. (2014) in the present study the ALL is investigated as an isolated structure. Clinically however, the ALL and its tensile properties have to be viewed in context with synergistically acting anatomical elements. Typically severe injuries will result in a traumatic destruction of the anterolateral capsule and the ALL. Isolated ALL ruptures are very unlikely, which lessens the clinical relevance of the low absolute values for load of failure (De Beule et al. 2014; Sonnery-Cottet et al. 2015).

Current publications already describe and discuss ALL reconstruction techniques without sufficient knowledge of the fundamental properties. Previous studies addressing the biomechanical properties of the anterolateral ligament have their focus on length changes during physiological motion of the knee. Claes et al. (2013); Dodds et al. (2014); Helito et al. (2013, 2014); Kittl et al. (2014); Parsons et al. (2015) whereas the information about length change is important for reconstruction techniques, tensile properties allow a better assessment of a ligament's significance. Dodds et al. (2011) this is the first study investigating the tensile properties of the ALL. The mean ultimate tension of 32.78 $\frac{N}{mm^2}$ (± 4.04 $\frac{N}{mm^2}$) shows a value that is comparable to other ligaments, e.g. ACL 37.80 $\frac{N}{mm^2}$ (± 3.80 $\frac{N}{mm^2}$) and MCL 38.60 $\frac{N}{mm^2}$ (± 4.80 $\frac{N}{mm^2}$). (Noyes et al. 1984; Moon et al. 2006; Quapp and Weiss 1998) however, because of the small cross-sectional area of the anteroateral ligament the ultimate load to failure of 49.90 N is only a fraction of values measured for ACL (1,725 N ± 269 N), (MCL 1,107 N ± 126 N) and PCL (1,051 N ± 237 N). The iliotibial tract displays a considerably lower ultimate tension of 19.1 N (± 2.9 N), but because of its dimensions a 15 times higher ultimate load to failure (769 N ± 99 N). All values reported above are based on findings described for a group of young specimen (ACL, IT: mean age 27 years; MCL, PCL: mean age unknown). Ligaments with a similar order of magnitude are the LCL (309 N ± 91 N) and the popliteofibular ligament complex (PFLC) (186 N ± 65 N)). The study for LCL and PFLC was performed on older specimen with a mean age of approximately 70 years. Table 2 gives an overview about tensile properties of various anatomic structures previously described. Table 2 gives an overview about tensile properties of various anatomic structures previously described.

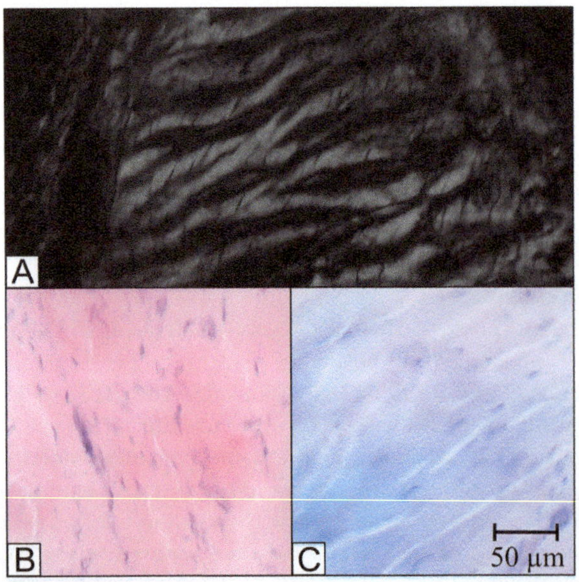

Figure 3 Histology of the ALL. Different histological illustrations of the ALL; **A**: Polarization with crimping; **B**: HE stain; **C**: Giemsa stain.

Noyes and Grood (1976), as well as Woo et al. (1991) have shown in separate studies, that the ultimate load to failure of the ACL in younger patients is 2.5 times higher than in older patients. In case a similar trend applies to the anterolateral ligament a value around 125 N may be possible. Wang et al. (2006) report an age-dependent modification of insertion sites leading to a decreasing load to failure. Furthermore this study has shown a strong

Table 2 Ultimate tension and ultimate load to failure of the ALL in comparison to other ligaments and possible grafts

Structure	Ultimate tension [MPa]	Ultimate load to failure [N]	Relation to ALL (load to failure) [%]
ALL	**32.78 ± 4.04**	**49.90 ± 14.62**	**100**
ACL[1] (Noyes et al. 1984)	37.80 ± 3.80	1,725 ± 269	3,457
PCL[2] (Noyes et al. 1984; Race and Amis 1994)	35.90 ± 15.20	739 - 1,627	1,481
MCL[3] (Moon et al. 2006; Quapp and Weiss 1998)	38.60 ± 4.80	1,107 ± 126	2,219
Distal sMCL[3] (Wijdicks et al. 2010)	-	557 ± 55	1,116
Proximal sMCL[3] (Wijdicks et al. 2010)	-	88 ± 36	176
POL[4] (Wijdicks et al. 2010)	-	256 ± 30	513
Deep MCL[3] (Wijdicks et al. 2010)	-	101 ± 10	202
LCL[5] (Sugita and Amis 2001)	-	309 ± 91	619
PFLC[6] (Sugita and Amis 2001)	-	186 N ± 65	373
ITB[7] (Noyes et al. 1984)	19.1 ± 2.9	769 ± 99	1,541
Fascia lata (Noyes et al. 1984)	78.7 ± 4.6	628 ± 35	1,259
Semitendinosus (Noyes et al. 1984)	88.5 ± 5.0	1,216 ± 50	2,437
Gracilis (Noyes et al. 1984)	111.5 ± 4.0	838 ± 30	1,679

[1]Anterior cruciate ligament, [2]posterior cruciate ligament, [3](superficial) medial collateral ligament, [4]posterior oblique ligament, [5]lateral collateral ligament, [6]popliteofibular ligament complex, [7]iliotibial band.

correlation between the cross-sectional area, thus representing the dimensions of the ALL, and the ultimate load to failure. The size of the ALL is expected to reduce with age, hence resulting in a decreasing maximum load. Other studies (Matthews et al. 1968; Moon et al. 2006; Viidik and Lewin 1966; Woo et al. 1986) have investigated how freezing of cadavers effects the tensile properties of ligaments. The results showed a concurrent worsening of the measured properties, thus implying that the *in vivo* features of the anterolateral ligament are rather underestimated in this study. Even if all possible limitations are taken into account the tensile properties the ALL are significantly lower than those of primary stabilizers of the knee, such as ACL, LCL and MCL. Further investigation is necessary to definitely conclude how the ALL contributes to ALRI. Based on the failure properties discovered in this study and recognizing the limitations of testing cadaveric tissues the ALL is to be considered a structure that acts synergistically with primary stabilizers, such as LCL, ACL and iliotibial band to support the knee. Furthermore, recommendations for reconstruction grafts can be proposed based on those findings. Claes at al. (2013) suggest an autologous graft of the gracilis tendon for an anatomical repair of the ALL. Notwithstanding, all autologous and artificial grafts choices displayed in Table 2 provide a sufficient load to failure to replace the ALL, but the ultimate tension of the gracilis tendon matches the ALL the least. Based on the preliminary data of this study other possible graft options, such as iliotibial band (ITB) or semitendinosus tendon split-offs appear more suitable. Besides choosing an appropriate graft for reconstruction of the ALL the development of a suitable technique is equally important. Lemaire et al. (1980) presented a surgical method coping with anterolateral instabilities using an ITB split-off. This approach has been adapted recently by Wagner et al. (2014). Essentially, these techniques use a ITB split-off. This split-off is shuttled underneath the LCL to create a dynamic stabilization of the joint in an anatomic course that is consistent with the axis of the ALL. This ITB-based approach is found in a similar manner in other techniques. Carson (1985), Österman et al. 1993, Wolff et al. (2005) approaches based on the semitendinosus tendon to address ALRI have also been discussed in literature (Ulmer et al. 2006; Zantop and Petersen 2010).

This study has several limitations. Apart from limitations that are generally associated with cadaveric measurements, such as post-mortem degeneration of tissue, age-dependency and effects of cadaver freezing, this study is based on measurements of only four cadaveric knee joints. However, the data of those four measurements shows little variances and is very consistent. Considering the fact that absolutely no data regarding the tensile properties of the ALL exists, but reconstruction methods are already being developed, this preliminary data suggests that further investigation of the biomechanical and especially tensile properties of the ALL is necessary, before continuing with the development of surgical techniques. Another limitation of this study is the determination of the cross-sectional area of explanted ligaments after load to failure testing. Tearing causes a constriction of the ligaments, which underestimates the cross-sectional area prior to testing. Furthermore the uniaxial direction of force tested in the measurement setup does not coincide with the physiological axes of the anterolateral ligament as a rotational stabilizer.

Conclusion

The anterolateral ligament is an anatomical structure with an ultimate load to failure of 49.90 N and an ultimate tension of 32.78 $\frac{N}{mm^2}$. Based on the findings of this study a definite conclusion regarding the significance of the ALL cannot be given, but our data strongly suggests that the ALL is not a primary stabilizer of the knee joint as the tensile strengths are significantly lower than those of primary stabilizers. Further fundamental biomechanical research is necessary before starting to clinically reconstruct the ALL.

Competing interests

The authors declare that they have no competing interests.

Authors' contributions

MZ and JR programmed the testing machine. MJF and PN dissected the cadaver knee joints. AB performed histologically examination. HOM and NPS constructed the machine mount. PW analyzed the data. All authors participated in the writing and proofreading of the manuscript. All authors read and approved the final manuscript.

Acknowledgements

The authors would like to thank the Deutsche Forschungsgemeinschaft (DFG) (WO 883/15-1 and WO 883/16-1), the MFG-Stiftung Baden-Wuerttemberg and the Deutsche Kniegesellschaft e.V. (DKG) for research grants and financial support. The article processing charge was funded by the German Research Foundation (DFG) and the Albert Ludwigs University Freiburg in the funding programme Open Access Publishing. Furthermore, the authors would like to thank Prof. Neuhuber and Dr. Buder at the University of Erlangen-Nuernberg for providing cadaver knee joints.

References

Arthrex I (2013) Anterolateral Ligament Reconstruction using SwiveLock. Video. [last downloaded 08/02/2014]. https://www.arthrex.com/resources/video/JOVv2r2KoE-v7gFCU0pqVw/anterolateral-ligament-reconstruction-using-swivelock

Baker CL, Norwood LA, Hughston JC (1983) Acute posterolateral rotatory instability of the knee. J Bone Joint Surgery Am Volume 65(5):614–8

Carson WG (1985) Extra-articular reconstruction of the anterior cruciate ligament: lateral procedures. Orthopedic Clinics North Am 16(2):191–211

Caterine S, Litchfield R, Johnson M, Chronik B, Getgood A (2014) A cadaveric study of the anterolateral ligament: re-introducing the lateral capsular ligament. Knee Surgery, Sports Traumatology, Arthroscopy: Official J ESSKA. doi:10.1007/s00167-014-3117-z

Claes S, Vereecke E, Maes M, Victor J, Verdonk P, Bellemans J (2013) Anatomy of the anterolateral ligament of the knee. J Anatomy 223(4):321–8. doi:10.1111/joa.12087

De Beule J, Vandenneucker H, Claes S, Bellemans J (2014) Can anterior cruciate ligament reconstruction be performed routinely in day clinic? Acta Orthopædica Belgica 80:391–396

Dodds AL, Gupte CM, Neyret P, Williams AM, Amis AA (2011) Extra-articular techniques in anterior cruciate ligament reconstruction: a literature review. J Bone Joint Surgery. Br Volume 93(11):1440–8. doi:10.1302/0301-620X.93B11.27632

Dodds AL, Halewood C, Gupte CM, Williams A, Amis AA (2014) The anterolateral ligament: Anatomy, length changes and association with the Segond fracture. Bone Joint J 96-B(3):325–31. doi:10.1302/0301-620X.96B3.33033

Helito CP, Demange MK, Bonadio MB, Tirico LEP, Gobbi RG, Pecora JR, Camanho GL (2013) Anatomy and Histology of the Knee Anterolateral Ligament. Orthopaedic J Sports Med 1(7):2325967113513546. doi:10.1177/2325967113513546

Helito, C P, Demange MK, Bonadio MB, Tirico LEP, Gobbi RG, Pecora JR, Camanho GL (2014) Radiographic landmarks for locating the femoral origin and tibial insertion of the knee anterolateral ligament. Am J Sports Med 42(10):2356–62. doi:10.1177/0363546514543770

Hughston JC, Andrews JR, Cross MJ, Moschi A (1976) Classification of knee ligament instabilities. Part II. The lateral. J Bone Joint Surg Am 58:173–179

Kittl C, Halewood C, Stephen JM, Gupte CM, Weiler A, Williams A, Amis AA (2014) Length change patterns in the lateral extra-articular structures of the knee and related reconstructions. Am J Sports Med 0363546514560993. doi:10.1177/0363546514560993

Lemaire M, Combelles F (1980) Technique actuelle de plastie ligamentaire pour rupture ancienne du ligament croise anterieur. Rev Chir Orthop 66:523–525

Matthews LS, Ellis D (1968) Viscoelastic properties of cat tendon: Effects of time after death and preservation by freezing. J Biomechanics 1(2):65–71. doi:10.1016/0021-9290(68)90008-0

Moon DK, Woo SL-Y, Takakura Y, Gabriel MT, Abramowitch SD (2006) The effects of refreezing on the viscoelastic and tensile properties of ligaments. J Biomechanics 39(6):1153–7. doi:10.1016/j.jbiomech.2005.02.012

Noyes FR, Grood ES (1976) The strength of the anterior cruciate ligament in humans and Rhesus monkeys. J Bone Joint Surgery. Am Volume 58(8):1074–82

Noyes FR, Butler DL, Grood ES, Zernicke RF, Hefzy MS (1984) Biomechanical analysis of human ligament grafts used in knee-ligament repairs and reconstructions. J Bone Joint Surgery. Am Volume 66(3):344–52

Österman K, Kujala UM, Kivimäki J, Österman H (1993) The MacIntosh lateral substitution reconstruction for anterior cruciate deficiency. Int Orthopaedics 17(4). doi:10.1007/BF00194183

Parsons EM, Gee AO, Spiekerman C, Cavanagh PR (2015) The biomechanical function of the anterolateral ligament of the knee. Am J Sports Med. doi:10.1177/0363546514562751

Quapp KM, Weiss JA (1998) Material Characterization of Human Medial Collateral Ligament. J Biomech Eng 120(6):757. doi:10.1115/1.2834890

Race A, Amis AA (1994) The mechanical properties of the two bundles of the human posterior cruciate ligament. J Biomechanics 27(1):13–24. doi:10.1016/0021-9290(94)90028-0

Rezansoff AJ, Caterine S, Spencer L, Tran MN, Litchfield RB, Getgood AM (2014) Radiographic landmarks for surgical reconstruction of the anterolateral ligament of the knee. Knee Surgery, Sports Traumatology, Arthroscopy: Official J ESSKA. doi:10.1007/s00167-014-3126-y

Segond P (1879) Recherches Cliniques et Expérimentales sur les épanchements Sanguins du Genou Par Entorse. Publications du Progr{è}s m{é}dical. Aux Bureaux du Progrès médical, Paris

Sonnery-Cottet B, Archbold P, Rezende FC, Neto AM, Fayard J-M, Thaunat M (2014) Arthroscopic Identification of the Anterolateral Ligament of the Knee. Arthroscopy Tech 3(3):389–92. doi:10.1016/j.eats.2014.02.009

Sonnery-Cottet B, Thaunat M, Freychet B, Pupim BHB, Murphy CG, Claes S (2015) Outcome of a Combined Anterior Cruciate Ligament and Anterolateral Ligament Reconstruction Technique With a Minimum 2-Year Follow-up. Am J Sports Med 0363546515571571. doi:10.1177/0363546515571571

Sugita T, Amis AA (2001) Anatomic and Biomechanical Study of the Lateral Collateral and Popliteofibular Ligaments. Am J Sports Med 29(4):466–472

Tanaka M, Vyas D, Moloney G, Bedi A, Pearle AD, Musahl V (2012) What does it take to have a high-grade pivot shift? Knee Surgery, Sports Traumatology, Arthroscopy: Official J ESSKA 20(4):737–42. doi:10.1007/s00167-011-1866-5

Terry GC, Norwood LA, Hughston JC, Caldwell KM (1993) How iliotibial tract injuries of the knee combine with acute anterior cruciate ligament tears to influence abnormal anterior tibial displacement. Am J Sports Med 21(1):55–60. doi:10.1177/036354659302100110

Ulmer MG, Rose T, Imhoff AB (2006) Bandverletzungen Am Kniegelenk - Teil II. Orthopädie und Unfallchirurgie up2date - 1, vol. 1. Thieme Verlag, Stuttgart, pp 404–405

Viidik A, Lewin T (1966) Changes in Tensile Strength Characteristics and Histology of Rabbit Ligaments Induced by Different Modes of Postmortal Storage. Acta Orthopaedica 37(2):141–155. doi:10.3109/17453676608993274

Wagner M, Weiler A (2014) Anterolaterale Stabilisierung. Arthroskopie 27(3):198–201. doi:10.1007/s00142-014-0819-7

Wang I-NE, Mitroo S, Chen FH, Lu HH, Doty SB (2006) Age-dependent changes in matrix composition and organization at the ligament-to-bone insertion. J Orthopaedic Research: Official Publ Orthopaedic Res Soc 24(8):1745–55. doi:10.1002/jor.20149

Wijdicks CA, Ewart DT, Nuckley DJ, Johansen S, Engebretsen L, Laprade RF (2010) Structural properties of the primary medial knee ligaments. Am J Sports Med 38(8):1638–46. doi:10.1177/0363546510363465

Wolff D, Bidermann T, Hempfling H, Bühren V (2005) Die extraartikuläre kniestabilisierung nach macintosh-eine alternative bei fehlgeschlagenem vorderen kreuzbandersatz? Zentralblatt für Chirurgie 130(04):333–337

Woo SL-Y, Hollis JM, Adams DJ, Lyon RM, Takai S (1991) Tensile properties of the human femur-anterior cruciate ligament-tibia complex: The effects of specimen age and orientation. Am J Sports Med 19(3):217–225. doi:10.1177/036354659101900303

Woo SL-Y, Orlando CA, Camp JF, Akeson WH (1986) Effects of postmortem storage by freezing on ligament tensile behavior. J Biomechanics 19(5):399–404. doi:10.1016/0021-9290(86)90016-3

Wroble RR, Grood ES, Cummings JS, Henderson JM, Noyes FR (1993) The role of the lateral extraarticular restraints in the anterior cruciate ligament-deficient knee. Am J Sports Med 21(2):257–263. doi:10.1177/036354659302100216

Zantop T, Petersen W (2010) [Modified Larson technique for posterolateral corner reconstruction of the knee]. Operative Orthopädie und Traumatologie 22(4):373–86. doi:10.1007/s00064-010-9030-9

Zens M, Ruhhammer J, Goldschmidtboeing F, Woias P, Feucht MJ, Mayr HO, Niemeyer P (2014) A New Approach to Determine Ligament Strain Using Polydimethylsiloxane Strain Gauges: Exemplary Measurements of the Anterolateral Ligament. J Biomech Eng 136(12):124504. doi:10.1115/1.4028837

28

The benefits and limitations of animal models for translational research in cartilage repair

Conor J. Moran[1,2,3], Ashwanth Ramesh[1,2,3], Pieter A. J. Brama[4], John M. O'Byrne[1,5], Fergal J. O'Brien[1,2,3] and Tanya J. Levingstone[1,2,3*]

Abstract

Much research is currently ongoing into new therapies for cartilage defect repair with new biomaterials frequently appearing which purport to have significant regenerative capacity. These biomaterials may be classified as medical devices, and as such must undergo rigorous testing before they are implanted in humans. A large part of this testing involves in vitro trials and biomechanical testing. However, in order to bridge the gap between the lab and the clinic, in vivo preclinical trials are required, and usually demanded by regulatory approval bodies. This review examines the in vivo models in current use for cartilage defect repair testing and the relevance of each in the context of generated results and applicability to bringing the device to clinical practice. Some of the preclinical models currently used include murine, leporine, ovine, caprine, porcine, canine, and equine models. Each of these has advantages and disadvantages in terms of animal husbandry, cartilage thickness, joint biomechanics and ethical and licencing issues. This review will examine the strengths and weaknesses of the various animal models currently in use in preclinical studies of cartilage repair.

Keywords: Tissue engineering, Collagen, In vivo, Osteochondral, Cartilage

Introduction

Cartilage defects have long caused significant morbidity for patients and present difficulty for surgeons attempting repair. Due to the avascular nature of the chondral surface and the specialised rigid extracellular matrix with a low cell density this tissue rarely regenerates by itself (Mankin 1982). There is significant ongoing research focused on halting the propagation of these defects and the eventual requirement for joint replacement. Current clinical procedures include bone marrow stimulation techniques, cartilage plug transplant, and expanded autologous chondrocyte implantation (Camp et al. 2014; Steadman et al. 2003; Brittberg et al. 1994; Peterson et al. 2003; Hangody et al. 2001). In recent years, the focus has moved to bioengineered materials and cell-seeded bioengineered scaffolds (Levingstone et al. 2014; Almeida et al. 2015; Hunziker et al. 2015). While in vitro testing and biomechanical analysis of biomaterials can provide much information about the safety, efficacy and potential for repair of these new biomaterials, in order to truly assess their regenerative capabilities, and the immune response associated with implantation, the use of animal models is required. Furthermore, regulatory bodies require in vivo animal studies to be carried out before new devices can be translated into clinical practice (Chu 2001; Hoemann et al. 2011; Hurtig et al. 2011). When carrying out animal studies the principles of the three R's; Reduction, Replacement and Refinement must applied (Russell & Burch 1959). The number of animals used should be reduced to the minimum required to achieve a valid statistically significant result. Wherever possible the use of animals should be replaced by other means, such as computer simulation, cadaveric, or in vitro testing, and the experiment must refined or altered in any way possible so as to decrease potential for suffering for all involved animals.

* Correspondence: tanyalevingstone@rcsi.ie
[1]Tissue Engineering Research Group, Department of Anatomy, Royal College of Surgeons in Ireland, 123 St. Stephen's Green, Dublin 2, Ireland
[2]Trinity Centre for Bioengineering, Trinity College Dublin, Dublin 2, Ireland
Full list of author information is available at the end of the article

Review

General considerations when selecting an appropriate animal model for the assessment of biomaterials strategies for cartilage repair

A range of factors require consideration when selecting an appropriate animal model for the assessment of biomaterial strategies for cartilage repair. Firstly a decision on small or large animal model is required is necessary: small animal models include rodents such as mice, rats and rabbits; while large animal models include dogs, goats, sheep, pigs and horses. Each has advantages and disadvantages, in the assessment of the clinical potential of new materials the model that most closely representing human anatomy and physiology of healing should be considered. Factors requiring consideration include, the size of the joint, the cartilage thickness, the depth and critical size of the defect (critical size implies a defect which will not heal spontaneously without any intervention), the age of skeletal maturity (better results in young patients regardless of treatment type), load distribution of the stifle, affordability and ease of animal handling. (Hunziker et al. 2002) Additionally, the defect position is closely related to its loading conditions and is therefore an important consideration. Although clinically most defects occur on the weight bearing medial condyle of the femur, many animal studies choose a partial-weight bearing site such as the trochlea, to improve the retention of the scaffold and cells implanted. (Hoemann et al. 2011). While many studies report improved cartilage repair in defects positioned in the trochlear over the femoral condyle (Orth et al. 2013a), conflicting results, where less defect repair occurs in the trochlea compared to the medial condyle have also been reported (Hoemann et al. 2011; Hoemann et al. 2005). In the clinical scenario most operators will follow surgery with a 4–6 week period of partial-weight bearing with full range of motion in the joint, slowly working up to full weight bearing (Vogt et al. 2013) even though short term studies have shown an accelerated rehab protocol can reduce pain and increase function (Vogt et al. 2013; Ebert et al. 2008) In the preclinical in vivo model weight bearing can be controlled by using external fixators and casts on the animals (Kojima et al. 2014; Roth et al. 1988). Confining animals to pens for the initial post-operative period has been shown to be effective in reducing post-operative joint load (Etterlin et al. 2014). Many studies favour uni-lateral (one treatment per animal) models (Marmotti et al. 2012; Nixon et al. 2015), however, bi-lateral models offer the advantages of allowing direct comparison of a treatment to a control within the same animal, thus counteracting the effect of host factors such as age, sex, weight, tissue characteristics, physical activity, or hormonal status and enabling a reduction in animal numbers (Orth et al. 2013b). Consideration of post-operative mobilisation is important in model selection and bi-lateral models are unsuitable when unloading of the treated joint is necessary or when gait analyses are to be performed. Guidelines have been set out in ASTM F 2451-05 for animal models suitable for the assessment of cartilage repair (Steadman et al. 2003). A comparison of the properties of various animal models used for the assessment of biomaterial approaches to cartilage defect repair is present in Table 1.

Small animal models

Rodent models

Small animal models can be very useful to give information about the residence time of an implant, and also to determine the type of repair tissue formed (ASTM F2451-05 2010). The availability of athymic, transgenic and knockout strains of both rats and mice means these models can be used to assess a multitude of factors including the use of strains of mice (DBA/1) in which osteoarthritis occurs spontaneously (Nordling et al. 1992) and athymic strains which can be used to assess allogenic and xenogeneic cells and tissues (Chu et al. 2010a). Rodents, such as mice and rats, have the advantage of being purpose bred to reduce biological variation, while being affordable, and easy to breed and maintain in-house. They thus act as a good bridge between in vitro and in vivo experiments to provide proof of concept data; however, their joints are small with very thin cartilage consisting of only a few cell layers (Chu et al. 2010a). Rodent models can provide useful subcutaneous models and intramuscular models for the assessment of the degradation rate and safety profile of biomaterials and implants generally 6–8 weeks in duration (Chu et al. 2010a). Rat models are not frequently used in the assessment of chondral defect repair due to the thinness of the cartilage layer (Gelse et al. 2003; Kuroda et al. 2006). However, a study by Choi et al. reports the use of chondral defects 1 mm in diameter and 0.15 mm deep on the femoral trochlear groove for assessment of growth factor releasing hydrogels (Choi et al. 2015). Additionally osteochondral defects of 1.5 mm (Dahlin et al. 2014) and 2 mm (Chung et al. 2014) diameter on the femoral condyle have been used for the assessment of biomaterial strategies (Singh et al. 2013). These models have limited potential in the determination of the clinical potential of new biomaterials as repair processes that are successful in restoring such small diameter defects may not be applicable in larger defect (Chu et al. 2010a). Rodents also have open growth plates throughout their maturity (Libbin & Rivera 1989) and therefore may have the increased intrinsic healing capacity of a juvenile. Additionally, the gait pattern and biomechanical loading environment in rodents varies significantly to that in humans. Rodents are therefore very limited in their

Table 1 A comparison of various models used in preclinical models for the assessment of biomaterial strategies for cartilage defect repair to the human knee joint

Species	Breed	Age of skeletal maturity	Adult weight	Cartilage thickness	Calcified cartilage layer thickness	Bone plate thickness	Critical size defect	References
Human		18–22 years	60–90 kg	2.4–2.6 mm	0.1 mm	0.2–0.5 mm	10 mm	Chevrier (Chevrier et al. 2015), ASTM (Dahlin et al. 2014)
Rabbit	New Zealand White	9 months	3–4 kg	0.16–0.75 mm	0.1–0.15 mm	0.4–0.5 mm	3 mm	Chevrier (Chevrier et al. 2015). ASTM (Dahlin et al. 2014)
Dog	Mongrel, Beagle	1–2 years	15–30 kg	0.95–1.3 mm	-	-	4 mm	Ahern (Ahern et al. 2009), ASTM (Dahlin et al. 2014)
Mini-pig	Gottingen Mini-pig, Yucatan, Lee-sung	10 months–1 year	20–40 kg	1.5 mm–2.0 mm	-	-	6 mm	Ahern (Ahern et al. 2009), ASTM (Dahlin et al. 2014)
Pig	Large White	2 years	250 kg	1.5 mm-2.0 mm	-	-	6 mm	Ahern (Ahern et al. 2009), ASTM (Dahlin et al. 2014)
Goat	Spanish, Dairy, Boer Cross, Saanan	2–3 years	40–70 kg	0.8–2 mm	0.2 mm	0.3 mm	6 mm	Patil (Patil et al. 2014), ASTM (Dahlin et al. 2014), Frisbie (Frisbie et al. 2009),
Sheep	Suffolk, Texel	2–3 years	35–80 kg	0.7–1.7 mm	0.2 mm	0.7 mm	7 mm	Chevrier (Chevrier et al. 2015), ASTM (Dahlin et al. 2014)
Horse	Mixed, Thoroughbred, Quarter Horse	2–4 years	500–600 kg	2.0–3.0 mm	0.2 mm	0.7 mm	9 mm	Chevrier (Chevrier et al. 2015), ASTM (Dahlin et al. 2014)

potential to be used as a translational model for cartilage surface repair in humans (Chu et al. 2010a).

Rabbit model

The rabbit model provides a more suitable small animal model for the assessment of cartilage repair as they have larger joints and are a good size for easy surgical procedures and specimen handling with a cartilage thickness of 0.25 mm–0.75 mm (Table 1) (Fig. 1.) (ASTM F2451–05 2010). Rabbits have been widely used for the assessment of cartilage repair in studies lasting up to 16 weeks, although some 1 year rabbit studies have been performed (Maruyama 1979; Brittberg et al. 1997; Fragonas et al. 2000; Yanai et al. 2005; Funayama et al. 2008; Luengo Gimeno et al. 2006; Chu et al. 1997; Levingstone et al. 2015). Rabbits offer many advantages as they are cost effective, easy to handle and to house. The femoral condyle is the most often used defect site for weight bearing models, especially those located inferioposteriorly (An & Freidman 1999). However, a comprehensive biokinematic study of rabbit gait pattern during hopping performed by Gushue et al. (Gushue et al. 2005) noted that, due to the wide variety of landing patterns of the hind limb during hopping, there are increased forces in the lateral tibiofemoral joint with a mean of 262.3 % body weight going through the medial side, and 303.8 % body weight in the lateral joint (Gushue et al. 2005). This correlates with previous studies showing increased bone mineral density at the lateral tibial plateau and balanced subchondral tissue volume (Messner et al. 2001; Wei et al. 1998). Additionally, the rabbit hind limbs are kept primarily in a fully flexed position as opposed to human weight bearing which is primarily on a knee locked in extension (Madry et al. 2015). Thus due to the differing biomechanics, caution is therefore advised when comparing results from rabbit studies to humans. Intercondylar groove defects have been used as partial weight bearing defects. (ASTM F2451–05 2010; Chu et al. 1997). Greater rates of repair may occur in rabbit articular cartilage models compared to other species due to higher metabolic activity and density of pluripotent stem cells near the defect site (Fig. 2) (ASTM F2451–05 2010). In addition, while the size of chondrocytes in human and rabbit articular cartilage do not differ significantly from each other (Hunziker 1999), the overall cell volume density is approximately 1.7 % in cartilage from the human medial femoral condyle (MFC) as opposed to 12.2 % in the adult rabbit. These amount to cell densities of 1800 and 7500 per mm^3 in humans and rabbits respectively (Hunziker 1999). The low cellularity of human hyaline cartilage thus contributes to the poor levels of repair observed while the increased density of chondrocytes in rabbits means there are more cells abutting the defect site for repair. The bone mineral density in the rabbit medial femoral condyle (MFC) is reported to be similar to that in humans at the bone plate (1.19 g/cm^3 and 1.17 respectively g/cm^3) but at a depth of 3 mm was 0.65 g/cm^3 compared to 0.36 g/cm^3 in humans. (Chevrier et al. 2015) Bone volume fraction was 58 ± 10 % in the rabbit MFC compared to 33 ± 13 % in humans (Chevrier et al. 2015). Rabbit stifle joints have different load characteristics and cartilage thickness compared to humans, making it difficult to investigate translation potential in this model.

Large animal models

Short (8–12 weeks) studies can be used to provide information regarding the biocompatibility, early cellular responsiveness and persistence and condition of the implant within the defect. Longer studies (6–12 months) are necessary to gain confidence in extent of success in the repair and regeneration of articular cartilage, including interface with adjacent cartilage and subchondral bone as well as the opposing articular surface (ASTM

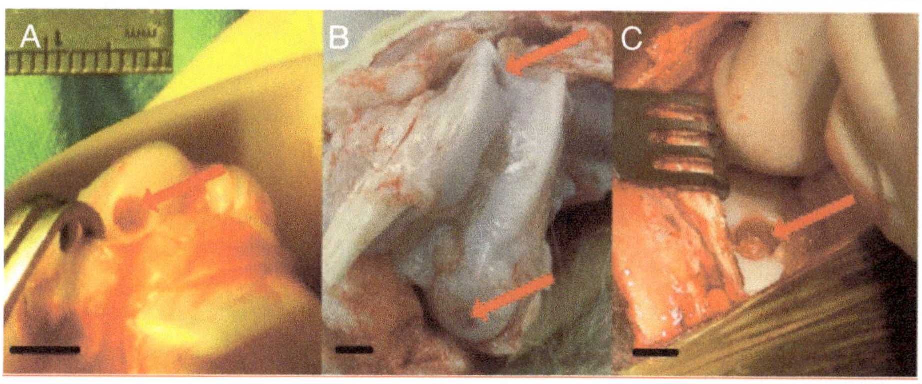

Fig. 1 Macroscopic image of distal femur of (**a**) rabbit, (**b**) goat and (**c**) horse showing (**a**) 3 mm, (**b**) 6 mm and (**c**) 9 mm defects created by drilling. This demonstrates the significant difference in the size of the joints involved and the size of the defects that can be created using these models. (Scale bar = 5 mm)

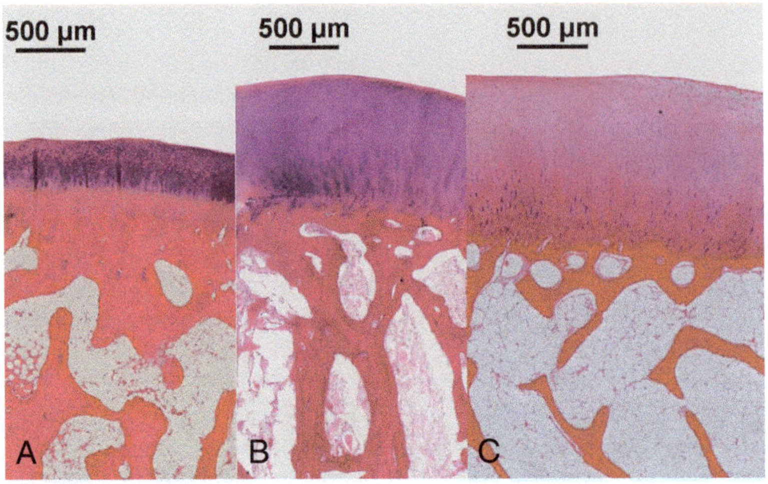

Fig. 2 H&E stained histology specimens of the distal femur of (**a**) rabbit (**b**) goat and (**c**) horse. These images demonstrate the histological similarity between the different models, but also the vast differences in the thickness of the cartilage at the joint surface. The chondrocyte distribution differences are also evident, with the rabbit cartilage being much more densely packed with chondrocytes than either goat or horse which could explain some better intrinsic healing of cartilage defects in rabbits

F2451–05 2010). A range of large animal models suitable for the assessment of cartilage repair have been investigated, including dogs (Engkvist 1979; Igarashi et al. 2012; Breinan et al. 2000), pigs (Hunziker et al. 2001; Lohan et al. 2013; Boopalan et al. 2011; Klein et al. 2009; Christensen et al. 2015), sheep (Kon et al. 2010a; Milano et al. 2010; Erggelet et al. 2009), goats (Getgood et al. 2012; Jurgens et al. 2013; Lu et al. 2006; Wang et al. 2007) and horses (Kon et al. 2010b; Frisbie et al. 2009; Hendrickson et al. 1994). When using any large animal model it is important to determine where on the joint the defect should be created based on the biomechanics of the joint. In humans, most cartilage defects occur on the weight bearing medial condyle this is thus the most common defect site used in cartilage repair studies (An & Freidman 1999). If using this defect type, the following should be considered in order to meet ASTM F2451-05 (ASTM F2451–05 2010).

1) The defect size should not exceed 15 to 20 % of the articulating surface or 50–60 % of the condylar width.
2) Due to the convex curvature of the defect sites the defect can differ from the centre to the margins.
3) It is necessary to consider the impact of articulation with both the meniscus and the tibial plateau.

Canine model

Dogs suffer from many of the cartilage pathologies found in humans like osteochondritis dissecans and osteoarthritis (Shortkroff et al. 1996) and veterinary surgeons regularly perform arthroscopies on canine stifles. As such, canine models are considered to be a good choice for cartilage repair studies (An & Freidman 1999). They accept rehabilitation regimens, cope well with immobilising the joint, and can be trained to walk on treadmills, and can co-operate in swimming and controlled weight bearing rehabilitation (Hurtig et al. 2011). The cartilage thickness, however, is significantly thinner than human cartilage even in medium to large dogs (range: 0.95–1.3 mm) (Table 1) and the reported diameter of critical size defects, at 4 mm, is considerably small even in the largest dogs (Ahern et al. 2009). Anatomical differences are present between canine and human knee joints with the existence of an extra intra-capsular, extra-articular, lateral long digital extensor tendon (LDET) which originates just inferior to the lateral edge of the patellar groove in the canine joint. Its function is dorsiflexion of the forefoot during knee flexion and is found in many quadrupeds (Proffen et al. 2012). Therefore, although canines deal well with the perioperative regimen, the canine knee joint does not model the human knee joint very closely Due to their longstanding status as companion and family pet, ethical issues also prevent their widespread use. In the UK and Ireland cats, dogs, horses, non-human primates and endangered species require a special justification for use to show no other species is suitable for the specified programme of work. It is therefore easier to get ethical approval for agricultural animals such as pigs, goats and sheep than canine models (An & Freidman 1999; Animals (Scientific Procedures) Act. Sect. 14 1986; Wolfensohn & Lloyd 2003).

Porcine model

Pigs (porcine) models are advantageous in the terms of their joint size, joint loading mechanics, weight (an adult sow can weigh up to 250 kg) (Wolfensohn & Lloyd 2003), lack of spontaneous healing of any significant defects, bone trabecular thickness and the arrangement of collagen network which resemble a human joint (Chu et al. 2010a). Nevertheless, these are large animals and require specialised husbandry and can be expensive to maintain in a research facility. They do not reach skeletal maturity until approximately two years and although researchers can utilise stock from commercial companies and farmers, most pigs will be slaughtered around the age of 6 months and therefore sourcing of skeletally mature animals of a similar age is often difficult. The alternative use of mature breeding animals makes sourcing of sufficient numbers, good health status and uniform age difficult because these animals are usually only replaced because of health problems on a one by one basis.

Mini-pigs are significantly smaller than full sized swine weighing roughly 40–70 kg as adults (Christensen et al. 2015; Wolfensohn & Lloyd 2003) and can thus provide some of the advantages of the pig model while overcoming some of the limitations (Schneider et al. 2011; Ebihara et al. 2012). The physiological parameters, such as blood count, blood clotting, electrolytes and liver enzymes, have been shown to be similar to values for humans (Chu et al. 2010a). A range of breeds of mini-pig have been utilised in the assessment of biomaterials for cartilage repair including Yucatan (Fisher et al. 2015), Gottingen (Schneider et al. 2011) and Lee-sung (Jiang et al. 2007) mini-pigs. Immature Yucatan mini-pigs are reported to have cartilage of 1–2 mm in thickness on the medial femoral condyle (Fisher et al. 2015). Histomorphometric analysis of peripheral bone in Gottingen mini-pigs has shown the bone apposition rate and trabecular thickness to be similar to human bone (Chu et al. 2010a), which is a significant factor when measuring the inflammatory response and toxicity of any implanted biomaterials. Mini-pigs of a defined type and known health status can be sourced from specialist laboratory suppliers but they are not skeletally mature until they reach 18–22 months of age (Chu et al. 2010a) and require specialist housing including specialised slatted flooring separate from a dry bedding area. Many studies thus use immature mini-pigs that have not reached skeletal maturity and thus the data reported has limited clinically relevance. Pigs will also turn any pasture into a mud bath by rooting for food and so can be expensive to maintain in a long term study (Wolfensohn & Lloyd 2003).

Caprine model

Two of the most commonly used models in research are ruminants, these are the caprine and ovine models. Goats are among the earliest animals domesticated by humans. They are farmed throughout the world and are used for a variety of products, including milk, meat and coat fibres (mohair and cashmere). They are, as a result, relatively easy to obtain when skeletally mature. The caprine (goat) femoral condyle and trochlear defect models have been used successfully for evaluation of new implants for treatment of partial thickness and osteochondral defects (Fig. 1) (Klein et al. 2009; Jurgens et al. 2013; Nukavarapu & Dorcemus 2013). Such models offer the advantages of joint size, cartilage thickness (although the ASTM F 2451–05 reports thicknesses of 1.5–2.0 mm, there are reports in the literature ranging from 0.8 mm (ASTM F2451–05 2010; Chu et al. 2010a; Brehm et al. 2006)) (Table 1), critical defect size (6 mm is the most commonly reported and will not spontaneously heal at 6 months) (Getgood et al. 2012; Ahern et al. 2009; Shahgaldi 1998; Jackson et al. 2001) and proportion of cartilage to bone and subchondral bone thickness being close to humans (Ahern et al. 2009; Jackson et al. 2001; Chu et al. 2010b). Subchondral bone trabecular structure in goats is similar to that in humans (Fig. 3) and bone mineral density has been reported to be 0.67 g/cm^3 (Gollehon et al. 1987). The caprine stifle

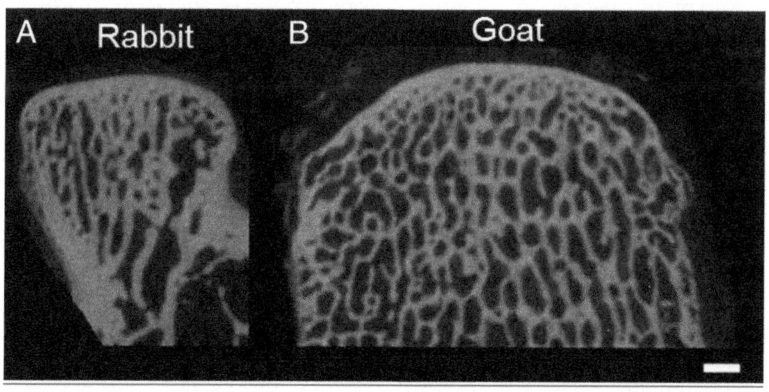

Fig. 3 2D micro-CT sections from rabbit (**a**) and goat (**b**) medial femoral condyles. These images demonstrate the similarity between the both models, with similar bone plate thickness and trabecular thickness in both cases. (Scale = 2 mm)

joint, like the human knee consists of tibiofemoral and patellofemoral articulations. In a direct comparative study of the stifle joint of cows, sheep, goats, dogs, pigs, and rabbits the goat stifle was found to have the closest anatomy to the human knee (Proffen et al. 2012). However, the femur has a deep long trochlear groove with prominent medial and lateral ridges. The femoral condyles are also distinct with a large intercondylar notch. The tibial plateau is convex and sloped posterolaterally with a prominent fibular styloid laterally roughly correlating to the fibular head and styloid process in humans (LaPrade et al. 2006). Additionally, the soft tissue structures which prevent abnormal joint movement specifically in the lateral compartment of the goat knee are similar to those in the human knee joint; these include lateral collateral ligament (LCL) complex, popliteus tendon and popliteofibular ligament. These structures act as primary stabilisers to prevent abnormal varus and tibial external rotation while also acting as secondary stabilisers, preventing anterior and posterior translation of the knee (Gollehon et al. 1987). Articular congruity at the tibiofemoral joint is poor in both humans and goats due to the convex surface of the tibial plateau, but goats have significantly thicker menisci, which contribute to increasing congruity between goats and humans (Patil et al. 2014). In the human knee flexion is limited to less than 30° in normal walking and stance phase however the goat stifle joint is flexed between 50°and 70° (Patil et al. 2014) meaning contact areas are different and must be considered.

Caprine cartilage is slightly thinner than the human distal femoral cartilage (Hoemann et al. 2011; ASTM F2451–05 2010) and the stiffness and elastic modulus of the caprine cartilage has been found to be greater than human articular cartilage (Patil et al. 2014). However in depth biomechanical analysis of the differences between the goat stifle joint and the human knee joint has shown that when the joint is loaded under conditions representing normal walking (ranging from 25 % body weight to 200 % body weight), most of the peak contact pressures in goat knees were comparable to those generated in human knees. (Patil et al. 2014) It did show, however the peak contact pressures in the caprine tibiofemoral joint at peak flexion are higher than normal human tibiofemoral contact pressure in the normal walking cycle, under twice body weight at peak flexion of normal walking (70°) goats reach a contact pressure of 12.57 MPa whereas in normal walking humans only flex to 30° and reach 4.93 MPa (Patil et al. 2014). Aside from this peak, the biomechanics and contact pressures of the goat walking cycle are broadly similar to the human equivalent. Goats are also relatively inexpensive to maintain, easy to handle, and the cartilage thickness allows for the creation of both chondral and osteochondral defects (Chu et al. 2010a). If adequate facilities are available to house them, then this model is feasible to conduct large animal studies to evaluate biological responses, durability, toxicology, lesion size and location analogous to human studies (Cook et al. 2014). Caprine models thus represent a good option for in vivo assessment of chondral and osteochondral defect repair.

Ovine model

The sheep (ovine) model is one commonly used for in vivo trials of materials for cartilage repair (Kon et al. 2010a; Milano et al. 2010; Guo et al. 2004). Weighing between 35 and 80 kg when skeletally mature at 2–3 years they transmit a scientifically relevant amount of weight through its tibiofemoral joint (Wolfensohn & Lloyd 2003). They have a cartilage thickness of roughly 0.4–1.7 mm at the medial condyle (ASTM F2451–05 2010; Ahern et al. 2009). The sheep stifle joint is a diarthrodal joint with four separate articulations: femoropatellar, femorotibial, femorofibular and tibiofibular. Like the goat, the sheep has a long trochlear groove formed by prominent medial and lateral trochlear ridges The femorotibial joint has a range of motion from 72+/−3° in full flexion to 145 +/− 5° in full extension (Allen et al. 1998). A large amount of research can be done using the ovine stifle joint as it has very similar cruciate ligaments to humans and large menisci as well as a similar LCL complex, popliteus tendon and popliteofibular ligament and can therefore be used in surgical training as well as device development (Madry et al. 2015; Allen et al. 1998). This also means second look arthroscopy can be performed by a skilled arthroscopist to review integration (Ahern et al. 2009).

Sheep are also readily available as they are commonly bred in agriculture and are relatively placid, tolerate stifle surgery well and are easily housed and maintained. They have, however, been reported to have a very variable articular cartilage thickness, between 0.4 and 1.7 mm on the MFC (Ahern et al. 2009), this variability can cause issues with study design and results. Bone mineral density in sheep MFC has been shown to be similar to that in humans, reportedly 1.19 g/cm^3. However at a depth of 3 mm the bone mineral density is reportedly 0.67 g/cm^3 compared to 0.36 g/cm^3 in humans. (Chevrier et al. 2015) The bone volume fraction in the MFC is reportedly higher in sheep than humans at 3 mm below the bone surface (42 ± 4 % and 33 ± 13 % respectively) (Chevrier et al. 2015). Contact pressures generated in sheep are largely comparable to those in humans, although while humans can reach a mean peak contact force of 5.4 times body weight ascending stairs (Taylor et al. 2004) the maximum in vivo contact force measured in sheep is 2.25 times body weight (Patil et al. 2014; Taylor et al. 2006).

Techniques that expose the subchondral bone such as the implantation of osteochondral repair scaffolds or osteochondral allografts, may induce subchondral bone cyst formation either through fluid intrusion or bony contusion. Increased formation of cysts in the subchondral bone have been reported in both goats and sheep models (von Rechenberg et al. 2003; Orth et al. 2012). This cyst formation can hamper subchondral bone repair (von Rechenberg et al. 2003; Pallante-Kichura et al. 2013). Other disadvantages include extra fat pad that can obscure the joint and the more labour intensive husbandry practices required for animal handling (Wolfensohn & Lloyd 2003) and the acquisition of animals from an agricultural background instead of bred for purpose, meaning their health status and genetic background will be less uniform. The use of goats and sheep in research is much less common than the use of rodents and thus specialised commercial products, such as antibodies, available to researchers utilising rodent models are not readily available for ruminants.

Equine model

Horse (equine) models offer several advantages in the investigation of cartilage repair strategies. Horses are animals primarily bred and kept for their athletic performance and, as a result, suffer regularly from cartilage injuries and joint diseases such as osteoarthritis and osteochondrosis. Hence performing pre-clinical evaluations on cartilage repair mechanisms may be of direct benefit to the species itself (Fig. 3.) (Malda et al. 2012). However candidates for entry to a study must be screened in advance for naturally occurring disease to avoid affecting results. Due to the large joint surface, arthroscopies are routine and can be used both for cartilage defect creation and repair, and longitudinal follow up on the process of cartilage repair at different time points. The equine model has critical size defects up to 9 mm, cartilage mean thickness of 2.0–3.0 mm and a vertically loaded stifle joint during gait, and so is beneficial for translatable cartilage studies and especially partial thickness defects which are the most relevant to human therapy (ASTM F2451–05 2010; Ahern et al. 2009; Malda et al. 2012). The horse is the largest animal model in use as a model for cartilage repair, commonly weighing around 500–600 kg, the joint is, therefore, adapted to withstand elevated loads, with a hardened subchondral bone and efficient joint force distribution (Chu et al. 2010a). Bone mineral density in the horse MFC is reportedly similar to that in humans at the bone plate (1.19 g/cm^3) but higher at a depth 3 mm (0.64 g/cm^3). Bone mineral density values were found to be similar to humans in the horse lateral trochlea at a depth of 3 mm (0.5 g/cm^3) (Chevrier et al. 2015). Bone volume fraction is reportedly higher in horse than in humans in the MFC (47 ± 8 %) at a depth and 3 mm. (Chevrier et al. 2015) Loading is of concern as continuous static loading of weight bearing condyles of the joint cannot be minimised, as a result the lateral trochlea of the femur where loading is intermittent is the most common location for cartilage defects (Ahern et al. 2009). In the horse model it is also common to use the carpus and the tibiotarsal joints and joints of the middle carpal bones for defect formation, as chondral injuries can be common here and the stifle joint is difficult to access for diagnostic imaging such as MRI due to the bulk of the upper hind limb. The stifle is however amenable to ultrasound in the hands of an experienced user (Fig. 4) (Hurtig et al. 2011; Ahern et al. 2009; Hurtig et al. 2001; Vachon et al. 1992; Rautiainen et al. 2013). While the horse is an appealing model in terms of cartilage thickness and joint morphology, a highly specialized and a well-equipped centre with well-trained personnel is required to carry out equine surgeries, and they require a large specialised habitat. These all lead to substantially increased costs involved in the study. In addition to practical considerations, horses are also subject to stringent licencing in some jurisdictions due to their historic status as a companion animal (Hurtig et al. 2011; Animals (Scientific Procedures) Act. Sect. 14 1986).

Operative factors influencing model selection

There are many reasons to choose one model over another (Table 2.), however surgical limitations of certain models play a large part in the selection of the appropriate group. Size is one of the main factors. In order to implant a biomaterial in a particular area the area must be of sufficient size to allow implantation. For example the knee joint of a rat has a cartilage thickness of 0.1 mm on the MFC, and in the mouse cartilage is only a few cell layers thick (Chu et al. 2010a) compared to between 0.8 and 2.0 mm on the MFC of the caprine stifle (ASTM F2451–05 2010; Chu et al. 2010a). To create a defect this small presents a technical difficulty for the operator meaning purely chondral defects are impossible and can lead to large inter-animal variation even when producing osteochondral defects meaning a much greater sample size would have to be used to achieve a statistically significant outcome contravening the 3 R's (Russell & Burch 1959).

Post-operative rehabilitation of cartilage repair in humans varies from centre to centre, it has been shown free movement and gradual increase in weight bearing improves outcomes, however, this is complex to ensure in animal models (Nishino et al. 2010; Assche et al. 2011). When using an in vivo model casts can be used to immobilise rat limbs (Kojima et al. 2014; Maldonado et al. 2013), however it is more common in large animals such as goats and sheep to keep them in small pens in the immediate post-operative period (Marmotti et al.

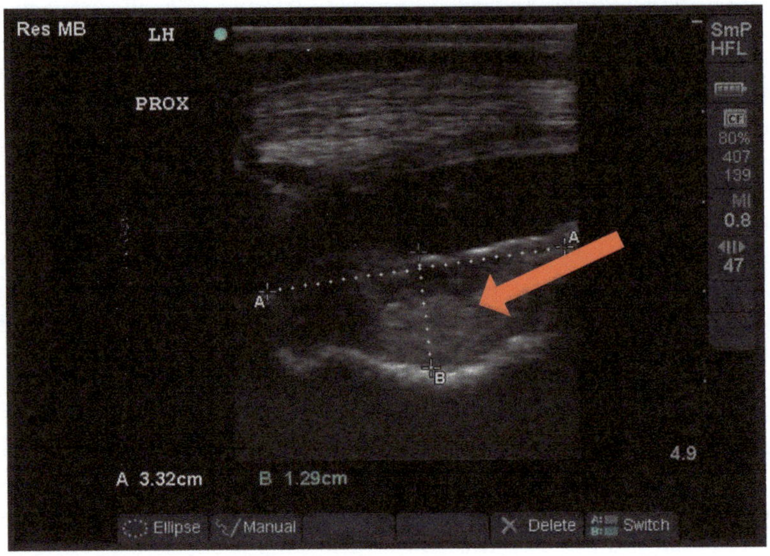

Fig. 4 Image of ultrasound of horse stifle taken one month post implantation of biomaterial scaffold (arrow) into naturally occurring osteochondral defect of trochlea of femur. This demonstrates the large defects occurring in the horse. The ability to image the implanted scaffold during the post-operative period is also a significant advantage to the large animal model

Table 2 Advantages and disadvantages of various in vivo models commonly used in the assessment of biomaterial strategies for cartilage defect repair

Species	Advantage	Disadvantage
Mouse	Low cost, manageable easily available Transgenic and athymic strains available Can be used in subcutaneous and intramuscular model for degradation rate and safety profile	Very small joints–in situ examination impossible
Rat	Low cost, easily available Athymic strains available Maintain in-house	Permanently open growth plates accelerating intrinsic healing Increased density of cells in cartilage causing more efficient healingPartial thickness defects impossible
Rabbit	Low costMaintain in-house	Increased intrinsic healing due to increased cell density Very different load characteristics Consistent partial thickness defects very difficult to achieve
Dog	Naturally occurring disease state Co-operate with rehabilitation regime	Thin cartilage Small critical size defect (4 mm) Complex ethical approval process
Pig	Biochemistry similar to humans Bone apposition rate and trabecular thickness similar to human Partial thickness defects possible	Expensive Difficult to obtain at skeletal maturity Specialised habitatTemperament
Goat	Anatomy and biomechanics similar to humans Partial thickness defects possible Easily availableLow maintenance	Subchondral cyst formation
Sheep	Anatomy similar to humans Partial thickness defects possible Easily availableLow maintenance	Subchondral cyst formation
Horse	Large defects similar to humans Partial thickness large diameter defects possible Naturally occurring defects Similar biomechanics in trochlear groove Second look arthroscopy possible	Expensive to acquire and maintain – specialised centre required Cannot avoid weight bearing on the joint during rehab phase if required Very dense subchondral boneMRI/CT impossible due to size

2013) to limit their mobilising. In some animals, such as horses, non-weight bearing is impossible, and can cause severe life-threatening illnesses. Horses will fully weight bear immediately post recovery, but if the defect area is on the patellofemoral joint rather than the tibiofemoral joint, a regimen of supervised walking building up to limited running can offload the patellofemoral joint in the post-operative phase.

Ex vivo factors influencing model selection

The chosen model affects the analysis that can the carried out, both during the study and post euthanasia at the study end point, and also the results that can be obtained. In smaller animals, it is possible to do in situ microcomputed tomography or magnetic resonance imaging on live animals, allowing good radiological scoring. Due to limited equipment availability this is more challenging for large animals. In large animals, the larger joint size allows for second look arthroscopy to be carried out during of the study. This can provide useful information about the repair tissue prior to the study endpoint. The use of large animal models results in larger tissue specimens for analysis. For example, in the horse model, the critical size defect is 9 mm. This poses some technical disadvantages as the dense subchondral bone requires longer decalcification times prior to histological staining. However, division of samples is possible without much difficulty, allowing for example, mechanical testing to be performed on one half and histological staining on the other. This doubles the amount of information collected from the experiment. Dividing a 6 mm (caprine) or 7 mm (ovine) can be a more daunting prospect and can leave artefact obscuring true results. These factors must be carefully considered at the outset of the study and the appropriate model chosen for the results and analyses required.

Conclusion

There is a significant pre-clinical gap to be bridged in the development of a device to ease suffering and halt joint degeneration before it can be used as a therapeutic clinically. Therefore, the selection of an appropriate preclinical in vivo model is important in ensuring successful translation to the clinic. The financial and labour costs involved in a large animal study can be prohibitive, and so for a proof of concept or degradation and safety profile it can be appropriate to use a small animal or rodent model before confirming effectiveness in a large animal study. It is also important to consider the different biomechanics and biokinematics of joints in quadrupeds and how the contact pressures on the weight bearing areas of the joint are affected along with stresses and strains on areas of joints not completely analogous to stresses and strains of the human knee. Therefore, in many ways, the caprine model is the most appropriate model for large scale large animal studies in cartilage surface defect repair, as the anatomy is closest to humans, they have similar biomechanics of their stifle joint to human knees, they have an adequate cartilage thickness allowing for partial and full thickness defects. Goats do not require specialised housing other than warm indoor bedding in winter and access to pasture in summer. In addition, goats are widely available as they are commonly used in agriculture. Pre-clinical studies are important to ensure safety and efficacy of biomaterials prior to widespread use, however, there are significant differences in the anatomy and biomechanics of different animal models and of humans. In order to enable the successful translation of biomaterials to the clinic, these differences must be recognised and considered in both study design and in comparing study outcomes.

Competing interests

No competing financial interests exist.

Authors' contributions

CM and TL conceived the review, CM, TL and AR drafted the paper. PB gave veterinary input, JOB gave clinical input and FOB gave scientific input. All authors critically revised the paper and approved the final manuscript.

Acknowledgements

The authors acknowledge Science Foundation Ireland/Health Research Board Translational Research Award (TRA/2011/19) for funding.

Author details

[1]Tissue Engineering Research Group, Department of Anatomy, Royal College of Surgeons in Ireland, 123 St. Stephen's Green, Dublin 2, Ireland. [2]Trinity Centre for Bioengineering, Trinity College Dublin, Dublin 2, Ireland. [3]Advanced Materials and Bioengineering Research (AMBER) Centre, RCSI & TCD, Dublin, Ireland. [4]Section of Veterinary Clinical Sciences, School of Veterinary Medicine, University College Dublin, Dublin, Ireland. [5]Cappagh National Orthopaedic Hospital, Finglas, Dublin 11, Ireland.

References

Ahern BJ, Parvizi J, Boston R, Schaer TP (2009) Preclinical animal models in single site cartilage defect testing: a systematic review. Osteoarthritis Cartilage 17(6):705–713

Allen MJ, Houlton JE, Adams SB, Rushton N (1998) The surgical anatomy of the stifle joint in sheep. Vet Surg 27(6):596–605

Almeida HV, Cunniffe GM, Vinardell T, Buckley CT, O'Brien FJ, Kelly DJ (2015) Coupling Freshly Isolated CD44 Infrapatellar Fat Pad-Derived Stromal Cells with a TGF-beta3 Eluting Cartilage ECM-Derived Scaffold as a Single-Stage Strategy for Promoting Chondrogenesis. Adv Healthc Mater 4(7):1043–53

An YH, Freidman RJ (1999) Animal Models in Orthopaedic Research. CRC Press, London

Animals (Scientific Procedures) Act. Sect. 14 (1986).

Assche DV, Caspel DV, Staes F, Saris DB, Bellemans J, Vanlauwe J et al (2011) Implementing one standardized rehabilitation protocol following autologous chondrocyte implantation or microfracture in the knee results in comparable physical therapy management. Physiother Theory Pract 27(2):125–136

ASTM F2451-05 (2010) Standard Guide for in vivo Assessment of Implantable Devices Intended to Repair or Regenerate Articular Cartilage., ASTM International

Boopalan PR, Arumugam S, Livingston A, Mohanty M, Chittaranjan S (2011) Pulsed electromagnetic field therapy results in healing of full thickness articular cartilage defect. Int Orthop 35(1):143–148

Brehm W, Aklin B, Yamashita T, Rieser F, Trub T, Jakob RP et al (2006) Repair of superficial osteochondral defects with an autologous scaffold-free cartilage construct in a caprine model: implantation method and short-term results. Osteoarthritis Cartilage 14(12):1214–1226

Breinan HA, Martin SD, Hsu HP, Spector M (2000) Healing of canine articular cartilage defects treated with microfracture, a type-II collagen matrix, or cultured autologous chondrocytes. J Orthop Res 18(5):781–789

Brittberg M, Lindahl A, Nilsson A, Ohlsson C, Isaksson O, Peterson L (1994) Treatment of deep cartilage defects in the knee with autologous chondrocyte transplantation. N Engl J Med 331(14):889–895

Brittberg M, Sjogren-Jansson E, Lindahl A, Peterson L (1997) Influence of fibrin sealant (Tisseel) on osteochondral defect repair in the rabbit knee. Biomaterials 18(3):235–242

Camp CL, Stuart MJ, Krych AJ (2014) Current concepts of articular cartilage restoration techniques in the knee. Sports health 6(3):265–273

Chevrier A, Kouao AS, Picard G, Hurtig MB, Buschmann MD (2015) Interspecies comparison of subchondral bone properties important for cartilage repair. J Orthop Res 33(1):63–70

Choi B, Kim S, Fan J, Kowalski T, Petrigliano F, Evseenko D et al (2015) Covalently conjugated transforming growth factor-beta1 in modular chitosan hydrogels for the effective treatment of articular cartilage defects. Biomaterials science 3(5):742–752

Christensen BB, Foldager CB, Olesen ML, Vingtoft L, Rölfing JHD, Ringgaard S et al (2015) Experimental articular cartilage repair in the Göttingen minipig: the influence of multiple defects per knee. J Exp Orthop 2(1):13

Chu CR (2001) Chondral and osteochondral injuries: mechanisms of injury and repair responses. Oper Tech Orthop 11(2):70–75

Chu CR, Dounchis JS, Yoshioka M, Sah RL, Coutts RD, Amiel D (1997) Osteochondral repair using perichondrial cells. A 1-year study in rabbits. Clin Orthop Relat Res 340:220–229

Chu CR, Szczodry M, Bruno S (2010a) Animal models for cartilage regeneration and repair. Tissue Eng B Rev 16(1):105–115

Chu CR, Szczodry M, Bruno S (2010b) Animal models for cartilage regeneration and repair. Tissue Eng Part B-Re 16(1):105–115

Chung JY, Song M, Ha CW, Kim JA, Lee CH, Park YB (2014) Comparison of articular cartilage repair with different hydrogel-human umbilical cord blood-derived mesenchymal stem cell composites in a rat model. Stem Cell Res Ther 5(2):39

Cook JL, Hung CT, Kuroki K, Stoker AM, Cook CR, Pfeiffer FM et al (2014) Animal models of cartilage repair. Bone Joint Res 3(4):89–94

Dahlin RL, Kinard LA, Lam J, Needham CJ, Lu S, Kasper FK et al (2014) Articular chondrocytes and mesenchymal stem cells seeded on biodegradable scaffolds for the repair of cartilage in a rat osteochondral defect model. Biomaterials 35(26):7460–7469

Ebert JR, Robertson WB, Lloyd DG, Zheng MH, Wood DJ, Ackland T (2008) Traditional vs accelerated approaches to post-operative rehabilitation following matrix-induced autologous chondrocyte implantation (MACI): comparison of clinical, biomechanical and radiographic outcomes. Osteoarthritis Cartilage 16(10):1131–1140

Ebihara G, Sato M, Yamato M, Mitani G, Kutsuna T, Nagai T et al (2012) Cartilage repair in transplanted scaffold-free chondrocyte sheets using a minipig model. Biomaterials 33(15):3846–3851

Engkvist O (1979) Reconstruction of patellar articular cartilage with free autologous perichondrial grafts. An experimental study in dogs. Scand J Plast Reconstr Surg 13(3):361–369

Erggelet C, Endres M, Neumann K, Morawietz L, Ringe J, Haberstroh K et al (2009) Formation of cartilage repair tissue in articular cartilage defects pretreated with microfracture and covered with cell-free polymer-based implants. J Orthop Res 27(10):1353–1360

Etterlin PE, Ytrehus B, Lundeheim N, Heldmer E, Osterberg J, Ekman S (2014) Effects of free-range and confined housing on joint health in a herd of fattening pigs. BMC Vet Res 10:208

Fisher MB, Belkin NS, Milby AH, Henning EA, Bostrom M, Kim M et al (2015) Cartilage repair and subchondral bone remodeling in response to focal lesions in a mini-pig model: implications for tissue engineering. Tissue Eng A 21(3–4):850–860

Fragonas E, Valente M, Pozzi-Mucelli M, Toffanin R, Rizzo R, Silvestri F et al (2000) Articular cartilage repair in rabbits by using suspensions of allogenic chondrocytes in alginate. Biomaterials 21(8):795–801

Frisbie DD, Lu Y, Kawcak CE, DiCarlo EF, Binette F, McIlwraith CW (2009) In vivo evaluation of autologous cartilage fragment-loaded scaffolds implanted into equine articular defects and compared with autologous chondrocyte implantation. Am J Sports Med 37(Suppl 1):71S–80S

Funayama A, Niki Y, Matsumoto H, Maeno S, Yatabe T, Morioka H et al (2008) Repair of full-thickness articular cartilage defects using injectable type II collagen gel embedded with cultured chondrocytes in a rabbit model. J Orthop Sci 13(3):225–232

Gelse K, von der Mark K, Aigner T, Park J, Schneider H (2003) Articular cartilage repair by gene therapy using growth factor-producing mesenchymal cells. Arthritis Rheum 48(2):430–441

Getgood AM, Kew SJ, Brooks R, Aberman H, Simon T, Lynn AK et al (2012) Evaluation of early-stage osteochondral defect repair using a biphasic scaffold based on a collagen-glycosaminoglycan biopolymer in a caprine model. Knee 19(4):422–430

Gollehon DL, Torzilli PA, Warren RF (1987) The role of the posterolateral and cruciate ligaments in the stability of the human knee. A biomechanical study. J Bone Joint Sur Am 69(2):233–242

Guo X, Wang C, Zhang Y, Xia R, Hu M, Duan C et al (2004) Repair of large articular cartilage defects with implants of autologous mesenchymal stem cells seeded into beta-tricalcium phosphate in a sheep model. Tissue Eng 10(11–12):1818–1829

Gushue DL, Houck J, Lerner AL (2005) Rabbit knee joint biomechanics: motion analysis and modeling of forces during hopping. J Orthop Res 23(4):735–742

Hangody L, Feczko P, Bartha L, Bodo G, Kish G (2001) Mosaicplasty for the treatment of articular defects of the knee and ankle. Clin Orthop Relat Res 391(Suppl):S328–S336

Hendrickson DA, Nixon AJ, Grande DA, Todhunter RJ, Minor RM, Erb H et al (1994) Chondrocyte-fibrin matrix transplants for resurfacing extensive articular cartilage defects. J Orthop Res 12(4):485–497

Hoemann CD, Hurtig M, Rossomacha E, Sun J, Chevrier A, Shive MS et al (2005) Chitosan-glycerol phosphate/blood implants improve hyaline cartilage repair in ovine microfracture defects. J Bone Joint Sur Am 87(12):2671–2686

Hoemann C, Kandel R, Roberts S, Saris DB, Creemers L, Mainil-Varlet P et al (2011) International Cartilage Repair Society (ICRS) recommended guidelines for histological endpoints for cartilage repair studies in animal models and clinical trials. Cartilage 2(2):153–172

Hunziker EB (1999) Biologic repair of articular cartilage. Defect models in experimental animals and matrix requirements. Clin Orthop Relat Res 367(Suppl):S135–S146

Hunziker EB, Driesang IM, Morris EA (2001) Chondrogenesis in cartilage repair is induced by members of the transforming growth factor-beta superfamily. Clin Orthop Relat Res 391 Suppl:S171-81

Hunziker EB, Quinn TM, Hauselmann HJ (2002) Quantitative structural organization of normal adult human articular cartilage. Osteoarthritis Cartilage 10(7):564–572

Hunziker EB, Lippuner K, Keel MJ, Shintani N (2015) An educational review of cartilage repair: precepts & practice - myths & misconceptions - progress & prospects. Osteoarthritis Cartilage 23(3):334–350

Hurtig M, Pearce S, Warren S, Kalra M, Miniaci A (2001) Arthroscopic mosaic arthroplasty in the equine third carpal bone. Veterinary surgery : VS 30(3):228–239

Hurtig MB, Buschmann MD, Fortier LA, Hoemann CD, Hunziker EB, Jurvelin JS et al (2011) Preclinical studies for cartilage repair: recommendations from the international cartilage repair society. Cartilage 2(2):137–152

Igarashi T, Iwasaki N, Kawamura D, Kasahara Y, Tsukuda Y, Ohzawa N et al (2012) Repair of articular cartilage defects with a novel injectable in situ forming material in a canine model. J Biomed Mater Res A 100(1):180–187

Jackson DW, Lalor PA, Aberman HM, Simon TM (2001) Spontaneous repair of full-thickness defects of articular cartilage in a goat model. A preliminary study. J Bone Joint Sur Am 83-a(1):53–64

Jiang CC, Chiang H, Liao CJ, Lin YJ, Kuo TF, Shieh CS et al (2007) Repair of porcine articular cartilage defect with a biphasic osteochondral composite. J Orthop Res 25(10):1277–1290

Jurgens WJ, Kroeze RJ, Zandieh-Doulabi B, van Dijk A, Renders GA, Smit TH et al (2013) One-step surgical procedure for the treatment of osteochondral defects with adipose-derived stem cells in a caprine knee defect: a pilot study. Bio Research open access 2(4):315–325

Klein TJ, Malda J, Sah RL, Hutmacher DW (2009) Tissue engineering of articular cartilage with biomimetic zones. Tissue Eng B Rev 15(2):143–157

Kojima S, Hoso M, Watanabe M, Matsuzaki T, Hibino I, Sasaki K (2014) Experimental joint immobilization and remobilization in the rats. J Phys Ther Sci 26(6):865–871

Kon E, Delcogliano M, Filardo G, Fini M, Giavaresi G, Francioli S et al (2010a) Orderly osteochondral regeneration in a sheep model using a novel nano-composite multilayered biomaterial. J Orthop Res 28(1):116–124

Kon E, Mutini A, Arcangeli E, Delcogliano M, Filardo G, Nicoli Aldini N et al (2010b) Novel nanostructured scaffold for osteochondral regeneration: pilot study in horses. J Tissue Eng Regen Med 4(4):300–308

Kuroda R, Usas A, Kubo S, Corsi K, Peng H, Rose T et al (2006) Cartilage repair using bone morphogenetic protein 4 and muscle-derived stem cells. Arthritis Rheum 54(2):433–442

LaPrade RF, Kimber KA, Wentorf FA, Olson EJ (2006) Anatomy of the posterolateral aspect of the goat knee. J Orthop Res 24(2):141–148

Levingstone TJ, Matsiko A, Dickson GR, O'Brien FJ, Gleeson JP (2014) A biomimetic multi-layered collagen-based scaffold for osteochondral repair. Acta Biomater 10(5):1996–2004

Levingstone TJ, Thompson E, Matsiko A, Schepens A, Gleeson JP, O'Brien FJ (2015) Multi-layered collagen-based scaffolds for osteochondral defect repair in rabbits. Acta Biomater In Press.

Libbin RM, Rivera ME (1989) Regeneration of growth plate cartilage induced in the neonatal rat hindlimb by reamputation. J Orthop Res 7(5):674–682

Lohan A, Marzahn U, El Sayed K, Bock C, Haisch A, Kohl B et al (2013) Heterotopic and orthotopic autologous chondrocyte implantation using a minipig chondral defect model. Ann Anat 195(5):488–497

Lu Y, Dhanaraj S, Wang Z, Bradley DM, Bowman SM, Cole BJ et al (2006) Minced cartilage without cell culture serves as an effective intraoperative cell source for cartilage repair. J Orthop Res 24(6):1261–1270

Luengo Gimeno F, Gatto S, Ferro J, Croxatto JO, Gallo JE (2006) Preparation of platelet-rich plasma as a tissue adhesive for experimental transplantation in rabbits. Thromb J 4:18

Madry H, Ochi M, Cucchiarini M, Pape D, Seil R (2015) Large animal models in experimental knee sports surgery: focus on clinical translation. J Exp Orthop 2(1):9

Malda J, Benders KE, Klein TJ, de Grauw JC, Kik MJ, Hutmacher DW et al (2012) Comparative study of depth-dependent characteristics of equine and human osteochondral tissue from the medial and lateral femoral condyles. Osteoarthritis Cartilage 20(10):1147–1151

Maldonado DC, Silva MC, Neto Sel R, de Souza MR, de Souza RR (2013) The effects of joint immobilization on articular cartilage of the knee in previously exercised rats. J Anat 222(5):518–525

Mankin HJ (1982) The response of articular cartilage to mechanical injury. J Bone Joint Surg Am 64(3):460–466

Marmotti A, Bruzzone M, Bonasia DE, Castoldi F, Rossi R, Piras L et al (2012) One-step osteochondral repair with cartilage fragments in a composite scaffold. Knee Surg Sports Traumatol Arthrosc 20(12):2590–2601

Marmotti A, Bruzzone M, Bonasia DE, Castoldi F, Von Degerfeld MM, Bignardi C et al (2013) Autologous cartilage fragments in a composite scaffold for one stage osteochondral repair in a goat model. Eur Cell Mater 26:15–31, discussion –2

Maruyama Y (1979) An experimental study on cartilage foramation in autogenous perichondrial transplantation in rabbits. Keio J Med 28(2):63–72

Messner K, Fahlgren A, Persliden J, Andersson BM (2001) Radiographic joint space narrowing and histologic changes in a rabbit meniscectomy model of early knee osteoarthrosis. Am J Sports Med 29(2):151–160

Milano G, Sanna Passino E, Deriu L, Careddu G, Manunta L, Manunta A et al (2010) The effect of platelet rich plasma combined with microfractures on the treatment of chondral defects: an experimental study in a sheep model. Osteoarthritis Cartilage 18(7):971–980

Nishino T, Ishii T, Chang F, Yanai T, Watanabe A, Ogawa T et al (2010) Effect of gradual weight-bearing on regenerated articular cartilage after joint distraction and motion in a rabbit model. J Orthop Res 28(5):600–606

Nixon AJ, Rickey E, Butler TJ, Scimeca MS, Moran N, Matthews GL (2015) A chondrocyte infiltrated collagen type I/III membrane (MACI((R)) implant) improves cartilage healing in the equine patellofemoral joint model. Osteoarthritis Cartilage 23(4):648–660

Nordling C, Karlsson-Parra A, Jansson L, Holmdahl R, Klareskog L (1992) Characterization of a spontaneously occurring arthritis in male DBA/1 mice. Arthritis Rheum 35(6):717–722

Nukavarapu SP, Dorcemus DL (2013) Osteochondral tissue engineering: current strategies and challenges. Biotechnol Adv 31(5):706–721

Orth P, Goebel L, Wolfram U, Ong MF, Graber S, Kohn D et al (2012) Effect of subchondral drilling on the microarchitecture of subchondral bone: analysis in a large animal model at 6 months. Am J Sports Med 40(4):828–836

Orth P, Meyer HL, Goebel L, Eldracher M, Ong MF, Cucchiarini M et al (2013a) Improved repair of chondral and osteochondral defects in the ovine trochlea compared with the medial condyle. J Orthop Res 31(11):1772–1779

Orth P, Zurakowski D, Alini M, Cucchiarini M, Madry H (2013b) Reduction of sample size requirements by bilateral versus unilateral research designs in animal models for cartilage tissue engineering. Tissue Eng Part C, Methods 19(11):885–891

Pallante-Kichura AL, Cory E, Bugbee WD, Sah RL (2013) Bone cysts after osteochondral allograft repair of cartilage defects in goats suggest abnormal interaction between subchondral bone and overlying synovial joint tissues. Bone 57(1):259–268

Patil S, Steklov N, Song L, Bae WC, D'Lima DD (2014) Comparative biomechanical analysis of human and caprine knee articular cartilage. Knee 21(1):119–125

Peterson L, Minas T, Brittberg M, Lindahl A (2003) Treatment of osteochondritis dissecans of the knee with autologous chondrocyte transplantation: results at two to ten years. J Bone Joint Sur Am 85-A(Suppl 2):17–24

Proffen BL, McElfresh M, Fleming BC, Murray MM (2012) A comparative anatomical study of the human knee and six animal species. Knee 19(4):493–499

Rautiainen J, Lehto LJ, Tiitu V, Kiekara O, Pulkkinen H, Brunott A et al (2013) Osteochondral repair: evaluation with sweep imaging with fourier transform in an equine model. Radiology 269(1):113–121

Roth JH, Mendenhall HV, McPherson GK (1988) The effect of immobilization on goat knees following reconstruction of the anterior cruciate ligament. Clin Orthop Relat Res 229:278–282

Russell WMS, Burch RL (1959) The Principles of Humane Experimental Technique. Methuen, London

Schneider U, Schmidt-Rohlfing B, Gavenis K, Maus U, Mueller-Rath R, Andereya S (2011) A comparative study of 3 different cartilage repair techniques. Knee Surg Sports Traumatol Arthrosc 19(12):2145–2152

Shahgaldi BF (1998) Repair of large osteochondral defects: load-bearing and structural properties of osteochondral repair tissue. Knee 5(2):111–117

Shortkroff S, Barone L, Hsu HP, Wrenn C, Gagne T, Chi T et al (1996) Healing of chondral and osteochondral defects in a canine model: the role of cultured chondrocytes in regeneration of articular cartilage. Biomaterials 17(2):147–154

Singh NK, Singh GR, Jeong DK, Lee SJ (2013) Healing of full-thickness articular cartilage defects treated with cultured autologous chondrogenic satellite cells isolated from chondral stem cell niche in rabbits. J Surg Res 183(2):629–638

Steadman JR, Briggs KK, Rodrigo JJ, Kocher MS, Gill TJ, Rodkey WG (2003) Outcomes of microfracture for traumatic chondral defects of the knee: average 11-year follow-up. Arthroscopy 19(5):477–484

Taylor WR, Heller MO, Bergmann G, Duda GN (2004) Tibio-femoral loading during human gait and stair climbing. J Orthop Res 22(3):625–632

Taylor WR, Ehrig RM, Heller MO, Schell H, Seebeck P, Duda GN (2006) Tibio-femoral joint contact forces in sheep. J Biomech 39(5):791–798

Vachon AM, McIlwraith CW, Powers BE, McFadden PR, Amiel D (1992) Morphologic and biochemical study of sternal cartilage autografts for resurfacing induced osteochondral defects in horses. Am J Vet Res 53(6):1038–1047

Vogt S, Angele P, Arnold M, Brehme K, Cotic M, Haasper C et al (2013) Practice in rehabilitation after cartilage therapy: an expert survey. Arch Orthop Trauma Surg 133(3):311–320

von Rechenberg B, Akens MK, Nadler D, Bittmann P, Zlinszky K, Kutter A et al (2003) Changes in subchondral bone in cartilage resurfacing–an experimental study in sheep using different types of osteochondral grafts. Osteoarthritis Cartilage 11(4):265–277

Wang DA, Varghese S, Sharma B, Strehin I, Fermanian S, Gorham J et al (2007) Multifunctional chondroitin sulphate for cartilage tissue-biomaterial integration. Nat Mater 6(5):385–392

Wei X, Rasanen T, Messner K (1998) Maturation-related compressive properties of rabbit knee articular cartilage and volume fraction of subchondral tissue. Osteoarthritis Cartilage 6(6):400–409

Wolfensohn S, Lloyd M (2003) Handbook of Laboratory Animal Management and Welfare, 3rd edn. Blackwell Publishing, Oxford

Yanai T, Ishii T, Chang F, Ochiai N (2005) Repair of large full-thickness articular cartilage defects in the rabbit: the effects of joint distraction and autologous bone-marrow-derived mesenchymal cell transplantation. J Bone Joint Sur British 87(5):721–729

A new subscapular sling operation to stabilize the shoulder. A cadaver study

P J Klungsøyr*, F Guldal, T Vagstad and J A Klungsøyr

Abstract

Introduction: A new arthroscopic shoulder stabilisation procedure is proposed, which for some patients could be an alternative to the arthroscopic Latarjet procedure.

Methods: The objective was to stabilize the shoulder by making a sling around the subscapularis tendon, using a hamstring graft and enhancing the anterior rim of the glenoid with the same graft. The anatomical feasibility of the surgical procedure was tested to establish the surgical method.

Results: Four surgeons performed the surgery on six cadavers. After the surgery the cadavers were dissected to visualize the result. The sling was placed according to the intention and the nerves in the area (axillary and musculocutaneus) were not at risk, nor had they altered position during the procedure.

Conclusion: The procedure is technically feasible and the risk of complications seems low. This procedure could be an alternative to the Latarjet procedure and to other operations used for anterior instability of the shoulder. A biomechanical study will be performed as the next stage of the development.

Clinical relevance: This procedure could be an alternative to the Latarjet procedure and to other operations used for anterior instability of the shoulder.

Trial registration: 2012/1978/REK sør-øst

Keywords: Shoulder instability; Arthroscopic sling procedure; Hamstring graft; Subscapularis tendon; Cadaver study

Background

The Latarjet procedure for anterior shoulder instability has today regained popularity. The main indication is instability with a glenoid bone defect, but it is increasingly used as a revision procedure following previous surgery and as the primary procedure in cases with weak anterior structures (Blomquist et al. 2012). The Latarjet operation yields good results, but also has complications (Hovelius et al. 2004, Shah et al. 2012, Griesser et al. 2013). It is currently the first choice for some shoulder surgeons. The Latarjet procedure is considered technically demanding, especially when performed arthroscopically, but even so it is routinely done arthroscopically in some centres (Lafosse et al. 2010, Shah et al. 2012). The learning curve for the arthroscopic operation is long, with significant reported and unreported complications (Butt and Charalambous 2013). Gracitelli et al. (2013) reported results of arthroscopic Latarjet procedure in cadavers in Brazil and found a high risk of complications. If the Latarjet operation fails, a revision procedure might be difficult because of the distorted anatomy and the increased risk of nerve complications. In this regard, the musculocutaneus nerve is at risk, since its position is altered during the operation when the conjoined tendon is pulled inferiorly (Freehill et al. 2013).

In this study, the objective was to develop a procedure that could be an alternative to the Latarjet procedure. The sling effect of the Latarjet around the inferior part of the subscapularis tendon and capsule hinders the anterior translation of the humeral head. In addition, the fixation of the coracoid bone onto the anterior rim of glenoid increases the glenoid size and thus increases the stability. The dynamic sling effect in Latarjet is described in biomechanical testing by Giles et al (2013). The effect seems to be enhanced by the coracoid bone block. The effect of the bone block has also been shown by Yamamoto et al. (2009). Wellmann et al. (2012) showed that the Latarjet

* Correspondence: pklungsoyr@gmail.com
Orthopaedic Department. Aalesund Hospital, Aalesund, Norway

procedure will lose anterior stability if the subscapularis tendon is torn.

The Resch method is theoretically an extra capsular tightening of the anterior capsule. To achieve this, Resch used a special portal going through the muscle belly of the subscapularis muscle, using a slalom technique to avoid injuring the conjoined tendon and the musculocutaneus nerve Resch.H et al. (1996). Even though the aim of Resch was not to do a subscapular tenodesis, we believe that the insertion of tacks may cause a partial tenodesis or sling effect. The posterior tendinous sheath of the subscapularis muscle and the fibrous structures around it are strongly connected to the anterior capsule and thus pulled towards the anterior rim of glenoid in the Resch procedure. When performing the Resch method we observed that the fixation of the plugs resulted in a reduced external rotation that could be partly a result of an effect on the subscapularis muscle. As the structures are gradually stretched out over time, the effect diminishes and this could explain the excellent primary results and the high numbers of late recurrences Cartus et al. (2007).

This study therefore proposes an arthroscopic operation that could be used in patients where the Bankart operation was judged to be insufficient and as a possible alternative to arthroscopic Latarjet. The proposed procedure should have less potential complications and a shorter learning curve. The hypothesis is that the sling effect can be created by a technically less demanding procedure, and can be made in a manner that would remove the need for a bone block.

Methods

The proposed procedure makes a sling around the upper part of the subscapularis tendon with a hamstring graft and at the same time increases the size of the soft tissue structures anteriorly with the same graft (Fig. 1) to increase the size of the glenoid cup. The increase in soft tissue on the anterior rim of the glenoid, as a widening of the cup, could prevent engagement of Hill-Sachs lesions. The sling would prevent the dislocation of the humeral head through the active and passive function of the subscapularis tendon in the sling. To achieve this, the sling should be placed around the upper part of the tendon and not the inferior part as in Latarjet. By placing the sling in such a manner, the inferior movement could possibly be more restricted. The Latarjet procedure has only one leg of the sling attached to the glenoid and does not, according to Wellmann et al. (2012), hinder the inferior movement. The proposed sling will have two legs and might prevent inferior movement by hindering the subscapularis tendon from sliding inferiorly and thus assisting in keeping the humeral head in place. The hamstring tendons are used as a strong and lasting tissue replacement in many locations, are easy to harvest and do not give much donor site discomfort. The intention was to use the semitendinosus tendon and do the procedure arthroscopically.

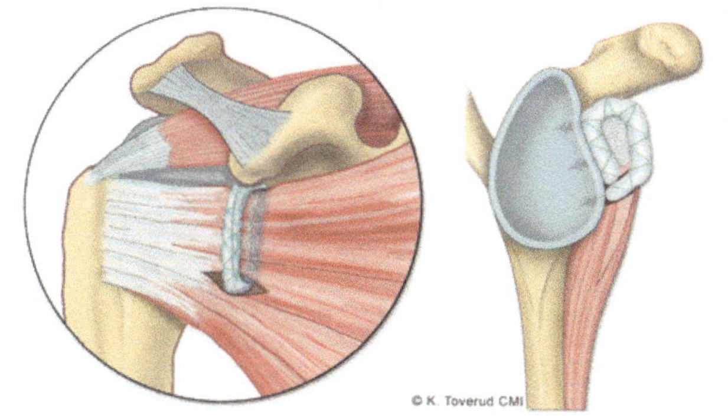

Fig. 1 Drawing of the sling

After the Regional Ethics Committee gave its approval, the procedure was tested on cadavers at the Smith and Nephew Surgical Skills Centre, York, North Yorkshire, United Kingdom. Four experienced shoulder surgeons used two working stations and six fresh frozen right shoulder cadavers including half of the upper arm. The specimen was fastened to a table with a scapula clamp in a Beach chair position. There was no available equipment for measuring exact movements, any translations or any form for biomechanical testing. The surgeons worked in pairs and rotated so all surgeries were not dependent on one surgeon. The centre provided already harvested hamstring tendons. Standard arthroscopic equipment and Bioraptor 2.9 anchors with two preloaded sutures were used. Three portals were introduced; posterior for the scope, anterior upper for instrumentation and inferior anterior for graft introduction. For the graft portal (3rd portal) an 11 mm portal, and for the upper, a standard 8 mm portal were used. Preoperatively the placement of the inferior anterior portal was discussed. We had experience with the Resch slalom technique and used this experience to go inferior with the portal at the same level as Resch used. By going through the tendinous part of the subscapularis tendon the risk of injuring the musculocutaneus nerve would be reduced. Since we intended to make a split mainly in the tendinous part and not in the muscular part of subscapularis tendon, the slalom technique was not used. The graft was doubled.

After placing the two first portals, the layer anterior to the subscapularis tendon (Fig. 2-a) was opened up. By doing this a small part of the rotator interval was opened. Blunt dissection with a trocar through the upper portal exposed the inferior anterior part of the tendon. Then the inferior anterior portal was introduced. First by using a trocar from outside and with coblation (radiofrequency) from inside. A longitudinal slit in the capsule and subscapularis

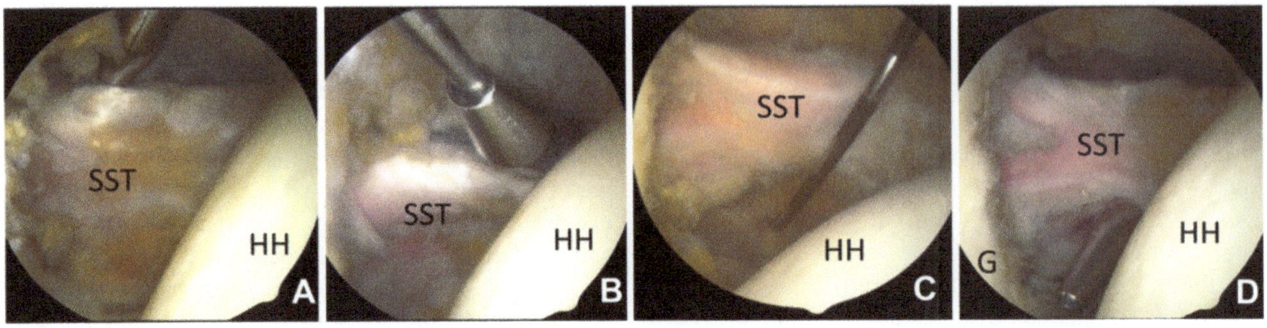

Fig. 2 Arthroscopic pictures showing the preparation of the subscapularis tendon. **a**: Dissecting the anterior surface of the tendon from the upper portal. **b**: From the inferior portal. **c**: The point of entry for the slit in the subscapularis tendon from inside. **d**: The trocar advanced through the slit. Abbreviations: SST: Subscapularis tendon. HH: Humeral head. G: Glenoid. P: Portal

tendon was made and the portal was introduced into the joint (Fig. 2-b,c and d). The anterior surface of the glenoid neck was cleared by coblation. An anchor with two pairs of sutures was introduced through the 3rd portal on the anterior rim of glenoid between 4 and 5 o'clock. Using a sliding knot, the end of the transplant was pulled in and fixed to the anterior glenoid rim (Fig. 3-a and b). The portal was then partly withdrawn anteriorly to the subscapularis and moved into the joint above the tendon. By the help of an extra suture on the outer end of the transplant it was pulled into the joint above the subscapularis tendon and out through the upper portal (Fig. 3-c). A new anchor was introduced (using the 3rd portal in its new position) at around 2 o'clock and the graft was slightly tightened and sutured to this anchor (Fig. 3-d and 4-a). The rest of the graft was pushed back into the joint and placed along the anterior glenoid rim, sutured with the second suture of the first and second anchor. Additional anchors could be inserted to make an even firmer fixation. As a result the end loop would be placed as an extra tissue wall on glenoid anteriorly, similar to a thick labrum (Fig. 4-b and c).

After the arthroscopic procedure, the shoulder was dissected to study the graft placement and the relation to the main nerves. The placement of the anterior inferior portal was evaluated. The deltoid was dissected away from its upper attachments and then the conjoined tendon was detached and reflected inferiorly so the graft, the slit, the subscapularis muscle-tendon and the actual nerves could be inspected.

Results

The procedure was performed in six cadavers with different combinations of surgeons and none encountered any major difficulties in performing the procedure. In the first cadaver, the lower anterior 3rd portal was made through the conjoined tendon (Fig. 5-a). On the following cadavers the skin incision was made 0.5 cm lateral to the line inferior from the tip of coracoid in the line of the upper arm and the portal 90 degrees on the frontal plane, which successfully avoided the conjoined tendon (Fig. 5-b). The distance from the anterior tip of coracoid to the portal was 2 cm in all. In none of the cadavers was the musculocutaneus nerve injured, nor was its position altered. The

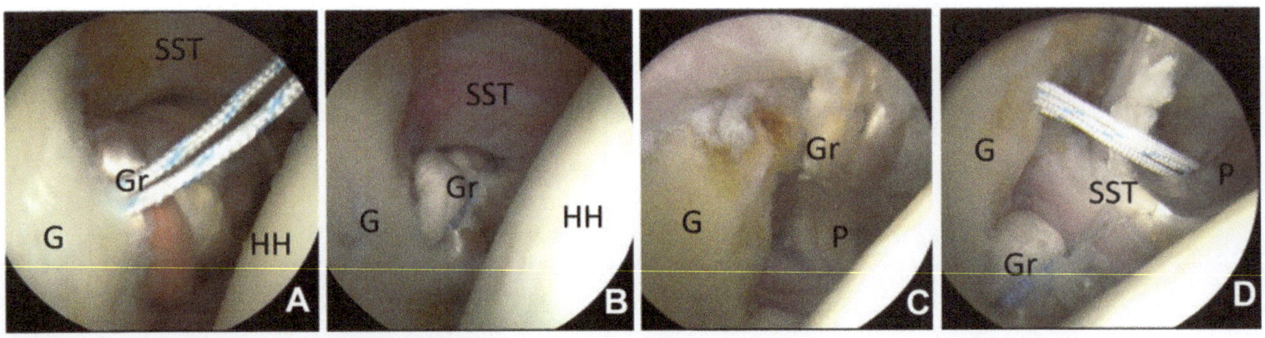

Fig. 3 Arthroscopic pictures showing the introduction of the graft. **a**: The graft has been pulled in towards the glenoid anchor through the portal. **b**: The portal is withdrawn. **c** and **d**: The portal is placed anterior and superior to the subscapularis tendon and the graft is pulled out through the upper portal. Abbreviations: SST: Subscapularis tendon. HH: Humeral head. G: Glenoid. Gr: Graft. P: Portal

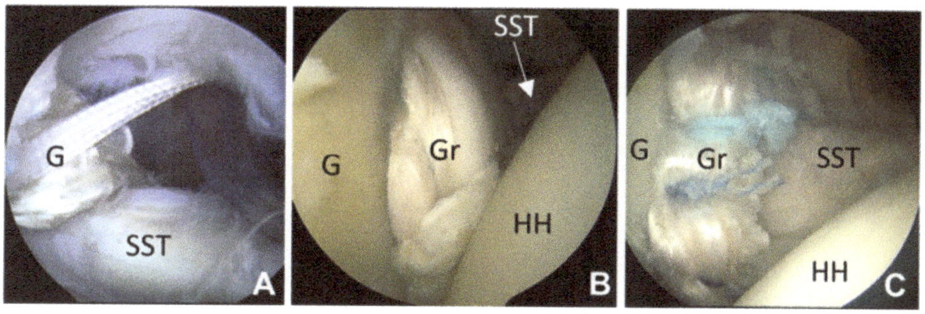

Fig. 4 Arthroscopic pictures of the final placement of the graft seen from inside. **a**: The upper leg is fixed to the glenoid with the first suture, the second suture goes into the upper portal. **b** and **c**: The upper part of the graft placed on the anterior ridge of glenoid. Abbreviations: SST: Subscapularis tendon. HH: Humeral head. G: Glenoid. Gr: Graft. P: Portal

axillary nerve was dissected and it was not at risk in any of the cadavers (Fig. 5-c). It was not possible to make accurate measurements of the distance from the nerves to the 3rd portal and from the end of the slit to the axillary nerve because of the condition of the tissue, extravasation of fluid and altered consistency of the tissue because of the handling before surgery. Since the axillary nerve crosses on the anterior surface of the subscapularis muscle it could be injured while doing the blunt dissection on the anterior surface of the muscle, but the distance between the medial end of the split in the tendon and the nearest location of the axillary nerve was measured to be at least 1.5 cm on all the cadavers. The width of the subscapularis tendon in the created sling was 1.5 to 2.5 cm. A substantial part of the tendon was thus included in the sling (Fig. 6-a and b). Since the tendon is rather flat the width of the graft inside the sling would also depend on the tension applied to the graft. The measurements were done with the arm tentatively in neutral rotation and in the line of the body. Although a rather short longitudinal split in the subscapularis tendon was made, the movement of the subscapularis tendon inside the sling was visualized arthroscopically.

One of the cadavers was unstable in all directions before the surgery because of a massive rupture of the rotator cuff, but with the subscapularis tendon intact. Prior to the procedure the head was dislocated inferiorly, but after the surgery the humeral head was in place and the joint was stable under quite forceful manual testing. In one of the cadavers with an intact rotator cuff, the upper cuff was released from the humerus, but still the sling kept the head up (Fig. 6-c). Since the set up was not designed for proper testing of the movements, exact measurements cannot be given. As far as could be tested manually, the external/internal rotation, flexion and abduction were not restricted in any of the cadavers after the operation. In all the cadavers the outward rotation was estimated as not less than 45 degrees. We did not dissect the suprascapular nerve posteriorly to the joint because we had not introduced any instruments or placed any anchors/screws which could possibly cause injury to this nerve. This complication is described by Gracitelli et al. (2013).

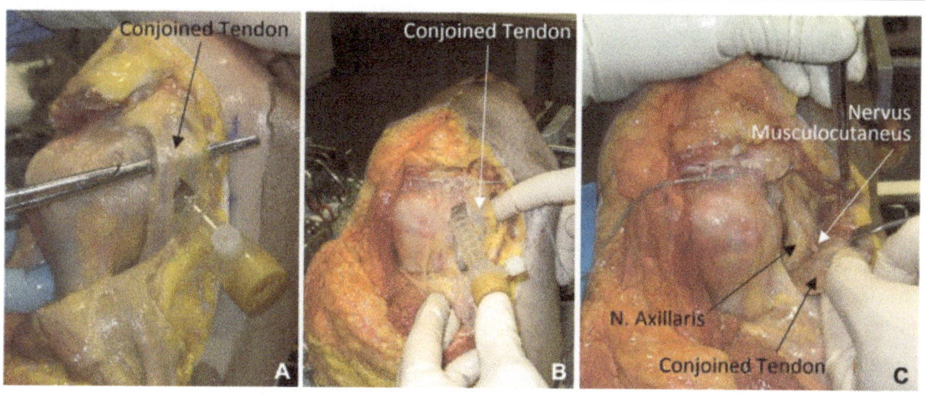

Fig. 5 Post-operative pictures. **a**: Portal placed through the conjoined tendon. **b**: Correct portal placement. **c**: The musculocutaneus nerve is seen in the reflected conjoined tendon/muscle. The axillary nerve is seen in the fatty tissue

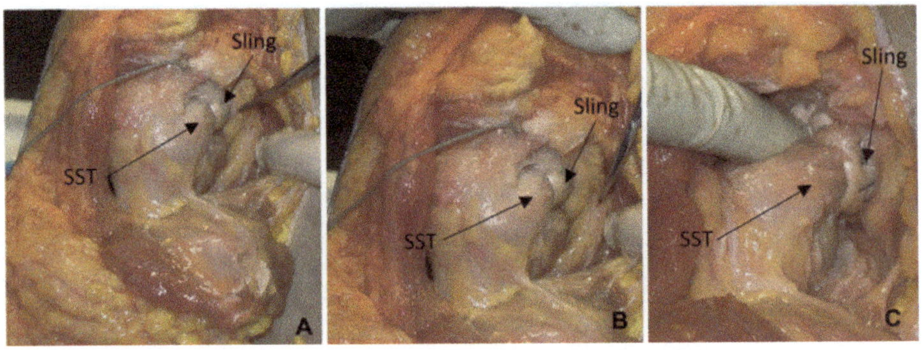

Fig. 6 Post-operative pictures: **a** and **b**: Placement of the sling. **c**: Supraspinatus and the anterior part of the inferior capsule is cut. The sling holds the head in the glenoid cavity. Abbreviation: SST: Subscapularis tendon

Discussion

The procedure could be performed without any major technical difficulties and no nerve injury was observed. All four surgeons did the surgery and there were no differences in performance. To avoid perforating the conjoined tendon we had to alter the placement of the inferior anterior portal, making it slightly more lateral. During the dissection after the arthroscopic procedure, it was noted that neither the musculocutaneous nor the axillary nerves were at risk, nor had they altered position. According to the reports of both open and arthroscopic Latarjet procedure there is always a change in the anatomical position of the musculocutaneus nerve that could represent a danger if a reoperation has to be performed later (Freehill et al. 2013). This will not be the case with the proposed procedure since the conjoined tendon is not being manipulated. During both the open and the arthroscopic Latarjet procedure there is always a manipulation of the area on the anterior surface of the subscapularis muscle close to the axillary nerve and there are also reports of injuries to the nerve (Shah et al 2012). Judged by findings during dissection, there is less risk of axillary nerve involvement in the proposed operation.

The procedure is probably technically easier to perform than the arthroscopic Latarjet. No more difficulties were noted in performing this operation than during an arthroscopic Bankart operation. Problems with bleeding are not generally encountered while clearing the anterior surface of the subscapularis tendon in the open Latarjet operations. By comparing the amount of dissection done in an arthroscopic Latarjet, it is expected that the proposed operation would have a lower risk of bleeding.

Wellmann et al (2012) showed that the sling effect of Latarjet hinders anterior movement, but the sling would not hinder inferior movement. Dines et al. (2013) also showed that the Latarjet procedure hindered the anterior translation of the humeral head while preserving the ROM. Our hypothesis is that a sling with two legs attached to the glenoid would better hinder the inferior movement as compared with the Latarjet sling with only one leg fixed to glenoid rim. The two legged sling could hinder the subscapularis muscle from being pulled inferiorly and since the subscapular muscle is a very important active stabiliser of the joint, this would hinder inferior movement and give additional stabilisation. The cadaver that had an intact subscapularis tendon with a massive cuff rupture was stabilized with the sling. The sling in that particular cadaver provided passive stabilisation so it may be that the upper sling could act as a stabiliser by both passive and active forces. Additional biomechanical testing must be performed. In another of the cadavers, the superior rotator cuff was completely severed, but it did not seem to reduce the stability when the sling was in place.

It is possible that the sling could cause degeneration and rupture of the subscapularis tendon and there could be atrophy of the muscle. Open operations with an L-shaped incision in the subscapular muscle will, according to some publications, lead to reduction in the strength and some atrophy of the subscapularis muscle (Paladini et al. 2012), but the present study suggests this problem is at least very much reduced when a subscapularis split has been made. Hiemstra et al. (2008) showed there was no difference in subscapularis function between open and arthroscopic stabilisation in a tendon splitting approach. Strength deficits existed in both the arthroscopic and the open groups when compared to the contralateral limb. We are not aware of any publication that has shown rupture of the inferior part of subscapularis muscle after Latarjet, where only a split has been made. According to Hinton et al. (1994) the insertion part of the subscapular muscle differs in the sense that the superior 60 % consists of tendon and the inferior 40 % mainly of muscle. It was also observed during dissection that there is gradual transition with increasing muscle and decreasing tendon structure moving inferiorly. Degeneration and rupture generally comes in the tendinous part of a muscle which could indicate that an upper sling as we made, could be more vulnerable for degenerations than an inferior sling. We are not aware of any literature discussing this problem in depth. Would our sling cause degeneration and eventually rupture of the subscapularis tendon? The insertion of the tendon was not injured and the sling should not strangulate the tendon. The sling will, according to our thesis, provide dynamic stability in abduction and external rotation through the subscapularis muscle function, but otherwise there would probably not be any tension on the tendon.

A systematic review by Griesser et al. (2013) of multiple medical databases included studies reporting outcomes with complication and reoperation rates following original or modified versions of the Bristow or Latarjet. The total complication rate was 30 %. Recurrent anterior dislocation and subluxation rates were 2.9 % and 5.8 %, respectively. The reoperation rate was 7 %. Mild loss of external rotation was common. Reoperation rates were lower following all-arthroscopic techniques, but there was a greater loss of postoperative external rotation with all-arthroscopic surgery. We cannot see that the proposed upper sling should cause more reduction in the external rotation than a Latarjet procedure. In some patients probably some reduction could be desirable to hinder instability.

Late mobilisation can cause reduced strength in internal rotation and thus early mobilization could be an advantage. To maintain the split in the tendon after the operation it may be essential to start early exercises. In Latarjet a slit is also made and any healing of that slit seems to be of less concern. Early mobilisation could affect the healing of the graft towards the anterior glenoid. This has to be considered before any in vivo operation. Suture anchors have achieved good healing between the capsule and glenoid in other shoulder operations. Post-operative rehabilitation would be similar to standard arthroscopic Bankart operations. In that case this operation should not cause more external rotation lag and subscapularis atrophy than the Latarjet procedure, except for the possibility that the upper sling in itself could cause more degeneration than the inferior sling. The labrum and capsule could also be included in the graft on the anterior rim of glenoid in the same way as Latarjet is often combined with a Bankart procedure.

This is an anatomic study of a new procedure. No biomechanical analysis has been performed. We had planned to do a second alternative of this operation by introducing a bone block with the tendon and fixate it to the lower anterior part of glenoid with sutures or screws and then proceed with the sling. This is possible through the same 11 mm portal. The bone block could be harvested from the tibia together with the tendon graft. To get enough experience with the present operation, it was decided not to do the second alternative. Giles et al. (2013) tested the importance of a sling on the inferior part of the tendon and capsule and found that the additional bone was important when there was a bone defect. The bone defect was quite substantial in their trial. It is possible that a sling around the upper and middle part of the tendon has a higher stability and could give good results without a bone block, since the sling around the upper part might hinder the anterior and inferior translation more effectively. Biomechanical testing is needed to establish this.

Today the Latarjet procedure is used in many hospitals as the primary operation when the anterior structures are weak and not fit for a Bankart operation. This tendency can probably be explained by the disappointing results of the Bankart operation in young patients (Blomquist et al.2012). Our sling could be a possible alternative in younger patients, and if it fails one still has the possibility of using the Latarjet procedure without any expected difficulties caused by the primary surgery. Cosmetically the proposed operation would give a better result, since the coracoid is not touched.

Conclusion

A tendon sling was made around the subscapularis tendon in an arthroscopic procedure on cadavers to prevent anterior instability in the shoulder. As part of this procedure a tissue wall was created anterior to the glenoid that also may help to prevent dislocation. The risk of injuring the two main nerves seems less than in the Latarjet procedure and possible future reoperation will probably have a lower risk of complications since the anatomy is not altered. From a technical perspective, this procedure could be performed safely in vivo. To know the actual effect of the sling, further testing in a biomechanical laboratory is needed, especially in cases with glenoid bone loss. The proposed procedure was feasible in cadavers and technically not demanding.

Clinical relevance

This procedure could probably be used on patients with a weak anterior capsule even though arthroscopic Bankart will still be widely used. In young patients with less bone loss, where the tendency in some hospitals today is to perform the Latarjet procedure, the proposed procedure could be an alternative. Whether it is applicable in cases with or without bone loss needs to be tested biomechanically. If a bone block is needed, this could be done by harvesting a bone block from the tibia, keeping the original attachment of the hamstring tendon, and doing the identical operation with the additional bone fixation.

Competing interests

A grant was provided by the Orthopaedic Research Fund, Aalesund Hospital, for the payment to Smith and Nephew and our travel expenses. Smith and Nephew Norway facilitated the research, but had no influence on the project and we have no obligations to them.

Authors' contribution

PJK, FG, TV and JAK took all part in the operations and writing the final manuscript. PJK put forward the original idea and wrote the draft. All authors read and approved the final manuscript.

Authors' information

Each author is a consultant in orthopaedic surgery at the Orthopaedic Department, Aalesund Hospital. Norway.

Acknowledgements

We appreciate help from Dr Engebretsen with manuscript editing, and comments from Dr C. Schrøder. We also appreciate Kari C.Toverud who made the illustration and Dr Paul Saunderson who has revised the English text.

References

Blomquist J, Solheim E, Liavaag S, Schroder CP, Espehaug B, Havelin LI, Shoulder instability surgery in Norway (2012) The first report from a multicenter register, with 1-year follow-up. Acta Orthop 83(2):165–170

Butt U, Charalambous CP (2013) Arthroscopic Coracoid Transfer in the Treatment of Recurrent Shoulder Instability: A Systematic Review of Early Results. Arthroscopy: The Journal of Arthroscopic and Related Surgery 29(4):774–779

Cartus C, Kartus J, Matis N, Forstner R, Resh H (2007) Long-term independent evaluation after arthroscopic extra-articular Bankart repair with absorbable tacks. J Bone Joint Surg Am 89(7):1442–1448

Dines JS, Dodson CC, McGarry MH, Oh JH, Altchek DW, Lee TQ (2013) Contribution of osseous and muscular stabilizing effects with the Latarjet procedure for anterior instability without glenoid bone loss. J Shoulder Elbow Surg 22:1689–1694

Freehill MT, Srikumaran U, Archer KR, McFarland EG, Petersen SA (2013) The Latarjet coracoid process transfer procedure: alterations in the neurovascular structures. J Shoulder Elbow Surg 22(5):695–700

Giles JW, Boons HW, Elkinson I, Faber KJ, Louis M, Ferreira LM, Johnson JA, Athwal GS (2013) Does the dynamic sling effect of the Latarjet procedure improve shoulder stability? A biomechanical evaluation. J Shoulder Elbow Surg 22:821–827

Gracitelli MEC, Ferreira N, Benegas E, Malavolta EA, Sunada EE, Assunção JH (2013) Arthroscopic latarjet procedure: safety evaluation in cadavers. Acta Ortop Bras 21(3):139–143

Griesser MJ, Harris JD, McCoy BW, Hussain WM, Jones MH, Bishop JY, Miniaci A (2013) Complications and re-operations after Bristow-Latarjet shoulder stabilization: a systematic review. J Shoulder Elbow Surg 22:286–292

Hiemstra LA, Sasyniuk TM, Mohtadi NGH, Fick GH (2008) Shoulder strength after open versus arthroscopic stabilization. Am J Sports Med 36(5):861–867

Hinton MA, Parker AW, Drez D, Altcheck D (1994) An anatomic study ofthe subscapularis tendon and hintonmyotendinous junction. J Shoulder ElbowSurg 3:224–229

Hovelius L, Sandstrøm B, Sundgren K, Saebø M (2004) One hundred eighteen Bristow_Latarjet repairs for recurrent anterior dislocation of the shoulder followed for fifteen years: Study 1-Clinical results. J Shoulder Elbow Surg 13:509–516

Lafosse L, Boyle S, Gutierrez-Aramberri M, Shah A, Meller R (2010) Arthroscopic Latarjet Procedure. Orthop Clin N Am 41:393–405

Paladini P, Merolla G, De Santis E, Campi F, Porcelli G (2012) Long-term subscapularis strength assessment after Bristow-Latarjet procedure: isometric study. J Shoulder Elbow Surg 21:42–47

Resch H, Wykypiel HF, Maurer H, Wambacher M (1996) The Anterior-Inferior (Transmuscular) Approach for Arthroscopic Repair of the Bankart Lesion: An Anatomic and Clinical Study. Arthroscopy: J Arthrosc Relat Surg 12(3):309–322

Shah AA, Butler RB, Romanowski J, Goel D, Karadagli D, Warner JJP (2012) Short-Term Complications of the Latarjet Procedure. J Bone Joint Surg Am 94:495–501

Wellmann M, De Ferrari H, Smith T, Petersen W, Siebert CH, Agneskirchner JD, Hurrschler C (2012) Biomechanical investigation of the stabilization principle of the Latarjet procedure. Arch Orthop Trauma Surg 132:377–386

Yamamoto N, Itoi E, Abe H, Kikuchi K, Seki N, Minagawa H, et al. Effect of an anterior glenoid defect on anterior shoulder stability: a cadaveric study. Am J Sports Med. 2009;37(5):949-54

Large animal models in experimental knee sports surgery: focus on clinical translation

Henning Madry[1,2,3], Mitsuo Ochi[4], Magali Cucchiarini[1,2*], Dietrich Pape[2,5,6] and Romain Seil[2,5,6]

Abstract

Large animal models play a crucial role in sports surgery of the knee, as they are critical for the exploration of new experimental strategies and the clinical translation of novel techniques. The purpose of this contribution is to provide critical aspects of relevant animal models in this field, with a focus on paediatric anterior cruciate ligament (ACL) reconstruction, high tibial osteotomy, and articular cartilage repair. Although there is no single large animal model strictly replicating the human knee joint, the sheep stifle joint shares strong similarities. Studies in large animal models of paediatric ACL reconstruction identified specific risk factors associated with the different surgical techniques. The sheep model of high tibial osteotomy is a powerful new tool to advance the understanding of the effect of axial alignment on the lower extremity on specific issues of the knee joint. Large animal models of both focal chondral and osteochondral defects and of osteoarthritis have brought new findings about the mechanisms of cartilage repair and treatment options. The clinical application of a magnetic device for targeted cell delivery serves as a suitable example of how data from such animal models are directly translated into in clinical cartilage repair. As novel insights from studies in these translational models will advance the basic science, close cooperation in this important field of clinical translation will improve current reconstructive surgical options and open novel avenues for regenerative therapies of musculoskeletal disorders.

Keywords: Musculoskeletal disorders; Large animal models; Sheep; Paediatric anterior cruciate ligament reconstruction; High tibial osteotomy; Articular cartilage repair; Osteoarthritis; Clinical studies; Mesenchymal stem cells; Magnetic-assisted delivery

Introduction

Large animal models play a crucial role in orthopaedic sports surgery, as they are critical for the exploration of new experimental strategies and the clinical translation of novel techniques (Espregueira-Mendes & Karahan 2014). On December 3rd, 2014, about 100 clinicians and basic scientists from Europe, North America, and Asia, met on the occasion of the Research Day of the Annual Congress of the *Société Française d'Arthroscopie* in Luxembourg to discuss requirements for such translational animal models (Table 1). This research day was organized together with the Cartilage Net of the Greater Region, a multinational forum for exploring basic scientific and translational research, development and clinical applications in the diverse field of articular cartilage.

The purpose of this contribution is to provide critical aspects of relevant animal models in experimental knee sports surgery, including paediatric anterior cruciate ligament (ACL) reconstruction, high tibial osteotomy, and articular cartilage repair. These three models discussed are based on the individual presentations (Table 1) and thought to provide a representative and clinically relevant, although by no means exhaustive selection of translational animal models in this field. This paper is aimed at the diverse community of those engaging in experimental orthopaedics, among which orthopaedic surgeons, biomaterial scientists, cell and molecular biologists, biochemists, biotechnologists, and biomechanical engineers. It intends to highlight new developments and to display how far knowledge gathered from these models is already (or will be in the near future) translatable in humans. An emphasis is placed on the "transferability" to patients.

* Correspondence: mmcucchiarini@hotmail.com
[1]Center of Experimental Orthopaedics, Saarland University Medical Center and Saarland University, Bldg 37, Kirrbergerstr. 1, D-66421 Homburg, Germany
[2]Cartilage Net of the Greater Region, Homburg, Germany
Full list of author information is available at the end of the article

Table 1 Lectures of the Research Day session on December 3rd, 2014 of the Annual Congress of the *Société Française d'Arthroscopie* in Luxembourg

Speaker	City	Country	Title of lectures
Magali Cucchiarini	Homburg	Germany	Recombinant adeno-associated viral vectors as efficient tools for musculoskeletal gene therapy
Christel Henrionnet	Vandoeuvre lès Nancy	France	Innovative and non-invasive evaluation of the quality of collagen scaffold functionalized by human mesenchymal stem cells before graft in cartilage lesion
Henning Madry	Homburg	Germany	Animal models for cartilage repair
Didier Mainard	Vandoeuvre lès Nancy	France	Hoffa ligament: a fat tissue with pro-inflammatory properties
Mitsuo Ochi	Hiroshima	Japan	Cartilage repair using magnets
Dietrich Pape	Luxembourg	Luxembourg	The preclinical sheep model of high tibial osteotomy
Astrid Pinzano	Vandoeuvre lès Nancy	France	Bioengineering and cartilage
Romain Seil	Luxembourg	Luxembourg	Large animal models for pediatric ACL reconstruction

General requirements for translational animal models in experimental orthopaedics and sports medicine

General requirements for large animal experiments in translational orthopaedic research are manifold: 1) the model needs to be comparable to the human species, 2) comparison data need to be available, 3) the results must be transferable, 4) surgery must be technically feasible, 5) a specialized animal facility must be available with acceptable related expenditures, 6) animals need to be affordable and available, 7) surgery should be ethically accepted, and finally 8) anaesthesia, surgery, and rehabilitation need to be tolerated by the selected animals. Nevertheless, for the human knee joint, no gold standard exists, as the models differ in many important structural and functional aspects compared with the clinical situation (Poole et al. 2010). There is no large animal model replicating the human knee joint perfectly (Aigner et al. 2010). In addition, the activity pattern of animals is different compared with the bipedal locomotion of humans. For example, their quadruped gait results in altered biomechanics compared to the human knee (Rudert et al. 2000), together with differences in the knee range of motion and resting positions. Also, the biomechanical properties of knee joint cartilage are species-specific (Simon 1971), resulting in significant differences of the mechanical properties (Athanasiou et al. 1991).

Review

Large animal models for paediatric anterior cruciate ligament reconstruction

The treatment of ligamentous ACL lesions in the paediatric population causes a therapeutic dilemma for physicians because of the lack of current international guidelines. To overcome this problem, a variety of experimental studies concerning the growth plates and paediatric ACL reconstruction have been performed in small and large animal models (Edwards et al. 2001; Guzzanti et al. 1994; Janarv et al. 1998; Ono et al. 1998; Meller et al. 2009a; Meller et al. 2009b; Meller et al. 2008a; Meller et al. 2008b; Seil et al. 2008; Stadelmaier et al. 1995). The complexity of paediatric ACL reconstruction makes the interpretation of this surgical technique and the transferability of its results to humans difficult when small animal models are used. However, there are strong similarities between the stifle joint and the human knee joint. From an anatomical point of view, these joints have asymmetric collateral as well as cruciate ligaments and menisci and the articulating surface is covered with articular cartilage (Dye 1987; Arnoczky & Marshall 1977; Bosch & Kasperczyk 1993). Based on our own experiments (Seil et al. 2008), the sheep model seems to be appealing for the above-mentioned study purpose. Merino sheep are easily available, they are easy to handle and are ethically better accepted than dogs or primates (Allen et al. 1998). Three gross anatomic features have the potential to interfere with ACL surgery and must be known by the surgeon to avoid potential pitfalls: the very narrow intercondylar notch of this species, the different -much more undulating- form of the distal femoral growth plate in comparison to the human knee and the range of motion of the stifle joint with spontaneous 30-40° extension deficit.

Paediatric ligamentous ACL injuries do rarely occur before the age of 8 or 9 years (Chotel et al. 2013). Therefore, a critical point to perform ACL reconstructions in growing sheep is the fact that surgery should be performed at a moment corresponding to the age where ligamentous ACL injuries in children appear to be the most frequent and problematic. In their early growth studies in humans, Bailey and Pinneau showed that at a skeletal age between 8 and 12 years, humans reach 79-92% of their adult height in females and 72-83% in males (Bayley & Pinneau 1952). In the absence of precise data from veterinary studies, sheep should therefore ideally be operated when they reach between 70% and 90% of the adult height. However, information on animals is rarely available (Salomon 2001). Studies on the longitudinal growth of the sheep forearm revealed that they reached 70% of their adult height at day 20 and 90% at day 167 (Salomon 2001). Supposing that these data could be transferred to the hind limb of this species, the use of 4-months old sheep appears justified, and grossly 4 cm of longitudinal hind limb growth could be expected at this age (Seil 2003). This sheep model was used to evaluate the risk for growth disturbances of transphyseal drilling and ACL reconstruction (Seil et al. 2008). Three technical variants were used. In group I, the ACL was resected and 5-mm tunnels were drilled and left empty in four-months-old Merino sheep. Unilateral ACL reconstruction using an autologous Achilles tendon graft and rigid button fixation was performed in group II. A double-stranded graft with a diameter of 5 mm was used in group II-A, and a single stranded graft with a diameter of 3 mm in group II-B. The tunnel diameter was 5 mm in both groups. Six months after the procedure, the combination of peripheral, posterolateral growth plate injuries and empty tunnels led to severe growth deformities on the femoral side with a shortening of the lateral femur of 8 mm (7–10 mm), a valgus deformity of 12.8° (12-14°) and a flexion deformity of 8.6° (5-15°). Histological examination revealed a strong bone bridge formation over the physis and an injury to the perichondral structures. Central growth plate lesions on the tibia did not induce growth abnormalities. Transphyseal ACL replacements did not cause clinically relevant growth disturbances, neither on the tibia, nor on the femur, even if the drilling injury damaged the perichondral structures on the posterolateral physis.

Clinical relevance for paediatric anterior cruciate ligament reconstruction

This study showed that the sheep model is useful to analyze the outcome of paediatric ACL reconstruction with open growth plates. In terms of risk for growth changes, we identified major differences between femoral and tibial growth plate injuries caused by tunnel drilling. On the tibial side the central positioning of the drill hole in the proximal tibial growth plate appeared to be safe in terms of growth abnormalities. On the femoral side, however, the eccentrically placed femoral tunnel is at risk to injure the periphery of the growth plate. In the paediatric knee, this may either occur during the drilling procedure, for instance if the posterior wall of the tunnel gets injured (posterior blow-out) or if the surgeon chooses to perform an extraepiphyseal graft placement during which this zone might be rasped for better graft adherence to the bone (Kocher et al. 2002). Injuries of the perichondral structures have shown to be at risk to develop major growth abnormalities due to an asymmetric remaining growth (Koman & Sanders 1999; Robert & Casin 2010; Kocher et al. 2002; Chotel & Seil 2013). In the Ogden classification, they are classified as type VI injuries and correspond to a localized peripheral bone bridge (Ogden 1981).

Furthermore, large animal models showed that filling the tunnels with tendon grafts prevented growth abnormalities in transphyseal ACL replacement procedures. Several other studies confirmed the suitability of this model for the study of paediatric ACL reconstruction (Meller et al. 2009a; Meller et al. 2009b; Meller et al. 2008a; Meller et al. 2008b).

The preclinical sheep model of high tibial osteotomy

HTO is an excellent alternative to knee arthroplasty, especially for younger and physically active patients with knee OA of the medial tibiofemoral compartment and varus malalignment (Brinkman et al. 2008; Pape et al. 2010; Lobenhoffer & Agneskirchner 2003a; Lobenhoffer & Agneskirchner 2014; W-Dahl et al. 2012; Prodromos et al. 2015). The weightbearing axis is shifted away from the medial compartment. Consequently, the load distribution between the medial and lateral compartments of the knee is altered (Van Thiel et al. 2011). Loading is transferred towards the lateral tibiofemoral compartment -especially when a valgus overcorrection is performed- and loading of the medial compartment is decreased (Agneskirchner et al. 2007). Preclinical large animal models of HTO can be used to test different types of osteotomies and to evaluate the effects of lower limb alignment on the reconstructive therapy of articular cartilage lesions and on the development and progression of OA. Traditionally, our experimental knowledge about osteotomies was chiefly based on cadaver studies (Agneskirchner et al. 2007; Lim et al. 2011), models of below-knee amputation or femur valgus osteotomy in guinea-pigs (Wei et al. 2001), on data from cartilage samples obtained from patients undergoing total knee replacement (Otsuki et al. 2008; Wei et al. 2001) and on CT-osteoabsorptiometric investigations in patients (Muller-Gerbl et al. 1992; Madry et al. 2010). More recently, the sheep has emerged as a suitable preclinical animal model of HTO (Pape & Madry 2013). In these studies, adult Merino sheep underwent an HTO of their tibiae. Either a medial open-wedge technique inducing a normal and an excessive valgus alignment or a closed-wedge technique inducing a varus alignment were applied (Table 2). Relevant steps of the surgical technique were essentially performed according to the clinical recommendations of osteotomy experts (Lobenhoffer & Agneskirchner 2003b). During the course of the surgeries, no intraoperative complications occurred, and the popliteal artery and femoral vein were never injured. Some species-specific complications emerged in the post-operative course (Table 3). These included instability of the osteotomy which occurred as a consequence of performing a classical monocortical fixation of the three proximal screws of the implant as in patients. Also, chronic patella dislocation was seen, caused by excessive valgus osteotomy and subsequently insufficient closure after medial arthrotomy, and

Table 2 Comparison of surgical anatomical parameters for HTO in sheep and humans (adapted from (Pape & Madry 2013) with permission)

Congenital anatomical differences	Sheep stifle joint	Human knee	Surgical consequence for the sheep HTO model
Tibial plateau width [mm]	46-56	60-70	Match screw length
			Narrow and strait plate design necessary
Tibia valga [°]	3.5	0	Valgus overcorrection more likely
Normal knee range of motion (transverse axis) [°]	0-35-72	0-0-140	Dorsal plate positioning after open wedge HTO is recommended due to increased loading of the posterior tibial plateau
tibial tuberosity dimension adding to the AP diameter of the tibial head [%]	30-35	10-15	Anterior plate misplacement more likely
Tibial tuberosity height distance in relation to joint line [mm]	10-15 mm	25-30 mm	Anterior plate misplacement more likely
Posterior slope of the posterior articular surface [°]	20 ± 3	0-10	Narrow and straight plate design necessary for posterior placement
Biomechanical properties of tibial head	Brittle cortical bone, together with little spongious bone	Elastic cortical bone with an exuberant amount of spongious bone	Bicortical proximal screw placement mandatory to avoid fracture/dislocation
			Biplanar osteotomy mandatory regardless of the desired direction of correction
Musculature of the hind limb	Voluminous on medial and lateral side of the femur	Remote from bony knee structures	Distal femoral and proximal lateral tibial osteotomy almost impossible to conduct, stay on the medial side of the proximal tibia for any desired correction angle
Trochlea ridge	Medial ridge extending further cranially and dorsally than lateral ridge	Lateral ridge extending further laterally and anteriorly	Higher propensity of patella instability after valgus correction

intraarticular infection. Taken these specific complications into account, the following surgical principles were identified as a prerequisite for solid bone healing and the maintenance of the correction in sheep: 1) a medial and longitudinal approach to the proximal tibia, 2) biplanar osteotomy to increase the initial rotatory stability regardless of the direction of correction (Pape et al. 2011), 3) application of a small, narrow but long implant with locking screws (e.g. small stature HTO plate; Synthes, Umkirch, Germany), 4) posterior plate placement to avoid slope changes, and 5) use of bicortical screws to account for the brittle bone of the tibial head and to avoid tibial head displacement (Tables 2 and 3). Thus, although successful HTO in sheep is complex and requires attention to these principles, the sheep represents because of its similarities with humans (Allen et al. 1998) an elegant model to induce axial malalignment in a clinically relevant environment, and osteotomy healing under challenging mechanical conditions (Pape & Madry 2013).

Table 3 Comparison of probabilities of potential pitfalls among sheep and humans (adapted from (Pape & Madry 2013) with permission)

Structure involved	Human	Sheep
Neurologic injuries	++	NR
Osteonecrosis of proximal fragment	++	NR
Fracture through proximal fragment with violation of joint space	++	NR
Infection	+	+++
Vessel injury	+	++
Subchondral bone cysts (tibial head) without screw perforation	NR	+
Compartment syndrome	+	NR
Non-union	+	NR
Loss of correction due to implant failure	#	+
Overcorrection	#	NR

"NR" not reported; + seldom, ++ infrequent, +++ frequent, # may depend on implant design (Song et al. 2010).

Clinical relevance for high tibial osteotomy

Published studies using this model have focused so far on the effect of axial alignment on the lateral tibiofemoral compartment. Specifically, effects on the articular cartilage and the development of OA, the lateral meniscus and the subchondral bone were investigated (Madry et al. 2013b; Madry et al. 2014b; Ziegler et al. 2013; Ziegler et al. 2014). The data first revealed interesting and specific topographical relationships that are present in the central region of lateral tibiofemoral compartment, regardless of correction. For example, there exists a correlation between the thickness of the articular cartilage layer and the subchondral bone. The important protective role of the lateral meniscus for the cartilage (Beaufils et al. 2006) is reflected in the correlation of thickness between the articular cartilage in the submeniscal periphery and the lateral meniscus. The clinical observation that cartilage lesions proceed much faster after lateral than after medial meniscectomy, and that the clinical outcomes of lateral meniscectomy are significantly worse than after medial meniscectomy underscore the delicate balance between the lateral meniscus and the articular cartilage (Bolano & Grana 1993; Hoser et al. 2001; Macnicol & Thomas 2000; Scheller et al. 2001; Heijink et al. 2012).

As valgus HTO leads to an increase in the pressure in the lateral compartment, the subsequent question was whether HTO results in structural changes in the lateral tibiofemoral osteochondral unit and lateral meniscus, and whether these changes depend in the extent of correction; reflective of the pressure in the lateral compartment. Importantly, the pressure increase in the lateral compartment following standard correction valgus HTO (with 4.5° tibial valgus) did not lead to mid-term morphological alterations in the lateral tibiofemoral compartment. In contrast, the higher increase in pressure following valgus overcorrection (with 9.5° tibial valgus) induced adaptive subchondral bone changes, reflected by an increased specific bone surface (BS/BV) in the subarticular spongiosa compared with unloading by varisation. Also, in the lateral menisci, a decrease in the number of cells in the red–red (peripheral) zone of the middle third was noted, however without structural changes (such as meniscal lesions). The lateral meniscus (Beaufils et al. 2006) is of specific importance, since the peak contact stress and maximum shear stress in the cartilage increased 200% more after a lateral than a medial meniscectomy under axial femoral compressive loads (Pena et al. 2006). Altogether, these results show that for the clinical situation, opening wedge HTO is a safe surgical procedure for the lateral tibial osteochondral unit and the lateral meniscus.

Animal models for cartilage repair

Animal models for articular cartilage repair are vital for basic scientific and translational studies (Hunziker 2009; Blaney Davidson et al. 2014). They need to reflect the different appearances and aetiologies of cartilage defects, which may be caused by OA, trauma, osteochondritis dissecans, and osteonecrosis (Madry et al. 2010). Such models may be used to study spontaneous cartilage repair or improved reconstructive surgical options. These currently include the removal or refixation of chondral or osteochondral fragments, autologous or allogeneic osteochondral transplantation, marrow stimulation, articular chondrocyte implantation, or HTO (Hunziker 2002; Madry et al. 2011). Importantly, the difference between focal, non-OA cartilage defects and the often ill-defined OA lesions needs to be appreciated (Figure 1). Focal defects are usually surrounded by a normal cartilaginous tissue, while OA lesions are often larger in size and thus may affect the entire joint surface and are of different depths (Madry et al. 2011; Pritzker et al. 2006). Animal models also play an important role in evaluating novel experimental treatments (Cucchiarini et al. 2014), such as application of bioinspired scaffolds or defined cell populations (Henderson & La Valette 2005; Deie et al. 2007; Bosch & Kasperczyk 1993; Frisbie et al. 2006b).

Focal cartilage defect models can be created in a variety of small and large animals, among which the mouse, rat, rabbit, dog, minipig, sheep, goat, and horse (Hunziker 1999b; Hunziker 1999a; Hunziker 2000; Hunziker 2009). Major considerations of focal articular cartilage defect models are summarized in Table 4. Here, not only the cartilage thickness is important, but also cartilage microstructure such as cellularity (Aigner et al. 2010; Poole et al. 2010), the age of animals, defect size, depth, anatomy, and subchondral bone plate thickness (Chevrier et al. 2015). For example, a full-thickness chondral defect does not extend into the subchondral bone, but merely ends at the junction of calcified cartilage and the subchondral bone plate (Figure 2) (Frisbie et al. 2006b; Hunziker 1999b; Madry et al. 2010).

Goat, sheep, minipigs, and horses are well suited to induce chondral defects (Hunziker 1999b; Hunziker 1999a; Hunziker 2000; Hunziker 2009). Particular attention has to be paid to a meticulous surgical technique when creating chondral defect models, as the defect should not extend into the subchondral bone (Frisbie et al. 2006b; Frisbie et al. 2006a; Drobnic et al. 2010). Reflecting this important point, displaying in a publication a photomicrograph of a histological section of the chondral defect resulting from the surgical technique applied in an *ex vivo* setting of the animal model might, in some cases, be helpful to see how deep the created lesion extends. The spontaneous repair of chondral defects is rather limited, as Hunziker and Rosenberg have shown that only a few cells from the synovial membrane migrate into the lesion over time (Hunziker & Rosenberg 1996). In contrast, when marrow stimulation is applied at the base of those defects by Pridie drilling (Smillie 1957; Pridie 1959), microfracture (Steadman et al. 2001), or abrasion arthroplasty (Johnson 2001), pluripotent progenitor cells from the subchondral bone marrow migrate into the defect, differentiate into chondrocytes, and form a cartilaginous repair tissue (Frisbie et al. 1999; Frisbie et al. 2003; Shapiro et al. 1993). Interestingly, articular cartilage repair depends also on the topographic location of the defect. Clinical investigations indicate

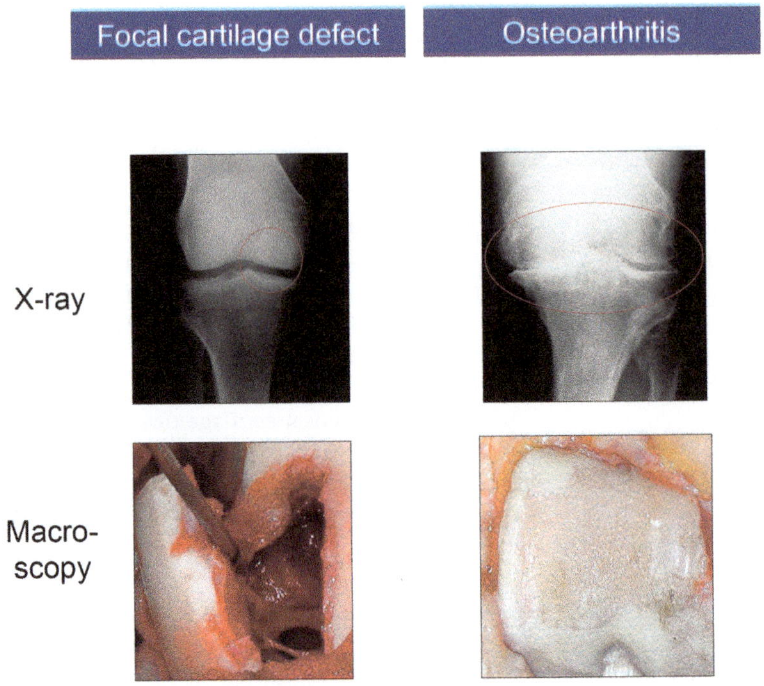

Figure 1 When contemplating on the use of animal models of articular cartilage defects, the important difference between focal, non-OA cartilage defects and OA lesions needs to be kept in mind. Focal defects are usually surrounded by a normal cartilaginous tissue (left side, shown is a lesion caused by osteochondritis dissecans of the human knee). The often ill-defined OA lesions are often larger in size and may affect the entire joint (right side, shown is a case of tricompartimental osteoarthritis of the human knee).

Table 4 Major considerations for focal articular cartilage defect models

Factor	Comments
Cartilage thickness	Generally increasing with the size of the animals. Depends on anatomic location within the joint
Subchondral bone plate thickness	Not always reflective of the size of the animals. Minipigs, for example, have a thin subchondral bone plate, while sheep have a thick subchondral bone plate
Age of animals	Adult animals are preferred as juvenile animals have a higher degree of spontaneous repair
Defect size	Can be determined as area of defect and placed in relation with the condylar width
Defect depth	Needs to be adapted to the osteochondral anatomy to reflect the desired defect type
Defect anatomy	Circular or rectangular patterns are commonly used
Defect location	Topographic differences within a joint exist for cartilage thickness, biochemical composition and repair potential
Knee resting position	Differs among animals, often lack of full extension as in humans
Gait patterns	Differs among animals, the sheep/goat/horse usually considered to best resemble be situation in humans

that the femoral condyles and the trochlear groove are the key locations where articular cartilage defects occur (Hjelle et al. 2002; Curl et al. 1997), and that small chondral lesions in the human femoral condyles repair better than in the trochlea (Kreuz et al. 2006b). This finding is not always reflected in the animal models. For example, articular cartilage repair in sheep is better at the trochlea than at the condyle, and therefore the repair pattern of the sheep trochlea is more reflective of the human femoral condyle (Orth et al. 2013c).

A recent focus has been to simultaneously investigate the subchondral bone in the context of osteochondral repair (Chen et al. 2011; Chen et al. 2009; Hoemann et al. 2012; Madry 2010; Goebel et al. 2012; Orth et al. 2013a; Orth et al. 2013b; Orth et al. 2012b). Data from large animal models have shown that subchondral bone changes such as the upward migration of the subchondral bone plate, intralesional osteophytes, subchondral bone cysts, and a generalized impairment of the osseous microarchitecture below the defect persist for a longer period of time than previously acknowledged (Orth et al. 2013a). Osteochondral defects, in contrast to partial- or full-thickness chondral defects, heal with the sequence of osteochondral repair (Orth et al. 2012a; Shapiro et al. 1993). Current translational studies have shown a variety of subchondral bone changes which are associated with

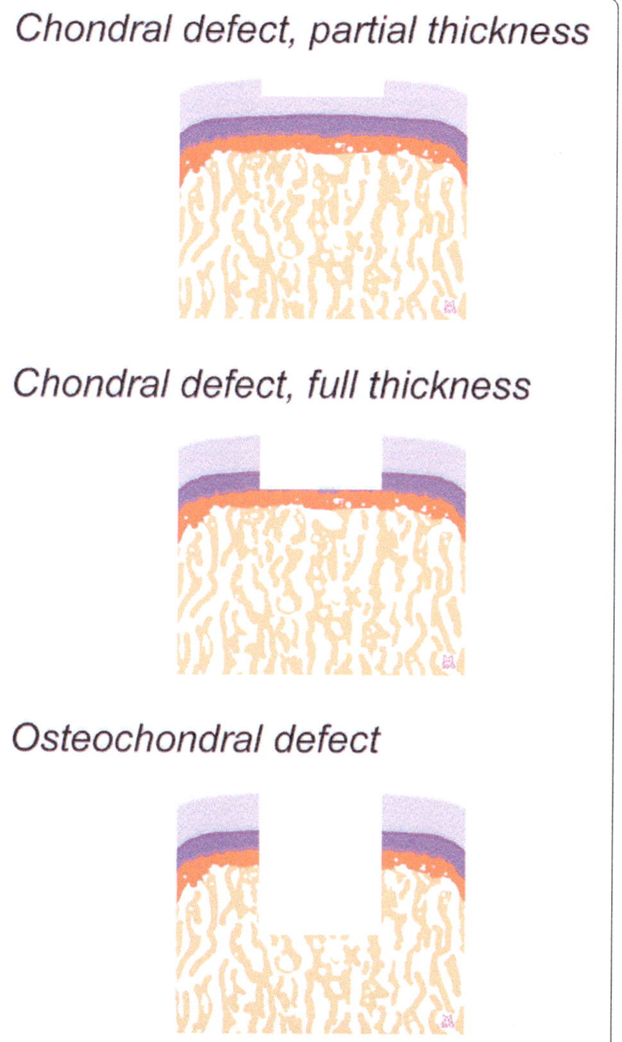

Figure 2 Classification of cartilage defects. Both partial- and full-thickness chondral defects involve, by definition, only the cartilage layer. Osteochondral defects extend through the subchondral bone plate into the subchondral bone. Light blue: articular cartilage; dark blue: calcified cartilage; dark orange: subchondral bone plate; orange: subarticular spongiosa.

osteochondral repair, among which the upward migration of the subchondral bone plate, the formation of intralesional osteophytes, the appearance of subchondral bone cysts, and generalized changes of the subchondral bone microarchitecture (Qiu et al. 2003; Orth et al. 2013a; Chen et al. 2009; Chen et al. 2011). These spatial and temporal alterations proceed in a defined manner (Orth et al. 2012a). Clinical studies in patients have identified similar changes of the subchondral bone below a cartilage lesion (Niemeyer et al. 2015; Bert 2015; Gomoll et al. 2010). These chiefly include the upward migration of the subchondral bone plate, intralesional osteophytes, and subchondral bone cysts (Orth et al. 2013a; Niemeyer et al. 2015; Bert 2015). Whether their development over the long-term shows a similar pattern as seen in animal models remains to be elucidated. Also, the relationship of these alterations to the degradation of the cartilaginous repair tissue remains elusive. While many animal studies did not find a correlation between the structural quality of the cartilaginous repair tissue and the advancement of the subchondral bone plate, our current understanding on the (long-term) clinical effect of such subchondral bone changes is even more limited (Niemeyer et al. 2015; Bert 2015; Sansone et al. 2015; Orth et al. 2013a; Cole et al. 2011; Vasiliadis et al. 2010; Brown et al. 2004; Kreuz et al. 2006a; Mithoefer et al. 2005; Saris et al. 2009; Dhollander et al. 2011; Henderson & La Valette 2005).

OA models are mainly established in the mouse, rat, guinea pig, rabbit, sheep, goat, and horse (Little & Zaki 2012). Notably, the Osteoarthritis Research Society International (OARSI) devoted an entire issue of their journal Osteoarthritis Cartilage for recommendations for the use of animal models in the study of OA (Johnstone et al. 1998; Agung et al. 2006). In general, utmost importance has to be given to the selection of the method for an OA induction, as this should reflect the clinical entity which is studied (Cook et al. 2010; Gerwin et al. 2010; Glasson et al. 2010; Kraus et al. 2010; Laverty et al. 2010; Little et al. 2010; McIlwraith et al. 2010). Moreover, the time of therapeutic intervention has to be carefully selected following or during OA induction.

To evaluate experimental osteochondral repair, a large variety of methods can be used and should be applied simultaneously. These include, but are not limited to macroscopic evaluation of the repair tissue and the treated joint (Goebel et al. 2012), non destructive structure evaluation by high field MRI (Goebel et al. 2014) and micro CT (Eldracher et al. 2014), biochemical (Kiss et al. 2014) and molecular biological evaluation of the repair tissue (Cucchiarini & Madry 2014), and histological (Orth et al. 2012c), and immunohistochemical evaluations (Madry et al. 2013a). Histological scoring remains the gold standard (Getgood et al. 2014). Here, both elementary and comprehensive histological scores are well suited to quantify the structure of cartilaginous repair tissue (Orth et al. 2012c). Interestingly, when evaluating osteochondral repair, only the Sellers and the Pineda score allow for an assessment of the osteochondral junction in subchondral bone (Sellers et al. 1997; Pineda et al. 1992). Close attention should be paid to sample size requirements, as a bilateral research design (where cartilage defects are established in both joints of the same animal) reduces sample sizes (Orth et al. 2013d). Recently, high field MRI at 9.4 Tesla has been shown to correlate with macroscopic and histological scoring (Goebel et al. 2014; Goebel et al. 2012). When performing micro CT analysis of the subchondral bone, a separation of the subchondral bone into subchondral bone plate and subarticular spongiosa, based on their anatomy, appears useful (Orth et al. 2012b). In the context of OA, similar principles apply, with the additional focus of the evaluation of the synovial membrane (Pastoureau et al. 2010).

Clinical application of a magnetic device for targeted cell delivery in cartilage repair

The clinical application of a magnetic device for targeted cell delivery in cartilage repair serves as a suitable example of how data from animal models are directly translated into clinical cartilage repair (Cucchiarini et al. 2014). Current cartilage repair techniques do suffer from two weak points (Johnstone et al. 2013). One weak point is that the number of mesenchymal stem cells (MSCs) obtained in the knee with an arthroscopic procedure is limited (Min et al. 2013). The simplest strategy to increase the number of the cells is the intra-articular injection of MSCs after increase of autologous MSCs by cultivation (Frisch et al. 2014). MSCs are the cell population of undifferentiated cells isolated from adult tissue that have the capacity to differentiate into mesodermal lineages, such as bone, cartilage, fat, muscle or other tissues (Johnstone et al. 1998; Johnstone & Yoo 1999). MSCs from the bone marrow can be cultured and differentiated into the desired lineage *in vitro* with the application of specific growth factors or bioactive molecules (Zellner et al. 2014). Intra-articular injection of too many MSCs, however, generated free bodies of scar tissue (Agung et al. 2006). A novel stem cell delivery system for cartilage repair using magnetically labelled MSCs and an external magnetic device was therefore developed, aiming at accumulating a relatively small number of MSCs to a desired location. Ferumoxides are dextran-coated superparamagnetic iron oxide nanoparticles approved by the US Food and Drug Administration (FDA) as a magnetic resonance contrast agent by intravenous injection for hepatic imaging of humans (Wang et al. 2001). By employing ferumoxides, it is easy to generate magnetically labelled MSCs. The ability to deliver magnetically labelled MSCs to a cartilage defect that is a desired place under arthroscopy was demonstrated in rabbit and swine knee joints using an external magnetic device at 0.6 Tesla (Kobayashi et al. 2008).

This result indicates that this minimally invasive system under arthroscopy can be applicable for a focal osteochondral defect in the knee joint. The next step was to examine if this external magnetic system is effective for OA. Here, the question was investigated if a cartilage layer on degenerated human cartilage could successfully be regenerated *in vitro* using this external magnetic system (Kobayashi et al. 2009). MSCs from human bone marrow were cultured and magnetically labelled. Degenerated human cartilage was obtained during total knee arthroplasty. The osteochondral fragments were attached to the sidewall of tissue culture flasks, and magnetically labelled MSCs were injected into the flasks. Using an external magnetic device, a magnetic force was applied for 6 h to the direction of the cartilage, and then the degenerated osteochondral fragment was cultured in chondrogenic differentiation medium for 3 weeks. In the control group, a magnetic force was not applied. Histological evaluated revealed that a new cell layer has formed on the surface of the degenerated cartilage. Positive staining of this cell layer with Toluidine blue, Safranin O, and with anti-type-II collagen immunostaining indicated that is contained a cartilage-like extracellular matrix. In the control group, such a cell layer was not observed. In conclusion, these findings demonstrate that the magnetic system can deliver MSCs onto degenerated human cartilage, which then form an abundant extracellular matrix *in vitro*. Another experimental study was conducted using minipigs to further demonstrate the effectiveness of this system for cartilage repair (Kamei et al. 2013). The safety of the cell application and the capability of the cell proliferation were also investigated and confirmed (Kamei et al. 2013). The first-in-men to apply this procedure to human with a cartilage defect will be started in 2015.

Another weak point is the overload of the focal area treated by marrow-stimulation as a result of early postoperative weight-bearing (Orth et al. 2012b). A novel approach to solve this problem is to reduce the load to the repaired area to protect immature tissue regenerated at the repaired area against destruction caused by overloading. A new distraction arthroplasty device was introduced (Meira, Nagoya, Japan), which allows the range of motion with knee joint distraction (Deie et al. 2007). After an experimental study using rabbits, this technique was applied to patients with OA. After drilling or microfracture under arthroscopy, the new external device was fixed with four 6-mm pins drilled into the distal femur and the proximal tibia. After the appropriate distractive tension was applied, the ROM and the post-distraction and pre-distraction tibiofemoral joint spaces at 30° of flexion were measured. Although this device is usually applied for 3 months, full weight bearing is allowed one month after surgery. Until now, this device has been demonstrated to function well to repair human articular cartilage defects.

Conclusions

The complexity of reconstructive surgical approaches for musculoskeletal disorders complicates the development of novel therapies. Large animal models continue to play a major role to translate new surgical techniques to patients. Although there is no single large animal model replicating the human knee joint perfectly, the sheep stifle joint shares strong similarities with the human knee joint. Large animal models for the treatment of ligamentous ACL lesions may help to overcome the therapeutic dilemma of how to treat such tears in the paediatric population. The newly developed preclinical large animal model of HTO can be applied to evaluate different types of osteotomies and to the effect of lower limb alignment on the reconstructive cartilage therapy. Animal models for cartilage repair need to precisely reflect the clinically very different aetiologies of articular cartilage defects, appearances and appropriate surgical options. This results in the currently large variety of different animal models for focal defects and OA. In the clinical situation, the combination of injection of magnetically labelled MSCs under magnetic field and external arthroplasty device may be an option to successfully treat large osteochondral defects or OA in the near future. As novel insights from studies using these translational models will advance the basic science, and close cooperation in this important field of clinical translation (Madry et al. 2014a) will improve current reconstructive surgical options, the clinical application of such innovative approaches will open novel avenues for regenerative therapies of musculoskeletal disorders.

Competing interests
The authors declare that they have no competing interests.

Authors' contributions
HM, MO, MC participated equally in drafting the manuscript in particular the cartilage defect section. HM, DP participated equally in drafting the manuscript in particular the osteotomy section. RS participated equally in drafting the manuscript in particular the section about the paediatric ACL reconstruction. All of the authors read and approved the final manuscript.

Acknowledgments
The authors thank the presenters, discussion moderators, and all the participants to the Symposium for their valuable input and contributions. We wish to confirm that there are no known conflicts of interests associated with this publication and there has been no financial support for this work that could have influenced its outcome.

Author details
[1]Center of Experimental Orthopaedics, Saarland University Medical Center and Saarland University, Bldg 37, Kirrbergerstr. 1, D-66421 Homburg, Germany. [2]Cartilage Net of the Greater Region, Homburg, Germany. [3]Department of Orthopaedic Surgery, Saarland University Medical Center and Saarland University, D-66421 Homburg/Saar, Germany. [4]Department of Orthopaedic Surgery, Graduate School of Biomedical Sciences, Hiroshima University, Hiroshima, Japan. [5]Department of Orthopaedic Surgery, Centre Hospitalier du Luxembourg, L-1460, Luxembourg, Luxembourg. [6]Sports Medicine Research Laboratory, Public Research Centre for Health, Luxembourg, Centre Médical de la Fondation Norbert Metz, 76 rue d'Eich, L-1460, Luxembourg, Luxembourg.

References
Agneskirchner JD, Hurschler C, Wrann CD, Lobenhoffer P (2007) The effects of valgus medial opening wedge high tibial osteotomy on articular cartilage pressure of the knee: a biomechanical study. Arthroscopy 23(8):852–861, doi:S0749-8063(07)00585-3 [pii] 10.1016/j.arthro.2007.05.018

Agung M, Ochi M, Yanada S, Adachi N, Izuta Y, Yamasaki T, Toda K (2006) Mobilization of bone marrow-derived mesenchymal stem cells into the injured tissues after intraarticular injection and their contribution to tissue regeneration. Knee Surg Sports Traumatol Arthrosc 14(12):1307–1314, doi:10.1007/s00167-006-0124-8

Aigner T, Cook JL, Gerwin N, Glasson SS, Laverty S, Little CB, McIlwraith W, Kraus VB (2010) Histopathology atlas of animal model systems - overview of guiding principles. Osteoarthritis Cartilage 18(Suppl 3):S2–6, doi:S1063-4584(10)00250-5 [pii] 10.1016/j.joca.2010.07.013

Allen MJ, Houlton JE, Adams SB, Rushton N (1998) The surgical anatomy of the stifle joint in sheep. Vet Surg 27(6):596–605, doi:S0161349998000672 [pii]

Arnoczky SP, Marshall JL (1977) The cruciate ligaments of the canine stifle: an anatomical and functional analysis. Am J Vet Res 38(11):1807–1814

Athanasiou KA, Rosenwasser MP, Buckwalter JA, Malinin TI, Mow VC (1991) Interspecies comparisons of *in situ* intrinsic mechanical properties of distal femoral cartilage. J Orthop Res 9(3):330–340, doi:10.1002/jor.1100090304

Bayley N, Pinneau SR (1952) Tables for predicting adult height from skeletal age: revised for use with the Greulich-Pyle hand standards. J Pediatr 40(4):423–441

Beaufils P, Hardy P, Chambat P, Clavert P, Djian P, Frank A, Hulet C, Potel JF, Verdonk R (2006) Adult lateral meniscus. Rev Chir Orthop Reparatrice Appar Mot 92(5 Suppl):2S169–162S194, doi:MDOI-RCO-09-2006-92-S5-0035-1040-101019-200518962 [pii]

Bert JM (2015) Arthroscopy 31(3):501–505, doi:S0749-8063(14)01029-9 [pii] 10.1016/j.arthro.2014.12.018

Blaney Davidson EN, van de Loo FA, van den Berg WB, van der Kraan PM (2014) How to build an inducible cartilage-specific transgenic mouse. Arthritis Res Ther 16(3):210, doi:ar4573 [pii] 10.1186/ar4573

Bolano LE, Grana WA (1993) Isolated arthroscopic partial meniscectomy. Functional radiographic evaluation at five years. Am J Sports Med 21(3):432–437

Bosch U, Kasperczyk WJ (1993) The healing process after cruciate ligament repair in the sheep model. Orthopade 22(6):366–371

Brinkman JM, Lobenhoffer P, Agneskirchner JD, Staubli AE, Wymenga AB, van Heerwaarden RJ (2008) Osteotomies around the knee: patient selection, stability of fixation and bone healing in high tibial osteotomies. J Bone Joint Surg Br 90(12):1548–1557, doi:90-B/12/1548 [pii] 10.1302/0301-620X.90B12.21198

Brown WE, Potter HG, Marx RG, Wickiewicz TL, Warren RF (2004) Magnetic resonance imaging appearance of cartilage repair in the knee. Clin Orthop Relat Res (422):214–223. doi:00003086-200405000-00036 [pii]

Chen H, Sun J, Hoemann CD, Lascau-Coman V, Ouyang W, McKee MD, Shive MS, Buschmann MD (2009) Drilling and microfracture lead to different bone structure and necrosis during bone-marrow stimulation for cartilage repair. J Orthop Res 27(11):1432–1438, doi: 10.1002/jor.20905

Chen H, Chevrier A, Hoemann CD, Sun J, Ouyang W, Buschmann MD (2011) Characterization of subchondral bone repair for marrow-stimulated chondral defects and its relationship to articular cartilage resurfacing. Am J Sports Med 39(8):1731–1740, doi:0363546511403282 [pii] 10.1177/0363546511403282

Chevrier A, Kouao AS, Picard G, Hurtig MB, Buschmann MD (2015) Interspecies comparison of subchondral bone properties important for cartilage repair. J Orthop Res 33(1):63–70, doi: 10.1002/jor.22740

Chotel F, Seil R (2013) Growth disturbances after transphyseal ACL reconstruction in skeletally immature patients: who is more at risk? Young child or adolescent? J Pediatr Orthop 33(5):585–586, doi:10.1097/BPO.0b013e31 8286c161 01241398-201307000-00022 [pii]

Chotel F, Seil R, Greiner P, Chaker MM, Berard J, Raux S (2013) The difficult diagnosis of cartilaginous tibial eminence fractures in young children. Knee Surg Sports Traumatol Arthrosc 22(7):1511–1516, doi:10.1007/s00167-013-2518-8

Cole BJ, Farr J, Winalski CS, Hosea T, Richmond J, Mandelbaum B, De Deyne PG (2011) Outcomes after a single-stage procedure for cell-based cartilage repair: a prospective clinical safety trial with 2-year follow-up. Am J Sports Med 39(6):1170–1179, doi:0363546511399382 [pii] 10.1177/0363546511399382

Cook JL, Kuroki K, Visco D, Pelletier JP, Schulz L, Lafeber FP (2010) The OARSI histopathology initiative - recommendations for histological assessments of osteoarthritis in the dog. Osteoarthritis Cartilage 18(Suppl 3):S66–79, doi:S1063-4584(10)00237-2 [pii] 10.1016/j.joca.2010.04.017

Cucchiarini M, Madry H (2014) Overexpression of human IGF-I via direct rAAV-mediated gene transfer improves the early repair of articular cartilage defects *in vivo*. Gene Ther 21(9):811–819, doi:gt201458 [pii] 10.1038/gt.2014.58

Cucchiarini M, Madry H, Guilak F, Saris DB, Stoddart MJ, Koon Wong M, Roughley P (2014) A vision on the future of articular cartilage repair. Eur Cell Mater 27:12–16, doi:vol027sa03 [pii]

Curl WW, Krome J, Gordon ES, Rushing J, Smith BP, Poehling GG (1997) Cartilage injuries: a review of 31,516 knee arthroscopies. Arthroscopy 13(4):456–460

Deie M, Ochi M, Adachi N, Kajiwara R, Kanaya A (2007) A new articulated distraction arthroplasty device for treatment of the osteoarthritic knee joint: a preliminary report. Arthroscopy 23(8):833–838, doi:S0749-8063(07)00237-X [pii] 10.1016/j.arthro.2007.02.014

Dhollander AA, De Neve F, Almqvist KF, Verdonk R, Lambrecht S, Elewaut D, Verbruggen G, Verdonk PC (2011) Autologous matrix-induced chondrogenesis combined with platelet-rich plasma gel: technical description and a five pilot patients report. Knee Surg Sports Traumatol Arthrosc 19(4):536–542, doi:10.1007/s00167-010-1337-4

Drobnic M, Radosavljevic D, Cor A, Brittberg M, Strazar K (2010) Debridement of cartilage lesions before autologous chondrocyte implantation by open or transarthroscopic techniques: a comparative study using post-mortem materials. J Bone Joint Surg Br 92(4):602–608, doi:92-B/4/602 [pii] 10.1302/0301-620X.92B3.22558

Dye SF (1987) An evolutionary perspective of the knee. J Bone Joint Surg Am 69(7):976–983

Edwards TB, Greene CC, Baratta RV, Zieske A, Willis RB (2001) The effect of placing a tensioned graft across open growth plates. A gross and histologic analysis. J Bone Joint Surg Am 83-A(5):725–734

Eldracher M, Orth P, Cucchiarini M, Pape D, Madry H (2014) Small subchondral drill holes improve marrow stimulation of articular cartilage defects. Am J Sports Med 42(11):2741–2750, doi:0363546514547029 [pii] 10.1177/0363546514547029

Espregueira-Mendes J, Karahan M (2014) Orthopaedic sports surgery: art or science? Knee Surg Sports Traumatol Arthrosc 22(5):959–960, doi:10.1007/s00167-014-2921-9

Frisbie DD, Trotter GW, Powers BE, Rodkey WG, Steadman JR, Howard RD, Park RD, McIlwraith CW (1999) Arthroscopic subchondral bone plate microfracture technique augments healing of large chondral defects in the radial carpal bone and medial femoral condyle of horses. Vet Surg 28(4):242–255

Frisbie DD, Oxford JT, Southwood L, Trotter GW, Rodkey WG, Steadman JR, Goodnight JL, McIlwraith CW (2003) Early events in cartilage repair after subchondral bone microfracture. Clin Orthop Relat Res 407:215–227

Frisbie DD, Cross MW, McIlwraith CW (2006a) A comparative study of articular cartilage thickness in the stifle of animal species used in human pre-clinical studies compared to articular cartilage thickness in the human knee. Vet Comp Orthop Traumatol 19(3):142–146, doi:06030142 [pii]

Frisbie DD, Morisset S, Ho CP, Rodkey WG, Steadman JR, McIlwraith CW (2006b) Effects of calcified cartilage on healing of chondral defects treated with microfracture in horses. Am J Sports Med 34(11):1824–1831

Frisch J, Venkatesan JK, Rey-Rico A, Madry H, Cucchiarini M (2014) Current progress in stem cell-based gene therapy for articular cartilage repair. Curr Stem Cell Res Ther. doi:CSCRT-EPUB-62443 [pii]

Gerwin N, Bendele AM, Glasson S, Carlson CS (2010) The OARSI histopathology initiative - recommendations for histological assessments of osteoarthritis in the rat. Osteoarthritis Cartilage 18(Suppl 3):S24–34, doi:S1063-4584(10)00247-5 [pii] 10.1016/j.joca.2010.05.030

Getgood A, Henson F, Skelton C, Brooks R, Guehring H, Fortier L, Rushton N (2014) Osteochondral tissue engineering using a biphasic collagen/GAG scaffold containing rhFGF18 or BMP-7 in an ovine model. J Exp Orthop 1 (13). doi: doi:10.1186/s40634-014-0013-x

Glasson SS, Chambers MG, Van Den Berg WB, Little CB (2010) The OARSI histopathology initiative - recommendations for histological assessments of osteoarthritis in the mouse. Osteoarthritis Cartilage 18(Suppl 3):S17–23, doi:S1063-4584(10)00238-4 [pii] 10.1016/j.joca.2010.05.025

Goebel L, Orth P, Muller A, Zurakowski D, Bucker A, Cucchiarini M, Pape D, Madry H (2012) Experimental scoring systems for macroscopic articular cartilage repair correlate with the MOCART score assessed by a high-field MRI at 9.4 T - comparative evaluation of five macroscopic scoring systems in a large
animal cartilage defect model. Osteoarthritis Cartilage 20(9):1046–1055, doi:S1063-4584(12)00839-4 [pii] 10.1016/j.joca.2012.05.010

Goebel L, Zurakowski D, Muller A, Pape D, Cucchiarini M, Madry H (2014) 2D and 3D MOCART scoring systems assessed by 9.4 T high-field MRI correlate with elementary and complex histological scoring systems in a translational model of osteochondral repair. Osteoarthritis Cartilage 22(10):1386–1395, doi:S1063-4584(14)01109-1 [pii] 10.1016/j.joca.2014.05.027

Gomoll AH, Madry H, Knutsen G, van Dijk N, Seil R, Brittberg M, Kon E (2010) The subchondral bone in articular cartilage repair: current problems in the surgical management. Knee Surg Sports Traumatol Arthrosc 18(4):434–447, doi:10.1007/s00167-010-1072-x

Guzzanti V, Falciglia F, Gigante A, Fabbriciani C (1994) The effect of intra-articular ACL reconstruction on the growth plates of rabbits. J Bone Joint Surg Br 76(6):960–963

Heijink A, Gomoll AH, Madry H, Drobnic M, Filardo G, Espregueira-Mendes J, Van Dijk CN (2012) Biomechanical considerations in the pathogenesis of osteoarthritis of the knee. Knee Surg Sports Traumatol Arthrosc 20(3):423–435, doi: 10.1007/s00167-011-1818-0

Henderson IJ, La Valette DP (2005) Subchondral bone overgrowth in the presence of full-thickness cartilage defects in the knee. Knee 12(6):435–440, doi:S0968-0160(05)00065-7 [pii] 10.1016/j.knee.2005.04.003

Hjelle K, Solheim E, Strand T, Muri R, Brittberg M (2002) Articular cartilage defects in 1,000 knee arthroscopies. Arthroscopy 18(7):730–734, doi: S0749806302000257 [pii]

Hoemann CD, Lafantaisie-Favreau CH, Lascau-Coman V, Chen G, Guzman-Morales J (2012) The cartilage-bone interface. J Knee Surg 25(2):85–97

Hoser C, Fink C, Brown C, Reichkendler M, Hackl W, Bartlett J (2001) Long-term results of arthroscopic partial lateral meniscectomy in knees without associated damage. J Bone Joint Surg Br 83(4):513–516

Hunziker EB (1999a) Articular cartilage repair: are the intrinsic biological constraints undermining this process insuperable? Osteoarthritis Cartilage 7 (1):15–28

Hunziker EB (2000) Articular cartilage repair: problems and perspectives. Biorheology 37(1–2):163–164

Hunziker EB (2002) Articular cartilage repair: basic science and clinical progress. A review of the current status and prospects. Osteoarthritis Cartilage 10(6):432–463, doi:10.1053/joca.2002.0801 S1063458402908010 [pii]

Hunziker EB (2009) The elusive path to cartilage regeneration. Adv Mater 21(32–33):3419–3424, doi: 10.1002/adma.200801957

Hunziker EB (1999) Biologic repair of articular cartilage. Defect models in experimental animals and matrix requirements. Clin Orthop (367 Suppl):S135-146

Hunziker EB, Rosenberg LC (1996) Repair of partial-thickness defects in articular cartilage: cell recruitment from the synovial membrane. J Bone Joint Surg Am 78(5):721–733

Janarv PM, Wikstrom B, Hirsch G (1998) The influence of transphyseal drilling and tendon grafting on bone growth: an experimental study in the rabbit. J Pediatr Orthop 18(2):149–154

Johnson LL (2001) Arthroscopic abrasion arthroplasty: a review. Clin Orthop (391 Suppl):S306-317

Johnstone B, Yoo JU (1999) Autologous mesenchymal progenitor cells in articular cartilage repair. Clin Orthop Relat Res (367 Suppl):S156-162

Johnstone B, Hering TM, Caplan AI, Goldberg VM, Yoo JU (1998) *In vitro* chondrogenesis of bone marrow-derived mesenchymal progenitor cells. Exp Cell Res 238(1):265–272, doi:S0014-4827(97)93858-1 [pii] 10.1006/excr.1997.3858

Johnstone B, Alini M, Cucchiarini M, Dodge GR, Eglin D, Guilak F, Madry H, Mata A, Mauck RL, Semino CE, Stoddart MJ (2013) Tissue engineering for articular cartilage repair–the state of the art. Eur Cell Mater 25:248–267, doi:vol025a18 [pii]

Kamei G, Kobayashi T, Ohkawa S, Kongcharoensombat W, Adachi N, Takazawa K, Shibuya H, Deie M, Hattori K, Goldberg JL, Ochi M (2013) Articular cartilage repair with magnetic mesenchymal stem cells. Am J Sports Med 41(6):1255–1264, doi:0363546513483270 [pii] 10.1177/0363546513483270

Kiss A, Cucchiarini M, Menger MD, Kohn D, Hannig M, Madry H (2014) Enamel matrix derivative inhibits proteoglycan production and articular cartilage repair, delays the restoration of the subchondral bone and induces changes of the synovial membrane in a lapine osteochondral defect model *in vivo*. J Tissue Eng Regen Med 8(1):41–49, doi: 10.1002/term.1495

Kobayashi T, Ochi M, Yanada S, Ishikawa M, Adachi N, Deie M, Arihiro K (2008) A novel cell delivery system using magnetically labeled mesenchymal stem cells and an external magnetic device for clinical cartilage repair. Arthroscopy 24(1):69–76, doi:S0749-8063(07)00755-4 [pii] 10.1016/j.arthro.2007.08.017

Kobayashi T, Ochi M, Yanada S, Ishikawa M, Adachi N, Deie M, Arihiro K (2009) Augmentation of degenerated human cartilage *in vitro* using magnetically labeled mesenchymal stem cells and an external magnetic device. Arthroscopy 25(12):1435–1441, doi:S0749-8063(09)00521-0 [pii] 10.1016/j.arthro.2009.06.009

Kocher MS, Saxon HS, Hovis WD, Hawkins RJ (2002) Management and complications of anterior cruciate ligament injuries in skeletally immature patients: survey of the Herodicus Society and The ACL Study Group. J Pediatr Orthop 22(4):452–457

Koman JD, Sanders JO (1999) Valgus deformity after reconstruction of the anterior cruciate ligament in a skeletally immature patient. A case report. J Bone Joint Surg Am 81(5):711–715

Kraus VB, Huebner JL, DeGroot J, Bendele A (2010) The OARSI histopathology initiative - recommendations for histological assessments of osteoarthritis in the guinea pig. Osteoarthritis Cartilage 18(Suppl 3):S35–52, doi:S1063-4584(10)00234-7 [pii] 10.1016/j.joca.2010.04.015

Kreuz PC, Erggelet C, Steinwachs MR, Krause SJ, Lahm A, Niemeyer P, Ghanem N, Uhl M, Sudkamp N (2006a) Is microfracture of chondral defects in the knee associated with different results in patients aged 40 years or younger? Arthroscopy 22(11):1180–1186

Kreuz PC, Steinwachs MR, Erggelet C, Krause SJ, Konrad G, Uhl M, Sudkamp N (2006b) Results after microfracture of full-thickness chondral defects in different compartments in the knee. Osteoarthritis Cartilage 14(11):1119–1125

Laverty S, Girard CA, Williams JM, Hunziker EB, Pritzker KP (2010) The OARSI histopathology initiative - recommendations for histological assessments of osteoarthritis in the rabbit. Osteoarthritis Cartilage 18(Suppl 3):S53–65, doi:S1063-4584(10)00244-X [pii] 10.1016/j.joca.2010.05.029

Lim HC, Bae JH, Song HR, Teoh SH, Kim HK, Kum DH (2011) High tibial osteotomy using polycaprolactone-tricalcium phosphate polymer wedge in a micro pig model. J Bone Joint Surg Br 93(1):120–125, doi:93-B/1/120 [pii] 10.1302/0301-620X.93B1.24767

Little CB, Zaki S (2012) What constitutes an "animal model of osteoarthritis"–the need for consensus? Osteoarthritis Cartilage 20(4):261–267, doi:S1063-4584 (12)00054-4 [pii] 10.1016/j.joca.2012.01.017

Little CB, Smith MM, Cake MA, Read RA, Murphy MJ, Barry FP (2010) The OARSI histopathology initiative - recommendations for histological assessments of osteoarthritis in sheep and goats. Osteoarthritis Cartilage 18(Suppl 3):S80–92, doi:S1063-4584(10)00235-9 [pii] 10.1016/j.joca.2010.04.016

Lobenhoffer P, Agneskirchner JD (2003a) Improvements in surgical technique of valgus high tibial osteotomy. Knee Surg Sports Traumatol Arthrosc 11(3):132–138, doi:10.1007/s00167-002-0334-7

Lobenhoffer P, Agneskirchner JD (2014) Osteotomy around the knee vs. unicondylar knee replacement. Orthopade 43(10):923-9. doi: 10.1007/s00132-014-3011-x

Macnicol MF, Thomas NP (2000) The knee after meniscectomy. J Bone Joint Surg Br 82(2):157–159

Madry H (2010) The subchondral bone: a new frontier in articular cartilage repair. Knee Surg Sports Traumatol Arthrosc 18(4):417–418, doi:10.1007/s00167-010-1071-y

Madry H, van Dijk CN, Mueller-Gerbl M (2010) The basic science of the subchondral bone. Knee Surg Sports Traumatol Arthrosc 18(4):419–433, doi:10.1007/s00167-010-1054-z

Madry H, Grun UW, Knutsen G (2011) Cartilage repair and joint preservation: medical and surgical treatment options. Dtsch Arztebl Int 108(40):669–677, doi: 10.3238/arztebl.2011.0669

Madry H, Kaul G, Zurakowski D, Vunjak-Novakovic G, Cucchiarini M (2013a) Cartilage constructs engineered from chondrocytes overexpressing IGF-I improve the repair of osteochondral defects in a rabbit model. Eur Cell Mater 25:229–247, doi:vol025a17 [pii]

Madry H, Ziegler R, Orth P, Goebel L, Ong MF, Kohn D, Cucchiarini M, Pape D (2013b) Effect of open wedge high tibial osteotomy on the lateral compartment in sheep. Part I: Analysis of the lateral meniscus. Knee Surg Sports Traumatol Arthrosc 21(1):39–48, doi: 10.1007/s00167-012-2176-2

Madry H, Alini M, Stoddart MJ, Evans C, Miclau T, Steiner S (2014a) Barriers and strategies for the clinical translation of advanced orthopaedic tissue engineering protocols. Eur Cell Mater 27:17–21, doi:vol027sa04 [pii]

Madry H, Ziegler R, Pape D, Cucchiarini M (2014b) Structural changes in the lateral tibiofemoral compartment after high tibial osteotomy. Orthopade 43(11):958–965, doi: 10.1007/s00132-014-3024-5

McIlwraith CW, Frisbie DD, Kawcak CE, Fuller CJ, Hurtig M, Cruz A (2010) The OARSI histopathology initiative - recommendations for histological assessments of osteoarthritis in the horse. Osteoarthritis Cartilage 18(Suppl 3): S93–105, doi:S1063-4584(10)00251-7 [pii] 10.1016/j.joca.2010.05.031

Meller R, Kendoff D, Hankemeier S, Jagodzinski M, Grotz M, Knobloch K, Krettek C (2008a) Hindlimb growth after a transphyseal reconstruction of the anterior cruciate ligament: a study in skeletally immature sheep with wide-open physes. Am J Sports Med 36(12):2437–2443, doi:0363546508322884 [pii] 10.1177/0363546508322884

Meller R, Willbold E, Hesse E, Dreymann B, Fehr M, Haasper C, Hurschler C, Krettek C, Witte F (2008b) Histologic and biomechanical analysis of anterior cruciate ligament graft to bone healing in skeletally immature sheep. Arthroscopy 24(11):1221–1231, doi:S0749-8063(08)00515-X [pii] 10.1016/j.arthro.2008.06.021

Meller R, Brandes G, Drogemuller C, Fritz F, Schiborra F, Fehr M, Hankemeier S, Krettek C, Hurschler C (2009a) Graft remodeling during growth following anterior cruciate ligament reconstruction in skeletally immature sheep. Arch Orthop Trauma Surg 129(8):1037–1046, doi: 10.1007/s00402-008-0784-6

Meller R, Haasper C, Westhoff J, Brand J, Knobloch K, Hankemeier S, Hesse E, Krettek C, Jagodzinski M (2009b) An animal model to study ACL reconstruction during growth. Technol Health Care 17(5–6):403–410, doi:FJ024610011H62Q0 [pii] 10.3233/THC-2009-0561

Min BH, Choi WH, Lee YS, Park SR, Choi BH, Kim YJ, Jin LH, Yoon JH (2013) Effect of different bone marrow stimulation techniques (BSTs) on MSCs mobilization. J Orthop Res 31(11):1814–1819, doi:10.1002/jor.22380

Mithoefer K, Williams RJ 3rd, Warren RF, Potter HG, Spock CR, Jones EC, Wickiewicz TL, Marx RG (2005) The microfracture technique for the treatment of articular cartilage lesions in the knee. A prospective cohort study. J Bone Joint Surg Am 87(9):1911–1920

Muller-Gerbl M, Putz R, Kenn R (1992) Demonstration of subchondral bone density patterns by three-dimensional CT osteoabsorptiometry as a noninvasive method for *in vivo* assessment of individual long-term stresses in joints. J Bone Miner Res 7(Suppl 2):S411–418, doi:10.1002/jbmr.5650071409

Niemeyer P, Uhl M, Salzmann GM, Morscheid YP, Sudkamp NP, Madry H (2015) Evaluation and analysis of graft hypertrophy by means of arthroscopy, biochemical MRI and osteochondral biopsies in a patient following autologous chondrocyte implantation for treatment of a full-thickness-cartilage defect of the knee. Arch Orthop Trauma Surg. doi:10.1007/s00402-015-2194-x

Ogden JA (1981) Injury to the growth mechanisms of the immature skeleton. Skeletal Radiol 6(4):237–253

Ono T, Wada Y, Takahashi K, Tsuchida T, Minamide M, Moriya H (1998) Tibial deformities and failures of anterior cruciate ligament reconstruction in immature rabbits. J Orthop Sci 3(3):150–155

Orth P, Cucchiarini M, Kaul G, Ong MF, Graber S, Kohn DM, Madry H (2012a) Temporal and spatial migration pattern of the subchondral bone plate in a rabbit osteochondral defect model. Osteoarthritis Cartilage 20(10):1161–1169, doi:S1063-4584(12)00863-1 [pii] 10.1016/j.joca.2012.06.008

Orth P, Goebel L, Wolfram U, Ong MF, Graber S, Kohn D, Cucchiarini M, Ignatius A, Pape D, Madry H (2012b) Effect of subchondral drilling on the microarchitecture of subchondral bone: analysis in a large animal model at 6 months. Am J Sports Med 40(4):828–836, doi:0363546511430376 [pii] 10.1177/0363546511430376

Orth P, Zurakowski D, Wincheringer D, Madry H (2012c) Reliability, reproducibility, and validation of five major histological scoring systems for experimental articular cartilage repair in the rabbit model. Tissue Eng Part C Methods 18(5):329–339, doi: 10.1089/ten.TEC.2011.0462

Orth P, Cucchiarini M, Kohn D, Madry H (2013a) Alterations of the subchondral bone in osteochondral repair–translational data and clinical evidence. Eur Cell Mater 25:299–316, doi:vol025a21 [pii]

Orth P, Cucchiarini M, Zurakowski D, Menger MD, Kohn DM, Madry H (2013b) Parathyroid hormone [1–34] improves articular cartilage surface architecture and integration and subchondral bone reconstitution in osteochondral defects *in vivo*. Osteoarthritis Cartilage 21(4):614–624, doi:S1063-4584(13) 00023-X [pii] 10.1016/j.joca.2013.01.008

Orth P, Meyer HL, Goebel L, Eldracher M, Ong MF, Cucchiarini M, Madry H (2013c) Improved repair of chondral and osteochondral defects in the ovine trochlea compared with the medial condyle. J Orthop Res 31(11):1772–1779, doi:10.1002/jor.22418

Orth P, Zurakowski D, Alini M, Cucchiarini M, Madry H (2013d) Reduction of sample size requirements by bilateral versus unilateral research designs in animal models for cartilage tissue engineering. Tissue Eng Part C Methods 19(11):885–891, doi: 10.1089/ten.TEC.2012.0699

Otsuki S, Nakajima M, Lotz M, Kinoshita M (2008) Hyaluronic acid and chondroitin sulfate content of osteoarthritic human knee cartilage: site-specific correlation with weight-bearing force based on femorotibial angle measurement. J Orthop Res 26(9):1194–1198, doi: 10.1002/jor.20571

Pape D, Madry H (2013) The preclinical sheep model of high tibial osteotomy relating basic science to the clinics: standards, techniques and pitfalls. Knee Surg Sports Traumatol Arthrosc 21(1):228–236, doi: 10.1007/s00167-012-2135-y

Pape D, Filardo G, Kon E, van Dijk CN, Madry H (2010) Disease-specific clinical problems associated with the subchondral bone. Knee Surg Sports Traumatol Arthrosc 18(4):448–462, doi:10.1007/s00167-010-1052-1

Pape D, Kohn D, van Giffen N, Hoffmann A, Seil R, Lorbach O (2011) Differences in fixation stability between spacer plate and plate fixator following high tibial osteotomy. Knee Surg Sports Traumatol Arthrosc 21(1):82–89, doi:10.1007/s00167-011-1693-8

Pastoureau PC, Hunziker EB, Pelletier JP (2010) Cartilage, bone and synovial histomorphometry in animal models of osteoarthritis. Osteoarthritis Cartilage

18(Suppl 3):S106–112, doi:S1063-4584(10)00232-3 [pii] 10.1016/j.joca.2010.05.024
Pena E, Calvo B, Martinez MA, Palanca D, Doblare M (2006) Why lateral meniscectomy is more dangerous than medial meniscectomy. A finite element study. J Orthop Res 24(5):1001–1010, doi: 10.1002/jor.20037
Pineda S, Pollack A, Stevenson S, Goldberg V, Caplan A (1992) A semiquantitative scale for histologic grading of articular cartilage repair. Acta Anat (Basel) 143(4):335–340
Poole R, Blake S, Buschmann M, Goldring S, Laverty S, Lockwood S, Matyas J, McDougall J, Pritzker K, Rudolphi K, van den Berg W, Yaksh T (2010) Recommendations for the use of preclinical models in the study and treatment of osteoarthritis. Osteoarthritis Cartilage 18(Suppl 3):S10–16, doi:S1063-4584(10)00241-4 [pii] 10.1016/j.joca.2010.05.027
Pridie KH (1959) A method of resurfacing osteoarthritic knee joints. Proceedings of the British Orthopaedic Association J Bone Joint Surg (Br) 41:618–619
Pritzker KP, Gay S, Jimenez SA, Ostergaard K, Pelletier JP, Revell PA, Salter D, van den Berg WB (2006) Osteoarthritis cartilage histopathology: grading and staging. Osteoarthritis Cartilage 14(1):13–29, doi:S1063-4584(05)00197-4 [pii] 10.1016/j.joca.2005.07.014
Prodromos CC, Amendola A, Jakob RP (2015) High tibial osteotomy: indications, techniques, and postoperative management. Instr Course Lect 64:555–565
Qiu YS, Shahgaldi BF, Revell WJ, Heatley FW (2003) Observations of subchondral plate advancement during osteochondral repair: a histomorphometric and mechanical study in the rabbit femoral condyle. Osteoarthritis Cartilage 11(11):810–820
Robert HE, Casin C (2010) Valgus and flexion deformity after reconstruction of the anterior cruciate ligament in a skeletally immature patient. Knee Surg Sports Traumatol Arthrosc 18(10):1369–1373, doi: 10.1007/s00167-009-0988-5
Rudert M, Moller HD, Schulze M, Wirth CJ (2000) Tissue engineering for therapy of osteochondral cartilage lesions. Zentralbl Chir 125(6):509–515
Salomon FV (2001) Personal Communication. Department of Veterinary Medicine, University of Leipzig, Leipzig, Germany
Sansone V, de Girolamo L, Pascale W, Melato M, Pascale V (2015) Long-term results of abrasion arthroplasty for full-thickness cartilage lesions of the medial femoral condyle. Arthroscopy 31(3):396–403, doi:S0749-8063(14)00841-X [pii] 10.1016/j.arthro.2014.10.007
Saris DB, Vanlauwe J, Victor J, Almqvist KF, Verdonk R, Bellemans J, Luyten FP (2009) Treatment of symptomatic cartilage defects of the knee: characterized chondrocyte implantation results in better clinical outcome at 36 months in a randomized trial compared to microfracture. Am J Sports Med 37(Suppl 1):10S–19S, doi:0363546509350694 [pii] 10.1177/0363546509350694
Scheller G, Sobau C, Bulow JU (2001) Arthroscopic partial lateral meniscectomy in an otherwise normal knee: Clinical, functional, and radiographic results of a long-term follow-up study. Arthroscopy 17(9):946–952, doi:S0749-8063(01)57748-8 [pii] 10.1053/jars.2001.28952
Seil R (2003) Die Ersatzplastik des vorderen Kreuzbandes bei offenen Wachstumsfugen - eine experimentelle Untersuchung. Saarland University, Homburg, Habilitation thesis
Seil R, Pape D, Kohn D (2008) The risk of growth changes during transphyseal drilling in sheep with open physes. Arthroscopy 24(7):824–833, doi:S0749-8063(08)00149-7 [pii] 10.1016/j.arthro.2008.02.007
Sellers RS, Peluso D, Morris EA (1997) The effect of recombinant human bone morphogenetic protein-2 (rhBMP-2) on the healing of full-thickness defects of articular cartilage. J Bone Joint Surg Am 79(10):1452–1463
Shapiro F, Koide S, Glimcher MJ (1993) Cell origin and differentiation in the repair of full-thickness defects of articular cartilage. J Bone Joint Surg Am 75(4):532–553
Simon WH (1971) Scale effects in animal jointsII. Thickness and elasticity in the deformability of articular cartilage. Arthritis Rheum 14(4):493–502
Smillie IS (1957) Treatment of osteochondritis dissecans. J Bone Joint Surg Br 39(2):248–260
Song EK, Seon JK, Park SJ, Jeong MS (2010) The complications of high tibial osteotomy: closing- versus opening-wedge methods. J Bone Joint Surg Br 92(9):1245–1252, doi:92-B/9/1245 [pii] 10.1302/0301-620X.92B9.23660
Stadelmaier DM, Arnoczky SP, Dodds J, Ross H (1995) The effect of drilling and soft tissue grafting across open growth plates. A histologic study. Am J Sports Med 23(4):431–435
Steadman JR, Rodkey WG, Rodrigo JJ (2001) Microfracture: surgical technique and rehabilitation to treat chondral defects. Clin Orthop (391 Suppl):S362-369
Van Thiel GS, Frank RM, Gupta A, Ghodadra N, Shewman EF, Wang VM, Bach BR, Verma NN, Cole BJ, Provencher MT (2011) Biomechanical evaluation of a high tibial osteotomy with a meniscal transplant. J Knee Surg 24(1):45–53
Vasiliadis HS, Danielson B, Ljungberg M, McKeon B, Lindahl A, Peterson L (2010) Autologous chondrocyte implantation in cartilage lesions of the knee: long-term evaluation with magnetic resonance imaging and delayed gadolinium-enhanced magnetic resonance imaging technique. Am J Sports Med 38(5):943–949, doi:0363546509358266 [pii] 10.1177/0363546509358266
Wang YX, Hussain SM, Krestin GP (2001) Superparamagnetic iron oxide contrast agents: physicochemical characteristics and applications in MR imaging. Eur Radiol 11(11):2319–2331, doi:10.1007/s003300100908
W-Dahl A, Robertsson O, Lohmander LS (2012) High tibial osteotomy in Sweden, 1998–2007. Acta Orthop. doi:10.3109/17453674.2012.688725
Wei L, Hjerpe A, Brismar BH, Svensson O (2001) Effect of load on articular cartilage matrix and the development of guinea-pig osteoarthritis. Osteoarthritis Cartilage 9(5):447–453, doi:10.1053/joca.2000.0411 S1063-4584(00)90411-4 [pii]
Zellner J, Kujat R, Koch M, Angele P (2014) Role of mesenchymal stem cells in meniscal repair. J Exp Orthop 1 (12). doi:10.1186/s40634-014-0012-y
Ziegler R, Goebel L, Cucchiarini M, Pape D, Madry H (2013) Effect of open wedge high tibial osteotomy on the lateral tibiofemoral compartment in sheep. Part II: standard and overcorrection do not cause articular cartilage degeneration. Knee Surg Sports Traumatol Arthrosc. doi:10.1007/s00167-013-2410-6
Ziegler R, Goebel L, Seidel R, Cucchiarini M, Pape D, Madry H (2014) Effect of open wedge high tibial osteotomy on the lateral tibiofemoral compartment in sheep. Part III: analysis of the microstructure of the subchondral bone and correlations with the articular cartilage and meniscus. Knee Surg Sports Traumatol Arthrosc. doi:10.1007/s00167-014-3134-y

Development and validation of a new method for locating patella sensory nerves for the treatment of inferior and superior knee pain

Emily Hu[1*], Jessica Preciado[1], Vinod Dasa[2] and Jason Mussell[3]

Abstract

Background: Radiofrequency ablation and percutaneous cryoneurolysis to relieve knee pain requires treating large areas to ensure coverage due to high variability in the sensory innervation of the knee and limitations of current methods for defining treatment targets. This study sought to define and validate a new treatment approach targeting the major sensory nerves of the superior patella and expand upon previous work to define a more efficient treatment approach targeting the sensory nerves of the inferior patella.

Methods: Transcutaneous electrical nerve stimulation and ultrasound were used to evaluate the location and relationship of the cutaneous nerves to the superior and inferior aspects of the knee in 25 healthy volunteers. Using information derived from these evaluations, investigators defined new linear target treatment areas, or treatment lines, using anatomical landmarks, which were validated against locations of sensory nerves through cadaveric dissection of 15 fresh specimens.

Results: The proposed treatment lines captured the vast majority of nerve branching variations during cadaveric validation.

Conclusion: This study defined treatment lines, identifiable using only anatomical landmarks, which effectively target the nerves responsible for superior and inferior knee pain and reduce the total treatment area and procedure time when administering treatments such as radiofrequency ablation and cryoneurolysis.

Keywords: Anterior knee pain; Infrapatellar nerves; Saphenous nerve; Femoral cutaneous nerves; Cryoneurolysis

Background

Nerve-targeting treatments for knee pain, such as radiofrequency ablation and percutaneous cryoneurolysis, require treating large areas to ensure coverage of the target nerve(s), due to high variability in the sensory innervation patterns of the knee and limited descriptions of these variations in the literature (Horner & Dellon 1994). Methods of localizing the nerves that contribute to patellar pain include ultrasound imaging and transcutaneous electrical nerve stimulation (TENS). Because the nerves that innervate the patella are normally small (0.5-3 mm in diameter), sonographic visualization can be difficult and time consuming (Gray 2012; Scott 2012). TENS requires searching the entire surface area of the anterior thigh using the TENS wand, which is time consuming as well and may be uncomfortable for the patient. A method of localizing the sensory nerves of the superior and inferior patella using only anatomical landmarks would improve treatment efficiency and tolerability.

Currently, there is no validated anatomical treatment approach that targets the branches of the anterior femoral cutaneous nerve (AFCN) and the lateral femoral cutaneous nerve (LFCN), which innervate the superior aspect of the patella and the surrounding tissue (Scott 2012).

* Correspondence: Emily.s.hu@gmail.com
[1]myoscience, Inc., 46400 Fremont Blvd, Fremont, CA 94538, USA
Full list of author information is available at the end of the article

A previous anatomical study in five embalmed cadavers mapped the course of the infrapatellar saphenous nerve (ISN) and medial cutaneous femoral nerve (MFCN), which are responsible for sensory innervation of the inferior aspect of the patella and the surrounding tissue (Le Corroller et al. 2011). Investigators found that the infrapatellar branches of the ISN and the MFCN are located within the area between 55 mm from the medial border of the patella and 44 mm from the medial border of the patellar tendon (Le Corroller et al. 2011). A "treatment box" which targets the branches of ISN and MFCN responsible for inferior patella pain may be defined using these anatomical landmarks as the medial and lateral borders, respectively, and the midline of the patella and top of the tibial tubercle as the superior and inferior borders, respectively. When utilizing this approach to located and treat these nerve branches, the entire length of the treatment box must be treated. This is a large area that includes locations that do not contain nerves of interest, increasing operator time and patient discomfort.

The present study was designed to 1) investigate the locations of the sensory nerves that innervate the superior and inferior patella; 2) using only bony landmarks, define a treatment approach which encompasses all variations of branching patterns of the AFCN, LFCN, MFCN, and ISN as identified using TENS and ultrasound; and 3) validate the accuracy of the treatment approach using cadaveric dissections. This study aims to break new ground by developing the first validated methodology for targeting the nerves that innervate the superior patella. In addition, this study will expand upon previous work targeting the nerves that innervate the inferior patella by defining a more efficient treatment approach.

Methods

TENS and ultrasound nerve location study in volunteers

The study protocol was approved by an ethics committee and informed consent was obtained from all individual participants included in the study. All procedures performed in studies involving human participants were in accordance with the ethical standards of the institutional and/or national research committee and with the 1964 Helsinki declaration and its later amendments or comparable ethical standards. Eligible subjects were healthy adults aged 18–60 years with no history of surgery, trauma, or altered anatomy in the measurement areas.

All subjects were examined in the supine position with the knees extended using the SonoSite M-Turbo® Ultrasound System with a 14 MHz linear transducer and the Braun Stimuplex® HNS 12. The ultrasound transducer was placed in the transverse plane with a short axis view of the nerve and held in minimal contact with the skin to ensure that the skin above the nerve was not compressed during measurement. Branches of nerves were identified on the ultrasound as small echogenic honeycomb-shaped structures under the fat layers and on top of the muscle fascia. Nerve branches were located and measured on one or both knees.

Innervation of the superior knee

To locate the AFCN and LFCN, a vertical line bisecting the anterior thigh along the sagittal plane was drawn from the center of the patella to the top of the femoral head at the iliac crease (Fig. 1). The vertical line and the width of the patella were measured. The surface of the thigh was traced with the TENS wand with an initial setting of 1.3 mA, 1.0 ms, and 2.0 Hz. The TENS current

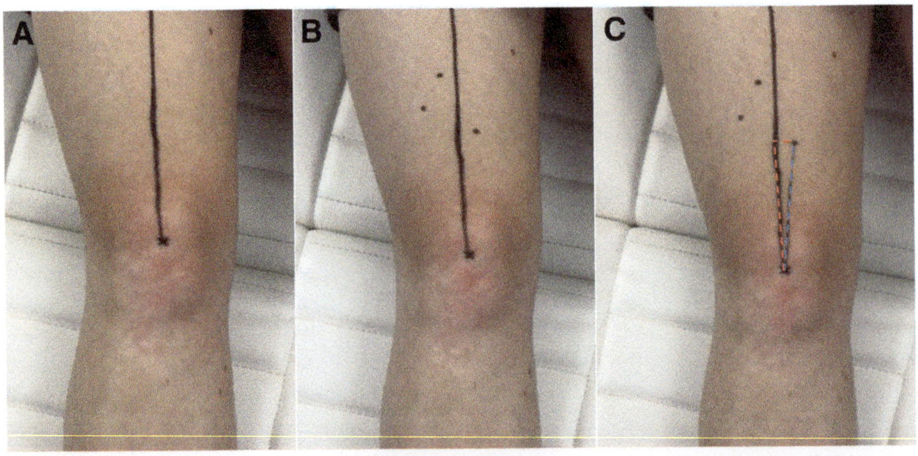

Fig. 1 AFCN and LFCN localization and measurement method. A vertical line bisecting the anterior thigh along the sagittal plane is drawn from the center of the patella to the top of the femoral head at the iliac crease (**a**). AFCN and LFCN branches which innervate the superior patella are located using TENS. Black dots on thigh indicate nerve locations (**b**). For each nerve location, the distance to and along the vertical center line is measured, denoted by the red dotted lines. A line is drawn from the nerve location to the center of the knee, denoted by the blue dotted line, and the angle between this line and the vertical center line is measured (**c**)

was increased in increments of 0.2 mA until the subject reported a sensation in or near the medial portion of the superior edge of the patella. Areas of maximal TENS response for the AFCN branches were located using subject feedback and recorded. These locations were retraced with incrementally lower currents to minimize the radius of stimulation and further specify the nerve location, until pain or sensation in the superior knee was no longer felt by the subject. The final nerve location was marked; this process was repeated for all areas of TENS response for the superior knee. The distance from each nerve location to the vertical center line was measured. A line was drawn from each nerve location to the center of the knee to form an angle with the vertical center line of the thigh, which was measured.

The area between two nerve locations was then traced with the TENS wand in order to discern which nerve locations arose from the same branch. If the subject reported identical sensations when the wand was passed between the nerve locations as when the wand was directly on the nerve locations, it was assumed that the locations were part of the same nerve branch. All nerve locations were confirmed and nerve depths measured using ultrasound. .

Innervation of the inferior knee

To locate the infrapatellar nerve branches innervating the inferior patella, a treatment box (Fig. 2) was drawn on the knee using the anatomical landmarks described by Le Corroller et al., and its dimensions measured (Le Corroller et al. 2011). The surface of the skin within the treatment box was traced with the TENS wand with an initial setting of 1.5 mA, 1.0 ms, and 2.0Hz. Nerve locations were identified using the same technique described for the femoral cutaneous nerves of the superior knee. Each nerve location was marked and its distance from the borders of the treatment box measured. The nerve location and measurement procedure was repeated for all areas of maximal TENS response within the treatment box and at additional infrapatellar nerve locations superior, inferior, and medial to the treatment box (Fig. 3).

After all nerve locations were identified, investigators used the same technique described for the femoral cutaneous nerves to discern which nerve locations arose from the same infrapatellar nerve branch. The infrapatellar nerve location was confirmed and nerve depth measured via ultrasound.

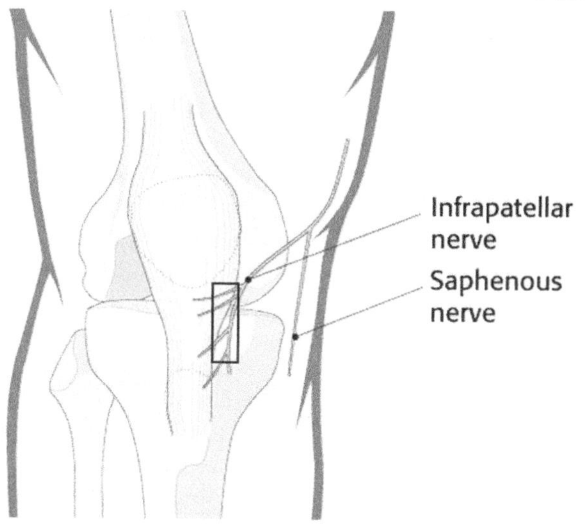

Fig. 2 Infrapatellar nerve "treatment box" targeting the ISN and MFCN as defined by Le Corroller. The medial and lateral borders of "treatment box" occur 55 mm medial from the medial border of the patella and 44 mm medial from the medial border of the patellar tendon, respectively. The midline of patella serves as the superior border, and the top of the tibial tubercle the inferior border. Treatment box is not drawn to scale

Cadaveric validation

After completion of data analysis from the TENS and ultrasound study, Investigators used the branching patterns that had been identified to propose two linear target treatment areas, or treatment lines, which would optimally target the nerves. These treatment lines were then validated through cadaveric dissection. Prior to dissection, the proposed treatment lines for the nerves innervating the superior and inferior patella were drawn on the skin. All cadavers were inspected to verify the presence of cutaneous nerves at the proposed treatment lines. Dissection began at the anterior superior iliac spine and continued to the region of the superior tibia, inferior to the tibial tubercle. To reveal the presence of the nerves, the skin and fat layers inferior to the treatment line for the femoral cutaneous nerves (superior patella) and medial to the treatment line for the infrapatellar nerves (inferior patella) were removed (Fig. 4).

Results

For the TENS and ultrasound nerve location study, volunteers were 25 healthy adults (12 females and 13 males) with a mean age of 39 ± 12 years and an average body mass index (BMI) of 27 (6) kg/m^2.

For the cadaveric validation, fifteen fresh human thigh/knee specimens from 10 cadavers (2 females, 8 males) were dissected. The cadavers were classified into 3 groups by BMI, which was approximated through visual estimation by the orthopedic surgeon performing the dissections. Three specimens were classified as lean (BMI <20 mg/kg^2), seven as average (BMI 20–30 mg/kg^2), and five as heavy (BMI >30 mg/kg^2).

Innervation of the superior knee

Nerve branches in the superior knee were located and measured in 22 subjects (10 bilateral and 12 unilateral).

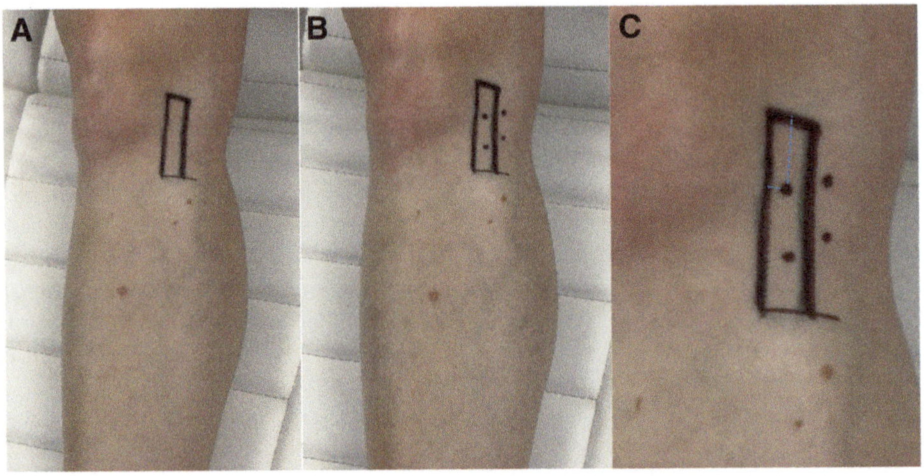

Fig. 3 ISN and MFCN localization and measurement method. Le Corroller's treatment box is drawn (**a**) and nerves are located using TENS within, superior, inferior, and medial to the treatment box. Black dots indicate nerve locations determined using TENS (**b**). The distance from each nerve location to the borders of the treatment box is then measured, indicated by the blue dotted lines (**c**)

Using data obtained from TENS and ultrasound nerve localization, investigators created a heat map depicting the population density of nerve branches within the measurement area (Fig. 5). Nerve locations were measured relative to the total length of the vertical center line connecting the center of the patella to the top of the femur. Nerves were identified superior to the center of the patella at a mean distance of 36 % ±13 % of the total length of the vertical center line. The mean distance of the maximum (i.e. furthest from the center of the patella) nerve location for each thigh was on average 45 % ± 13 % along the length of the vertical center line. In 56 % (18/32) of thighs, all nerve locations were found on or medial to the vertical center line and the lines connecting each nerve location to the center of the patella were located between 25° medial and 10° lateral to the center of the knee.

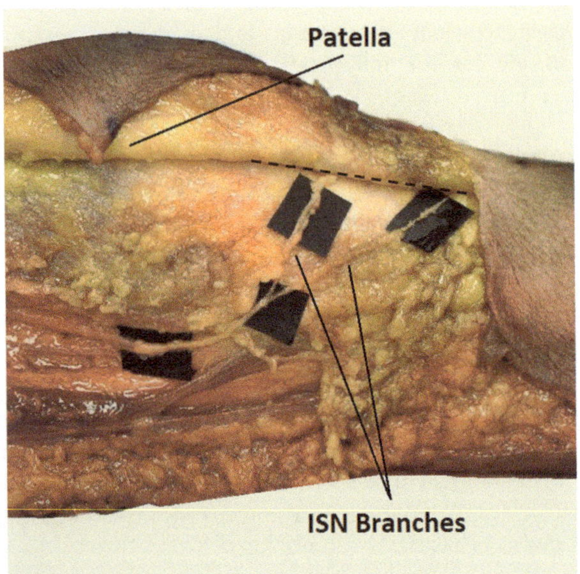

Fig. 4 Infrapatellar nerves of the left thigh. Two branches of the ISN cross the treatment line to provide sensory innervation to the inferior knee. Dotted line denotes treatment line

At least one nerve branch was found in 91 % (29/32) and two nerve branches in 50 % (16/32) of thighs. When two branches were identified, they were a mean of 2.7 ± 1.2 cm apart; in all cases, the distance between the branches of the nerves innervating the superior knee was less than the width of the patella at all points along the nerve branches.

The majority (57 %) of nerve locations determined using TENS occurred superior to the center of the patella at a distance of 20–40 % along the length of vertical center line; therefore, it was determined that treatment would be optimally located at a distance of 1/3 along the vertical length of the thigh superior to the knee. At this distance from the center of the patella, the medial and later borders of the patella represent the lines 25° medial and 10° lateral to the center of the knee. Therefore, a proposed horizontal treatment "line" drawn at a distance of 1/3 the vertical length of the thigh superior to the knee and connecting the medial and lateral orders of the patella would encompass the largest occurrence of femoral cutaneous nerves innervating the superior knee (Fig. 6). The proposed horizontal treatment line was validated through cadaveric dissection and was found to intersect the femoral cutaneous nerves in 93 % (14/15) of the cadaver specimens.

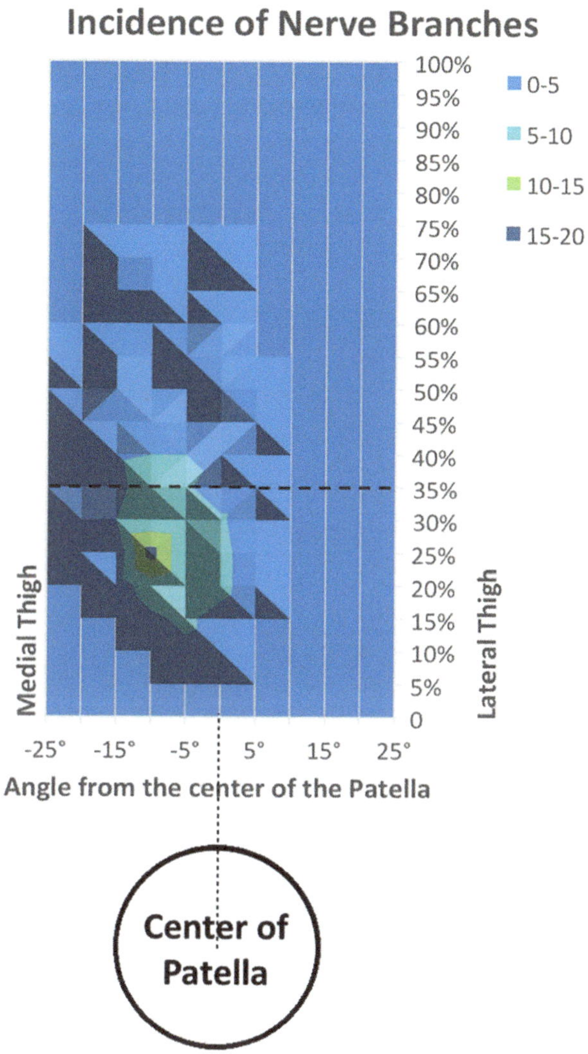

Fig. 5 Heat map of the occurrence of the branches of the femoral cutaneous nerve using the left leg where x = 0, y = 0 is the center of the patella. The x-axis represents the angle from the nerve branch to the vertical midline of the patella; the y-axis represents the percent distance of the nerve branch along the thigh; and the z-axis indicates the number of nerve branches occurring at each location. The majority of nerve locations determined using TENS occur at the light blue and green regions of the map. The dotted black line denotes the proposed treatment line

Innervation of the inferior knee

Nerve branches in the inferior knee were located and measured in 24 subjects (19 bilateral and 5 unilateral). Knees were assessed for the number of branches innervating the inferior knee located within the measurement area; there were 14 % (6/43) of knees with one branch, 72 % (31/43) with two branches, 7 % (3/43) with three branches, and 7 % (3/43) for whom no branch patterns could be discerned within the measurement area. Most (83 %; 15/18) subjects had the same number of nerve branches innervating the inferior knee on both lower extremities; there was one subject for whom nerve locations were identified but branching patterns could not be confirmed. Although it is possible that the remaining 17 % of subjects had an asymmetrical number of branches, it is more likely that additional infrapatellar branches of the MFCN or ISN could not be detected by TENS due to their small size. For many subjects, including those with a symmetrical number of nerve branches on both extremities, nerve locations were not necessarily identical on each side. In 37 % (7/19) of assessed bilateral knees, there was a 20 % or greater difference in the distance from the superior border of the treatment box defined using Le Corroller's methodology for one or more branches of the infrapatellar nerve between the subject's right and left lower extremity.

For the 24 subjects (43 knees) measured, the most superior infrapatellar nerve branch was located an average distance of 45 % ± 30 % of the length of the treatment box inferior to the superior border of the treatment box (Fig. 7). The most inferior infrapatellar nerve branch was located an average distance of 15 % ± 25 % of the length

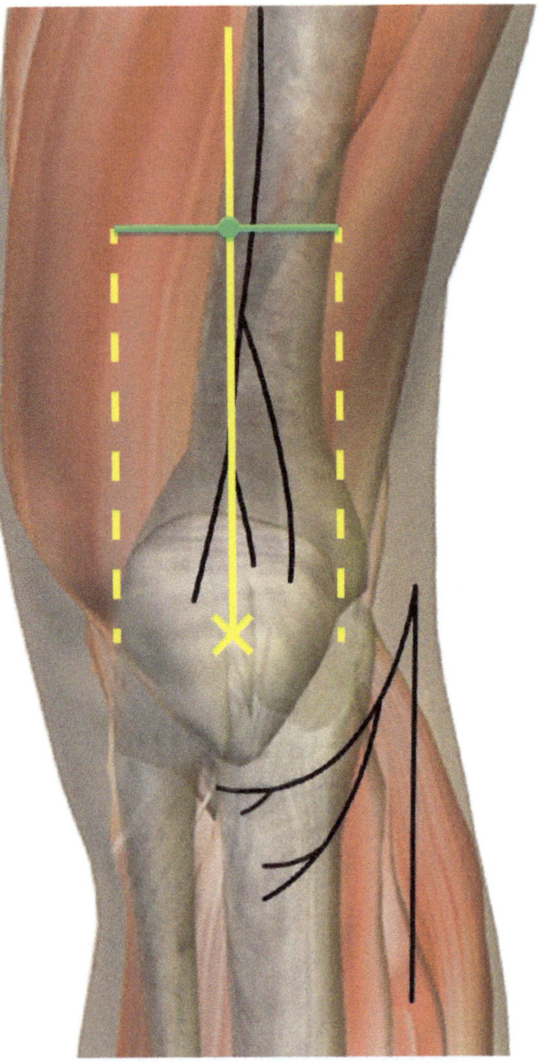

Fig. 6 Proposed treatment line for the superior knee. Green line denotes the treatment line. Yellow X denotes the center of the patella. Yellow solid line denotes the vertical midline of the patella. Yellow dotted lines denote the lateral and medial treatment line boundaries, the lateral and medial borders of the patella, respectively. Picture not drawn to scale

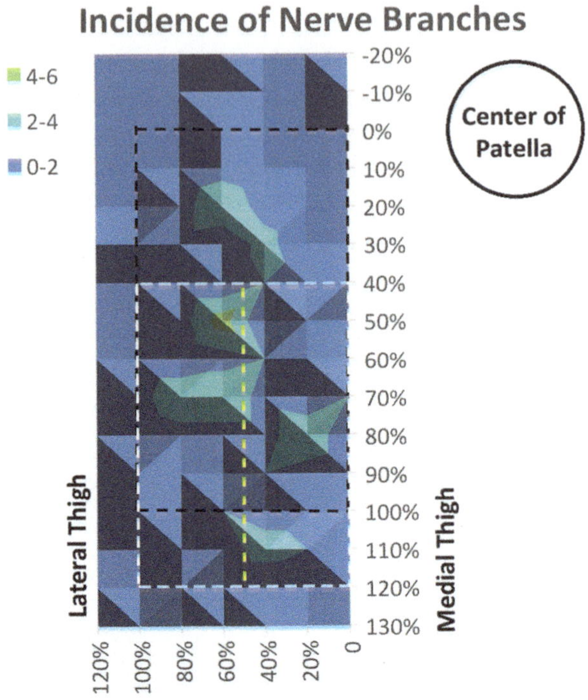

Fig. 7 Heat map of the occurrence of the infrapatellar branches of the MFCN and ISN on the right knee. The x-axis represents the percentage of the width of the treatment box lateral to the patella; the y-axis represents the percentage of the length of the treatment box inferior to the patella; and the z-axis indicates the number of nerve branches occurring at each location. The superior, inferior, medial, and lateral boundaries of the treatment box as determined by Le Corroller are defined as y = 0, y = 100, x = 0, and x = 100, respectively, and are denoted by the dotted black box. The majority of nerve locations determined using TENS occur within the area bound by the dotted white box. The dotted yellow line denotes the proposed treatment line

of the treatment box superior to the lower border of the treatment box.

Eighty percent of all identifiable infrapatellar nerve branches were located within 40–120 % the length of the treatment box inferior to the upper border (denoted by the white dotted box in Fig. 7). Anatomical landmarks that correlated to these locations were identified as the lower pole of the patella (upper bound) and immediately inferior to the tibial tubercle (lower bound). Thus, a vertical treatment line originating at 50 mm medial to the lower pole of the patella and connecting to the lower pole of the patella at a point just inferior to the tibial tubercle in a straight line would encompass 80 % of the nerve branches innervating the anteromedial aspect of the inferior knee (Fig. 8). The proposed vertical treatment line was validated through cadaveric dissection and was found to intersect the infrapatellar nerves in 93 % (14/15) of the cadaver specimens.

Discussion

This study is the first to describe a new approach to more efficiently locate and treat the sensory nerves of the superior and inferior knee to relieve pain. Using data derived from TENS and ultrasound localization, investigators defined two treatment lines that can be identified using only anatomical landmarks to target the sensory nerves innervating the superior and inferior knee.

For the nerves of the superior knee, the horizontal treatment line is defined at a distance of 1/3 the vertical length of the thigh superior to the knee and connects the medial and lateral borders of the patella. In cases where the proposed horizontal treatment line does not capture the target nerves, as indicated by an insufficient reduction in superior knee pain, treatment should be extended medially past the medial edge of the patella, as the majority of femoral cutaneous nerve branches occur medial to the

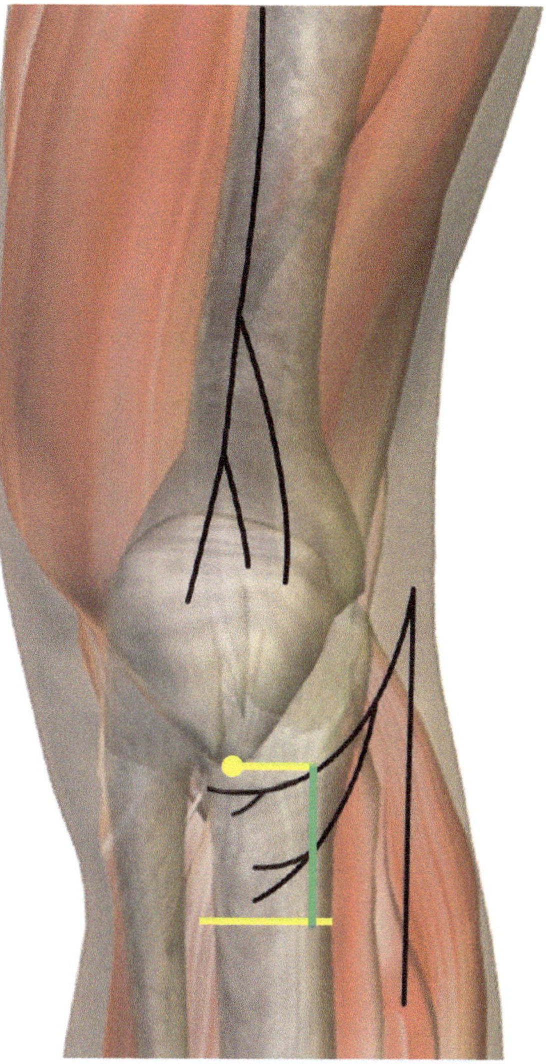

Fig. 8 Treatment line for the inferior knee. Picture not drawn to scale. Yellow solid lines denote the superior and inferior borders of the treatment line, the lower pole of the patella and the tibial tubercle, respectively. Green line denotes treatment line, a vertical line which is located 5 cm medial to the lower pole of the patella

vertical centerline of the thigh. The present study was the first to define and validate a treatment line to target the major sensory nerves of the superior patella using anatomical landmarks. This novel approach obviates the need for additional location instrumentation and captures the vast majority of variations in the branching patterns of the targeted sensory nerves in the superior knee.

In addition, this study refined a basic approximation for targeting nerves of the inferior knee developed by Le Correller et al. and validated the new method with a larger sample of cadaver specimens (15 fresh versus 5 embalmed cadavers) than were used by Le Correller et al. (Le Corroller et al. 2011). Results from the TENS location on live volunteers and cadaveric dissections in the present study corroborate findings of previous studies on the innervation and branching patterns in the inferior knee, and confirm that a vertical treatment line at the specified landmarks should allow for the successful treatment of inferior knee pain in most individuals (Kalthur et al. 2015; Kartus et al. 1999; Scott 2012; Tifford et al. 2000). In cases where this line does not capture all targeted branches, suboptimal results for treating inferior knee pain could be improved by extending treatment superiorly along the treatment line to the center of the patella and inferiorly to 1 cm below the tibial tubercle, as a small percentage of nerve branches cross the treatment line at the level of the patella or inferior to the tibial tuberosity. The location of this treatment line is consistent with findings by Kalthur et al., who found that that the infrapatellar nerve branches were located between the lower pole of the patella to under the tibial tubercle in 65.6 % of cases, with the remaining 15.6 % and 18.7 % of cases located near the patella and tibial tuberosity, respectively (Kalthur et al. 2015). In the present study, two branches innervating the inferior knee were located within the measurement area in 72 % of knees, with a single branch in 14 % and three branches in 7 % of knees. These findings are consistent with those of a previous cadaver study, which found that the infrapatellar saphenous nerve had a single branch, two branches, and three branches innervating the inferior patella in 25 %, 62 %, and 10 % of knees, respectively (Kartus et al. 1999).

These treatment lines allow for the treatment of various types of indications, including the treatment of osteoarthritis knee pain in the anterior and medial knee and treatment prior to knee surgery to reduce post-operative pain. In a surgical setting, the sensory innervation of the anterior knee described within this paper covers the workhorse anterior midline knee incision used in surgeries such as total knee replacement. Other potential uses for these treatment lines include treatment of neuropathic pain associated with conditions such as diabetes. However, due to anatomical variability and unpredictability, treating the entirety of the treatment line(s) in all patients may be worthwhile to ensure that all potential branches are targeted. If branches responsible for knee pain remain untreated, clinical results may not be as robust. Further clinical studies are needed to confirm whether treatment of all nerves branches which cross the treatment line is required to provide a meaningful clinical benefit for patients or if treatment of a subset of branches is sufficient.

Limitations of this study include its relatively small sample size of 25 live volunteers and 10 cadaver dissections, with a disproportionately low representation of individuals with BMIs greater than 40 (which compromise the majority of chronic knee pain patients). However, looking at the variation between the existing BMI subgroups and their local anatomies, we anticipate the anatomy in the higher BMI patients to follow the same pattern as those from < 20 to 40. While we would expect a larger subcutaneous adipose layer, the underlying nerve would follow the same course along the fascia and retinaculum since this is independent of the thickness of the adipose tissue. The limiting factor of treatment within this group may be the technology's ability to reach deeper nerves rather than expecting a variation in nerve location an anatomy. Further research could include additional cadaver dissections to cover a larger variety of BMIs.

Another limitation of this study was that it excluded subjects with prior knee surgeries, distortions (including scar tissue), or neuropathies in the measurement area as the impact of these conditions on local anatomy variation was unclear. Treating nerves in areas of previous surgery or trauma may be difficult. Clinicians will need to ensure that treatment is proximal to any potential neuroma formation to adequately disrupt transmission of the pain signal, and that the nerve path relative to the treatment line landmarks has not changed as a result of surgery or trauma. Other difficulties may include distorted local anatomy such as bone deformities which could render the treatment line landmarks ineffective. Scar tissue could present multiple difficulties in isolating and distinguishing the targeted nerve using imaging such as ultrasound as well as effectively treating the nerve once found. Further research is needed to assess the impact of deformities, common surgical approaches, and local trauma on nerve location and potential response to treatment.

Conclusions

This study increases knowledge of the anatomical relationships between the knee region and the cutaneous nerves that innervate it. Despite common variations in the innervation and branching of the femoral, medial, and lateral femoral cutaneous nerves and saphenous nerves, anatomical treatment lines were defined using the results of this study to efficiently and effectively locate and target the sensory nerves implicated in superior and inferior knee pain. The cadaver study confirmed that TENS is a highly accurate method of locating the target nerves on live subjects, as the treatment lines intersected all of the nerves innervating the knee regions most commonly associated with knee pain in 93 % of cadaver specimens. Applying treatment along these treatment lines should effectively target the nerves responsible for superior and inferior knee pain and reduce the total treatment area and procedure time when administering treatments such as radiofrequency ablation and cryoneurolysis.

Abbreviations

AFCN: Anterior femoral cutaneous nerve; BMI: Body mass index; ISN: Infrapatellar saphenous nerve; LFCN: Lateral femoral cutaneous nerve; MFCN: Medial cutaneous femoral nerve; TENS: Transcutaneous electrical nerve stimulation.

Competing interests

Emily Hu and Jessica Preciado are paid employees of and own stock in myoscience, Inc. Vinod Dasa is a paid consultant of myoscience, Inc., Bioventus, Ferring Pharmaceuticals, and Cropper Medical. Jason Mussell is a paid consultant of myoscience, Inc.

Authors' contributions

The TENS and Ultrasound Nerve Location Study in Volunteers was designed by EH and JP and executed by EH. The data analysis and development of the treatment lines were performed by EH. All authors participated in the design and execution of the cadaveric validation. EH performed the statistical analysis and drafted the manuscript. All authors read and approved the final manuscript.

Acknowledgments

We thank Amy Bronstone who provided technical writing services on behalf of myoscience, inc.

Author details

[1]myoscience, Inc., 46400 Fremont Blvd, Fremont, CA 94538, USA. [2]Department of Orthopedics, Louisiana State University, 1542 Tulane Avenue, Box T6-7, New Orleans, LA 70112, USA. [3]Department of Cell Biology and Anatomy, Louisiana State University, 1901 Perdido Street, Room 6123A, New Orleans, LA 70112, USA.

References

Gray AT (2012) Altas of Ultrasound-guided Regional Anesthesia, 2nd edn. Saunders, Philadelphia

Horner G, Dellon AL (1994) Innervation of the human knee joint and implications for surgery. Clin Orthop Relat Res 301:221–226

Kalthur SG, Sumalatha S, Nair N, Pandey AK, Sequeria S, Shobha L (2015) Anatomic study of infrapatellar branch of saphenous nerve in male cadavers. Ir J Med Sci 184:201–6

Kartus J, Ejerhed L, Eriksson BI, Karlsson J (1999) The localization of the infrapatellar nerves in the anterior knee region with special emphasis on central third patellar tendon harvest: a dissection study on cadaver and amputated specimens. Arthroscopy 15:577–586

Le Corroller T, Lagier A, Pirro N, Champsaur P (2011) Anatomical study of the infrapatellar branch of the saphenous nerve using ultrasonography. Muscle Nerve 44:50–54

Scott WN (2012) Anatomy. In: Insall and Scott Surgery of the Knee, 5th edn. Churchill Livingstone, Philadelphia

Tifford CD, Spero L, Luke T, Plancher KD (2000) The relationship of the infrapatellar branches of the saphenous nerve to arthroscopy portals and incisions for anterior cruciate ligament surgery an anatomic study. Am J Sports Med 28:562–567

Permissions

All chapters in this book were first published in JEO, by Springer; hereby published with permission under the Creative Commons Attribution License or equivalent. Every chapter published in this book has been scrutinized by our experts. Their significance has been extensively debated. The topics covered herein carry significant findings which will fuel the growth of the discipline. They may even be implemented as practical applications or may be referred to as a beginning point for another development.

The contributors of this book come from diverse backgrounds, making this book a truly international effort. This book will bring forth new frontiers with its revolutionizing research information and detailed analysis of the nascent developments around the world.

We would like to thank all the contributing authors for lending their expertise to make the book truly unique. They have played a crucial role in the development of this book. Without their invaluable contributions this book wouldn't have been possible. They have made vital efforts to compile up to date information on the varied aspects of this subject to make this book a valuable addition to the collection of many professionals and students.

This book was conceptualized with the vision of imparting up-to-date information and advanced data in this field. To ensure the same, a matchless editorial board was set up. Every individual on the board went through rigorous rounds of assessment to prove their worth. After which they invested a large part of their time researching and compiling the most relevant data for our readers.

The editorial board has been involved in producing this book since its inception. They have spent rigorous hours researching and exploring the diverse topics which have resulted in the successful publishing of this book. They have passed on their knowledge of decades through this book. To expedite this challenging task, the publisher supported the team at every step. A small team of assistant editors was also appointed to further simplify the editing procedure and attain best results for the readers.

Apart from the editorial board, the designing team has also invested a significant amount of their time in understanding the subject and creating the most relevant covers. They scrutinized every image to scout for the most suitable representation of the subject and create an appropriate cover for the book.

The publishing team has been an ardent support to the editorial, designing and production team. Their endless efforts to recruit the best for this project, has resulted in the accomplishment of this book. They are a veteran in the field of academics and their pool of knowledge is as vast as their experience in printing. Their expertise and guidance has proved useful at every step. Their uncompromising quality standards have made this book an exceptional effort. Their encouragement from time to time has been an inspiration for everyone.

The publisher and the editorial board hope that this book will prove to be a valuable piece of knowledge for researchers, students, practitioners and scholars across the globe.

List of Contributors

Justus-Martijn Brinkman and Ronald J van Heerwaarden
Department of Orthopaedics, Limb deformity reconstruction unit, Sint Maartensclinic, Woerden, The Netherlands

Christof Hurschler
Labor für Biomechanik und Biomaterialien, Orthopädische Klinik der Medizinischen Hochschule Hanover, Hanover, Germany

Jens Agneskirchner and Philip Lobenhoffer
Sportsclinic Germany, Hanover, Germany

René M Castelein
Department of Orthopedics, University Medical Centre Utrecht, Utrecht, The Netherlands

John J Wilson, Connie Chamberlain, Geoffrey S Baer, Marcus Greatens and Nicole Kamps
Division of Sports Medicine, Department of Orthopedics and Rehabilitation, University of Wisconsin School of Medicine and Public Health, 1685 Highland Avenue, Madison, Wisconsin 53705, USA

Kenneth S Lee
Department of Radiology, University of Wisconsin School of Medicine and Public Health, Madison, Wisconsin 53705, USA

Ryan DeWall
Department of Biomedical Engineering, University of Wisconsin School of Medicine and Public Health, Madison, Wisconsin 53705, USA
Department of Radiology, University of Wisconsin School of Medicine and Public Health, Madison, Wisconsin 53705, USA

Juan Carlos Jacinto-Tinajero, Brenda Marquina and Jorge Barrios-Payán
Experimental Pathology and Surgery Departments, National Institute of Medical Sciences and Nutrition "Salvador Zubiran", Mexico city, Mexico

Daniel Ascencio
Plastic Surgery, Angeles Hospital, Mexico city, Mexico

Maria Concepcion Gutierrez
Experimental Biology Department, Metropolitan University, Mexico city, Mexico

Miguel Gomez Lim
Department of Genetic Engineering in Plants, National Politechnique Institute Center of Research and Advanced Studies, Irapuato, Mexico

Rogelio Hernández Pando
Experimental Pathology and Surgery Departments, National Institute of Medical Sciences and Nutrition "Salvador Zubiran", Mexico city, Mexico
Department of Pathology, National Institute of Medical Sciences and Nutrition 'Salvador Zubirán', Section of Experimental Pathology, Mexico city, DF 14000, Mexico

Claudio Rosso
Center for Advanced Orthopaedic Studies, Beth Israel Deaconess Medical Center and Harvard Medical School, Boston, MA, USA
Orthopaedic Department, University Hospital Basel and University of Basel, Basel, Switzerland
Altius Swiss Sportsmed Center, Rheinfelden, Switzerland

Andreas M Mueller
Center for Advanced Orthopaedic Studies, Beth Israel Deaconess Medical Center and Harvard Medical School, Boston, MA, USA
Orthopaedic Department, University Hospital Basel and University of Basel, Basel, Switzerland

Brett McKenzie, Vahid Entezari and Ara Nazarian
Center for Advanced Orthopaedic Studies, Beth Israel Deaconess Medical Center and Harvard Medical School, Boston, MA, USA

Andrea Cereatti and Ugo Della Croce
Information Engineering Unit, POLCOMING Department, University of Sassari, Sassari, Italy

Arun J Ramappa and Joseph P DeAngelis
Department of Orthopaedic Surgery, Beth Israel Deaconess Medical Center, Harvard Medical School, 330 Brookline Avenue, Stoneman 10, Boston, MA 02215, USA

Yoshihiro Kusayama, Yasushi Akamatsu, Ken Kumagai, Hideo Kobayashi, Masato Aratake and Tomoyuki Saito
Department of Orthopaedic Surgery, Yokohama City University School of Medicine, 3-9 Fukuura, Kanazawa-ku, Yokohama 236-0004, Japan

Tian Wang
Surgical & Orthopaedic Research Laboratories, Prince of Wales Clinical School, University of New South Wales, Clinical Science Bldg, Prince of Wales Hospital, Gate 6, Avoca Street, 2031 Sydney, Australia Graduate School of Biomedical Engineering, University of New South Wales, Sydney, NSW, Australia

Jonathon R Ball
Royal North Shore Hospital, St Leonards, NSW, Australia

Mattew H Pelletier and William R Walsh
Surgical & Orthopaedic Research Laboratories, Prince of Wales Clinical School, University of New South Wales, Clinical Science Bldg, Prince of Wales Hospital, Gate 6, Avoca Street, 2031 Sydney, Australia

Francesca Vannini
Orthopaedic Clinic and Movement Analysis Laboratory, Rizzoli Orthopaedic Institute, Via di Barbiano n. 1/10, 40136 Bologna, Italy

Berardo Di Matteo and Giuseppe Filardo
Orthopaedic Clinic and Biomechanics Laboratory, Rizzoli Orthopaedic Institute, Via di Barbiano n. 1/10, 40136 Bologna, Italy

Deborah J Gorth and Lachlan J Smith
Department of Neurosurgery, Perelman School of Medicine, University of Pennsylvania, 424 Stemmler Hall, 3450 Hamilton Walk, Philadelphia, PA 19104, USA
Department of Orthopaedic Surgery, Perelman School of Medicine, University of Pennsylvania, 424 Stemmler Hall, 3450 Hamilton Walk, Philadelphia, PA 19104, USA
Translational Musculoskeletal Research Center, Veterans Affairs Medical Center, 3900 Woodland Avenue, Philadelphia, PA 19104, USA

John T Martin, George R Dodge and Robert L Mauck
Department of Orthopaedic Surgery, Perelman School of Medicine, University of Pennsylvania, 424 Stemmler Hall, 3450 Hamilton Walk, Philadelphia, PA 19104, USA
Translational Musculoskeletal Research Center, Veterans Affairs Medical Center, 3900 Woodland Avenue, Philadelphia, PA 19104, USA

Dawn M Elliott
Department of Biomedical Engineering, College of Engineering, University of Delaware, 125 E. Delaware Ave, Newark, DE 19716, USA

Neil R Malhotra
Department of Neurosurgery, Perelman School of Medicine, University of Pennsylvania, 424 Stemmler Hall, 3450 Hamilton Walk, Philadelphia, PA 19104, USA
Department of Orthopaedic Surgery, Perelman School of Medicine, University of Pennsylvania, 424 Stemmler Hall, 3450 Hamilton Walk, Philadelphia, PA 19104, USA

Andreas Nilsson
Department of Orthopaedics, Institute of Clinical Sciences, Sahlgrenska Academy, University of Gothenburg, Sahlgrenska University Hospital, Guldhedsgatan 10 A, 413 46 Gothenburg, Sweden

Qiuxia Zhang and Jorma Styf
Department of Orthopaedics, Institute of Clinical Sciences, Sahlgrenska Academy, University of Gothenburg, Sahlgrenska University Hospital, Guldhedsgatan 10 A, 413 46 Gothenburg, Sweden Department of Orthopaedics, Sahlgrenska University Hospital, Gothenburg, Sweden

Peter Angele
University Medical Center Regensburg, Franz-Josef-Strauss-Allee 11, 93053 Regensburg, Germany
Sporthopaedicum Regensburg/Straubing, Hildegard von Bingen Strasse 1, 93053 Regensburg, Germany

Richard Kujat, Matthias Koch and Johannes Zellner
University Medical Center Regensburg, Franz-Josef-Strauss-Allee 11, 93053 Regensburg, Germany

Bernardo Crespo, Katharine J Wilson and Shannon M Pomeroy
Steadman Philippon Research Institute, 181 W. Meadow Dr. Suite 1000, Vail 81657 CO, USA

Cathrine Aga
Department of Orthopaedic Surgery, Oslo University Hospital and Faculty of Medicine, University of Oslo, Oslo, Norway

Robert F LaPrade
Steadman Philippon Research Institute, 181 W. Meadow Dr. Suite 1000, Vail 81657 CO, USA
The Steadman Clinic, Vail, CO, USA

Lars Engebretsen
Department of Orthopaedic Surgery, Oslo University Hospital and Faculty of Medicine, University of Oslo, Oslo, Norway
Oslo Sports Trauma Research Center, Oslo, Norway

Coen A Wijdicks
Department of Biomedical Engineering, Steadman Philippon Research Institute, 181 W. Meadow Dr. Suite 1000, Vail 81657 CO, USA

D Tan Nguyen, Sietske Dellbrügge, Leendert Blankevoort and Niek C van Dijk
Department of Orthopedic Surgery, Orthopaedic Research Center Amsterdam, Academic Medical Center, University of Amsterdam, P.O. Box 22660, 1100 DD Amsterdam, The Netherlands

Paul P Tak
Division of Clinical Immunology and Rheumatology, Academic Medical Center, University of Amsterdam, Amsterdam, The Netherlands
GlaxoSmithKline, Stevenage, U.K and University of Cambridge, Cambridge, UK

Savio L-Y Woo
Department of Bioengineering, Musculoskeletal Research Center, University of Pittsburgh, Pittsburgh, USA

Alan Getgood
The Fowler Kennedy Sport Medicine Clinic 3M Centre, The University of Western Ontario, London, Ontario N6A 3K7, Canada

Frances Henson
Department of Veterinary Medicine, University of Cambridge, Cambridge, UK

Carrie Skelton, Roger Brooks and Neil Rushton
The University of Cambridge Orthopaedic Research Unit, Cambridge, UK

Hans Guehring
Merck Serono GmbH, Darmstadt, Germany

Lisa A Fortier
Department of Clinical Sciences, Cornell University, Ithaca, USA

Páll Sigurgeir Jónasson, Lars Ekström, Jón Karlsson and Adad Baranto
Department of Orthopaedics, Institute of Clinical Sciences at Sahlgrenska Academy, University of Gothenburg and Sahlgrenska University Hospital, Gothenburg, Sweden

Anna Swärd
Östersund Hospital, Östersund, Sweden

Mikael Sansone and Mattias Ahldén
Orthocenter/IFK-KLINIKEN, Sports Medicine Clinic, Gothenburg, Sweden

Claudia Schlundt, Georg N Duda and Katharina Schmidt-Bleek
Julius Wolff Institut and Center for Musculoskeletal Surgery, Charité - Universitätsmedizin Berlin, Augustenburger Platz 1, 13353 Berlin, Germany
Berlin-Brandenburg Center for Regenerative Therapies, Charité - Universitätsmedizin Berlin, Augustenburger Platz 1, 13353 Berlin, Germany

Hanna Schell
Julius Wolff Institut and Center for Musculoskeletal Surgery, Charité - Universitätsmedizin Berlin, Augustenburger Platz 1, 13353 Berlin, Germany

Stuart B Goodman
Department of Orthopaedic Surgery and (by courtesy) Bioengineering, Stanford University Medical Center Outpatient Center, 450 Broadway St., M/C 6342, 94063 Redwood City, CA, USA

Gordana Vunjak-Novakovic
Department of Biomedical Engineering and Department of Medicine, Columbia University, 622 west 168th Street, VC12-234, 10032 New York, NY, USA

Elizaveta Kon and Giuseppe Filardo
Nano-Biotechnology Laboratory, Rizzoli Orthopaedic Institute, Via di Barbiano n. 1/10, 40136 Bologna, Italy

Francesco Perdisa, Giulia Venieri and Maurilio Marcacci
Biomechanics Laboratory, Rizzoli Orthopaedic Institute, Via di Barbiano n. 1/10, 40136 Bologna, Italy

Páll Sigurgeir Jónasson
SportsMed, Gothenburg, Sweden

Lars Ekström, Jón Karlsson and Adad Baranto
Department of Orthopaedics, Institute of Clinical Sciences at Sahlgrenska Academy, University of Gothenburg, and Sahlgrenska University Hospital, Gothenburg, Sweden

Hans-Arne Hansson
Institute of Biomedicine, Sahlgrenska Academy, University of Gothenburg, Gothenburg, Sweden

Mikael Sansone and Leif Swärd
Orthocenter/IFK-Kliniken, Gothenburg, Sweden

Marco Giordano, Francesco Falciglia, Alessia Poggiaroni, Angelo Gabriele Aulisa and Pietro Savignoni
Orthopaedics and Traumatology Division, Bambino Gesù Children's Hospital, Institute of Scientific Research, Piazza San Onofrio 4, I-00165 Rome, Italy

Vincenzo Guzzanti
Orthopaedics and Traumatology Division, Bambino Gesù Children's Hospital, Institute of Scientific Research, Piazza San Onofrio 4, I-00165 Rome, Italy
University of Cassino (FR), Cassino, Italy

Magali Cucchiarini
Center of Experimental Orthopaedics, Saarland University Medical Center and Saarland University, Bldg 37, Kirrbergerstr. 1, D-66421 Homburg, Germany
Cartilage Net of the Greater Region, Homburg, Germany

Christel Henrionnet, Didier Mainard and Astrid Pinzano
Cartilage Net of the Greater Region, Homburg, Germany
Ingénierie Moléculaire et Physiopathologie Articulaire, Unité Mixte de Recherches 7365 Centre National de la Recherche Scientifique, Université de Lorraine, F-54505 Vandoeuvre Lès Nancy, France

Henning Madry
Center of Experimental Orthopaedics, Saarland University Medical Center and Saarland University, Bldg 37, Kirrbergerstr. 1, D-66421 Homburg, Germany
Cartilage Net of the Greater Region, Homburg, Germany
Department of Orthopaedic Surgery, Saarland University Medical Center and Saarland University, D-66421 Homburg/Saar, Germany

Jerry Natenstedt and Jenny Dankelman
Department of Biomechanical Engineering, Faculty of Mechanical, Materials and Maritime Engineering, Delft University of Technology, Mekelweg 2, Delft 2628 CD, The Netherlands

Aimee C Kok
Department of Orthopedic Surgery, Academic Medical Centre, Meibergdreef 9, Amsterdam, AZ 1105, The Netherlands

Gabrielle JM Tuijthof
Department of Biomechanical Engineering, Faculty of Mechanical, Materials and Maritime Engineering, Delft University of Technology, Mekelweg 2, Delft 2628 CD, The Netherlands

Department of Orthopedic Surgery, Academic Medical Centre, Meibergdreef 9, Amsterdam, AZ 1105, The Netherlands

Bjørn Borsøe Christensen, Casper Bindzus Foldager, Morten Lykke Olesen, Louise Vingtoft and Jan Hendrik Duedal Rölfing
Orthopedic Research Laboratory, Aarhus University Hospital, Nørrebrogade 44, building 1A, 1. Floor, Aarhus, Denmark

Steffen Ringgaard
MR Research Center, Aarhus University Hospital, Skejby, Denmark

Martin Lind
Department of Sports Traumatology, Department of orthopedic surgery, Aarhus University Hospital, Aarhus, Denmark

Carlo Henning, Gabriel Poglia, Murilo Anderson Leie and Carlos Roberto Galia
Department of Orthopaedics, Hospital de Clínicas de Porto Alegre, Medicine School, Universidade Federal do Rio Grande do Sul, Rua Ramiro Barcelos, 2350, Zip Code 90035-003 Porto Alegre Rio Grande do Sul, Brazil

Silvia Pianigiani and Walter Pascale
IRCCS Istituto Ortopedico Galeazzi, via via R. Galeazzi 4, 20161 Milan, Italy

Jos Vander Sloten
KU Leuven, Biomechanics Section, Celestijnenlaan 300 - bus 2419, Leuven, Belgium

Luc Labey
KU Leuven, Mechanical Engineering Technology TC, Kleinhoefstraat 4, Geel, Belgium

Bernardo Innocenti
BEAMS Department, Université Libre de Bruxelles, Av. F. Roosevelt, 50 CP165/56, Bruxelles, Belgium
Arnaud Diffo Kaze, Stefan Maas, Danièle Waldmann, Andreas Zilian,
Faculty of Science, Technology and Communication, University of Luxembourg, 6, rue R. Coudenhove-Kalergi, L-1359 Luxembourg, Luxembourg

Klaus Dueck and
Department of Orthopedic Surgery, Centre Hospitalier de Luxembourg, L-1460 Luxembourg, Luxembourg

Dietrich Pape
Sports Medicine Research Laboratory, Public Research Centre for Health, Luxembourg, Centre Médical de la Fondation Norbert Metz, 76, rue d'Eich, L-1460 Luxembourg, Luxembourg

Nikolas K. Knowles
Roth | Mcfarlane Hand and Upper Limb Centre, Surgical Mechatronics Laboratory, St. Josephs Health Care, 268 Grosvenor St., London N6A 4V2, ON, Canada
Department of Biomedical Engineering, The University of Western Ontario, 1151 Richmond St., N6A3K7 London, ON, Canada

Michael Gladwell and Louis M. Ferreira
Roth | Mcfarlane Hand and Upper Limb Centre, Surgical Mechatronics Laboratory, St. Josephs Health Care, 268 Grosvenor St., London N6A 4V2, ON, Canada
Schulich School of Medicine and Dentistry, The University of Western University, 1151 Richmond St., N6A3K7 London, ON, Canada

Romain Seil and Dietrich Pape
Department of Orthopaedic Surgery, Centre Hospitalier Luxembourg, Clinique d'Eich. 78, rue d'Eich, L-1460 Luxembourg, Luxembourg
Sports Medicine Research Laboratory, Luxembourg Institute of Health, 78 rue d'Eich, L-1460 Luxembourg, Luxembourg

Frederick K Weitz
Department of Pediatric Surgery, University of Tampere, Teiskontie 35, 33521 Tampere, Finland

Martin Zens
Albert-Ludwigs-University Freiburg, Department of Microsystems Engineering (IMTEK), Design of Microsystems, Georges-Koehler-Allee 102, 79110 Freiburg i. Brsg., Germany
University Medical Center Freiburg, Department of Orthopaedics and Trauma Surgery, Hugstetter Str. 55, 79106 Freiburg i. Brsg., Germany

Matthias J Feucht, Anke Bernstein, Hermann O Mayr, Norbert P Südkamp and Philipp Niemeyer
University Medical Center Freiburg, Department of Orthopaedics and Trauma Surgery, Hugstetter Str. 55, 79106 Freiburg i. Brsg., Germany

Johannes Ruhhammer and Peter Woias
Albert-Ludwigs-University Freiburg, Department of Microsystems Engineering (IMTEK), Design of Microsystems, Georges-Koehler-Allee 102, 79110 Freiburg i. Brsg., Germany

Conor J. Moran, Ashwanth Ramesh, Fergal J. O'Brien and Tanya J. Levingstone
Tissue Engineering Research Group, Department of Anatomy, Royal College of Surgeons in Ireland, 123 St. Stephen's Green, Dublin 2, Ireland
Trinity Centre for Bioengineering, Trinity College Dublin, Dublin 2, Ireland
Advanced Materials and Bioengineering Research (AMBER) Centre, RCSI & TCD, Dublin, Ireland

Pieter A. J. Brama
Section of Veterinary Clinical Sciences, School of Veterinary Medicine, University College Dublin, Dublin, Ireland

John M. O'Byrne
Tissue Engineering Research Group, Department of Anatomy, Royal College of Surgeons in Ireland, 123 St. Stephen's Green, Dublin 2, Ireland
Cappagh National Orthopaedic Hospital, Finglas, Dublin 11, Ireland

P J Klungsøyr, F Guldal, T Vagstad and J A Klungsøyr
Orthopaedic Department. Aalesund Hospital, Aalesund, Norway

Henning Madry
Center of Experimental Orthopaedics, Saarland University Medical Center and Saarland University, Bldg 37, Kirrbergerstr. 1, D-66421 Homburg, Germany
Cartilage Net of the Greater Region, Homburg, Germany
Department of Orthopaedic Surgery, Saarland University Medical Center and Saarland University, D-66421 Homburg/Saar, Germany

Mitsuo Ochi
Department of Orthopaedic Surgery, Graduate School of Biomedical Sciences, Hiroshima University, Hiroshima, Japan

Magali Cucchiarini
Center of Experimental Orthopaedics, Saarland University Medical Center and Saarland University, Bldg 37, Kirrbergerstr. 1, D-66421 Homburg, Germany
Cartilage Net of the Greater Region, Homburg, Germany

Dietrich Pape and Romain Seil
Cartilage Net of the Greater Region, Homburg, Germany
Department of Orthopaedic Surgery, Centre Hospitalier du Luxembourg, L-1460, Luxembourg, Luxembourg
Sports Medicine Research Laboratory, Public Research Centre for Health, Luxembourg, Centre Médical de la Fondation Norbert Metz, 76 rue d'Eich, L-1460, Luxembourg, Luxembourg

Emily Hu and Jessica Preciado
myoscience, Inc., 46400 Fremont Blvd, Fremont, CA 94538, USA

Vinod Dasa
Department of Orthopedics, Louisiana State University, 1542 Tulane Avenue, Box T6-7, New Orleans, LA 70112, USA

Jason Mussell
Department of Cell Biology and Anatomy, Louisiana State University, 1901 Perdido Street, Room 6123A, New Orleans, LA 70112, USA